CLINICAL ANATOMY
AND MANAGEMENT OF
LOW BACK PAIN

L. G. F. Giles MSc, DC(C), PhD

Reader
Department of Public Health and Tropical Medicine,
James Cook University of North Queensland, Townsville, Queensland, Australia
Chief Executive Officer and Research Director
National Centre for Multidisciplinary Studies of Back Pain,
Townsville General Hospital, Townsville, Queensland, Australia
Honorary Clinical Scientist
Townsville General Hospital, Townsville, Queensland, Australia

and

K. P. Singer MSc, PT, PhD

Associate Professor
School of Physiotherapy,
Curtin University of Technology,
Shenton Park, Western Australia, Australia
Honorary Research Fellow
Departments of Radiology, Neuropathology and Bioengineering,
Royal Perth Hospital, Perth, Western Australia, Australia

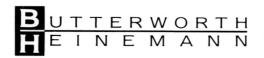
BUTTERWORTH
HEINEMANN

Butterworth-Heinemann
Linacre House, Jordan Hill, Oxford OX2 8DP
225 Wildwood Avenue, Woborn,
MA 01801 - 2041

A division of Reed Educational and Professional Publishing Ltd

A member of the Reed Elsevier plc group

OXFORD   AUCKLAND   BOSTON
JOHANNESBURG   MELBOURNE   NEW DELHI

First published 1997
Reprinted 2001
© Reed Educational and Professional Publishing Ltd 1997

British Library Cataloguing in Publication Data
A catalogue record for this book is available from the British Library.

Library of Congress Cataloguing in Publication Data
A catalogue record for this book is available from the Library of Congress.

ISBN 0 7506 2395 0   Coventry University

Composition by Genesis Typesetting, Rochester, Kent
Printed in India by Ajanta Offset, New Delhi

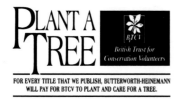

FOR EVERY TITLE THAT WE PUBLISH, BUTTERWORTH-HEINEMANN
WILL PAY FOR BTCV TO PLANT AND CARE FOR A TREE.

Contents

Contributors

Harold S. Amonoo-Kuofi MB, ChB, PhD
Professor of Clinical Anatomy, Department of
Anatomy College of Medicine and King Khalid
University Hospital, Riyadh, Saudi Arabia

Mohammed G.Y. El-Badawi MB, BCh, MS, MD
Professor of Anatomy, College of Medicine, Suez
Canal University, Ismailia, Egypt

Kim Burton PhD, DO, MERgS
Director Spinal Research Unit, University of
Huddersfield, UK

S.H. Burns DC(C), FCCS(C)
Private Practice of Chiropractic, Saskatoon,
Saskatchewan, Canada

Robert Clarke DO
Associate Osteopath and Research Associate, Spinal
Research Unit, University of Huddersfield, UK

C.M. Crawford BAppSc(Chiro), GradDip(Neurosci),
FCCS(C)
Research Fellow, James Cook University of North
Queensland, Townsville, Australia

Henry Vernon Crock MD, MS, FRCS, FRACS
Honorary Senior Lecturer, Orthopaedic Department,
Royal Post Graduate Medical School, Hammersmith
Hospital, London

Stephen J. Edmondston Dip PT, Adv Dip PT, PhD
Lecturer, School of Physiotherapy, Curtin University,
Perth WA, Australia

Robert L. Elvey BAppSc, PGDipMT
Senior Lecturer, School of Physiotherapy, Curtin
University, Perth WA, Australia

Mats Grönblad MD, PhD
Associate Professor and Senior Lecturer in Physical
Medicine and Rehabilitation, University of Helsinki,
Finland

Basil James BSc, MBBCh, FRANZCP, FRACP,
FRSPsych
Professor of Psychiatry and Behavioural Sciences,
Queensland, Australia

J. Randy Jinkins MD, FACR
Director of Neuroradiology, University of Texas
Health Science Center at San Antonio, Texas, USA

Shinichi Kikuchi MD, PhD
Professor and Chairman, Department of
Orthopaedic Surgery, Fukushima City, Japan

Bruce R. Knolmayer MD
Department of Orthopedics, Georgetown University
Medical Center, USA

Robert McAlindon MD
Department of Orthopedics, Georgetown University
Medical Center, USA

Tim McClune DO
Associate Osteopath and Research Associate, Spinal
Research Unit, University of Huddersfield, UK

Frank McDonald
Clinical Psychologist, Department of Psychiatry,
Townsville General Hospital, Townsville,
Queensland, Australia

D.R. Mierau BSPE, DC(C), MSc(Orth), FCCS(C)
Private Practice of Chiropractic, Saskatoon
Saskatchewan, Canada

K.L. Moore PhD, FIAC, FRSM
Professor Emeritus, Department of Anatomy and
Cell Biology, Faculty of Medicine, University of
Toronto, Canada

Kjell Olmarker MD PhD
Associate Research Professor, Department of
Orthopaedics, Sahlgren University Hospital,
Gothenburg, Sweden

Mark J. Pearcy BSc(Mech Eng), PhD (Bioeng)
Professor of Biomedical Engineering, School of
Mechanical, Manufacturing and Medical
Engineering, Queensland University of Technology,
Queensland, Australia

Lindsay J. Rowe MAppSc(Chiro), BMed,
DACBR(C), FACCR(Aus), FICC
Department of Medical Imaging, John Hunter
Hospital, Newcastle, Australia

Bjorn Rydevik MD, PhD
Associate Professor of Orthopaedic Surgery,
Department of Orthopaedics, Sahlgren University
Hospital, Gothenburg, Sweden

Paul Shekelle MD, PhD
West Los Angeles Veterans Affairs Medical Center,
University of California, Los Angeles, School of
Medicine, Rand, USA

J.R. Taylor MB, ChB, PhD, FAFRM(Sci)
Adjunct Professor, Curtin University of Technology,
Principal Research Fellow, Royal Perth Hospital,
Perth WA, Australia

Johanna Virri MSc
Junior Investigator, University of Helsinki, Finland

Charlotte Walker BSc(Hon), BSc(Ost)
Associate Osteopath and Research Associate, Spinal
Research Unit, University of Huddersfield, UK

Sam W. Wiesel MD
Professor and Chairman, Department of
Orthopedics, Georgetown University Medical
Center, USA

Hizedo Yoshizawa MD, PhD
Professor and Chairman, Department of
Orthopaedic Surgery, Fujita Health University,
School of Medicine, Japan

Foreword

My theme for this foreword is 'Back to the Basics'. Since World War II, and particularly in the past decade, there has been an explosion in the technology available to diagnose and treat low back pain, yet it is a sobering reality that the rate of disability and costs for care have risen disproportionately to the growth in the World's population. There is no doubt that advances in diagnostic imaging techniques, such as MRI and CT scanning, have vastly improved the clinician's capacity to less invasively identify pathology which threatens neurologic function. Also, there is no doubt that these advances have improved the care of people with major structural deformity such as scoliosis, and the outcome of the treatment of major pathologies including primary osseous and neurologic neoplasms, fractures and some infections, as well as the care of those with clearly manifest disc herniations and spinal stenosis. Realistically, these conditions account for a small minority of low back disorders.

During the past decade there also has been a major societal reappraisal of how health care is financed, and how quality is measured. This is most evident in the United States where market place forces have promoted a very rapid growth in managed care. The challenge increasingly posed to providers is to explicitly demonstrate the value of the services rendered, where value is measured by quality of the outcome, quality of the service, and cost. When value is measured in these explicit terms, the care of low back pain often is found wanting. For example, there is a growing literature which shows the cost of spinal fusion for many degenerative disorders is higher than alternative care, and the outcomes as measured by relief of symptoms and function, as well as a high rate of complications, suggest the procedure has marginal value.

The evident paradox is that as powerful technology has evolved, value, as seen by the majority of users, has marginally improved. In this context the current volume, *Clinical Anatomy and Management of Low*

Back Pain, seems particularly relevant because it gets back to the basics. Although the focus is on manipulative care, this series fully recognizes optimization of care for low back disorders requires the input of multiple disciplines, particularly when a condition is chronic or disabling. The authors recognize that the multiple disciplines need a common language built around the traditional and newer understanding of patho-anatomy, as well as psychosocial events which shape our individual response to pain stimuli, and how this influences functional capacity. In short, this is a worthy effort to develop a systematic approach to diagnosis and treatment which leads to continuous improvement in quality, hopefully at no greater, or even reduced costs.

What are some of the critical underpinning concepts which will improve the value of care for those with back disorders?

The practitioner needs to understand gross anatomy, and histopathology. More important is the clinical acumen to differentiate whether 'abnormal' anatomy is the likely cause of symptoms, or simply a feature of aging. For example, a narrowed L5–S1 disc space seen on plane radiographs is surely associated with histologic change of degeneration, yet the presence of this finding predicts little about the likely cause of pain. Even more perplexing is the observation that significant disc protrusions are identified in over 30% of people who never have experienced back pain. The back to the basics message, a good history and physical examination, are far more important in the vast majority of people with acute back pain than the most sophisticated imaging tests.

Similarly, a systematic approach to treatment and management is critical for all who engage in the care of patients. On one hand, allopathic physicians finally are becoming aware that manipulative treatment has scientifically proven efficacy. On the other hand, those engaged in manipulative treatment must recognize when the patient's pathology is not amenable to that type of treatment. It is debatable whether manipulation can impact positively, or negatively, those with frank lumbar disc herniations; even more debatable is the impact on spinal stenosis. Certainly it is critical that all think of, and recognize, causes for symptoms which can be adversely affected by manipulation, such as tumours, infections, occult fractures, significant osteoporosis, impending cauda equina syndrome, fixed deformities, or back pain of visceral aetiology. Similarly, it is important to recognize that those patients where non-operative treatment has failed, and whose pathology is amenable to surgical treatment, are better served by referral to surgeons expert in their management. Although complications of manipulation are rare, recognition and appropriate referral is also essential. This basic interplay between professions can always be best focused when the basic question is asked, 'What is best for the patient?'

As manipulation continues to grow as a focus for conservative management, there is the need to clearly define in the continuum of low back disorders where manipulation is effective, and where it is not. The scientific evidence to date demonstrates substantial efficacy only for acute (less than six weeks' duration) back disorders. Similar to all treatment methods, the substantiation of value cannot be done by testimony, isolated case reports, or by the hardly convincing statement, 'In my experience, it works'.

Instead, carefully constructed prospective randomized clinical trials with independent observation will be required. Outcome measures should focus on quality (functional, as well as pain reduction), and cost. Another approach is the application of quality improvement methods, whereby systems thinking and explicit protocols are used to measure the effects on a variety of outcome measures, for example utilization of health care service, functional measures, and cost.

I am heartened that the Editors and writers of this volume have addressed these issues built around the basic model of interdisciplinary collaboration and a systematic approach to the management of lumbar spinal disorders. I believe the significant advances will be less based on great advances in technology, and more on the application of systematically applied scientific and clinical knowledge. In short, it is back to the basics.

Professor John W. Frymoyer MD
Dean of Medicine
The University of Vermont

Preface

Our intention in compiling this new text series is to provide an international perspective on the rational approach to managing mechanical spinal pain. We present a comprehensive review and analysis of clinically relevant information on the basic sciences leading to diagnosis and treatment of mechanical spinal disorders, with a chapter dedicated to contra-indications for spinal manipulation.

This text highlights the value of a team approach to appreciating the complexity of spinal pain and a range of treatment approaches. Contemporary contributions from: epidemiology, anatomy, pathology, physiology, psychology, clinical medicine, orthopaedics, chiropractic, osteopathy and physiotherapy are presented in this volume. Each section, written by experienced academic clinicians, provides a summary of pertinent material which will lead to an improved understanding of the causes of mechanical back pain. Management strategies, based on routine assessment techniques, are proposed using clinical reasoning sequences. This text does not attempt to endorse a single therapy, rather to highlight the common approach to mechanical treatment which may be provided by chiropractic, osteopathy and physiotherapy practitioners.

Our goal is to present this information in a manner which will benefit both the undergraduate and postgraduate student of mechanical therapy, as well as all clinicians who seek a comprehensive review of mechanical spinal pain. In the belief that quality illustrations facilitate the message, careful selection of material and detailed captions have been prepared to complement the text. A second objective is to encourage greater communication between the clinical schools interested in this important subject. Through this, we hope to contribute to a stronger scientific basis for spinal care.

The text is organized so that it can be approached in several ways, according to the needs of the reader. The clinician who wishes a quick overview of clinical assessment concepts and techniques should consult Section IV: Diagnosis and Management. This includes: imaging procedures for mechanical back complaints, the psychological assessment of back pain, medicinal and surgical approaches to back pain and separate chapters on the assessment and management strategies provided by chiropractors, osteopaths and physiotherapists.

Section I introduces the reasoning behind this text, together with an epidemiological review of mechanical back pain. Section II presents the clinical anatomy and pathology of the lumbosacral spine, with specific chapters on: lumbar intervertebral discs and vertebrae, zygapophysial joints, blood supply, muscle and ligaments, sacroiliac joints and the thoracolumbar junction. Section III presents spinal clinical neuroanatomy and neurophysiology of the lumbosacral spine in such chapters as: innervation of spinal structures, mechanisms of inflammation in spinal tissues, stenosis, pathoanatomic basis of somatic and autonomic syndromes originating in the lumbosacral spine, and biomechanics of the lumbosacral spine.

Section V presents definitions to assist the reader with terms used throughout the text and these are complemented in some cases with illustrations.

Our general approach to both the clinical and scientific aspects of mechanical back pain is to provide a contemporary review of the literature and to present logical examples of clinical reasoning behind three disciplines of mechanical therapy. Despite the need to validate theories behind mechanical intervention and to show long-term efficacy of these therapies, this text also sets out our challenge, as clinician-scientists, to promote communication between all interested parties. Back pain is multifaceted and it demands the sharing of ideas and knowledge to improve the management offered to our patients.

LGF Giles
KP Singer

Acknowledgements

The support of clinical and technical staff at the University of Western Australia's Departments of Anatomy and Human Biology, Pathology and Radiology, and the Institute of Forensic Pathology, Brisbane, is noted with appreciation. This work was supported in part by grants from my Alma Mater, the Canadian Memorial Chiropractic College, Toronto, Foundation for Chiropractic Education and Research, USA, and the Australian Spinal Research Foundation Ltd.

LGFG

The support of colleagues at Royal Perth Hospital and the Department of Anatomy and Human Biology at the University of Western Australia is noted with appreciation. This work was supported in part by grants from the National Health and Medical Research Council of Australia.

KPS

Section

I

Introduction and Epidemiology

1

Introduction

L.G.F. Giles

Erect posture and low back pain of mechanical origin in homo sapiens

Some authors have attributed low back pain which is due to spinal joint dysfunction to homo sapiens' bipedal posture (Cailliet, 1968), although this is not universally accepted (Farfan, 1978). When osseous and/or soft tissue anomalies occur, normal circumstances no longer prevail, and such spinal joints are predisposed to abnormal mechanical stresses.

Humans are the only living creatures to have mastered the upright posture while standing and ambulating (Rickenbacher *et al.*, 1985), and this is the result, and measure, of mankind's successful struggle with gravity (Schede, 1961). In order to meet the dynamic functional demands required of the spine (Leger, 1959), transition to the erect posture required the human spine to have a double S-shape in the sagittal plane with a sharp bend between the sacrum and the lumbar spine which begins to develop before birth, although it is only during the first 3 years of childhood that the typical curves are gradually formed and, by puberty, they become established (Lafferty *et al.*, 1977; Rickenbacher *et al.*, 1985).

Phylogenetic studies have led to the realization that the bipedal posture, has meant making the fifth lumbar and first sacral vertebrae wedge shaped in the median plane, with a greater thickness anteriorly (Lippert, 1970), spinous processes of reduced size from the fourth lumbar to first sacral segments (Farfan, 1978), and positioning the base of the adult sacrum at an acute angle of approximately 41 degrees to the horizontal (Lafferty *et al.*, 1977; Rickenbacher *et al.*, 1985). Other changes include turning the angle of the hip joints through 90 degrees, inclination of the neck of the femur, torsion of the femoral shaft and

the tibia, and formation of the unique human foot with its arch (Lippert, 1970; Benninghoff, 1980; Rickenbacher *et al.*, 1985).

In normal posture (Figure 1.1), the line of weight is the perpendicular through the centre of gravity (Joseph, 1960). The importance of this line lies in its relationship to the transverse axes of rotation of the joints of the vertebral column and the lower limbs,

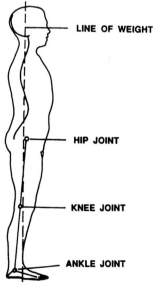

LINE OF WEIGHT

HIP JOINT

KNEE JOINT

ANKLE JOINT

Figure 1.1 Outline of a man to show the relation of the line of weight to the ankle, knee and hip joints and its probable relation to the curves of the vertebral column. (Reproduced with permission from Joseph, J. (1960) *Man's Posture: Electromyographic Studies.* Charles C. Thomas, Illinois, p. 14.)

since the body tends to fall forwards or backwards due to gravity according to whether the line of weight passes in front of or behind these axes respectively (Joseph, 1960).

Posture and movement are related to the musculature of the back which has two functions: (i) to hold the central supporting organ of the body (the spinal column) in its proper shape and position, and (ii) to supply the force for its movement; the muscles situated near the body's surface and far from the midline are highly effective motor agents, whereas the muscles situated adjacent to the spinal column are mainly concerned with maintenance of posture (Rickenbacher *et al.*, 1985).

Poor posture, in which the head is thrust forward with excessive spinal curves in the sagittal plane, sloping or hunched shoulders, protruding abdomen and hyperextended knees (Garlick, 1990) (Figure 1.2B) may be habitual or occupational (Mennell, 1960), and can be related to poor muscle tone. Chronic postural strain can cause myofascial pain (Keim and Kirkaldy-Willis, 1987).

Because of the permanent lumbar lordosis, lower lumbar joints are always subjected to a shearing force, so the lower two or three lumbar zygapophysial joints

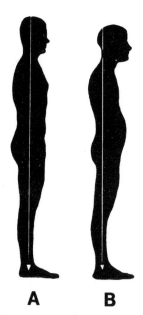

A   **B**

Figure 1.2 (A) Good posture due to good muscle tone and (B) bad posture which develops when poor muscle tone is present. (Modified from Feldenkrais, M. (1949) *Body and mature behaviour.* New York, International Universities Press Inc., p. 104) (Reproduced with permission from Giles, L.G.F. (1991) A review and description of some possible causes of low back pain of mechanical origin in *homo sapiens. Proceedings of the Australasian Society for Human Biology*, **4**, 193–212.)

have developed a more coronal orientation than have the higher lumbar zygapophysial joints (which have a more sagittal orientation) to provide protective support against this shear (Farfan, 1978).

The human spine is a very complicated structure, considered by some to be a masterpiece of engineering (Keith, 1923; Farfan, 1978). According to Fahrni (1966), others consider the spine to be a very defective and inefficient mechanism. It is probably a mechanically sound mechanism which is badly abused by its owner (Fahrni, 1966). This has caused some authors to attribute low back pain associated with mechanical dysfunction (Cailliet, 1968) to man's bipedal posture (Friberg, 1948; Rasch and Burke, 1967; Gross, 1979). However, in a comparative study of man compared with other anthropoids, Farfan (1978) concluded that the overall mechanical advantage of the lumbar spine's anatomical arrangements provides an overabundance of power to attain the erect posture and that the lumbar spine does not deserve to be described as a weak structure, under normal circumstances. Many mechanisms exist to provide some protection during normal movements. For example, during flexion of the lumbar spine, the lumbar lordosis is never reversed due to the inherent wedging of the lower lumbar intervertebral discs and vertebral bodies with their greater thickness anteriorly, thereby reducing the range of flexion. Although motion of the lumbar spine is under the control of active spinal musculature, further protective support is achieved from the complex ligamentous system (Farfan, 1978; Putz, 1992). Some ligaments have a dual role; for example the ligamenta flava are not only involved in resisting excess separation of the vertebral laminae but also protect the neural elements from adjacent osseous structures, such as the laminae and zygapophysial joints, in parts of the spinal and intervertebral (foramen) canals. The epidural and epiradicular adipose tissue affords an adequate reserve cushion for protection of neural and vascular structures within the spinal and intervertebral canals under normal circumstances.

Two main factors make the lumbosacral spine vulnerable to abnormal mechanical stresses, i.e. apparent disregard for maintaining good posture and protection of the spine from injury, which may lead to degenerative joints and dysfunction (Gracovetsky *et al.*, 1981), and congenital or acquired anomalies of osseous and soft tissues (Garlick, 1990).

Spinal injuries

The apparent inability to protect the spine from injury is an enormously complex issue which can be summarized as being due to unexpected trauma, or a poor understanding of spinal ergonomics and correct posture; these issues are beyond the scope of this volume.

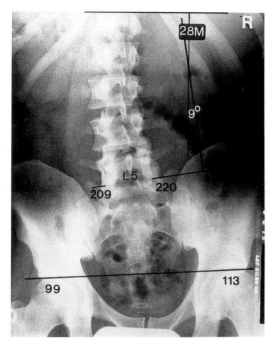

Figure 1.3 Erect posture radiograph of a 28-year-old male showing several anomalies: (i) a left leg length discrepancy of 14 mm, (ii) a hypoplastic left ilium above the hip joint (compared to the right), (iii) bilateral sacralization of the first segment of the sacrum, and (iv) asymmetry in the length of the laminae of the first sacral segment. L5 = fifth lumbar vertebra. R = right side of patient. The pelvic obliquity has resulted in a 9 degree postural scoliosis between the first lumbar and first sacral segments, as measured by Cobb's (1948) method. (Reproduced with permission from Giles, L.G.F. (1991) A review and description of some possible causes of low back pain of mechanical origin in *homo sapiens. Proceedings of the Australasian Society for Human Biology*, 4, 193–212.)

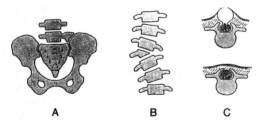

A   **B**   **C**

Figure 1.4 Three congenital anomalies of the spine are shown as an example: (A) hypertrophied transverse process forming a false joint with the ilium; (B) hemivertebra, an occasional cause of scoliosis; (C) two examples of spina bifida. In both, the neural arch is deficient posteriorly – the lower drawing shows spina bifida occulta which is the much commoner and less severe defect, with the skin and soft tissues intact; the upper drawing shows the overlying soft tissues are also deficient and the spinal theca bulges backwards to form a meningocele. (Reproduced with permission from Adams, J.C. (1981) *Outline of Orthopaedics*. Churchill Livingstone, Edinburgh, 9th edition.)

Anomalies

(i) Anomalies outside the spine, such as a significant leg length inequality, with or without pelvic osseous anomalies, and pelvic obliquity and postural scoliosis (Rush and Steiner, 1946; Stoddard, 1959; Gofton and Trueman, 1967; Giles and Taylor, 1981; Friberg, 1987) (Figure 1.3), and (ii) spinal osseous anomalies (Figure 1.4) or soft tissue anomalies, such as the tethered cord (Chapter 13) which may cause scoliosis (Roth, 1981), and conjoined nerve roots (Okuwaki *et al.*, 1991) should be considered in relation to low back pain.

A radiographic example of spina bifida occulta of the first sacral segment is given in Figure 1.5, which shows that the fifth lumbar spinous process is elongated in its superior to inferior dimension.

Pain

Back pain associated with anomalous lumbosacral transitional vertebrae is referred to as Bertolotti's syndrome and it is postulated by Elster (1989) that, in this syndrome, hypermobility and altered stresses become concentrated in the spine at the level immediately above a lumbar transitional vertebra due to biomechanical aberrations, resulting in pain. Anomalous variations of the lumbar and sacral bony anatomy are common and are detectable in about one-half of the population (Keim and Kirkaldy-Willis, 1987) and include some of those shown in Figure 1.4 which may result in pain, i.e. (i) overdevelopment of the fifth lumbar transverse process on one or both sides of the spine with a false joint between the hypertrophied process and the ilium, (ii) persistence of the first sacral segment as a separate vertebra (lumbarization of the first sacral vertebra), (iii) complete or incomplete incorporation of the fifth lumbar vertebral body into the sacrum (sacralization of the fifth lumbar vertebra), (iv) spina bifida occulta in which the walls of the vertebral canal fail to meet posteriorly during development which can be associated with bulging backwards of the theca (meningocele) (Adams, 1981), (v) facet asymmetry (tropism) (Keim and Kirkaldy-Willis, 1987), and (vi) hemivertebra.

Facet tropism, which occurs in approximately 20% of people (Cihak, 1970), is thought to be of clinical significance because it adds rotational stresses to the zygapophysial joints (see Chapter 5) (Keim and Kirkaldy-Willis, 1987). Mild forms of spina bifida occulta are considered to be of little practical importance by some (Adams, 1981; Keim and Kirkaldy-Willis, 1987) but are considered to be significant by others (Avrahami *et al.*, 1994). On viewing 500 lumbosacral plain film radiographs and 1000 myelographic examinations of patients with low back pain and root signs, Barzo *et al.* (1993) showed

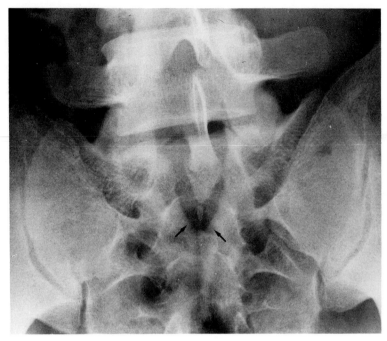

Figure 1.5 Spina bifida occulta of the first sacral segment (arrows) and an elongated superior to inferior dimension of the spinous process of the fifth lumbar vertebra.

transitional lumbosacral vertebrae in 8.4% of patients and in only 4.6% of a normal population.

Most soft tissue structures of the lumbosacral spine have a good nociceptive nerve supply, so that pain will warn of incorrect spinal movements and strains. This, coupled with the previously mentioned structural adaptations, indicates that the human lumbar spine seems highly advanced along the evolutionary scale (Farfan, 1978) but, in spite of this, low back pain, with or without sciatica, is second only to the common cold in its frequency (Lewinnik, 1983; Bronfort and Jochumsen, 1984; Deyo and Tsui-Wu, 1987). Low back pain affects up to 80–88% of the population at some time during their adult lives (Cailliet, 1968; Nachemson, 1971, 1976, 1977; Haldeman, 1980; Friedman, 1984; Kirkaldy-Willis and Cassidy, 1985; Jayson, 1986; Murtagh, 1994) with a high prevalence in adults, beginning in adolescence (Althoff *et al.*, 1992). It is a main cause of disability and expense from work-related conditions (Langworthy, 1993; Basler, 1994) and is a main cause of absence from work (Meade *et al.*, 1990). This places an enormous economic burden upon many world communities and in the United States of America it costs the community in excess of $100 billion per annum (Frymoyer and Cats-Baril, 1991) with the cost continuing to escalate (Werneke *et al.*, 1993). The cost to the Australian community is approximately $10 billion per annum and it is known that the epidemic increase of sickness in low back pain

syndromes is actually threatening the social welfare system in societies with socialized medicine (Allan and Waddell, 1989; Nachemson, 1991). In spite of this, back pain research has received very little academic attention, out of all proportion to the frequency of this complaint in the adult working population (Editorial, Lancet, 1990). Low back pain is the most frequent cause of limitation of activity in persons younger than 45 years and uses an enormous volume of medical services (Deyo, 1983).

Despite the spine's excellent design (Keith, 1923; Farfan, 1978; Giles, 1991), with its normal lumbar and cervical lordoses and thoracic kyphosis being well adapted to the function of the vertebral column, any major aberrations in these spinal curves are mechanically unsound (Rickenbacher *et al.*, 1985). Muscle weakness due to lack of exercise or disease can affect the spinal curves and cause postural defects leading to faulty spinal joint mechanics and low back pain (Garlick, 1990). It is well known that radiologically 'normal' but painful spines (Benson, 1983; El-Khoury and Renfrew, 1991) may have painful pathological changes which cannot be demonstrated radiologically (Dixon, 1980). It is suggested that pain in these cases may be due to mechanical irritation of various pain sensitive soft tissue structures which cannot be visualized by imaging procedures but can be found at post mortem by histological studies, although it is not possible to correlate histopathological findings in cadavers with pain.

On the other hand, many individuals with radiological abnormalities of spinal joints remain pain free and even frank disc herniations in the lumbosacral spine may be noted during imaging of completely asymptomatic individuals (Hitselberger and Witten, 1968; Wiesel *et al.*, 1984; Boden *et al.*, 1990). Therefore, the relation between these radiological abnormalities and clinical symptoms is not understood (Isherwood and Antoun, 1980; Vanharanta *et. al.*, 1985). Many spinal structures probably play a role in pain production, and all innervated structures in the motion segment are possible sources of pain (Haldeman, 1977; Nachemson, 1985).

Magnitude of the problem of low back pain

Low back pain, although sometimes due to other causes, can result from alterations from normal biomechanics in the vertebral column and constitutes a major health problem (Ham and Cormack, 1979; Loeser *et al.*, 1990); hence it is desirable to understand as much as possible about the clinical anatomy of intervertebral and zygapophysial joints (Ham and Cormack, 1979), as well as sacroiliac joints. Frequently the cause of low back pain is not known (Yong-Hing and Kirkaldy-Willis, 1983; Frymoyer, 1988) and our understanding of the problem is very limited. According to Dixon (1976), in nine out of 10 instances low back pain is transient, it is related to some posture or strain, and recovery can take place in a short time. However, chronic back pain and its associated disabilities represent a significant health problem (Kepes and Duncalf, 1985) of daunting proportions (Anderson, 1980; Wood and Bradley, 1980; Spengler *et al.*, 1986; Nachemson, 1994) in which physical signs are often totally lacking (Mellin, 1986).

According to Haldeman (1977), two important factors compound the problem of back pain mechanisms: (a) back pain may have a multifactorial aetiology, and (b) there may be several types of back pain which closely mimic each other. Baldwin (1977) states that part of the problem lies in the fact that the low back region is extremely complex, both anatomically and functionally. We await further elucidation of the pathophysiology of the back problem since the pathological aetiology of many varieties of back pain remains undiscovered (Pearcy *et al.*, 1985; Tajima and Kawano, 1986). However, most painful conditions of the lumbar spine affect the two lower lumbar mobile segments (Ehni, 1977) which degenerate earlier (Butler *et al.*, 1990).

In spite of many attempts to provide a rationale for clinicians to properly order diagnostic examinations and prescribe treatments that maximize the quality and efficiency of patient care (The North American Spine Society, 1991; Skelton *et al.*, 1995) the complex problem of low back pain continues unabated (Pelz and Haddad, 1989). Many psychological factors are believed to contribute to the development, exacerbation, and/or maintenance of chronic low back pain (Kinney *et al.*, 1991) and, when evaluating patients with chronic low back pain, it is necessary to understand clinical findings in relation to issues of everyday functioning, such as employment, activities of daily living, and social adjustment (Millard and Jones, 1991) (see Chapter 19). The answer to the complex issue of back pain may well depend upon multidisciplinary co-operation and, as Frymoyer *et al.* (1991) state, centres for spinal care will emerge as part of larger health care systems.

Motion (mobile) segment and its parts

Lewin *et al.* (1961), and Hirsch *et al.* (1963) pointed out that the basic anatomical and functional unit of the vertebral column is the articular triad consisting of the fibrocartilaginous intervertebral joint and the two synovial zygapophysial joints. The motion (mobile) segment of Junghanns (Schmorl and Junghanns, 1971) consists of all the space between two vertebrae where movement occurs: the intervertebral disc with its cartilaginous plates, the anterior and posterior longitudinal ligaments, the zygapophysial joints with their fibrous joint capsules and the ligamenta flava, the contents of the spinal canal and the left and right intervertebral canals, and the supraspinous and interspinous ligaments (Figure 1.6).

The intervertebral joints in the spine are primarily responsible for (a) the flexibility of the spine, allowing a variety of movements such as flexion, extension, lateral bending, and axial rotation, and (b) load transmission and shock absorption, as a result of the mechanical properties of the disc (Lovett, 1905; Shah, 1980).

The mobile segment (Schmorl and Junghanns, 1971) is conveniently subdivided into anterior and posterior elements (Andersson, 1983) and it is claimed, on the basis of clinical and experimental observations, that degeneration of the intervertebral disc and associated osteoarthritis of the zygapophysial joints can cause low back pain (Kirkaldy-Willis and Farfan, 1982; Keim and Kirkaldy-Willis, 1987). According to Butler *et al.* (1990), disc degeneration occurs before zygapophysial joint osteoarthritis, which may be secondary to mechanical changes in the loading of the zygapophysial joints. Miller *et al.* (1988) found lumbar disc degeneration first appears in the 11–19 year age range in males, and 1 decade later in females, with 97% of all lumbar discs exhibiting degeneration by 50 years of age. It has also been suggested that intervertebral disc herniation is associated with vertebrogenic pain and the auto-

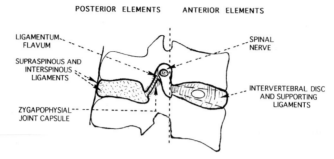

Figure 1. 6 The motion (mobile) segment. (Modified from Schmorl, G. and Junghanns, H. (1971) *The Human Spine in Health and Disease,* 2nd edition. Grune and Stratton, New York, p 37.)

nomic syndrome (Jinkins *et al.*, 1989; Giles, 1992a) (see Chapter 17). The importance of spinal osseous and soft tissue anomalies has also been stressed by various authors (Elster, 1989; Giles, 1991). Also, pain of vascular origin, due to vascular deformation and venous stasis within blood vessels of the spinal and intervertebral canals, has been suggested by Giles (1973), Hoyland *et. al.* (1989) and Giles and Kaveri (1990). Some authors stress psychological factors because diagnostic procedures may well not provide a precise diagnosis in cases where pain is due to mechanical dysfunction of joints (Hoehler and Tobis, 1983). Such pain may be experienced in the absence of degenerative joint disease, or other pathologic changes, as a result of traction on normal pain sensitive structures, for example, the joint capsules (Mehta and Sluijter, 1979; Budd, 1981), or pinching and tractioning of the highly vascular and innervated intra-articular synovial folds within the zygapophysial joints (Kos and Wolf, 1972; Giles and Taylor, 1982; Kirkaldy-Willis, 1984; Giles *et al.*, 1986; Giles, 1987, 1989) (see Chapter 5).

The sacroiliac joints

The sacroiliac joints have frequently been associated with low back pain of mechanical origin (Bourdillon, 1970; Bernard and Kirkaldy-Willis, 1987; Kirkaldy-Willis, 1988; Cassidy and Mierau, 1992) and play a very significant role in this type of back pain with or without referred pain to the leg (Bernard and Kirkaldy-Willis, 1987) (see Chapter 11).

Diagnostic problems

Back pain may originate from different spinal tissues, such as muscles, ligaments, dura mater, vertebrae, intervertebral discs, zygapophysial joints (Ahmed

et al., 1993) and other spine related joints such as sacroiliac joints (Lewis, 1985; Kirkaldy-Willis, 1988; Huskisson, 1990). Moreover, one of the major difficulties involved in evaluating a patient with low back pain of mechanical origin, with or without sciatica, is that the painful structure or structures are not amenable to direct scrutiny, so a tentative diagnosis is usually arrived at for an individual by taking a case history and employing a format similar to the briefly outlined examination and laboratory procedures, indicated in Chapter 20. However, in spite of following routine examination procedures, one often merely eliminates frank pathologies and the cause of low back pain of mechanical origin often remains obscure (Margo, 1994), especially when dysfunction and degenerative pathology of spinal and sacroiliac joints occurs. Thus, in severe cases, injections of anaesthetic, with or without steroid suspension, are sometimes used to augment the clinical evaluation (El-Khoury and Renfrew, 1991; Walker and Cousins, 1994), for example to determine whether pain originates in the zygapophysial or sacroiliac joint(s). Imaging procedures such as plain film radiography, myelography, computerized tomography (CT), magnetic resonance imaging (MRI) and bone scans (Chapter 18) have diagnostic limitations. Specifically, diagnostic problems relate to (a) inadequacies in the precise knowledge of the anatomy of the lumbosacral spine, (b) there being multifactorial causes of pain at a given level of the spine in some cases, and (c) the limitations of many diagnostic procedures. Also, there is often disagreement on which imaging procedures have diagnostic validity for back pain of mechanical origin, for example in the use of flexion-extension plain film radiography (Dvorak *et al.*, 1991). In addition, roentgenographic diagnosis often proves difficult because of the anatomical complexity of the spine (Le-Breton *et al.*, 1993).

Furthermore, some diagnostic and therapeutic chemical agents may be harmful, for example when such agents injected into intervertebral discs extravasate into the epidural space (Weitz, 1984; Adams *et al.*,

1986; MacMillan *et al.*, 1991) causing complications due to contact between these chemical agents and neural structures (Eguro, 1983; Dyck, 1985; Merz, 1986; Watts and Dickhaus, 1986). Therefore, such diagnostic tests should only be performed to provide reliable information about a patient's condition and if the result is likely to influence the patient's management (Modic and Herzog, 1994).

In many cases of acute low back pain with sciatica, intervertebral disc prolapse has been described as being the pathological cause (Mixter and Barr, 1934; Rothman and Simeone, 1975; Crock, 1976) but, according to Wiesel *et al.* (1984), herniated lumbar intervertebral discs are often asymptomatic, especially when a spinal canal's dimensions are normal (Heliovaara *et al.*, 1986). Herniated nucleus pulposus does not necessarily produce radiculopathy and may only cause vague low back pain (Yussen and Swartz, 1993). Many authorities believe that disc herniation has been over emphasized as the principal source of back pain and that advocating early surgery, even for patients with appropriate pathology such as herniated nucleus pulposus, is not recommended given the favourable history of natural recovery for the majority of these patients (Lehmann *et al.*, 1993). Spontaneous recovery of intervertebral disc herniation is well known (Fager, 1994) and Saal and Saal (1989) obtained a 90% good outcome with 'aggressive' non-operative treatment. In a 10-year prospective investigation to evaluate the use of quality-based standardized diagnostic and treatment protocols, Wiesel *et al.* (1994) showed that the number of surgeries performed decreased by 67%, the operative success rate increased dramatically, and there was a 60% reduction in expenditures for lost time and replacement wages. It is likely that lumbar zygapophysial joint pain is a common condition which is frequently overlooked, as has been the case with cervical zygapophysial joint pain (Wedel and Wilson, 1985; Bogduk and Marsland, 1988). The prevalence of zygapophysial joint pain should not be overlooked (Aprill and Bogduk, 1992). In patients presenting with local tenderness in the low back, muscle spasm, and low back pain referred to the back of the thigh, to the mid-calf, or to the ankle, it is often thought that the pain arises from the zygapophysial joints (Kirkaldy-Willis, 1983; Kirkaldy-Willis and Cassidy, 1984). The alleviation of the pain by injection of local anaesthetic, with or without steroid suspension, into the joints, under fluoroscopic control, supports this diagnosis according to Mooney and Robertson (1976), Carrera (1979), Destouet *et al.* (1982), Kirkaldy-Willis and Tchang (1983), Aprill (1986), Lewinnek and Warfield (1986), and El-Khoury and Renfrew (1991), although Jackson (1992) disagrees.

It has been known for many years that back pain of mechanical origin is far more prevalent than back pain with an aetiology of frank demonstrable pathology (Beaumont and Paice, 1992; Day *et al.*, 1994). The most common cause of mechanical back pain is dysfunction of spinal intervertebral joints due to injury, accounting for approximately 72% of back pain, while lumbar spondylosis accounts for approximately 10% of painful backs (Murtagh, 1991, 1994). However, many other causes of low back pain, with or without progressive radiculopathy, should be considered, for example juxtafacet synovial cysts (Tatter and Cosgrove, 1994).

The importance of the thoracolumbar zygapophysial joints in certain cases of low back pain of mechanical origin has been noted by Maigne (1974) and should always be considered in the differential diagnosis. The particular histological morphology of the thoracolumbar junction has been extensively reviewed by Singer (1994) (see Chapter 12). That sciatica is not a diagnostic end-point but rather a label for a pain syndrome that encompasses a long differential diagnosis, should always be remembered (Young, 1993; Herr and Williams, 1994).

The continuing interest shown in recent years in low back pain syndromes by epidemiologists, pathologists, rheumatologists, bioengineers, and biomedical researchers and other clinicians reflects the magnitude of the problem. In spite of this multidisciplinary interest, it is still only rarely possible to validate a diagnosis in cases of mechanical back pain (White and Gordon, 1982; Paterson, 1987, 1994) because it is not possible to establish the pathological basis of such pain in 80–90% of cases (Chila *et al.*, 1990; Pope and Novotny, 1993). This leads to diagnostic uncertainty and suspicion that some patients have a 'compensation neurosis' or other psychosocial problem.

Limitations of investigative methods

Routine plain film radiographs provide only a shadow of the truth as detailed anatomy and early pathology cannot be perceived by this method and the same can be said for CT, MRI and bone scans, although some of these procedures provide additional and different information to that provided by plain film radiographs. For example, MRI has proved to be a valuable diagnostic tool in the initial evaluation of the patient with discogenic pain and may reveal the different stages of deterioration and the levels of affected intervertebral discs (Horton and Daftari, 1992). It should be noted that, although MRI may be useful for nuclear anatomy, it is not helpful for symptomatology (Buirski and Silberstein, 1993). Magnetic resonance imaging can also assess spinal cord anatomy and pathology, ligamentous integrity (Brightman *et al.*, 1992), particularly the integrity of the anterior and posterior longitudinal ligaments (McArdle *et al.*, 1986), epidural fat, cerebrospinal fluid and marrow space (Lauterbur, 1973) and, used in conjunction with CT and plain film radiography, it can also aid in the evaluation of bony injuries (Brightman *et al.*, 1992). Also, certain areas of the spine and its related joints are more difficult to examine radiologically. For example, routine plain film radiological demonstration of the zygapophysial joints is not easy, because only one plane of the curved or 'biplanar' (Taylor and Two-mey, 1986) articular surface presents itself tangentially to the X-ray beam (Reichmann, 1973; Park, 1980). Therefore, spinal radiographs can be informative but have limitations (Carroll, 1987), and there is often a discrepancy between the degree of pain and the severity of radiographic changes (Stockwell, 1985). For example, disabling zygapophysial joint facet syndromes can be associated with normal or nearly normal plain film radiographs (Eisenstein and Parry, 1987).

Table 1.1. *Some possible causes of mechanical low back pain with or without leg pain*

Nerve root conditions

- Adhesions between dural sleeves and (a) the joint capsule with nerve root fibrosis (Jackson, 1966; Sunderland, 1968) and (b) intervertebral disc herniation
- Intervertebral disc degeneration (Nachemson, 1969) and fragmentation (Schiotz and Cyriax, 1975), or nucleus pulposus extrusion (Mixter and Barr, 1934) causing nerve root compression, or nerve root 'chemical radiculitis' (Marshall and Trethewie, 1973)
- Lumbosacral arachnoiditis (Spiller *et al.*, 1903; Peek *et al.*, 1993)

Zygapophysial joint conditions

- Joint derangement due to ligamentous and capsular instability (Hadley, 1964; Cailliet, 1968; Macnab, 1977)
- Joint capsule tension, encroachment of the intervertebral foramen lumen; impingement of the articular process tip against the pedicle above and the lamina below (Hadley, 1964)
- Joint degenerative changes, e.g. 'meniscal' incarceration (Schmorl and Junghanns, 1971), traumatic synovitis due to 'pinching' of synovial folds (Kirkaldy-Willis, 1983; Giles, 1989), synovial fold tractioning against the pain-sensitive joint capsule (Hadley, 1964; Giles, 1982), and osteoarthrosis (Eisenstein and Parry, 1987)
- Joint effusion with capsular distension which may (a) exert pressure on a nerve root (Mennell, 1960; Dory, 1981; Maldague *et al.*, 1981), (b) cause capsular pain (Jackson, 1966), or (c) cause nerve root pain by direct diffusion (Haldeman, 1977)
- Joint capsule adhesions (Farfan, 1980; Giles, 1989)

Intervertebral disc conditions

- Significant disc herniation into the spinal and intervertebral canals
- Spondylosis (Weinstein *et al.*, 1977; Vernon-Roberts and Pirie, 1977; Kramer, 1990). Significant anterolateral disc herniation with vertebral body osteophytes compromising neural structures (Nathan, 1962, 1968, 1987; Jinkins *et al.*, 1989; Giles, 1992a; Jinkins, 1993)

Miscellaneous conditions

- Spinal and intervertebral canal stenosis (Sachs and Fraenkel, 1900; Verbiest, 1955; Kirkaldy-Willis and McIvor, 1976; McRae, 1977; Weinstein *et al.*, 1977; Kirkaldy-Willis *et al.*, 1978; Dorwart *et al.*, 1983; Amonoo-Kuofi *et al.*, 1988; Giles and Kaveri, 1990; 1991; Rydevik *et al.*, 1990; Herzog *et al.*, 1991; Giles, 1992b,c; Pedowitz *et al.*, 1992; Giles, 1994)
- Intervertebral canal venous stasis (Giles, 1973; Sunderland, 1980; Giles and Kaveri, 1990)
- Myofascial genesis of pain (trigger areas) (Travell and Rinzler, 1952; Bonica, 1957; Simons and Travell, 1983)
- Hypertension in the bone marrow of the vertebral body or in the juxtachondral space of osteoarthritic intervertebral joints (Arnoldi, 1972, 1976; Arnoldi *et al.*, 1971, 1972, 1975; Astrom, 1975; Lemperg and Arnoldi, 1978; Foley and Kirkaldy-Willis, 1979; Hanai, 1980; Spencer *et al.*, 1981; Kiaer *et al.*, 1988, 1989, 1990; Moore *et al.*, 1991)
- Adhesions between the dural sac anteriorly and the adjacent posterior longitudinal ligament (Parke and Watanabe, 1990)
- Arachnoiditis (Peek *et al.*, 1993)
- Sacroiliac joint mechanical dysfunction and strain (Barbor, 1964; Turek, 1984; Lewis, 1985; Bernard and Kirkaldy-Willis, 1987; Kirkaldy-Willis, 1988; Cassidy and Mierau, 1992)
- Thoracic/thoracolumbar junction degenerative changes (Maigne, 1974, 1980; Singer, 1989; Singer and Giles, 1990)
- Osseous spinal and pelvic anomalies (e.g. transitional vertebra(e), spina bifida occulta, hemivertebra(e) (Ghormley, 1958; Adams, 1981; Stevens, 1968; Anderson, 1976; Nachemson, 1976; Witt *et al.*, 1984; Elster, 1989; Giles, 1991; Avrahami *et al.*, 1994)
- Significant (1 cm or more) leg length inequality and pelvic obliquity (Rush and Steiner, 1946; Stoddard, 1959; Nichols, 1960; Bourdillon, 1970; Sicuranza *et al.*, 1970; Clarke, 1972; Yates, 1976; Giles, 1981; Giles and Taylor, 1981; Hazelman and Bulgen, 1981; Subotnick, 1981; Reid and Smith, 1984; Friberg, 1987; Tjernstrom *et al.*, 1993; Jenner and Barry, 1995)
- Hip joint osteoarthrosis being associated with leg length inequality of >9 mm (Dixon and Campbell-Smith, 1969; Gofton, 1971; JP Gofton, 1989 personal communication; Gofton and Trueman, 1967; Pauwels, 1976; Morscher, 1977)

[Modified from Giles, L.G.F. (1989) *Anatomical Basis of Low Back Pain*. Williams and Wilkins, Baltimore.]

Some possible causes of mechanical low back pain with or without leg pain

Two commonly recognized tissue sources for low back pain are spinal joints and paravertebral muscles (Gillette *et al.*, 1993a). Studies have shown that noxious mechanical and chemical stimulation of diverse paraspinal tissues produces low back and hip pain which can radiate into the proximal leg (Gillette *et al.*, 1993b).

Table 1.1 briefly summarizes some possible causes of low back pain of mechanical origin, with or without leg pain, and provides a summary of some literature references over the years in order to provide a historical background to this complex issue.

Figure 1.7 summarizes some well-established causes of low back pain, with or without leg pain, which are due to the thoracolumbar and lumbosacral spines, and some of the adjacent soft tissue structures, as well as pelvic lesions. The sympathetic chain, lesions of which can cause reflex sympathetic dystrophy (see Chapter 17), is not shown.

Summary

It is not our intention to list all the causes of pelvic pain in this text on low back pain of mechanical origin.

In order to understand a low back pain sufferer's signs and symptoms, it is necessary to understand clearly the normal erect posture and the complex anatomy of the lumbosacral spine. Therefore, in this chapter, human erect posture has been considered prior to the following chapters which review the basic anatomy of the lumbosacral spine. The anatomy will be followed by a detailed review and study of possible pathological changes which may be associated with degenerative joint disorders. While it is not possible to correlate histopathological findings in cadavers with pain, the histological findings described in Chapters 2, 4, 5, 6, 12, 13, 14, 15, 16 identify some possible causes of joint degenerative changes which may be associated with low back pain of mechanical origin.

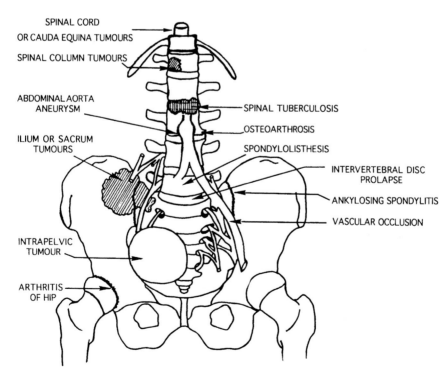

Figure 1.7 Some causes of pain in the low back or leg, which must be considered in differential diagnosis. (Modified from Adams, J.C. (1981) *Outline of Orthopaedics*, 9th edition. Churchill Livingstone, Edinburgh, p. 208 and Giles, L.G.F. (1989) *Anatomical Basis of Low Back Pain*. Williams and Wilkins, Baltimore.)

References

Adams, J.C. (1981) *Outline of Orthopaedics*, 9th edition. Churchill Livingstone, Edinburgh, p. 208.

Adams, M.A., Dolan, P., and Hutton W.C. (1986) The stages of disc degeneration as revealed by discogram. *J. Bone Joint Surg.*, **68B**, 36.

Ahmed, M., Bjurholm, A., Kreicbergs, A. *et al.* (1993) Sensory and autonomic innervation of the facet joint in the rat lumbar spine. *Spine*, **18**, 2121–2126.

Allan, D.B. and Waddell, G. (1989) An historical perspective on low back pain and disability. *Acta Orthop. Scand.*, (Suppl 234)

Althoff, I., Brinckmann, P., Frobin, W. *et al.* (1992) An improved method of stature measurement for quantitative determination of spinal loading. *Spine*, **17**, 682–693.

Amonoo-Kuofi, H.S., El-Badawi, M.G. and Fatani, J.A. (1988) Ligaments associated with lumbar intervertebral foramina. 1. L1 to L4. *J. Anat.*, **156**, 177–183.

Anderson, J.A.D. (1976) Back pain in industry. In *The Lumbar Spine and Back Pain* (M.I.V. Jayson, ed.), Sector Publishing, London, pp. 29–46.

Anderson, J.A.D. (1980) Back pain and occupation. In *The Lumbar Spine and Back Pain* (M.I.V., Jayson, ed.), 2nd edn. Pitman Medical, Kent, pp. 57–82.

Andersson, G.B.J. (1983) The biomechanics of the posterior elements of the lumbar spine. *Spine*, **8**: 326.

Aprill, C. (1986) Lumbar facet joint arthrography and injection in the evaluation of painful disorders of the low back (abstract). Presented at a meeting of the International Society for the Study of the Lumbar Spine, Dallas.

Aprill, C. and Bogduk, N. (1992) The prevalence of cervical zygapophyseal joint pain. *Spine*, **17**, 744–747.

Arnoldi, C.C. (1972) Intravertebral pressures in patients with lumbar pain: a preliminary communication. *Acta Orthop. Scand.*, **431**, 109–117.

Arnoldi, C.C. (1976) Intraosseous hypertension: a possible cause of low back pain? *Clin Orthop.*, **115**, 30–34.

Arnoldi, C.C., Lemperg, R.K. and Linderholm, H. (1971) Immediate effects of osteotomy of the intramedullary pressure of the femoral head and neck in patients with degenerative osteoarthritis. *Acta Orthop. Scand.*, **42**, 351–365.

Arnoldi, C.C., Linderholm, H. and Mussbichler, H. (1972) Venous engorgement and intraosseous hypertension in osteoarthritis of the hip. *J. Bone Joint Surg.*, **54B**, 409–421.

Arnoldi, C.C., Lemperg, R.K. and Linderholm, H. (1975) Intraosseous hypertension and pain in the knee. *J. Bone Joint Surg.*, **57B**, 360–363.

Astrom, J. (1975) Peroperative effect of fenestration upon intraosseous pressure in patients with osteoarthritis of the hip. *Acta Orthop. Scand.*, **46**, 963–967.

Avrahami, E., Frishman, E., Fridman, Z. *et al.* (1994) Spina bifida occulta of S1 is not an innocent finding. *Spine*, **19**, 12–15.

Baldwin, K.W. (1977) A critique of the low back pain problem. In *Approaches to the Validation of Manipulation Therapy*. (A.A. Buerger and J.S. Tobis,, eds), Charles C. Thomas, Springfield, IL, pp. 303–307.

Barbor, R. (1964) A treatment for chronic low back pain. *Excerpta Medica International Congress* Series, **107**, 661–664.

Barzo, P., Voros, E. and Bodosi, M. (1993) A lumbosacralis atmeneti csigolyak koroki szereperol (Bertolotti syndroma). *Orv. Hetil.* **134**, 2537–2540.

Basler, H.D. (1994) Chronifizierungsprozesse von Ruckenschmerzen. *Ther. Umsch.*, **51**, 395–402.

Beaumont, B. and Paice, E. (1992) Back pain. *Occas. Pap. R. Coll. Gen. Pract.*, **58**, 36–38.

Benninghoff, G. (1980) *Lehrbuch der Anatomie des Menschen*. 1. Bd. Allgemeine Anatomie, Cytrologie und Bewegungsapparat, 13.Aufl. Bearb. von J Staubesand. Urban and Schwarzenberg, München Berlin Wien.

Benson, D.R. (1983) The spine and neck. In *Musculoskeletal Diseases of Children* (M.E. Gershwin and D.L. Robbins, eds), Grune and Stratton, New York, p. 469.

Bernard, T.N. and Kirkaldy-Willis, W.H. (1987) Recognising specific characteristics of nonspecific low back pain. *Clin. Orthop. Rel. Res.*, **217**, 96.

Boden, S.D., Davis, D.O., Dina, T.S. *et al.* (1990) Abnormal magnetic-resonance scans of the lumbar spine in asymptomatic subjects. *J. Bone Joint Surg.*, **72A**, 403–408.

Bogduk, N. and Marsland, A. (1988) The cervical zygapophyseal joints as a source of neck pain. *Spine*, **13**, 610–617.

Bonica, J.J. (1957) Management of myofascial pain syndromes in general practice. *JAMA*, **164**, 732–738.

Bourdillon, J.F. (1970) *Spinal Manipulation*. William Heinemann Medical Books, London.

Brightman, R.P., Miller, C.A., Rea, G.L. *et al.* (1992) Magnetic resonance imaging of trauma to the thoracic and lumbar spine. *Spine*, **17**, 541–550.

Bronfort, G. and Jochumsen, O.H. (1984) The functional radiographic examination of patients with low back pain. A study of different forms of variations. *J. Manipulative Physiol. Ther.*, **7**, 89–97.

Budd, K. (1981) The use of non-pharmaceutical methods in the treatment of arthritic pain. *Clin. Rheum. Dis.*, **7**, 437–454.

Buirski, G. and Silberstein, M. (1993) The symptomatic lumbar disc in patients with low-back pain. *Spine*, **18**, 1808–1811.

Butler, D., Trafimow, J. H., Andersson, G. B. J. *et al.* (1990) Disc degenerate before facets. *Spine*, **15**, 111–113.

Cailliet, R. (1968) *Low Back Pain Syndrome*, 2nd edn. F.A. Davis, Philadelphia.

Carrera, G.F. (1979) Lumbar facet arthrography and injection in low back pain. *Wisc. Med. J.*, **78**, 35–37.

Carroll, G.J. (1987) Spectrophotometric measurement of proteoglycans in osteoarthritic synovial fluid. *Ann. Rheum. Dis.*, **46**, 375–379.

Cassidy, J.D. and Mierau, D.R. (1992) Pathophysiology of the sacroiliac joint. In *Principles and Practice of Chiropractic*, 2nd edn (S. Haldeman, ed.), Appleton and Lange, Norwalk, pp. 211–224.

Chila, A.G., Jeffries, R.R. and Levin, S.M. (1990) Is manipulation for your practice? *Patient Care*, May 15, 77–92.

Cihak, R. (1970) Variations of lumbosacral joints and their morphogenesis. *Acta Universitatis Carolinae Medica*, **16**, 145–165.

Clarke, G.R. (1972) Unequal leg length: an accurate method of detection and some clinical results. *Rheumatol. Phys. Med.* **11**, 285–390.

Cobb, J.R. (1948) Outline for the study of scoliosis. Instructional course lectures. *Am. Acad. Orthop. Surg.*, **5**, 261–275.

Crock, H.V. (1976) Isolated lumbar disk resorption as a cause of nerve root canal stenosis. *Clin. Orthop.*, **115**, 109–115.

Day, L.J., Bovill, E.G., Trafton, P.G. *et al.* (1994) Orthopedics. In *Current Surgical Diagnosis and Treatment* (L.W. Way, ed.), Appleton Lange,Connecticut, pp. 1011-1104.

Destouet, J.M., Gilula, L.A., Murphy, W.A. *et al.* (1982) Lumbar facet joint injection: indication, technique, clinical correlation and preliminary results. *Radiology,* **145**, 321-325.

Deyo, R.A. (1983) Conservative therapy for low back pain. *JAMA,* **250**, 1057-1062.

Deyo, R.A. and Tsui-Wu, Y.-J. (1987) Descriptive epidemiology of low back pain and its related medical care in the United States. *Spine* **12**, 264-268.

Dixon, A.St. (1976) Diagnosis of low back pain - sorting the complainers. In *The Lumbar Spine and Back Pain* (M. Jayson, ed.) Sector Publishing, London, pp. 77-92.

Dixon, A.St. (1980) Diagnosis of low back pain - sorting the complainers. In *The Lumbar Spine and Back Pain* 2nd edn, (M. Jayson, ed.), Pitman Medical, Kent, pp. 135-156.

Dixon, A.St. and Campbell-Smith, S. (1969) Long leg arthropathy. *Ann. Rheum. Dis.,* **28**, 359-365.

Dorwart, R.H., Vogler, J.B. and Helms, C.A. (1983) Spinal stenosis. *Radiol. Clin. North Am.,* **21**, 301-325.

Dory, M.A. (1981) Arthrography of the lumbar facet joints. *Radiology,* **140**, 23-27.

Dvorak, J., Panjabi, M.M., Novotny, J.E. *et al.* (1991) Clinical validation of functional flexion-extension roentgenograms of the lumbar spine. *Spine,* **16**, 943-945.

Dyck, P. (1985) Paraplegia following chemonucleolysis. *Spine,* **10**, 359.

Editorial (1978) Apophyseal joints and back pain. *Lancet,* **2**, 247.

Editorial (1990) Chiropractors and low back pain. *Lancet,* July, 28, 220.

Eguro, H. (1983) Transvers myelitis following chemonucleolysis. *J. Bone Joint Surg.,* **65A**, 1328.

Ehni, G. (1977) Historical writings on spondylotic caudal radiculopathy and its effect on the nervous system. In *Lumbar Spondylosis: Diagnosis, Management and Surgical Treatment* (P.R. Weinstein, G. Ehni and C.B. Wilson, eds), Year Book Medical Publishers, Chicago, pp. 1-12.

Eisenstein, S.M. and Parry, C.R. (1987) The lumbar facet arthrosis syndrome. Clinical presentation and articular surface changes. *J. Bone Joint Surg.,* **69B**, 3-7.

El-Khoury, G.Y. and Renfrew, D.L. (1991) Percutaneous procedures for the diagnosis and treatment of lower back pain: diskography. Facet joint injection, and epidural injection. *AJR,* **157**, 685-691.

Elster, A.D. (1989) Bertolotti's syndrome revisited. *Spine,* **14**, 1373-1377.

Fager, C.A. (1994) Observations on spontaneous recovery from intervertebral disc herniation. *Surg. Neurol.,* **42**, 282-286.

Fahrni, W.H. (1966) *Backache Relieved Through New Concepts of Posture.* Charles C. Thomas, Springfield, IL, pp. V, 13.

Farfan, H.F. (1978) The biomechanical advantage of lordosis and hip extension for upright man as compared with other anthropoids. *Spine,* **3**, 336-345.

Farfan, H.F. (1980) The scientific basis of manipulative procedures. *Clin. Rheum. Dis.,* **6**, 159-178.

Feldenkrais, M. (1949) *Body and Mature Behaviour.* International Universities Press, New York, p. 104.

Foley, R.K. and Kirkaldy-Willis, W.H. (1979) Chronic venous hypertension in the tail of the Wistar rat. *Spine,* **4**, 251-257.

Friberg, O. (1987) The statics of postural pelvic tilt scoliosis; a radiographic study on 288 consecutive chronic LBP patients. *Clin. Biomech.,* **2**, 211-219.

Friberg, S. (1948) Anatomical studies on lumbar disc degeneration. *Acta Orthop. Scand.,* **17**, 224-230.

Friedman, W.A. (1984) New techniques for treatment of disk disease. *Geriatrics,* **39**, 41-53.

Frymoyer, J.W. (1988) Back pain and sciatica. *N. Engl. J. Med.,* **318**, 291-300.

Frymoyer, J.W. and Cats-Baril, W.L. (1991) An overview of the incidences and costs of low back pain. *Orthop. Clin. North Am.,* **22**, 263-271.

Frymoyer, J.W., Ducker, T.B., Hadler, N.M. *et al.* (1991) The future of spinal treatment. In *The Adult Spine: Principles and Practice* (J.W. Frymoyer, ed.), Raven Press, New York, pp. 43-52.

Garlick, D. (1990) *The Lost Sixth Sense. A Medical Scientist Looks at the Alexander Technique.* Biological and Behavioural Sciences Printing Unit, The University of NSW, Kensington, NSW.

Ghormley, R.K. (1958) An etiologic study of back pain. *Radiology,* **70**, 649-652.

Giles, L.G.F. (1973) Spinal fixation and viscera. *J. Clin. Chiroprac. Arch.,* **3**, 144-165.

Giles, L.G.F. (1981) Lumbosacral facetal 'joint angles' associated with leg length inequality. *Rheumatol. Rehabil.,* **20**, 233-238.

Giles, L.G.F. (1982) *Leg Length Inequality with Postural Scoliosis: Its Effect on Lumbar Apophyseal Joints.* M.Sc thesis, University of Western Australia, Perth, Western Australia.

Giles, L.G.F. (1987) *The Anatomy of Human Lower Lumbar and Lumbo-Sacral Zygapophysial Joint Inferior Recesses with Particular Reference to their Synovial Fold Innervation.* Ph.D thesis, Department of Anatomy and Human Biology, University of Western Australia, Nedlands, Western Australia.

Giles, L.G.F. (1989) *Anatomical Basis of Low Back Pain.* Williams and Wilkins, Baltimore.

Giles, L.G.F. (1991) A review and description of some possible causes of low back pain of mechanical origin in *homo sapiens. Proc. Aust. Soc. Hum. Biol.,* **4**, 193-212.

Giles, L.G.F. (1992a) Paraspinal autonomic ganglion distortion due to vertebral body osteophytosis: a cause of vertebrogenic autonomic syndromes? *J. Manipulative Physiol. Ther.,* **15**, 551-555.

Giles, L.G.F. (1992b) Pathoanatomic studies and clinical significance of lumbosacral zygapophyseal (facet) joints. *J. Manipulative Physiol. Ther.,* **15**, 36-40.

Giles, L.G.F. (1992c) Ligaments traversing the intervertebral canals of the human lower lumbosacral spine. *Neuro-Orthop.,* **13**, 25-38.

Giles, L.G.F. (1994) A histological investigation of human lower lumbar intervertebral canal (foramen) dimensions. *J. Manipulative Physiol. Ther.,* **17**, 4-14.

Giles, L.G.F. and Kaveri, M.J.P. (1990) Some osseous and soft tissue causes of human intervertebral canal (foramen) stenosis. *J. Rheumatol.,* **17**, 1471-1481.

Giles, L.G.F. and Taylor, J.R. (1981) Low back pain associated with leg length inequality. *Spine,* **6**, 510-521.

Giles, L.G.F. and Taylor, J.R. (1982) Intra-articular synovial protrusions in the lower lumbar apophyseal joints. *Bull. Hosp. J. Dis.,* **42**, 248-255.

Giles, L.G.F., Taylor, J.R. and Cockson, A. (1986) Human

zygapophyseal joint synovial folds. *Acta Anat.*, **126**, 110–114.

Gillette, R.G., Kramis, R.C. and Roberts, W.J. (1993a) Spinal projections of cat primary afferent fibers innervating lumbar facet joints of multifidus muscle. *Neurosci. Lett.*, **157**, 67–71.

Gillette, R.G., Kramis, R.C. and Roberts, W.J. (1993b) Characterization of spinal somatosensory neurons having receptive fields in lumbar tissues of cats. *Pain*, **54**, 85–98.

Gofton, J.P. (1971) Studies in osteoarthritis of the hip: Part IV. Biomechanics and clinical considerations. *CMAJ*, **104**, 1007–1011.

Gofton, J.P. and Trueman, G.E. (1967) Unilateral idiopathic osteoarthritis of the hip. *Can. Med. Assoc. J.*, **87**, 1129–1132.

Gracovetsky, S., Farfan, H.F. and Lamy, C. (1981) The mechanism of the lumbar spine. *Spine.* **6**, 249–262.

Gross, D. (1979) Multifactorial diagnosis and therapy for low back pain. In *Advances in Pain Research and Therapy*, Vol 3. Raven Press, New York, pp. 671–683.

Hadley, L.A. (1964) *Anatomico-Roentgenographic Studies of the Spine*. Charles C. Thomas, Springfield, IL.

Haldeman, S. (1977) Why one cause of back pain? In *Approaches to the Validation of Manipulation Therapy* (A.A. Buerger and T.S. Tobis, eds), Charles C. Thomas, Springfield, IL, pp. 187–197.

Haldeman, S. (1980) The spine as a neuro-musculoskeletal organ. In *A Comprehensive Interdisciplinary Approach to the Management of Spinal Disorders*, Haldeman Interprofessional Conference on the Spine, Las Vegas.

Ham, A.W. and Cormack, D.H. (1979) *Histology*, 8th edn. J.B. Lippincott, Philadelphia, pp. 476, 642.

Hanai, K. (1980) Dynamic measurement of intraosseous pressure in lumbar spinal vertebrae with reference to spinal canal stenosis. *Spine*, **5**, 568–574.

Hazelman, B. and Bulgen, D. (1981) Low back pain. *Int. Med. Rheum. Dis.*, **1**, 486–491.

Heliovaara, M., Vanharanta, H., Korpi, J. *et al.* (1986) Herniated lumbar disc syndrome and vertebral canals. *Spine*, **11**, 433–435.

Herr, C.H. and Williams, J.C. (1994) Supralevator anorectal abscess presenting as acute low back pain and sciatica. *Ann. Emerg. Med.*, **23**, 132–135.

Herzog, R.J., Kaiser, J.A., Saal, J.A. *et al.* (1991) The importance of posterior epidural fat pad in lumbar central canal stenosis. *Spine*, **16**, S228–S233.

Hirsch, C., Ingelmark, B.E. and Miller, M. (1963) The anatomical basis for low back pain. *Acta Orthop. Scand.*, **33**, 1–17.

Hitselberger, W.E. and Witten, R.M. (1968) Abnormal myelograms in asymptomatic patients. *J. Neurosurg.*, **28**, 204.

Hoehler, F.K. and Tobis, J.S. (1983) Psychological factors in the treatment of back pain by spinal manipulation. *Br. J. Rheumatol.*, **22**, 206–212.

Horton, W.C. and Daftari, T.K. (1992) Which disc as visualized by magnetic resonance imaging is actually a source of pain? *Spine*, **17**, S164–S171.

Hoyland, J.A., Freemont, A.J. and Jayson, M.I.V. (1989) Intervertebral foramen venous obstruction. A cause of periradicular fibrosis? *Spine*, **14**, 558–568.

Huskisson, E.C. (1990) Back pain. In *Clinical Medicine*, 2nd edn (P.J. Kumar and M.L. Clark, eds), Baillière Tindall, London, p. 410.

Isherwood, I. and Antoun, N.M. (1980) CT scanning in the assessment of lumbar spine problems. In *The Lumbar Spine and Back Pain* (M.I.V. Jayson, ed.), 2nd edn. Pitman Medical, Kent, pp. 247–264.

Jackson, R. (1966) *The Cervical Syndrome*, 3rd edn. Charles C. Thomas, Springfield, IL.

Jackson, R.P. (1992) The facet syndrome. Myth or reality. *Clin. Orthop.*, **279**, 110–121.

Jayson, M.I.V. (1986) The inflammatory component of mechanical back problems. *Br. J. Rheumatol.*, **25**, 210–213.

Jenner, J.R. and Barry, M. (1995) Low back pain. *BMJ*, **310**, 929–932.

Jinkins, J.R. (1993) The pathoanatomic basis of somatic and autonomic syndromes originating in the lumbosacral spine. *Neuroimaging Clin. North Am.*, **3**, 443–463.

Jinkins, J.R., Whittemore, A.R. and Bradley, W.G. (1989) The anatomic basis of vertebrogenic pain and the autonomic syndrome associated with lumbar disk extrusion. *AJNR*, **10**, 219–231.

Joseph, J. (1960) *Man's Posture: Electromyographic Studies*. Charles C. Thomas, Springfield, IL, p. 14.

Keim, H.A. and Kirkaldy-Willis, W.H. (1987) *Clinical symposia. Low back pain* **39**, Ciba-Geigy Corp., New Jersey.

Keith, A. (1923) Man's posture: its evolution and disorders. *BMJ*, **3247**, 499–502.

Kellgren, J.H. (1939) On the distribution of pain arising from deep somatic structures with charts of segmental pain areas. *Clin. Sci.*, **4**, 35–46.

Kepes, E.R. and Duncalf, D. (1985) Treatment of backache with spinal injections of local anaesthetics, spinal and systemic steroids. A review. *Pain*, **22**, 33–47.

Kiaer, T., Gronlund, J. and Sorensen, K.H. (1988) Subchondral PO_2, PCO_2, pressure, pH and lactate in human osteoarthritis of the hip. *Clin. Orthop.*, **229**, 149–155.

Kiaer, T., Gronlund, J. and Sorensen, K.H. (1989) Intraosseous pressure and partial pressures of oxygen and carbon dioxide in osteoarthritis semin. *Arthritis Rheum.*, **18**, 57–60.

Kiaer, T., Pedersen, N.W., Kristensen, K.D. *et al.* (1990) Intraosseous pressure and oxygen tension in avascular necrosis and osteoarthritis of the hip. *J. Bone Joint Surg.*, **72B**, 1023–1030.

Kinney, R.K., Gatchel, R.J. and Mayer, T.G. (1991) The SCL-90R evaluated as an alternative of the MMPI for psychological screening of chronic low-back pain patients. *Spine*, **16**, 940–942.

Kirkaldy-Willis, W.H. (1983) The pathology and pathogenesis of low back pain. In *Managing Low Back Pain* (W.H. Kirkaldy-Willis, ed.), Churchill Livingstone, New York, pp. 23–43.

Kirkaldy-Willis, W.H. (1988) The site and nature of the lesion. In *Managing Low Back Pain*, 2nd edn (W.H. Kirkaldy-Willis ed.), Churchill Livingstone, New York, pp. 133–154.

Kirkaldy-Willis, W.H. (1984) The relationship of structural pathology to the nerve root. *Spine*, **9**, 49–52.

Kirkaldy-Willis, W.H. and Cassidy, J.D. (1984) Toward a more precise diagnosis of low back pain. In *Spine Update, 1984. Perspectives in Radiology, Orthopaedic Surgery, and Neurosurgery* (H.K. Genant, ed.). Radiology Research and Education Foundation, San Francisco, pp. 5–16.

Kirkaldy-Willis, W.H. and Cassidy, J. (1985) Spinal manipulator in the treatment of low back pain. *Can. Fam. Physician*, **31**, 535–540.

Kirkaldy-Willis, W.H. and Farfan, H.F. (1982) Instability of the lumbar spine. *Clin. Orthop.*, **165**, 110-123.

Kirkaldy-Willis, W.H. and McIvor, G.W.D. (1976) Lumbar spinal stenosis - editorial comment. *Clin. Orthop.*, **115**, 2-3.

Kirkaldy-Willis, W.H. and Tchang, S. (1983) Diagnosis. In *Managing Low Back Pain* (W.H. Kirkaldy-Willis, ed.), Churchill Livingstone, New York, pp. 109-127.

Kirkaldy-Willis, W.H., Wedge, J.H., Yong-Hing, K. *et al.* (1978) Pathology and pathogenesis of lumbar spondylosis and stenosis. *Spine*, **3**, 319-328.

Kos, J. and Wolf, J. (1972) Les Menisques Intervertebraux et leur Role Possible dans les Blocages Vertebraux. *Ann. Med. Phys.*, **XV**, 203-217.

Kramer, J. (1990) *Intervertebral Disk Diseases: Causes, Diagnosis, Treatment and Prophylaxis*, 2nd edn, Georg Thieme Verlag, New York, Stuttgart, p. 1.

Lafferty, J.F., Winter, W.G. and Gambaro, S.A. (1977) Fatigue characteristics of posterior elements of vertebrae. *J. Bone Joint Surg. (Am)*, **59**, 154-158.

Lauterbur, P.C. (1973) Image formation by induced local interactions: examples employing nuclear magnetic resonance. *Nature*, **242**, 190-191.

Langworthy, R. (1993) Evaluation of impairment related to low back pain. *J. Med. Syst.*, **17**, 253-256.

Le-Breton, C., Meziou, M., Laredo, J. D. *et al.* (1993) Sarcomes pagetiques rechidiens. A propos de huit observations. *Rev. Rhum. Ed. Fr.*, **60**, 16-22.

Leger, W. (1959) *Die Form der Wirbelsäule*, Enke, Stuttgart.

Lehmann, T.R., Spratt, K.F. and Lehmann, K.K. (1993) Predicting long-term disability in low back injured workers presenting to a spine consultant. *Spine*, **18**, 1103-1112.

Lemperg, R.K. and Arnoldi, C.C. (1978) The significance of intraosseous pressure in normal and diseased states with special reference to the intraosseous pain - engorgement syndrome. *Clin. Orthop.*, **136**, 143-156.

Lewin, T., Moffett, B. and Viidik, A. (1961) The morphology of the lumbar synovial intervertebral arches. *Acta Morphol. Neerlando-Scandinavica*, **4**, 299-319.

Lewinnik, G.E. (1983) Management of low back pain and sciatica. *Int. Anesthesiol. Clin.*, **21**, 61-78.

Lewinnik, G.E. and Warfield, C.A. (1986) Facet joint degeneration as a cause of low back pain. *Clin. Orthop.*, **213**, 216-222.

Lewis, T.L.T. (1985) Pelvis, pain in. In *French's Index of Differential Diagnosis* (D.F. Hart, ed.), 12th edn, Wright, London, pp. 660-661.

Lewit, K. (1985) *Manipulative Therapy in Rehabilitation of the Motor System*. Butterworths, London.

Lippert, H. (1970) Probleme der Statik und Dynamik von Wirbelsäule und Rückenmark. In *Wirbelsäule und Nervensystem* (D. Trostdort and H.S.T. Stender, eds), Thieme, Stuttgart, S, pp. 9-15.

Loeser, J.D., Bigos, S.J., Fordyce, W.E. *et al.* (1990) Low back pain. In *The Management of Pain* Vol 2. (J.J. Bonica, ed.), Lea and Febiger, Philadelphia, pp. 1148-1483.

Lovett, R.W. (1905) The mechanism of the normal spine and its relation to scoliosis. *N. Engl. J. Med.*, **153**, 349-359.

MacMillan, J., Schaffer, J.L. and Kambin, P. (1991) Routes and incidence of communication of lumbar discs with surrounding neural structures. *Spine*, **16**, 167-171.

Macnab, I. (1977) *Backache*. Williams and Wilkins, Baltimore.

Maigne, R. (1974) The dorso-lumbar origin of certain cases of low lumbar pain: the role of interapophysary articulations and the posterior branches of the spinal nerves. *Rev. Rheum. Malad. Osteoarticulares* **41**, 781-789.

Maigne, R. (1980) Low back pain from thoracolumbar origin. *Arch. Phys. Med. Rehabil.*, **61**, 389-394.

Maldague, B., Mathurin, P. and Malghem, J. (1981) Facet joint arthrography in lumbar spondylosis. *Radiology*, **140**, 29-36.

Margo, K. (1994) Diagnosis, treatment and prognosis in patients with low back pain. *Am. Fam. Phys.*, **49**, 171-179.

Marshall, L.L. and Trethewie, E.R. (1973) Chemical irritation of nerve root in disc prolapse. *Lancet*, **2**, 320.

McArdle, C.B., Crofford, M.J., Mirfakhraee, M. *et al.* (1986) Surface coil MR of spinal trauma: preliminary experience. *AJNR*, **7**, 885-893.

McRae, D.L. (1977) Radiology of the lumbar spinal canal. In *Lumbar Spondylosis. Diagnosis, Management and Surgical Treatment* (P.R. Weinstein, G .Ehni and C.B. Wilson, eds), Year Book Medical Publishers, Chicago, pp. 92-114.

Meade, T.W., Dyer, S., Brown, W. *et al.* (1990) Low back pain of mechanical origin: randomised comparison of chiropractic and hospital outpatient treatment. *BMJ*, **300**, 1431-1437.

Mehta, M. and Sluijter, M.E. (1979) The treatment of chronic back pain. *Anesthesia*, **34**, 768-775.

Mellin, G. (1986) Chronic low back pain in men 54-63 years of age. *Spine*, **11**, 421-426.

Mennell, J.McM. (1960) *Back Pain. Diagnosis and Treatment using Manipulative Techniques*, 1st edn, Little, Brown, Boston.

Merz, B. (1986) The honeymoon is over: spinal surgeons begin to divorce themselves from chemonucleolysis. *JAMA*, **256**, 317.

Millard, R.W. and Jones, R.H. (1991) Construct validity of practical questionnaires for assessing disability of low-back pain. *Spine*, **16**, 835-838.

Miller, J.A.A., Schmatz, C. and Schultz, A.B. (1988) Lumbar disc degeneration: correlation with age, sex, and spine level in 600 autopsy specimens. *Spine*, **13**, 173-178.

Mixter, W.J. and Barr, J.S. (1934) Rupture of the intervertebral disc with involvement of the spinal canal. *N. Engl. J. Med.*, **211**, 210-215.

Modic, M.T. and Herzob, R.J. (1994) Imaging corner. Spinal imaging modalities. What's available and who should order them? *Spine*, **19**, 1764-1765.

Mooney, V. and Robertson, J. (1976) The facet syndrome. *Clin. Orthop.*, **115**, 149-156.

Moore, M.R., Brown, C.W., Brugman, J.L. *et al.* (1991) Relationship between vertebral intraosseous pressure, pH, PO_2, PcO_2, and magnetic resonance imaging spinal inhomogeneity in patients with back pain. An *in vivo* study. *Spine (Suppl)*, **16**, S239-S242.

Morscher, E. (1977) Etiology and pathophysiology of leg length discrepancies. In *Leg Length Discrepancy. The Injured Knee* Vol. l, (Progress in Orthopedic Surgery) (D.S. Hungerford, ed.), Springer-Verlag, New York, pp. 9-19.

Murtagh, J. (1991) Low back pain. *Aust. Fam. Phys.*, **20**, 320-326.

Murtagh, J.E. (1994) The non pharmacological treatment of back pain. *Australian Prescriber* **17**, 9-12.

Nachemson, A.L. (1969) Intradiscal measurements of pH in patients with lumbar rhizopathies. *Acta Orthop. Scand.*, **40**, 23–42.

Nachemson, A.L. (1971) Low-back pain - its etiology and treatment. *Clin. Med.*, **78**, 18–24.

Nachemson, A.L. (1976) The lumbar spine: an orthopaedic challenge. *Spine*, **1**, 59–71.

Nachemson, A.L. (1977) Pathophysiology and treatment of back pain. A critical look at different types of treatment. In *Approaches to the Validation of Manipulation Therapy* (A.A. Buerger and J.S. Tobis, eds), Charles C. Thomas, Springfield, IL, pp. 42–57.

Nachemson, A.L. (1985) Advances in low-back pain. *Clin. Orthop.*, **200**, 266–278.

Nachemson, A.L. (1991) Spinal disorders. Overall impact on society and the need for orthopedic resources. *Acta Orthop. Scand.*, **62**, 17–22.

Nachemson, A.L. (1994) Chronic pain - the end of the welfare state? *Quality of Life Research*, **3**, S11–S17.

Nathan, H. (1962) Osteophytes of the vertebral column. *J. Bone Joint Surg.*, **44A**, 243–268.

Nathan, H. (1968) Compression of the sympathetic trunk by osteophytes of the vertebral column in the abdomen: an anatomical study with pathological and clinical considerations. *Surgery*, **63**, 609–625.

Nathan, H. (1987) Osteophytes of the spine compressing the sympathetic trunk and splanchnic nerves in the thorax. *Spine*, **12**, 527–532.

Nichols, P.J.R. (1960) Short-leg syndrome. *BMJ*, **1**, 1863–1865.

Okuwaki, T., Kunogi, J. and Hasue, M. (1991) Conjoined nerve roots associated with lumbosacral spine anomalies. *Spine*, **16**, 1347–1349.

Park, W.M. (1980) The place of radiology in the investigation of low back pain. *Clin. Rheum. Dis.*, **6**, 93–132.

Parke, W.W. and Watanabe, R. (1990) Adhesions of the ventral lumbar dura: an adjunct source of discogenic pain? *Spine*. **15**, 300–303.

Paterson, J.K. (1987) A survey of musculoskeletal problems in general practice. *Manuelle Medizin*, **3**, 40–48.

Paterson, J.K. (1994) 'I can tell': an impediment to progress in musculoskeletal medicine. *J. R. Soc. Med.*, **87**, 648–649.

Pauwels, F. (1976) *Biomechanics of the Normal and Diseased Hip* (translation of German, 1973 edition), Springer-Verlag, Berlin.

Pearcy, M., Portek, I. and Shepherd, J. (1985) The effect of low back pain on lumbar spinal movements measured by three-dimensional X-ray analysis. *Spine,* **10**, 150–153.

Pedowitz, R.A., Garfin, S.R., Massie, J.B., *et al.* (1992) Effects of magnitude and duration of compression on spinal nerve root conduction. *Spine*, **17**, 194–199.

Peek, R.D., Thomas, J.C. and Wiltse, L.L. (1993) Diagnosis of lumbar arachnoiditis by myelography. *Spine*, **18**, 2286–2289.

Pelz, D.M. and Haddad, R.G. (1989) Radiologic investigation of low back pain. *CMAJ*, **140**, 289–295.

Pope, M.H. and Novotny, J.E. (1993) Spinal biomechanics. *J. Biomech. Eng.*, **115**, 569–574.

Putz, R. (1992) The detailed functional anatomy of the ligaments of the vertebral column. *Ann. Anat.*, **174**, 40–47.

Rasch, P.J. and Burke, R.K. (1967) *Kinesiology and Applied Anatomy*, 3rd edn, Lea and Febiger, Philadelphia, p. 375.

Reichmann, S. (1973) Radiography of the lumbar intervertebral joints. *Acta Radiol.*, **14**, 161–170.

Reid, D.C. and Smith, B. (1984) Leg length inequality: a review of etiology and management. *Physiotherapy Canada*, **36**, 177–182.

Rickenbacher, J., Landolt, A.M. and Theiler, K. (1985) *Applied Anatomy of the Back*. Springer-Verlag, Berlin, pp. 93, 184–186.

Roth, M. (1981) Idiopathic scoliosis from the point of view of the neurologist. *Neuroradiology*, **21**, 133–138.

Rothman, R.H. and Simeone, F.A. (1975) Lumbar disc disease. In *The Spine* (R.H. Rothman and F.A. Simeone, eds), W.B. Saunders,Philadelphia, p. 442.

Rush, W.A. and Steiner, H.A. (1946) A study of lower extremity length inequality. *Am. J. Roentgenol.*, **56**, 616–623.

Rydevik, B., Holm, S., Brown, M.D. *et al.* (1990) Diffusion from the cerebrospinal fluid as a nutritional pathway for spinal nerve roots. *Acta Physiol. Scand.*, **138**, 247–248.

Saal, J.A. and Saal, J.S. (1989) Nonoperative treatment of herniated lumbar intervertebral disc with radiculopathy: an outcome study. *Spine*, **14**, 431–437.

Sachs, E.S. and Fraenkel, J. (1900) Progressive ankylotic rigidity of the spine. *J. Nerv. Ment. Dis.*, **27**, 1.

Schede, F. (1961) *Grundlagen der Körperlichen Erziehung*. Enke, Stuttgart.

Schiotz, E.H. and Cyriax, J. (1975) *Manipulation Past and Present*. William Heinemann Medical Books, London.

Schmorl, G. and Junghanns, H. (1971) *The Human Spine in Health and Disease*, 2nd edn, Grune and Stratton, New York, pp. 22, 37, 148, 197.

Shah, J.S. (1980) Structure, morphology and mechanics of the lumbar spine. In *The Lumbar Spine and Back Pain* (M.I.V. Jayson, ed.), 2nd edn. Pitman Medical, Kent,pp. 359–406.

Sicuranza, B.J., Richards, J. and Tisdall, L.H. (1970) The short leg syndrome in obstetrics and gynecology. *Am. J. Obstet. Gynecol.*, **107**, 217–219.

Simons, D.G. and Travell, J. (1983) Common myofascial origins of low back pain. *Postgrad. Med.*, **73**, 55–108.

Singer, K P. (1989) Variation at the human thoracolumbar transitional junction with particular reference to the posterior elements. Ph.D. Thesis, The University of Western Australia.

Singer, K.P. (1994) The anatomy and biomechanics of the thoracolumbar junction. In *Modern Manual Therapy* (J.D. Boyling and N. Palastanga, eds), Churchill Livingstone, Edinburgh, pp. 85–98.

Singer, K.P. and Giles. L.G.F. (1990) Manual therapy considerations at the thoracolumbar junction: an anatomical and functional perspective. *J. Manipulative Physiol. Ther.*, **13**, 83–88.

Skelton, A.M., Murphy, E.A., Murphy, R.J.L. and O'Dowd, T.C. (1995) General practitioner perceptions of low back pain patients. *Fam. Pract.*, **12**, 44–48.

Spencer, D.L., Ray, R.D., Spigos, D.G. *et al.* (1981) Intraosseous pressure in the lumbar spine. *Spine*, **6**, 159–161.

Spencer, D., Miller, J. and Bertolini, J. (1984) The effects of the intervertebral disc space narrowing on the contract forces between the nerve root and a simulated disc protrusion. *Spine*, **9**, 442–446.

Spengler, D.M., Bigos, S.J., Martin, N.A. *et al.* (1986) Back injuries in industry: a retrospective study. 1. Overview and cost analysis. *Spine*, **11**, 241–245.

Spiller, W.G., Musser, J.H. and Martin, E. (1903) Arachnoidal cysts. *University of Pennsylvania Medical Bulletin,* 16, 27–30.

Stevens, J. (1968) Pain and its clinical management. *Med. Clin. North Am.,* 52, 55–71.

Stockwell, R. A. (1985) *A Pre-clinical view of osteoarthritis.* A Sir John Struthers Lecture. The Medical School, Teviot Place, Edinburgh.

Stoddard, A. (1959) *Manual of Osteopathic Technique.* Hutchinson Medical Publications, London, p. 212.

Subotnick, S.I. (1981) Limb length discrepancies of the lower extremities (the short leg syndrome). *J. Orthop. Sports Phys. Ther.,* 3, 11–16.

Sunderland, S. (1968) *Nerves and Nerve Injuries.* Churchill Livingstone, Edinburgh.

Sunderland, S. (1980) The anatomy of the intervertebral foramen and the mechanisms of compression and stretch of nerve roots. In *Modern Developments in the Principles and Practice of Chiropractic* (S. Haldeman, ed.). Appleton-Century-Crofts, New York, pp. 45–64.

Tajima, N. and Kawano, K. (1986) Cryomicrotomy of the lumbar spine. *Spine,* 11, 376–379.

Tatter, S.B. and Cosgrove, G.R. (1994) Hemorrhage into a lumbar synovial cyst causing an acute cauda equina syndrome. Case report. *J. Neurosurg.,* 81, 449–452.

Taylor, J.R. and Twomey, L. (1986) Age changes in lumbar zygapophysial joints: observations on structure and function. *Spine,* 11, 739–745.

The North American Spine Society *AD HOC* Committee on Diagnostic and Therapeutic Procedures (1991) Common diagnostic and therapeutic procedures of the lumbosacral spine. *Spine,* 16, 1161–1167.

Travell, J. and Rinzler, S.H. (1952) Myofascial genesis of pain. *Postgrad. Med.,* 11, 425–434.

Tjernstrom, B., Olerud, S. and Karlstrom, G. (1993) Direct leg lengthening. *J. Orthop. Trauma,* 7, 543–551.

Turek, S.L. (1984) *Orthopaedics. Principles and their Application,* Volume 2, 4th edition, J.B. Lippincott Co., Philadelphia.

Vanharanta, H., Korpi, J., Heliovaara, M. *et al.* (1985) Radiographic measurements of lumbar spinal canal size and their relation to back mobility. *Spine,* 10, 461–466.

Verbiest, H. (1955) Further experiences on the pathological influence of a developmental narrowness of the bony lumbar vertebral canal. *J. Bone Joint Surg.,* 37B, 576.

Vernon-Roberts, B. and Pirie, C.J. (1977) Degenerative changes in the intervertebral disc of the lumbar spine and their sequelae. *Rheumatol. Rehabil.,* 16, 13–21.

Walker, S. and Cousins, M.J. (1994) Failed back surgery syndrome. *Aust. Fam. Phys.,* 23, 2308–2314.

Watts, C. and Dickhaus, E. (1986) Chemonucleolysis: a note of caution. *Surg. Neurol.,* 26, 236.

Wedel, D.J. and Wilson, P.R. (1985) Cervical facet arthrography. *Regional Anaesthesia,* 10, 7–11.

Weinstein, P.R., Ehni, G. and Wilson, C.B. (1977) Clinical features of lumbar spondylosis and stenosis. In *Lumbar Spondylosis, Diagnosis, Management and Surgical Treatment* (P.R. Weinstein, G. Ehni and C.B. Wilson, eds). Year Book Medical Publishers, Chicago, pp. 115–133.

Weitz, E.M. (1984) Paraplegia following chymopa pain injection. *J. Bone Joint Surg.,* 66A, 1131.

Werneke, M.W., Harris, D.E. and Lichter, R.L. (1993) Clinical effectiveness of behavioural signs for screening chronic low-back pain patients in a work-oriented physical rehabilitation program. *Spine,* 18, 2412–2418.

White, A.A. and Gordon, S.L. (1982) Synopsis: workshop on idiopathic low back pain. *Spine,* 7, 141–149.

Wiesel, S.W., Tsourmas, N., Feffer, H.L. *et al.* (1984) A study of computer-assisted tomography: 1. The incidence of positive CAT scans in an asymptomatic group of patients. *Spine,* 9, 549–551.

Witt, I., Vestergaard, A. and Rosenklink, A. (1984) A comparative analysis of X-ray findings of the lumbar spine in patients with and without lumbar pain. *Spine,* 9, 298–300.

Wood, P.H.N. and Badley, E.M. (1980) Back pain in the community. *Clin. Rheum. Dis.,* 6, 3–16.

Yates, A. (1976) Treatment of back pain. In *The Lumbar Spine and Back Pain* (M. Jayson, ed.), Sector Publishing, London, pp. 341–353.

Yong-Hing, K. and Kirkaldy-Willis, W.H. (1983) The pathophysiology of degenerative disease of the lumbar spine. *Orthop. Clin. North Am.,* 14, 491–504.

Young, W.B. (1993) The clinical diagnosis of lumbar radiculopathy. *Semin. Ultrasound CT MR,* 14, 385–388.

Yussen, P.S. and Swartz, J.D. (1993) The acute lumbar disc herniation: imaging diagnosis. *Semin Ultrasound CT MRI,* 14, 389–398.

2

The epidemiology of low back pain

Paul Shekelle

Understanding the epidemiology of low back pain is complicated by the effort of trying to understand what it is one is trying to measure and how it is to be measured. Ignoring the problem of defining exactly where anatomically 'low back pain' is located, we must consider what constitutes low back pain: any pain in the low back, no matter how mild or of brief duration, ever? Pain longer than a certain period, such as a day or a week? Pain severe enough to miss work: again over what time period? Pain significant enough to seek medical attention? Added to this definition problem is a measurement problem. There is no way to measure pain other than to ask the patient. If the patient is not asked contemporaneously about the pain, then there is the possibility of recall bias for past events. Lastly, one needs to decide in which group of persons to study the epidemiology of back pain. Depending on the circumstances, one might be interested in knowing about back pain among industrial workers, or among persons living in a particular community, or even an entire country. Ideally, what the clinician would like to know is the epidemiology of back pain in a well-defined population in which the pain was severe enough to cause a clinically meaningful decrement in the patient's functional activity, which lasted for some minimum length of time, say a day or two. Unfortunately, to gather such data would require that a defined population without any history of functional back problems be measured at near daily intervals with a sensitive measure of pain and functional health status, over a long period of time. Such data are not available. There have, however, been studies which approximate to a greater or lesser extent this ideal, and in this chapter I will attempt to piece together the data that are available to help provide a current picture of the epidemiology of low back pain.

First, I will define some common epidemiological terms. '*Incidence*' is a rate, and refers to the number of persons with new back pain occurring over a given time period among a known number of persons who were previously without back pain. '*Prevalence*' is a proportion, and refers to the number of persons who have back pain at any given time in a known population. Some investigations have measured the '*point prevalence*', meaning the proportion of persons who have back pain at any given moment, and the '*lifetime prevalence*', meaning the number of persons who have had back pain ever, even if they do not have it now. '*Risk factors*' are characteristics of demographics, genetics, lifestyle, occupation, behaviour, the environment, and other variables that affect the onset of back pain. In the case of back pain, some risk factors are probably 'risk markers', in that their role in the development of back pain is probably not causal (that is, they may be associated with both the occurrence of back pain and some other factor, possibly unknown, which is truly causal). '*Prognostic factors*' are variables which affect the course or outcome of back pain. Studies of risk factors, or the aetiology of back pain, come from observational studies which measure these variables before the diagnosis and treatment of back pain. Prognostic factors come from studies of the course of back pain patients after diagnosis and treatment. Figure 2.1 presents these concepts in graphic form. Risk and prognostic factors can be studied through cross-sectional studies, which measure at a single point in time the presence or absence of back pain and the presence or absence of the risk/prognostic factors of interest (history, cigarette smoking, etc.); through case-control studies, which identify persons with back pain, match these persons to others without back pain, and then compare between the two groups for the presence or absence of risk/prognostic variables; or through cohort studies, where groups of persons with and without certain risk factors are assembled, and then the groups are followed forward in time to see if they develop back

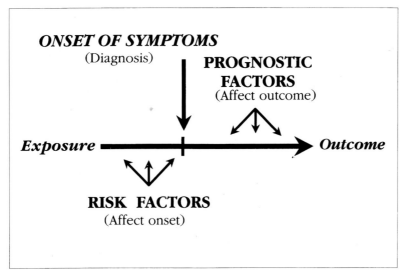

Figure 2.1 Distinguishing between risk and prognosis. (Reproduced with permission from Bombardier, C. (1994) *Spine*, **19 (18s)**, 2048.)

pain. Each type of study has its strengths and weaknesses, but in general a prospective cohort study is less susceptible to bias than the other two types. In many studies, it is not possible to distinguish whether risk factors or prognostic factors have been measured, and therefore they will be considered together. Risk and prognostic factor studies frequently report their results in terms of the odds ratio for a particular factor being associated with low back pain. The odds ratio is the odds of persons with the factor having back pain divided by the odds of persons without the factor having back pain, and is a commonly used measure of association. An '*adjusted' odds ratio* is an odds ratio for a given factor controlling for all other known confounding or associated factors. Another common way to report the association between a factor and low back pain is the *relative risk*, which is calculated by dividing the incidence of back pain amongst the persons with the factor by the incidence of back pain amongst the persons without the factor. For rare diseases, the odds ratio and the relative risk are approximately the same. For common illnesses, like low back pain, the odds ratio will always be greater than the corresponding relative risk. Case-control studies, by their design, only permit the calculation of odds ratios. To estimate a relative risk, a cohort study is needed.

Frequency of back pain

Table 2.1 presents some of the studies over the past 20 years that have reported measures of the fre-

quency of back pain. These studies have been performed in different countries, at different times, using different definitions of back pain and measuring back pain in different ways. All of these make direct comparisons from one study to another problematic. Still, some conclusions may be drawn. First is that most of the data about the epidemiology of back pain come from North America, the UK and the Scandinavian countries. We know very little about the epidemiology of back pain in most other parts of the world. Secondly, back pain is very common. Estimates of the yearly incidence range from 1.4 to 4.9%, point prevalence ranges from around 10 to over 50%, and lifetime prevalence ranges from about 14 to over 70%. Even the conservative estimates of the frequency of back pain mean that in most countries millions of people are affected. Thirdly, the estimate of the frequency probably depends upon how you measure it. For example, the lifetime prevalence for 'any occurrence' of low back pain in one study was 75% (Heliovaara, 1989b), but when defined in another study as 'back pain on most days for at least two weeks' the lifetime prevalence was just 13.8% (Deyo, 1987). Comparing these two studies is made difficult because, although in each study an individual's response to a survey question was the measure of back pain, the severity of that pain is clearly different. Lastly, because of major differences between studies, it is not possible to tell whether or not the frequency of low back pain has been changing over time. A recent systematic review of the Scandinavian literature on back pain reached the same conclusion (Leboeuf-Yde, 1996).

Table 2.1 *Epidemiologic studies of low back pain*

Community-based studies

Reference/year	Country of origin	Population	Sample size	How low back pain was defined	Findings
Hirsch (1969)	Sweden	Random sample of adult women in Gothenburg	692	Interview about only back symptoms	Lifetime prevalence approaches 70%
Lawrence (1969)	UK	Random sample from several communities in England	1 522	Answers to detailed history of symptoms	Point prevalence = 15%
Nagi (1973)	USA	Random sample of non-elderly adults in Columbus, Ohio	1 135	Interview about being 'often bothered' by back pain	Point prevalence = 18%
Bjelle (1981)	Sweden	Random sample of adults	45 000	Answers to personal interview about 'suffering from any long term illness, any complaint following accident, any handicap or other debility'	Prevalence = 6%
Svensson (1982)	Sweden	Random sample of men 40–47 years of age in Gothenberg	940	Interview about 'occurrence of LBP'	Lifetime prevalence = 61%
Biering-Sorensen (1983)	Denmark	Non-elderly adult population of a suburb of Denmark	928	Mail survey asking about any low back pain in past 12 months	Lifetime prevalence of LBP = 60–80%; 1 year incidence among 30 year olds = 11%
Cunningham (1984)	USA	Adult respondents to NHANES I (representative of USA)	2 494	Answers to detailed medical history about ever having pain in the back on most days lasting at least 1 month	Prevalence = 17.2%
Reisbord (1985)	USA	Random sample of the non-elderly adult population of Dayton, Ohio	2792	Survey question about presence of frequent back pain during previous year	Prevalence = 18%
Taylor and Curran (1985)	USA	Random sample of adult population who can be reached by telephone	1 254	Answer to question about 'how many days in the past year have you had LBP'	Prevalence 1 or more days = 56%; more than 30 days = 14%
Abenhaim (1987)	Canada	Population of Quebec	2.7 million	At least one day of compensated absence from work	Cumulative 1 year incidence = 1.4%
Deyo (1987)	USA	Adult respondents to NHANES II (representative of USA)	10 404	Affirmative answer to survey questions about LBP lasting for at least 2 weeks	Lifetime prevalence = 13.8%; 10.3% of respondents had back pain in previous year
Svensson (1988)	Sweden	Random sample of women 38–64 years of age in Gothenburg	1 410	Answers to mail survey about all conditions of pain, ache, stiffness, or fatigue localized to the low back	Point prevalence = 35%; lifetime prevalence = 66%

Author (year)	Country	Population	Method	n	Results
Brattberg (1989)	Sweden	Random sample of adults living in a county in Sweden	Answers to mail or telephone survey about 'any pain or discomfort'	827	Total prevalence = 31%; LBP of < 1 month = 8%; LBP of > 6 months = 20%
Heliovaara (1989)	Finland	Random sample of Finnish adults over age 30	Answers to survey about lifetime occurrence of LBP	7 217	LBP ever = 75%; six or more episodes = 45%; LBP in previous month = 21%
Bredkjaer (1991)	Denmark	Random sample of Danish adults	Answers to personal interview about LBP of > 6 months of LBP in previous 2 weeks	4 753	Prevalence of LBP > 6 months = 12%; prevalence of LBP in past 2 weeks = 23%
Walsh (1992)	UK	Random sample of adults living in eight geographic areas	Answers to survey about LBP of greater than 1 day in past year, or ever	2 667	1 year period prevalence = 36%; lifetime prevalence = 58%
Shekelle (1995a)	USA	Random sample of adults living in six geographic areas. Representative of the non-elderly USA population	Any health care visit for the patient-reported symptom of back pain	3 105	22% of persons had at least one back pain visit over a 3 to 5-year period
Papageorgiou (1995)	UK	Adults registered to two family practices in Manchester	Answers to survey about pain of greater than 1 day in past month; and question about LBP ever	7 699	1 month period prevalence = 39%; prevalence of LBP ever = 59%

Special population studies

Author (year)	Country	Population	Method	n	Results
Frymoyer (1980)	USA	All patients of a large family practice	Any medical visit for LBP	3 920	10.2% of all patients had at least one LBP visit within 3 years
Crook (1984)	Canada	Households on the rosta of a group family practice	Answers to telephone survey about being 'often troubled' or having 'noteworthy' pain in past 2 weeks	827	Point prevalence = 4.2%
Venning (1987)	Canada	All nurses at 10 facilities	Back complaint reported to employee health office	4 306	Annual incidence = 4.9%
Von Korff (1988)	USA	Enrollees of a large Health Maintenance Organization in Seattle	Answers to mail survey about back pain problems in the prior 6 months	1 016	Prevalence = 41%
Bergenudd (1988)	Sweden	Cohort of persons living in Malmo who were 55 years of age at the time of the study	Answers to health survey about pain, pain drawing	575	Point prevalence = 29%
Tuomi (1991)	Finland	Municipal workers 44–58 years of age	Answers to survey	4 255	Incidence over 4 years of LBP and sciatica was between 12% and 21% depending on gender and type of work; prevalence varied from 22% to 32%.
Rundcrantz (1991)	Sweden	Dentists	Answers to survey	359	Prevalence of LBP among males = 35%; among females = 49%

Table 2.1 *Continued*

Reference/year	Country of origin	Population	Sample size	How low back pain was defined	Findings
Rotgloz (1992)	Israel	Pharmaceutical factory workers	208	LBP by report to physician-directed questionnaire	66% of workers reported LBP; 17% reported pain lasting > 3 wk'
Salminen (1992)	Finland	14-year-old school children	1 503	Answers to survey	Lifetime prevalence = 30%
Anderson (1992)	USA	Oakland bus drivers	128	Medical interview and physical examination, pain on examination	Any low back pain on examination = 66%
Bigos (1992)	USA	Manufacturing workers	3 020	Back injury incident report or claim	4-year cumulative incidence rate = 9.2%
Moffett (1993)	UK	Student nurses	199	Daily recording of pain drawing	64% of nurses reported at least 1 day of LBP over 20-month period; 37% had back pain of at least 3 days
Chiou(1994)	China	Medical centre nurses	3 159	Answers to survey	Point prevalence of 13.9%; lifetime prevalence of 78%
Ebrall (1994)	Australia	Male adolescents in secondary school	610	Current LBP or recall of any back pain ever	17% reported current LBP; 57% reported current or past LBP

LBP = low back pain
NHANES = National Health and Nutrition Examination Survey

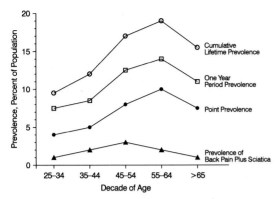

Figure 2.2 Low back pain prevalence according to age. Only episodes lasting at least 2 weeks were considered. 'Sciatica' was defined as pain that radiated to the legs and that increased with cough, sneeze or deep breathing. (Reproduced with permission from Deyo, R (1987) *Spine*, **12(3)**, 265.)

Based on these data, it is reasonable to conclude that back pain has an annual incidence in the adult population of around 2–5%, that the point prevalence for back pain is around 15–25%, and the lifetime prevalence for any back pain ever is probably well over 50% of the population. Longer or more severe episodes of back pain occur less frequently. Back pain with sciatica occurs with a lifetime prevalence of around 5–10%. The prevalence of low back pain rises with increasing age, and then falls after age 65 (Figure 2.2). Why the cumulative incidence of low back pain falls after age 65 is unknown, but may be related to recall bias among persons over the age of 65, differential mortality among persons with and without back pain (persons with back pain may die at a younger age due to other illnesses), or a cohort effect (persons currently over age 65 have always had a lower prevalence of back pain than persons born more recently, for unexplained reasons).

Risk and prognostic factors

The literature on risk and prognostic factors has been exhaustively reviewed several times since Andersson's seminal 1981 article (Heliovaara, 1989a; Pope, 1989; Garg, 1992). Little evidence has been produced to alter the conclusions of previous reviews. Table 2.2 summarizes many of the primary studies reporting data on risk and prognostic factors for low back pain. As in studies of the frequency of back pain, most of our information about risk and prognostic factors comes primarily from North America and the Scandinavian countries. Table 2.3 lists the principal studied risk and prognostic factors by their strength of association with back pain, which is a combination of the consistency of the evidence and the magnitude of the association. What follows is a best evidence synthesis of the data supporting various postulated risk and prognostic factors.

Strongly associated factors

The factor which has the strongest association with back pain is *history of previous back pain*. No other factor approaches a prior history of back pain in terms of the strength or magnitude of the association with future back pain. In eight prospective cohort studies or case-control studies of low back pain, the prior history of low back pain had an adjusted odds ratio predicting back pain ranging from 1.3 to 16.5, with most studies reporting adjusted odds ratios of between 3 and 5. In most of these studies, prior history was the most significant association predicting back pain. This is probably because recurrence of back pain is so common that back pain may be thought of as a chronic illness with intermittent symptomatic periods. As previously shown in Figure 2.2, there is an increasing prevalence of back pain with *increasing age*, reaching its maximum in the fifth and sixth decades, and then declining thereafter. There is a twofold increase in prevalence of back pain between persons in their sixth decade as compared to persons in their third decade. Several studies have shown that factors such as *depression, job dissatisfaction*, and *emotional distress* are as strongly (or even more strongly) associated with low back pain than job ergonomics and baseline measures of spinal function (Bongers, 1993). In the Boeing study (Bigos, 1991b), low job enjoyment and high distress scores on the Minnesota Multiphasic Personality Inventory were two of the strongest predictors of subsequent report of low back pain symptoms, with relative risks of 1.7 and 1.4, respectively. In another prospective cohort study, low job satisfaction was the third most important variable in predicting subsequent back injury report (after history of previous injury and smoking status – Ready, 1993). Several job factors have been strongly associated with back pain. The most important of these is *heavy or repetitive lifting*, particularly if combined with bending and twisting. Lifting has been associated with over 50% of worker's reported back injuries, and a history of heavy or repetitive lifting is seen twice as often in persons with back pain as in persons without back pain. An early prospective cohort study (Chaffin, 1973) found the incidence of low back pain to be twice as high in persons working jobs that have heavy spinal loading requirements compared with other jobs. A more recent prospective cohort study (Riihimaki, 1994) found that carpenters were 50% more likely than office workers to report low back pain during 3 years of

Table 2.2 *Risk/prognostic factors for low-back pain*

Reference/year/ country of origin	Study type	Study subjects	Factors studied	Findings
Battie (1989a) USA	Prospective cohort	3020 aircraft manufacturing workers	Cardiovascular fitness; smoking; demographic factors	Smoking, but not cardiovascular fitness, was associated with LBP over a 4-year follow up
Battie (1989b) USA	Prospective cohort	3020 aircraft manufacturing workers	Isometric lifting strength; demographic factors	No association between isometric lifting strength and LBP over a 4-year follow up
Battie (1990a) USA	Prospective cohort	3020 aircraft manufacturing workers	Anthropometric and clinical measures; demographic factors	Back symptoms on straight leg raising in both men and women, age and weight in women, and age and history of back problems in men were the only factors associated with LBP over 4 years of follow up.
Battie (1990b) USA	Prospective cohort	3020 aircraft manufacturing workers	Spinal flexibility	No association between spinal flexibility and future back pain reporting over a 4-year follow up
Bigos (1991b) USA	Prospective cohort	1576 aircraft manufacturing workers	Work perceptions and psychosocial factors; history of prior back problems; demographic factors	Current back pain, job dissatisfaction, and emotional distress had the strongest association with LBP over a 4-year follow up
Boshuizen (1993) Netherlands	Cross-sectional	4054 working men between ages 25–55	Cigarette smoking; occupation	Moderate association between smoking and LBP
Cady (1979) USA	Prospective cohort	1900 fire-fighters	Physical capacities	Increased fitness was associated with a decreased number of worker's compensation claims for back injury over a 3-year follow up
Chaffin (1973) USA	Prospective cohort	411 workers in jobs requiring some manual labour	Job lifting strength rating (LSR) calculated for each job taking into account the amount lifted and distance of the object from the person for two-handed sagittal plane lifting	Load lifting was associated with increased LBP over 1 year of follow up
Daltroy (1991) USA	Case-control	228 cases, 228 controls, postal workers	Job classification, ergonomic factors, demographics, worker's compensation history	History of a back injury claim, younger age, recent job change, and history of non-back injury claim were associated with LBP
Deyo (1989) USA	Cross-sectional	10 404 respondents representative of the USA	Smoking and obesity	Heavy smoking and obesity were independently associated with LBP
Dueker (1994) USA	Prospective cohort	230 applicants for heavy manual labour work	Isokinetic trunk strength; lifting strength	No association between isokinetic trunk evaluation and LBP over a 6-year follow up
Ebrall (1994b) Australia	Case-control	38 schoolboys between ages 12 and 19	Anthropometric dimensions	Four of 13 measurements (sitting height, pelvic height, suprapelvic height and upper body segment) were associated with low back pain
Harber (1994) USA	Prospective cohort	179 nurses	Worksite factors; prior back pain; psychosocial factors; training	Only prior significant back pain episode was associated with LBP over an 18-month follow up
Heliovaara (1991) Finland	Cross-sectional	5673 Finnish adults between 30 and 64 years of age	Occupational physical stress, occupational mental stress, anthropomorphics, sociodemographic factors	Age, prior traumatic back injury, occupational physical and mental stress, and cigarette smoking were associated with LBP
Leino et al. (1987) Finland	Prospective cohort	902 factory workers	Muscle function	No association between muscle function and LBP over a 10-year follow up

Study	Study design	Sample	Factors measured	Results
Leino et al. (1988) Finland	Prospective cohort	502 factory workers	Physical load	A weak association between physical workload and LBP over a 5-year follow up
Leino and Magni (1993) Finland	Prospective cohort	607 factory workers	Stress and depressive symptoms	Depressive symptoms were associated with LBP over a 5-year follow up
Leino (1993) Finland	Prospective cohort	607 factory workers	Leisure time physical activity; sociodemographic factors	Moderate inverse relationship between physical activity and low back morbidity over 5-year follow up
Mostardi (1990) USA	Prospective cohort	171 nurses	Isokinetic lifting strength; medical history	No association with LBP over 2-year follow up
Nissinen (1994) Finland	Prospective cohort	894 Finnish fourth grade children	Anthropomorphics	Modest association between sitting height and trunk asymmetry with the occurrence of LBP over a 3-year follow up
Nuwayhid (1993) USA	Case-control	415 cases, 109 controls, fire-fighters	Ergonomic factors, demographics, psychosocial factors	Certain job characteristics were associated with LBP
Pietri (1992) France	Prospective cohort	1118 commercial travellers	Lifestyle and work factors	Time spent driving a car, carrying loads, standing for long periods, smoking, and psychosomatic factors were associated with LBP over a 1-year follow up
Punnett (1991) USA	Case-control	95 cases, 124 controls, automobile assembly workers	Ergonomic factors, demographics, medical history, non-work physical activities	Trunk flexion and trunk twist or lateral bend were associated with LBP
Ready (1993) Canada	Prospective cohort	131 nurses	Fitness and lifestyle factors	Prior compensation for a back injury, smoking, and job satisfaction were most strongly associated with LBP over an 18-month period
Riihimaki (1989) Finland	Prospective cohort	419 labourers	Demographics; anthropomorphic and physical capacities; medical history; X-ray findings	Previous history of back symptoms had the greatest association with sciatic pain over a 5-year follow up, body mass index, smoking, and abdominal muscle strength did not
Rossignol (1993) Canada	Prospective cohort	205 male aircraft assembly workers	'Spinal health indicators'; demographics; medical history; psychosocial factors at work and home	Limitation of performing at work, or in activities of daily living, and a history of compensation were all independently associated with back pain over 1-year follow up
Ryden (1989) USA	Case-control	84 cases, 168 controls, hospital employees	Demographics, anthropomorphics, psychosocial factors, medical history and examination	History of LBP was significantly associated with current LBP; smoking was not
Virta (1993) Finland	Case-control	46 pairs of adults aged 45–64	Spondylolisthesis	Women with spondylolisthesis have slightly more mild back symptoms than women without spondylolisthesis. No difference in men
Venning (1987) Canada	Prospective cohort	4024 nurses at 10 facilities	Job category, lifting requirements, demographics, anthropomorphics, medical history	Service area, lifting, job category, and previously reported back injury were all associated with the reporting of LBP during 1-year follow up
Zwerling (1993) USA	Case-control	8183 postal workers; 154 subjects with LBP and 942 controls	Job classification, gender, age, history of back injury, pre-existing disability, body mass index, history of work-related injury, history of psychiatric disorder, history of substance abuse	Only heavy job classification and history of disability were associated with LBP

Table 2.3 *Risk/prognostic factors for low back pain*

Strongly associated

Prior history of back injury
Age
Job satisfaction/emotional distress
Heavy or repetitive lifting/heavy physical work
Prolonged sitting or standing

Moderately associated

Vibration
Smoking
Obesity
Height
Physical fitness

Weakly associated or not associated

Gender
Anthropometry
Lumbar mobility
Trunk strength
Radiographic structural abnormalities

observation. Lastly, *static work postures (prolonged sitting or standing)* are associated with an increased prevalence of low back pain, with estimates of the adjusted odds ratio being around 2.

Moderately associated factors

Exposure to *vibration* has been the subject of several studies, and in some cross-sectional studies it is one of the factors most strongly associated with low back pain (Frymoyer, 1980). Estimates of the relative risk for the association between vibration and low back pain have been around 2. However, prospective evaluations have been few. A systematic review concluded that long-term exposure to whole body vibration is probably 'harmful to the spinal system' but called for better quality studies before drawing any firm conclusions (Hulshof, 1987). Several prospective studies and many cross-sectional studies have reported an association between *cigarette smoking* and low back pain. Most report a relative risk in the range of 1.5. Some studies have failed to confirm this association. While a recent systematic review could not conclude that there was clear proof for a causal effect of cigarette smoking on low back pain (Leboeuf-Yde, 1996), there are plenty of other good reasons to recommend patients cease smoking, as noted by Lahad (1994). *Obesity* has been found in several cross-sectional studies and some, but not all, prospective studies, to be associated with low back pain. Although a causal relationship is not proven, as for cigarette smoking there exist plenty of good data

to recommend weight reduction to back pain patients. Taller *body height* was related in one prospective study to the incidence of sciatica, but not to other low back syndromes, with a barely statistically significant odds ratio of 1.2 (Heliovaara, 1991). In other studies low back pain was more common in taller persons. *Physical fitness* was studied prospectively in fire-fighters; a 10-fold increase in the incidence of low back injuries was found between the least fit tertile and the most fit tertile (Cady, 1979). A second prospective study of back pain amongst nurses failed to confirm this association (Ready, 1993). Lahad (1994) concluded that exercise is effective at preventing low back pain, but that the effect was modest.

Weakly associated or not associated factors

There is no clear association between gender and the frequency of low back pain. With the possible exceptions of obesity and height, there have been several negative prospective studies of other anthropomorphic measurements, and any association, if it exists at all, is probably very weak. There is evidence that reduced spinal mobility or flexibility is not associated with an increased incidence of low back pain, and there have been several negative prospective studies of trunk strength and back pain. With few exceptions, structural abnormalities seen on lumbosacral radiographs (osteoarthritis, degenerative changes, spondylolisthesis, sacralization, etc.) have not consistently been shown to predispose a person toward low back pain. Severe osteoporosis, because of its association with macro- or microvertebral fractures, is probably the most common radiographic finding which is associated with low back pain.

Health care utilization and cost

As opposed to the uncertainty about whether the occurrence of low back pain is increasing or not, there is no doubt that the frequency and cost of the use of health services for low back pain is increasing dramatically. Studies from both the USA and the UK show that the rate of sickness days due to back pain and the rate of lumbar spine surgery have been rising rapidly in the past decade (Figure 2.3). While rates of back surgery and disability are rising, in the USA non-surgical hospitalizations for low back pain have decreased by 73% between 1979 and 1990 (Taylor, 1994), and the number of physician office visits has increased (from 12 million to 15 million annually; with the proportion of office visits for low back pain remaining remarkably stable for the past decade: Hart, 1995).

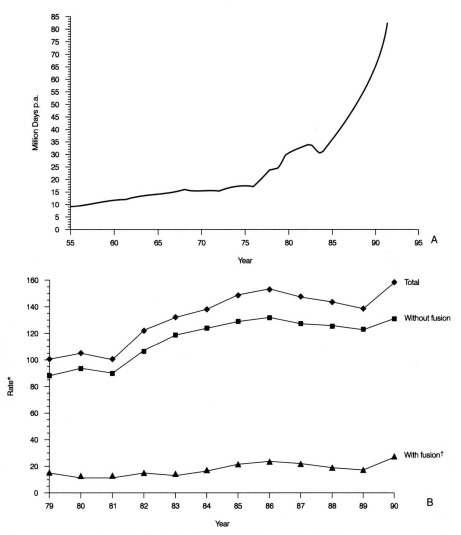

Figure 2.3 Sickness benefit for low back pain in Britain (A) and (B) low back surgery rates per 100 000 adults, overall and by procedure, 1979–1990. (A reproduced with permission from Deyo, R. (1993) *spine*, **18(15)**, 2155; B reproduced with permission from Deyo, R. (1994) *spine*, **19(11)**, 1209.)

The rate of lumbar surgery varies greatly amongst different countries. Cherkin and colleagues (1994) assessed the rate of back surgery in countries from North America, Scandinavia, Europe, Australia and New Zealand. Their results, displayed in Figure 2.4, show five-fold variations in the rate of back surgery, with the lowest rates observed in Scotland and England, and the highest rates in the USA. The rate of back surgery in the USA was 40% higher than the next highest country (the Netherlands). The rate of back surgery in these countries was strongly associated with differences in the supply of orthopaedic surgeons and neurosurgeons.

In the USA there is also marked regional variation in the rate of low back surgery. Amongst the counties that compose the state of Washington, rates of surgery for low back pain varied from 11.5/100 000 to 172/100 000; a difference of nearly 15-fold (Volinn, 1992). The ability to account for this variation through differences between counties in occupations, socio-economic conditions, surgeon density, available hospital beds, the primary payer of care, and health care availability was limited. It is likely that 'practice style' of the physicians in the various communities contributes greatly to the differences in surgical rates. Similar variations have been seen across large geographic areas of the USA. The annual rate of back surgery varies over 30%, from a low of 113 to a high of 171 operations per 100 000 adults in the West and South, respectively (Taylor, 1994). Lastly, geographic

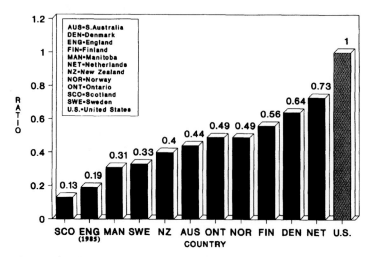

Figure 2.4 Ratios of back surgery rates in selected countries to back surgery rate in the USA (1988–1989). (Reproduced with permission from Deyo, R. (1994) *Spine*, **19(11)**, 1203.)

variations have also been shown in the USA for the occurrence of any back pain visit to a health professional (Shekelle, 1995a). In that study, geographic region of the country was a stronger predictor of a back pain visit than were patient sociodemographic factors such as age, gender, employment status, education, and occupation.

Persons with back pain may seek care in the USA from a variety of providers. In two studies that examined this issue, general practitioners, chiropractors, and orthopaedists were the most commonly sought providers by patients with back pain (Deyo 1987; Shekelle 1995b). In both studies, marked regional variations again were seen in the frequency with which patients sought care from different providers.

With all of this increase in health care use, it is no surprise that the costs associated with low back pain are both large and rising. The total annual US workers' compensation costs for 1977 was estimated at $4.6 billion (Andersson, 1991). By 1989, this figure had risen to $11.4 billion (Webster, 1994). Between 1980 and 1986 there was an estimated 241% increase in the total recoverable cost of low back pain (Webster, 1990). Low back pain is the most important component of workers' compensation costs. In the most recent analysis of the experience of the largest US underwriter of such insurance (Webster, 1994), the mean cost of a low back pain case was $8321 (in 1989 US dollars), which was more than twice the amount of the mean cost of all workers' compensation claims. This is also reflected by the percentage of low back cases to total cases in terms of numbers and costs. While low back cases accounted for 16% of the total number of cases, the total cost of low back cases accounted for 33% of the total costs of all cases.

Additionally, the median cost of a low back pain case was $396, indicating that the distribution of costs was substantially skewed. Twenty-five percent of the low back pain cases accounted for 96% of the costs. Lastly, between 1986 and 1989, the mean cost per case rose almost twice as fast as the consumer price index, the mean cost of indemnity payments per case rose at over twice the rate of the mean national wage, and the mean cost per case rose somewhat faster than the mean increase in overall medical care costs. Experiences such as these cause increased payments by employers for workers' compensation insurance, which is then passed on either to the consumer in the form of higher prices or to the worker in the form of lower direct economic compensation.

Summary

Low back pain is common, with an annual incidence in the adult population of between 2 and 5%, a point prevalence of 15–25%, and a lifetime prevalence of probably well over 50%. A history of previous back pain, increasing age up to late middle age, depression, job dissatisfaction, emotional distress, heavy or repetitive lifting and static work postures are the factors most strongly associated with the occurrence of low back pain. However, these factors taken together explain relatively little of the variation in the occurrence of low back pain between different populations. The health care cost and disability due to low back pain are rising at alarming rates. Low back pain is the most important component of workers' compensation costs. Most of the health care costs associated with low back pain are due to extraordinary costs for a small percentage of patients.

References

Abenhaim, L. and Suissa, S. (1987) Importance and economic burden of occupational back pain: a study of 2,500 cases representative of Quebec. *J. Occup. Med.*, **29(8)**, 670-4.

Anderson, R. (1992) The back pain of bus drivers: prevalence in an urban area of California. *Spine*, **17(12)**, 1481-488.

Andersson, G.B. (1981) Epidemiologic aspects on low-back pain in industry. *Spine*, **6(1)**, 53-60.

Andersson, G.B.J., Pope, M.H., Frymoyer, J.W., *et al.* (1991) Epidemiology and cost. In *Occupational low back pain: Assessment, treatment, and Prevention.* (Pope, M. H., Frymoyer, J. W., Andersson, G. B. J., et al., Eds), Mosby Year Book, St. Louis, MO.

Battie, M. C., Bigos, S. J., Fisher, L. D., *et al.* (1989a) A prospective study of the role of cardiovascular risk factors and fitness in industrial back pain complaints. *Spine*, **14(2)**, 141-147.

Battie, M. C., Bigos, S. J., Fisher, L. D., *et al.* (1989b) Isometric lifting strength as a predictor of industrial back pain reports. *Spine*, **14(8)**, 851-856.

Battie, M. C., Bigos, S. J., Fisher, L. D., *et al.* (1990a) Anthropometric and clinical measures as predictors of back pain complaints in industry: A prospective study. *Journal of Spinal Disorders*, **3(3)**, 195-204.

Battie, M. C., Bigos, S. J., Fisher, L. D., *et al.* (1990b) The role of spinal flexibility in back pain complaints within industry: A prospective study. *Spine*, **15(8)**, 768-773.

Bergenudd H, and Nilsson B. (1988) Back pain in middle age; occupational workload and psychologic factors: An epidemiologic survey. *Spine*, **13(1)**, 58-60.

Biering-Sorensen, F. (1982) Low back trouble in a general population of 30-, 40-, 50-, and 60-year-old men and women. *Dan Med Bull*, **29(6)**, 289-299.

Biering-Sorensen, F. (1983) A prospective study of low back pain in a general population. *Scand J Rehab Med*, **15**, 71-79.

Bigos, S. J., Battie, M. C., and Fisher, L. D. (1991a.) Methodology for evaluating predictive factors for the report of back injury. *Spine*, **16(6)**, 669-670.

Bigos, S. J., Battie, M. C., Spengler, D. M., *et al.* (1991b) A prospective study of work perceptions and psychosocial factors affecting the report of back injury. *Spine*, **16(1)**, 1-6.

Bigos, S. J., Battie, M. C., Spengler, D. M., *et al.* (1992) A longitudinal, prospective study of industrial back injury reporting. *Clin Orthop*, **279**, 21-34.

Bjelle A, Allander E, and Lundquist B. (1981.) Geographic distribution of rheumatic disorders and working conditions in Sweden. *Scand J Soc Med*, **91**, 119-126.

Bombardier, C., Kerr, M., Shannon, H., *et al.* (1994) A guide to interpreting epidemiologic studies on the etiology of back pain. *Spine*, **19(18S)**, 2047S-2056S.

Bongers, P. M., de Winter, C. R., Kompier, M. A., *et al.* (1993) Psychosocial factors at work and musculoskeletal disease. *Scand J Work, Environ Health*, **19**, 297-312.

Boshuizen, H. C., Verbeek, J. H., Broersen, J., *et al.* (1993) Do smokers get more back pain? *Spine*, **18(1)**, 35-40.

Brattberg G, Thorslund M, and Wikman A. (1989) The prevalence of pain in a general population. The results of a postal survey in a county of Sweden. *Pain*, **37**, 215-222.

Bredkjaer S. R. (1991) Musculoskeletal disease in Denmark: The Danish Health and Morbidity Survey 1986-87. *Acta Orthop Scand*, **62(Suppl 241)**, 10-12.

Cady, L. D., Bischoff, D. P., O'Connell, E. R., *et al.* (1979) Strength and fitness and subsequent back injuries in firefighters. *J Occup Med*, **21(4)**, 269-272.

Chaffin, D. B., and Park, K. S. (1973) A longitudinal study of low-back pain as associated with occupational weight lifting factors. *Am Ind Hyg Assoc J*, **34**, 513-525.

Chaffin, D. B. (1974) Human strength capability and low-back pain. *J Occup Med*, **16(4)**, 248-254.

Cherkin, D. C., Deyo, R. A., Loeser, J. D., *et al.* (1994) An international comparison of back surgery rates. *Spine*, **19(11)**, 1201-1206.

Chiou, W., Wong, M., and Lee, Y. (1994) Epidemiology of low back pain in Chinese nurses. *Int J Nurs Stud*, **31(4)**, 361-368.

Crook J, Rideout E, and Browne G. (1984) The prevalence of pain complaints in a general population. *Pain*, **18**, 299-314.

Cunningham L S, and Kelsey J L. (1984) Epidemiology of musculoskeletal impairments and associated disability. *Am J Public Health*, **74(6)**, 574-579.

Daltroy, L. H., Larson, M. G., Wright, E. A., *et al.* (1991) A case-control study of risk factors for industrial low back injury: Implications for primary and secondary prevention programs. *Am J Ind Med*, **20**, 505-515.

Deyo, R.A., and Tsui-Wu, Y. (1987) Descriptive epidemiology of low-back pain and its related medical care in the United States. *Spine*, **12(3)**, 264-268.

Dueker, J. A., Ritchie, S. M., Knox, T. J., *et al.* (1994) Isokinetic trunk testing and employment. *JOM*, **36(1)**, 42-48.

Ebrall, P. (1994a) The epidemiology of male adolescent low back pain in a north suburban population of Melbourne, Australia. *J Manip Physiol Ther*, **17(7)**, 447-453.

Ebrall, P. S. (1994b.) Some anthropometric dimensions of male adolescents with idiopathic low back pain. *J Manip Physiol Ther*, **17(5)**, 296-301.

Fordyce, W. E., Bigos, S. J., Battie, M. C., *et al.* (1992) MMPI Scale 3 as a predictor of back injury report: What does it tell us? *The Clinical Journal of Pain*, **8**, 222-226.

Frymoyer, J. W., Pope, M. H., Costanza, M. C., *et al.* (1980) Epidemiologic studies of low-back pain. *Spine*, **5(5)**, 419-423.

Garg, A., and Moore, J. S. (1992) Epidemiology of low-back pain in industry. *Occu Med*, **7(4)**, 593-608.

Harber, P., Pena, L., Hsu, P., *et al.* (1994) Personal history, training, and worksite as predictors of back pain of nurses. *Am J Ind Med*, **25**, 519-526.

Hart, L. G., Deyo, R. A., and Cherkin, D. C. (1995) Physician office visits for low back pain. *Spine*, **20(1)**, 11-19.

Heliovaara, M. (1989a) Risk factors for low back pain and sciatica. *Ann Med*, **21**, 257-264.

Heliovaara, M., Sievers, K., Impivaara, O., *et al.* (1989b) Descriptive epidemiology and public health aspects of low back pain. *Ann Med*, **21**, 327-333.

Heliovaara, M., Makela, M., Knekt, P., *et al.* (1991) Determinants of sciatica and low-back pain. *Spine*, **16(6)**, 608-613.

Hirsch, C., Jonsson, B., and Lewin, T. (1969) Low-back symptoms in a Swedish female population. *Clin Orthop*, **63**, 171-176.

Hulshof, C., and van Zanten, B. V. (1987) Whole-body vibration and low-back pain. *Int Arch Occup Environ Health*, **59**, 205-220.

Lahad, A., Malter, A. D., Berg, A. O., *et al*. (1994) The effectiveness of four interventions for the prevention of low back pain. *J Am Med Assoc*, **272(16)**, 1286–1291.

Lawrence J S. (1969) Disc degeneration: Its frequency and relationship to symptoms. *Ann Rheum Dis*, **28**, 121–137.

Leboeuf-Yde, C. (1996) Does smoking cause LBP? Reviewing the epidemiologic literature for causality. *J Manip Physiol Ther.*19, 99–108.

Leboeuf-Yde, C., and Lauritsen, J. M. (1995) The prevalence of low back pain in the literature: A structured review of 26 Nordic studies from 1954 to 1993. *Spine*, **20**, 2112–2118.

Leino, P., Aro, S., and Hasan, J. (1987) Trunk muscle function and low back disorders: A ten-year follow-up study. *J Chron Dis*, **40(4)**, 289–296.

Leino, P., Hasan J, and Karppi, S. (1988) Occupational class, physical workload, and musculoskeletal morbidity in the engineering industry. *Br J Ind Med*, **45**, 672–681.

Leino, P., and Magni, G. (1993) Depressive and distress symptoms as predictors of low back pain, neck-shoulder pain, and other musculoskeletal morbidity: A 10-year follow-up of metal industry employees. *Pain*, **53** 89–94.

Leino, P. (1993) Does leisure time physical activity prevent low back disorders? A prospective study of metal industry employees. *Spine*, **18(7)**, 863–871.

Moffett, J. K., Hughes, G., and Griffiths, P. (1993) A longitudinal study of low back pain in student nurses. *Int J Nurs Stud*, **30(3)**, 197–212.

Mostardi, R. A., Noe, D. A., Kovacik, M. W., *et al*. (1992) Isokinetic lifting strength and occupational injury: A prospective study. *Spine*, **17(2)**, 189–193.

Nagi, S. Z., Riley, L. E., and Newby, L. G. (1973) A social epidemiology of back pain in a general population. *J Chron Dis*, **26**, 769–779.

Nissinen, M., Heliovaara, M., Seitsamo, J., *et al*. (1994) Anthropometric measurements and the incidence of low back pain in a cohort of pubertal children. *Spine*, **19(12)**, 1367–1370.

Nuwayhid, I. A., Stewart, W., and Johnson, J. V. (1993) Work activities and the onset of first-time low back pain among New York city fire fighters. *Am J Epidemiol*, **137(5)**, 539–548.

Papageorgiou, A. C., Croft, P. R., Ferry, S., *et al*. (1995) Estimating the prevalence of low back pain in the general population: Evidence from the South Manchester Back Pain Survey. *Spine*, **20(17)**, 1889–1894.

Pietri, F., Leclerc, A., Boitel, L., *et al*. (1992) Low-back pain in commercial travelers. *Scand J Work, Enviro Health*, **18**, 52–58.

Pope, M. (1989.) Risk indicators in low back pain. *Ann Med*, **21**, 387–392.

Punnett, L., Fine, L. J., Keyserling, W. M., *et al*. (1991) Back disorders and nonneutral trunk postures of automobile assembly workers. *Scand J Work, Environ Health*, **17**, 337–346.

Raspe H. Back pain. (1993) In *Epidemiology of the Rheumatic Diseases*. (Silman A. J., Hochberg M. C., Eds). Oxford University Press, pp.330–374.

Ready, A. E., Boreskie, S. L., Law, S. A., *et al*. (1993) Fitness and lifestyle parameters fail to predict back injuries in nurses. *Can J Appl Phys*, **18(1)**, 80–90.

Reisbord, L. S., and Greenland, S. (1985) Factors associated with self-reported back-pain prevalence: A population-based study. *J Chron Dis*, **38(8)**, 691–702.

Riihimaki, H., Wickstrom, G., Hanninen, K., *et al*. (1989) Predictors of sciatic pain among concrete reinforcement workers and house painters – a five-year follow-up. *Scand J Work Environ Health*, **15**, 415–423.

Riihimaki, H., Viikari-Juntura, E., Moneta, G., *et al*. (1994) Incidence of sciatic pain among men in machine operating, dynamic physical work, and sedentary work: A three-year follow-up. *Spine*, **19(2)**, 138–142.

Rossignol, M., Lortie, M., and Ledoux, E. (1993) Comparison of spinal health indicators in predicting spinal status in a 1-year longitudinal study. *Spine*, **18(1)**, 54–60.

Rotgoltz, J., Derazne, E., Froom, P., *et al*. (1992) Prevalence of low back pain in employees of a pharmaceutical company. *Is J Med Sci*, **28(8–9)**, 615–618.

Rundcrantz, B., Johnsson, B., and Moritz, U. (1991) Pain and discomfort in the musculoskeletal system among dentists. *Swed Dent J*, **15**, 219–228.

Ryden, L. A., Molgaard, C. A., Bobbitt, S., *et al*. (1989) Occupational low-back injury in a hospital employee population: An epidemiologic analysis of multiple risk factors of a high-risk occupational group. *Spine*, **14(3)**, 315–320.

Salminen, J., Pentti, J., and Terho, P. (1992) Low back pain and disability in 14-year-old schoolchildren. *Acta Paediatr*, **81**, 1035–1039)

Shekelle, P. G., Markovich, M., and Louie R. (1995a) An epidemiologic study of episodes of back pain care. *Spine*, **20(15)**, 1668–1673.

Shekelle, P. G., Markovich, M., and Louie, R. (1995b) Factors associated with choosing a chiropractor for episodes of back pain care. *Med Care*, **33(8)**, 842–850.

Svensson, H. (1982) Low back pain in forty to forty-seven year old men. II. Socio-economic factors and previous sickness absence. *Scand J Rehab Med*, **14**, 55–60.

Svensson H, Andersson G B J, Johansson S, et al. (1988.)A retrospective study of low-back pain in 38- to 64-year-old women: Frequency of occurrence and impact on medical services. *Spine,* 13(5):548–52.

Taylor, V. M., Deyo, R. A., Cherkin, D. C., *et al*. (1994) Low back pain hospitalization: Recent United States trends and regional variations. *Spine*, **19(11)**, 1207–1213.

Taylor, H., and Curran, N. M. (1985) The Nuprin Pain Report. Louis Harris, New York.

Tsai, S. P., Bernacki, E. J., and Dowd, C. M. (1991) The relationship between work-related and non-work-related injuries. *J Community Health*, **16(4)**, 205–212.

Tuomi, K., Ilmarinen, J., Eskelinen, L., *et al*. (1991) Prevalence and incidence rates of diseases and work ability in different work categories of municipal occupations. *Scand J Work, Environ Health*, **17(Suppl 1)**, 67–74.

Venning, P. J., Walter, S. D., and Stitt, L. W. (1987) Personal and job-related factors as determinants of incidence of back injuries among nursing personnel. *J Occup Med*, **29(10)**, 820–825.

Viikari-Juntura, E., Vuori, J., Silverstein, B., *et al*. (1991) A life-long prospective study on the role of psychosocial factors in neck-shoulder and low-back pain. *Spine*, **16(9)**, 1056–1061.

Volinn, E., Mayer, J., Diehr, P., *et al*. (1992) Small area analysis of surgery for low-back pain. *Spine*, **17(5)**, 575–579.

Von Korff M, Dworkin S F, Resche L L, *et al*. (1988) An epidemiologic comparison of pain complaints. *Pain,* **32**, 173–183.

Walsh, K., Cruddas, M., and Coggon, D. (1992) Low back

pain in eight areas of Britain. *J Epidemiol Community Health*, **46**, 227-230.

Weber, B. S., and Snook, S. (1990) The cost of compensable low back pain. *J Occup Med*, **32**, 13-15).

Webster, B. S., and Snook, S. H. (1994) The cost of 1989 workers' compensation low back pain claims. *Spine*, **19(10)**, 1111-1116.

Zwerling, C., Ryan, J., and Schootman, M. (1993) A case-control study of risk factors for industrial low back injury: The utility of preplacement screening in defining high-risk groups. *Spine*, **18(9)**, 1242-1247.

Section

II

Anatomy and Pathology

3

Introductory graphic anatomy of the lumbosacral spine

L.G.F. Giles

Brief introduction

The human vertebral column is a remarkable structure consisting of many parts, which should be considered as an integrated unit (Morris, 1973; Hilton, 1980), the 'spinal organ'. It combines strength and flexibility by alternately interposing rigid bony vertebrae with deformable cartilaginous discs (Taylor and Twomey, 1980) which live because of movement (Kraemer *et al.*, 1985). The intervertebral disc acts as a shock absorber between adjacent vertebral bodies; its gelatinous nucleus pulposus (the remnant of the notochord) efficiently dissipates mechanical stress (Keim and Kirkaldy-Willis, 1987).

In the average adult, the entire spine is about 70 cm long in the male and 60 cm long in the female (Bullough and Boachie-Adjei, 1988) including a length of approximately 18 cm for the lumbar spine. However, the length of the spine varies throughout a 24-hour period, a phenomenon termed diurnal or circadian changes, with height greater in the morning than in the evening in young adults. A daily height change of up to 1% has been recorded (DePuky, 1935; Tyrrell *et al.*, 1985; Wing *et al.*, 1992) with approximately 8 mm (40%) of the height gain occurring in the lumbar spine, representing approximately 2 mm per lumbar intervertebral disc (Wing *et al.*, 1992). Normally there are five lumbar vertebrae, each of which comprises two principal parts: (a) the anterior vertebral body, which is composed of spongy bone covered by a thin layer of compact bone, and (b) the posterior vertebral arch with its processes (Koreska *et al.*, 1977) (Figures 3.1 and 3.2). The basic functional unit consists of an articular triad: two true

diarthrodial synovial zygapophysial joints and the corresponding amphiarthrodial cartilaginous joint between the vertebral bodies (Lewin *et al.*, 1961; Keim and Kirkaldy-Willis, 1987).

Graphic examples

Graphic examples of a partly macerated human spine extending from the thoracolumbar junction to the sacrum in an 83-year-old male are shown in Figures 3.1–3.3 and its corresponding 45 degree oblique radiographic projection is shown in Figure 3.4. An embalmed human spine (T10–S1) from a 52-year-old male, which has been bisected in the sagittal (median) plane, is shown in Figure 3.5 with its corresponding radiographic projections in Figure 3.6. Some histological sections from the eleventh thoracic (T11) vertebra to the lumbosacral joint are included in order to give a more comprehensive graphic understanding of the anatomy of the lumbosacral spine, with its adjacent lower thoracic and sacroiliac joints. Greater detail is given for lower thoracic and sacroiliac joints in Chapters 12 and 11, respectively. The following chapters provide detailed descriptions of each part of the lumbosacral spine and its associated structures.

An anterior view of the partly macerated lumbosacral spine is shown in Figure 3.1.

An oblique view radiograph of the partly macerated spine is shown in Figure 3.4 to demonstrate the pars interarticularis (isthmus) for each vertebra and the radiograph has been reproduced to emphasize the zygapophysial (facet) joints of this spine.

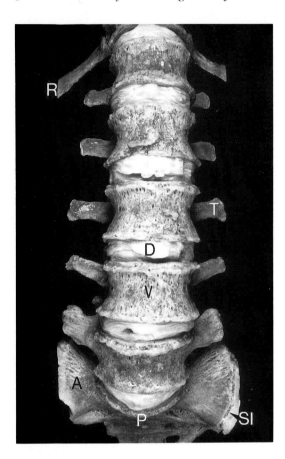

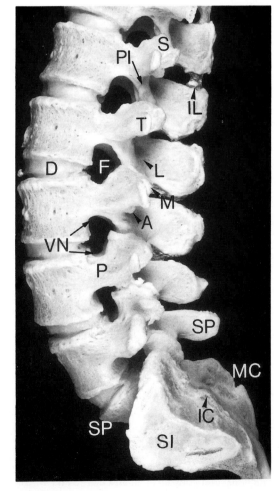

Figure 3.1 Anterior view of a partly macerated lumbosacral spine from an 83-year-old male. The vertebral bodies (V) are separated by intervertebral discs (D) which show a pattern of various directions taken by the collagen fibres of the anulus fibrosus. A = sacral ala; R = part of right twelfth rib; SI = part of the sinuous sacroiliac joint; P = sacral promontory; T = transverse process.

Figure 3.2 Lateral view of the specimen in Figure 3.1. A = accessory process; D = intervertebral disc; F = 'foramen' of intervertebral canal; IC = intermediate crest (articular tubercles); IL = interspinous ligament remains; L = lamina; M = mamillary process; MC = median sacral crest (spinous tubercles); P = pedicle; PI = pars interarticularis (or isthmus) region; SP = spinous process; S = superior articular process of first lumbar (L1) vertebra; SI = sacroiliac articulation; SP = sacral promontory; T = transverse process; VN = vertebral notches (superior and inferior, respectively).

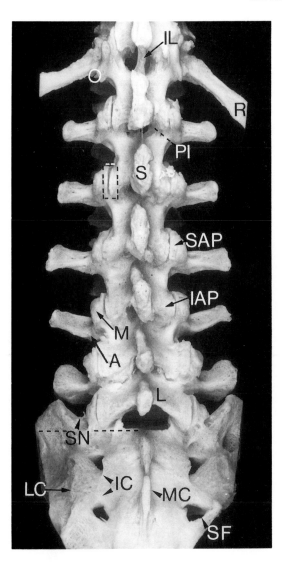

Figure 3.4 A 45 degree oblique radiographic view of the lumbosacral spine highlighting the left (LT) zygapophysial joints (Z) with their facets (F). The inferior (IAP) and superior (SAP) articular processes are shown. D = intervertebral disc space; L = lamina of opposite side seen on cross section; P = pedicle; PI = pars interarticularis; S = sacral superior articular process; SP = spinous process; T = transverse process.

Figure 3.3 Posterior view of the specimen shown in Figures 3.1 and 3.2. A = accessory process; IAP = inferior articular process; IC = intermediate crest; IL = interspinous ligament remains; LC = lateral crest (transverse tubercles); M = mamillary process; MC = median sacral crest; PI = pars interarticularis (or isthmus); broken line; R = part of right twelfth rib with costovertebral joint; S = spinous process; SAP = superior articular process; SF = sacral foramen (dorsal); SN = superior sacral notch. Broken line rectangle shows part of a synovial zygapophysial (facet) joint. Tropism is seen between the left and right paired zygapophysial joints at the L2–3 and L3–4 spinal levels in particular. Advanced osteoarthrotic osseous changes are noted involving some of the zygapophysial joints, for example at L4–5 bilaterally and on the right side at T12–L1 and L1–2. Osteophytic lipping (circle) of the left and right costovertebral (synovial) joints. The dotted reference line shows the approximate level of the histological section in Figure 3.20 which was prepared from an embalmed specimen.

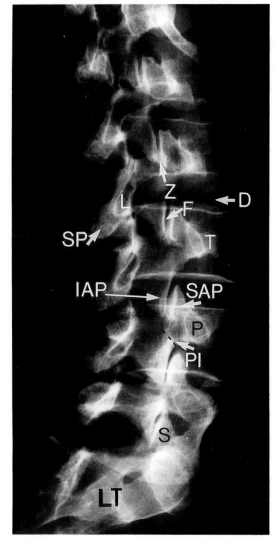

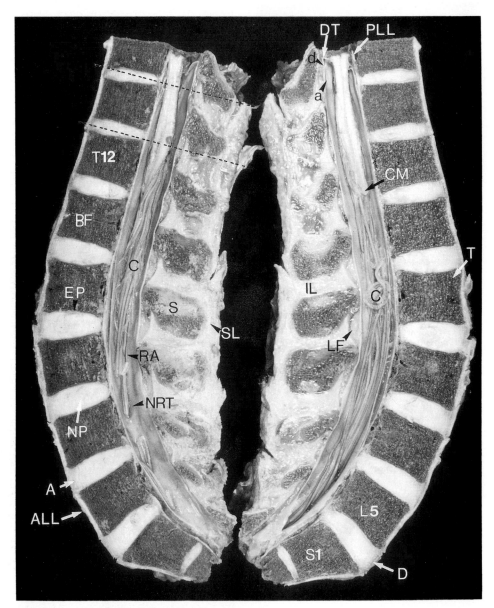

Figure 3.5 A bisected embalmed human spine (T10–S1/2) from a 52-year-old male. A = anulus fibrosus fibres; ALL = Anterior longitudinal ligament; BF = basivertebral vein foramen; C = cauda equina nerve root trunks; CM = conus medullaris; D = intervertebral disc; DT = dural tube within the spinal canal showing its dura mater (d) and arachnoid mater (a), the pia mater terminating at the end of the conus medullaris and fusing into a long slender filament, the filum terminale; EP = endplate of vertebra; IL = interspinous ligament; L5 = fifth lumbar vertebral body; LF = ligamentum flavum; NP = nucleus pulposus; NRT = nerve root trunks passing within the dural tube towards the intervertebral canal; PLL = posterior longitudinal ligament; RA = radicular arteries; S = spinous process; SL = supraspinous ligament; S1 = first sacral segment; T = trabeculae running vertically and transversely within the cancellous bone of the vertebral body which is surrounded by a shell of compact bone. T12 = twelfth lumbar vertebral body.

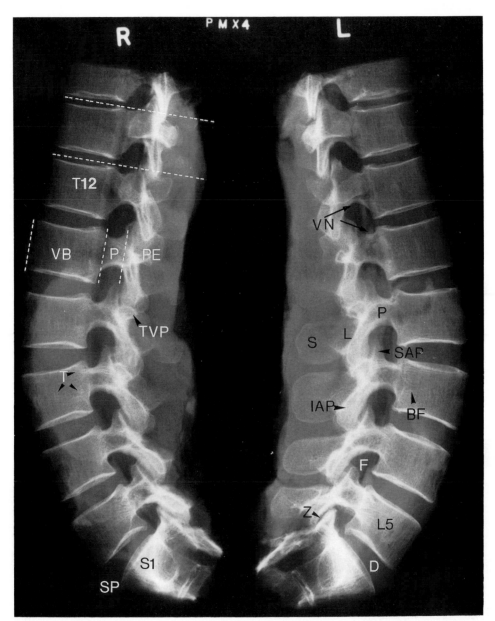

Figure 3.6 Radiograph of the bisected spine shown in Figure 3.5. BF = basivertebral vein foramen; D = intervertebral disc space; F = intervertebral canal 'foramen'; IAP = inferior articular process; L = lamina; L5 = fifth lumbar vertebral body; P = pedicle; S = spinous process; SAP = superior articular process; S1 = first sacral segment; SP = sacral promontory; T = trabeculae; T12 = twelfth lumbar vertebral body; TVP = transverse process; VN = vertebral notches superiorly and inferiorly, respectively; Z = zygapophysial synovial joint between the superior and inferior articular process facets. The three functional components of a vertebra, i.e. vertebral body (VB), pedicles (P) and the posterior elements (PE), are shown by the broken white lines which are parallel to the anterior and posterior margins of L1 vertebra. The broken white lines passing through the T10 and T11 intervertebral discs relate to similar lines on Figure 3.5 and give the approximate region from which a block of osteoligamentous tissues was sectioned from another spine to produce the superior to inferior radiographic view shown in Figure 3.7.

Note the numerous radicular arteries (RA) accompanying the nerve root trunks of the cauda equina as these pass caudally through the dural tube to their respective intervertebral canals in Figure 3.5. The nerve roots are bathed in cerebrospinal fluid from the spinal cord to the intervertebral foramen. The broken parallel lines at T11 (Figures 3.5 and 3.6) show the approximate region from which a block of osteoligamentous tissues was sectioned from another spine, then radiographed in the superior to inferior position as shown in Figure 3.7.

The left half of the bisected spine shown radiographically in Figure 3.6 clearly demonstrates how the superior to inferior dimension of the fourth and fifth spinous processes is considerably less than that of the second and third spinous processes. This enables a normal lordosis to develop. These lateral radiographic views also show how the plane of the zygapophysial joints is more coronal in the lower spine, thus enabling the joint facets to be seen in lateral projection. The more cephalad zygapophysial joints of the lumbar spine are more coronally orientated, which prevents them from being seen in the lateral projection. The more coronal orientation of the lower lumbar zygapophysial joints helps to resist postero-anterior shearing stresses at these levels.

It is interesting to note from Figure 3.6 that the intervertebral canal (foramen) between the fifth lumbar (L5) and first sacral segments (S1) is the smallest of the lumbar intervertebral foramina even though the fifth lumbar spinal nerve is the largest of the lumbar spinal nerves (Brailsford, 1929; Mitchell, 1934; Epstein, 1960).

A superior to inferior radiographic view of the osteoligamentous block of tissues associated with the T11 vertebra from a different spine is shown in Figure 3.7 which is representative of the spinal level shown in Figures 3.5 and 3.6. A histological section cut through the rib head level of this vertebra is shown in Figure 3.8.

The trabeculae within the cancellous bone can be seen forming an irregular mosaic pattern which is particularly obvious within the vertebral body (Figure 3.8). The trabeculae give strength to the vertebral bodies, and the intertrabecular spaces are filled with blood which also helps to transmit the weights associated with load-bearing (White and Panjabi, 1978). It should be remembered that the cancellous (spongy) bony tissue of the spine contains spaces filled with red marrow, the cells of which produce blood cells (haemopoiesis) (Tortora and Grabowski, 1993).

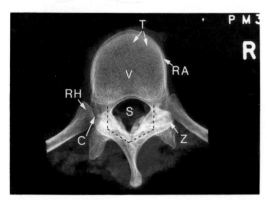

Figure 3.7 Superior view radiograph of a thoracic vertebra at the T11 level with parts of the left and right ribs. C = costovertebral (synovial) joint; RA = ring apophysis of cortical bone; RH = rib head; S = spinal canal; V = vertebral body showing trabecular pattern due to the small bony trabeculae (T) which run in various planes within the cancellous bone (spongiosa); Z = zygapophysial synovial joint. The osseous neural arch (broken line) which surrounds the neural structures is attached to the back of the vertebral body by the pedicles which form part of the arch. This is representative of the T11 spinal region shown in Figure 3.5. A histological section from the rib head level of the vertebra in this figure is shown in Figure 3.8.

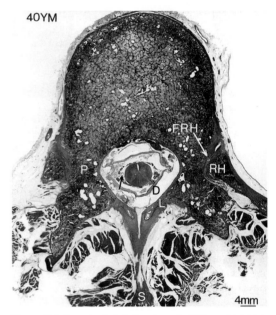

Figure 3.8 Superior to inferior view of a 200 μm thick histological section cut through the rib head level of the vertebra shown in Figure 3.7 which was from a 40-year-old male. Note the contents of the spinal canal where the spinal cord is protected within the dural tube (D). The black arrow shows a denticulate ligament between the anterior and posterior nerve roots which helps to protect the cord against shock and sudden displacement as it floats within the cerebrospinal fluid. FRH = facet, with hyaline articular cartilage, for rib head; L = lamina; P = pedicle; RH = rib head with hyaline articular cartilage; S = spinous process with muscles on its left and right sides. Note the synovial fold projecting into the right costovertebral joint 'cavity' from its posterior margin.

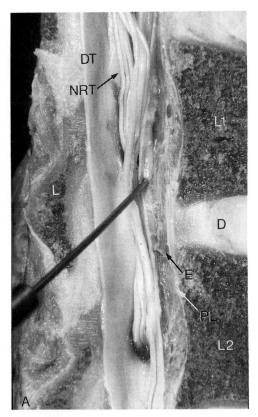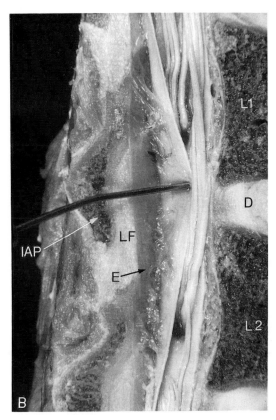

Figure 3.9 A,B. Block of spinal osteoligamentous tissues from the upper lumbar spine of a 52-year-old female, cut in the sagittal plane, showing parts of the first (L1) and second (L2) vertebral bodies with adjacent intervertebral discs (D), IAP = inferior articular process (see Figure 3.5 for lower power orientation). A: NRT = Nerve root trunks of the cauda equina within the dural tube (DT) passing caudally towards the intervertebral canals. The metal probe reflects the dural tube (DT) to show the epidural membrane (E) between the dura and the posterior longitudinal ligament (PL); L = lamina. B: The metal probe shows the epidural membrane (E) between the reflected dura and the ligamentum flavum (LF).

In Figure 3.5 the conus medullaris, which is covered in pia mater which terminates at the end of the conus medullaris and fuses into the filum terminale internum (Dorwart and Genant, 1983), is shown within the upper lumbar part of the dural tube which, under normal circumstances, is protected within the spinal canal by the epidural fat which surrounds it. The cauda equina nerve root trunks passing caudally through the dural tube to their respective intervertebral canals are shown in Figure 3.5 and in another specimen as shown in Figures 3.9 A and B. In these figures, an epidural membrane is also interposed between the dura and ligamentum flavum (Hasue *et al.*, 1983) (Figure 3.9).

In Figure 3.10 a metal probe has been inserted beneath the arachnoid membrane to show its relatively delicate structure when compared to the dural membrane. The vascular nerve root trunks of the cauda equina, which exit through the intervertebral

canal at the L2–3 level, and lower, have been partially displaced from within the opened dural tube, in order to demonstrate clearly the arachnoid membrane at this level.

A block of spinal osteoligamentous tissues, which includes the lumbosacral articular triad from a 51-year-old female, is shown in Figure 3.11 with its corresponding radiographs in Figures 3.12 and 3.13.

A histological section cut approximately through the middle of the zygapophysial joint of this osteoligamentous block of tissue (see Figure 3.12) is shown in Figure 3.14.

Ligaments traversing the lumbosacral *exit zone*, as seen in sections cut in the horizontal plane, are shown in Figures 3.14 and 3.15. These particular ligaments are a constant finding at the lumbosacral level *exit zone* (see Figure 6.3 and Chapter 7) and have been described by Bachop and co-workers (1981a,b, 1984), Amonoo-Kuofi *et al.* (1988a,b) and Giles (1992) and others (see Chapter 7).

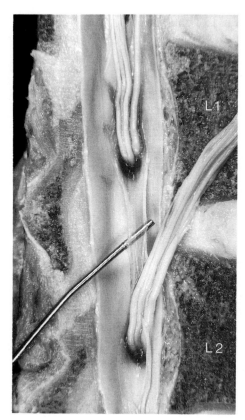

Figure 3.10 The vascular nerve root trunks of the cauda equina passing to the L2–3 intervertebral canal and lower, have been partially displaced from within the opened dural tube in order to show the arachnoid membrane which has been elevated by a metal probe.

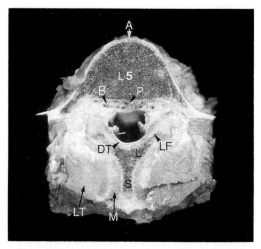

Figure 3.11 A block of osteoligamentous tissues cut in the horizontal plane from a 51-year-old female, showing the fifth lumbar vertebral body (L5), the spinal canal containing the dural tube (DT) with some nerve roots of the cauda equina. The dural tube is surrounded by epidural fat which contains Batson's venous plexus (B) and the epidural membrane. A = anterior longitudinal ligament; L = lamina; LF = ligamentum flavum; LT = longissimus thoracis muscle (part of erector spinae, i.e. sacrospinalis muscle); M = multifidus muscle; P = posterior longitudinal ligament; S = spinous process of L5 vertebra.

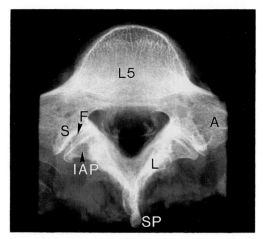

Figure 3.13 Superior to inferior radiographic view of the osteoligamentous block shown in Figures 3.11 and 3.12. Note the fifth vertebral body (L5), the spinal canal, parts of the ala (A) of the sacrum, the left and right lamina (L) joining at the lamina junction, the L5 spinous process (SP) and the left and right zygapophysial joints. Each zygapophysial joint is formed by the superior articular process (S) of the sacrum and its facet (F) and the inferior articular process of L5 (IAP) and its facet, with associated soft tissue structures. Due to the thickness of this specimen, various structures are superimposed, e.g. spinous process (SP) of L5 and the spinous tubercle of the first sacral segment and the L5 and S1 laminae.

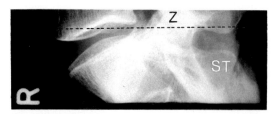

Figure 3.12 Lateral radiographic view of the osteoligamentous block shown in Figure 3.11 which shows the lumbosacral intervertebral joint and the zygapophysial synovial joints (Z) comprising the articular triad. The dotted line shows the approximate level of the 200 μm thick histological section shown in Figure 3.14. ST = spinous tubercle of the first sacral segment.

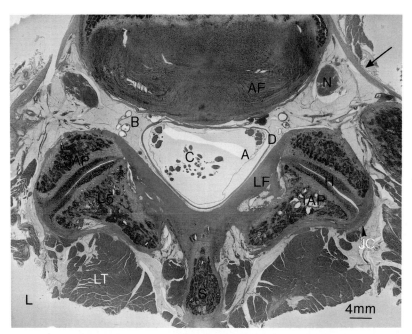

Figure 3.14 A 200 μm thick histological section cut in the horizontal plane at aproximately the level shown in Figure 3.12 (51-year-old female). Note the spinal canal which contains the dural tube with its dural (D) and arachnoid (A) membranes. The dural tube is surrounded by epidural fat in which are seen parts of Batson's venous plexus (B) and the epidural membrane (not visible as such). The left and right intervertebral canals leading off the spinal canal contain adipose tissue, large neural structures (N) (i.e. spinal ganglion and nerve roots) and blood vessels. The small diameter recurrent meningeal nerves are not visible. The zygapophysial joint capsule is formed by the ligamentum flavum (LF) medially and by the fibrous joint capsule (JC) laterally. LT = longissimus thoracis muscle. The sacral superior articular process (SAP) and the inferior articular process (IAP) of the fifth lumbar vertebra have facets lined with hyaline articular cartilage (H). AF = anulus fibrosus fibres of the lumbosacral intervertebral disc; S = spinous process; L = left side. Arrow = transforaminal ligament traversing the exit zone of the intervertebral canal. (Ehrlich's haematoxylin and light green counterstain.)

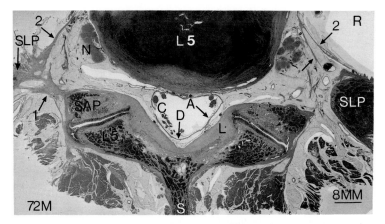

Figure 3.15 A 200 μm thick histological section cut in approximately the horizontal plane from a 72-year-old male. Note the cauda equina (C) within the dural sac with its dural (D) and arachnoid (A) membranes. The spinal nerves (N) are shown in close proximity to the ligaments (1 and 2) traversing the exit zone of the intervertebral canal. These ligaments pass from the superior articular process (SAP) joint capsule (1) to the sacral lateral process (SLP) and continue (2) to the lateral border of the L5 intervertebral disc and first sacral body. L5 (black) = inferior articular process of the fifth lumbar vertebra; L5 (white) = fifth intervertebral disc; R = right side. (Ehrlich's haematoxylin and light green counterstain.) (Reproduced with permission from Giles, L.G.F. (1992) Ligaments traversing the intervertebral canals of the human lower lumbosacral spine. *Neuro-Orthopedics*, **13**, 25–38.)

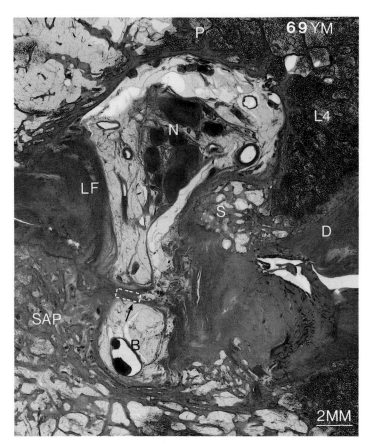

Figure 3.16 A 200 mm thick section cut in the parasagittal plane across the left L4-5 intervertebral canal of a 69-year-old male. The arrow shows a ligament traversing the lower part of the intervertebral canal, within the foramen and bisecting it. The depth of the ligament within the intervertebral canal is 4 mm. The region shown within the rectangle was resected from an adjacent unmounted section and is shown highly magnified in Figure 3.17. B = blood vessels; D = intervertebral disc; L = ligamentum flavum; L4 = fourth lumbar vertebral body; N = spinal nerve compex; P = pedicle; S = spur posterolaterally and inferiorly on L4 body; SAP = sacral superior articular process. (Ehrlich's haematoxylin and light green counterstain.) (Reproduced with permission from Giles, L.G.F. (1992) Ligaments traversing the intervertebral canals of the human lower lumbosacral spine. *Neuro-Orthopedics*, **13**, 25-38.)

Ligaments traversing the *mid-zones* of the L4-5 and L5-S1 intervertebral canals were found in 61% of sagittally cut L4-5 intervertebral canals, and in 43% of sagittally and horizontally cut L5-S1 intervertebral canals (Giles, 1992). An example of a ligament traversing the mid-zone of an L4-5 intervertebral canal, in an almost horizontal plane, is shown in Figure 3.16.

This ligament did not compromise the large neural structures in Giles' (1992) study. Thin histological sections cut at the area shown in the rectangle in Figure 3.16 exhibited nerves and blood vessels within the ligamentous tissue (Figure 3.17) which contains elastic fibres.

The average length, width and depth projected into the intervertebral canal of these horizontal ligaments at the mid-zones of the L4-5 and L5-S1 levels is shown in Table 3.1, which also shows the corresponding ranges.

Ligaments also traverse the mid-zone of intervertebral canals in a vertical plane, an example of which is shown in Figure 3.18.

Part of the transforaminal ligament shown in Figure 3.18 was resected from an adjacent unstained 100 μm

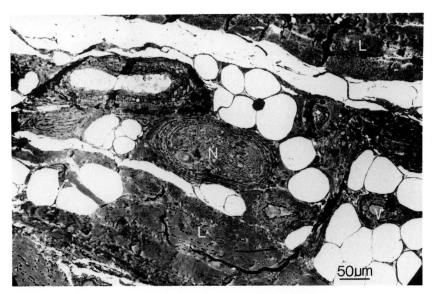

Figure 3.17 A thin section cut at a thickness of 1 μm. Note the small myelinated nerve (N), with an average diameter of approximately 117.2 μm, which is located within the ligament (L) shown in the rectangle in Figure 3.16. There are also several vascular structures (V) within the ligament which contains some elastic fibres. (Richardson's stain.) (Reproduced with permission from Giles, L.G.F. (1992) Ligaments traversing the intervertebral canals of the human lower lumbosacral spine. *Neuro-Orthopedics,* **13**, 25–38.)

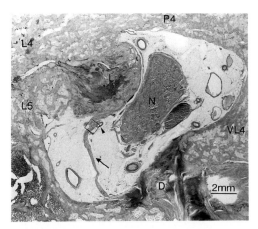

Figure 3.18 Parasagittal section, 100 μm thick, across the left L4–5 intervertebral foramen of a 79-year-old male. A ligament (arrow) traverses the intervertebral canal from the ligamentum flavum (L) to the intervertebral disc fibres (D). The vertebral body of the fourth lumbar vertebra (VL4) and its pedicle (P4) are shown with the adjacent superior articular process of the fifth lumbar vertebra (L5). N = neural complex. The region shown within the square was resected from an adjacent unmounted section and is shown in Figure 3.19 which includes part of the adjacent blood vessel (arrow head). (Ehrlich's haematoxylin and light green counterstain). (Reproduced with permission from Giles, L.G.F., Allen, D.E. and Horne, F. (1991). Thin histological sections prepared from large thick sections: a new technique. *Biotech. Histochem.,* **66**, 273–276.)

Table 3.1 *Average dimensions of ligaments traversing the mid-zones of L4–5 and L5–S1 canals in the horizontal plane (sections cut in the parasaggital plane)*

Horizontal ligaments	Average length mm	Average width mm	Average depth mm
L4–5	5.7	1.1	1.8
RANGE	3.1–9.8	0.4–1.9	1.0–3.0
L5–S1	6.6	1.2	1.7
RANGE	5.0–8.4	0.4–1.2	1.0–3.0

(Reproduced with permission from Giles, L.G.F. (1992) Ligaments traversing the intervertebral canals of the human lower lumbosacral spine. *Neuro-Orthopedics,* **13**, 25–38.)

thick histological section, re-embedded, and cut at a section thickness of 1 μm to determine its cellular structure.

The 1 μm thick sections showed that elastic fibres are present (their morphology and their staining is similar to the elastic interna of the adjacent blood vessel) (Figure 3.19).

The average length, width, and depth projected into the intervertebral canal of these vertical ligaments at the mid-zones of the L4–5 and L5–S1 levels is shown in Table 3.2, which also shows the corresponding ranges.

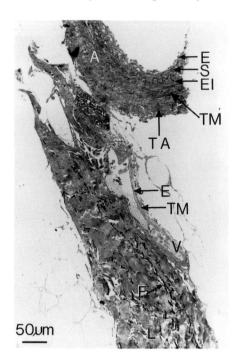

50 µm

Figure 3.19 Section of the area in the square shown in Figure 3.18 cut at 1 µm from an adjacent 100 µm thick LVNC section. Note the elastic fibres (F) in the ligamentum flavum (L) and in the wall of the artery (A). The histological composition of the artery is shown (E = endothelium; S = subendothelial layer; EI = elastic interna; TM = tunica media; TA = tunica adventitia) as well as that of a vein (V) containing blood cells. The blood vessels seen within the transforaminal ligament were not visible in the 100 µm thick section. (Richardson's stain.) (Reproduced with permission from Giles, L.G.F., Allen, D.E. and Horne, F. (1991) Thin histological sections prepared from large thick sections: a new technique. *Biotech. Histochem.*, **66**, 273–276.)

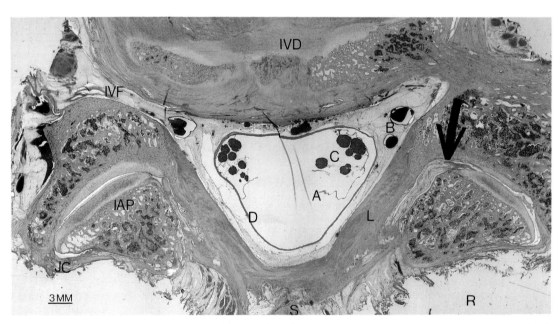

Figure 3.20 A 200 µm thick histological section cut slightly obliquely in the horizontal plane through the left and right lumbosacral zygapophysial joint inferior recesses. The black arrow indicates a large fat-filled vascular intra-articular synovial fold projecting into the medial part of the right zygapophysial joint from below. A = arachnoid membrane; B = Batson's venous plexus; C = cauda equina nerve root trunks; D = dural membrane; IAP = inferior articular process of L5; IVD = intervertebral disc; IVF = intervertebral canal (foramen); JC = fibrous joint capsule; L = ligamentum flavum; R = right side of spine; S = spinous process remains. (Modified from Giles, L.G.F. and Taylor, J.R. (1982) Intra-articular synovial protrusions in the lower lumbar apophyseal joints. *Bull. Hosp. Joint Dis.*, **XLII**, 248–255.)

Table 3.2 *Average dimensions of ligaments traversing the mid-zones of L4–5 and L5–S1 canals in the vertical plane (sections cut in the parasaggital plane)*

Vertical ligaments	Average length mm	Average width mm	Average depth mm
L4–5	6.5	1.3	2.6
RANGE	3.7–9.2	0.5–2.5	1.0–4.0
L5–S1	6.6	1.2	2.0
RANGE	3.6–9.5	0.2–1.5	0.4–2.2

(Reproduced with permission from Giles, L.G.F. (1992) Ligaments traversing the intervertebral canals of the human lower lumbosacral spine. *Neuro-Orthopedics*, **13**, 25–38.)

The thin histological sections showed that this ligament contains elastic fibres, blood vessels and small diameter myelinated nerves.

The transforaminal ligaments are described by Bogduk and Twomey (1991) as consisting of narrow bands of collagen fibres that traverse the outer end of the intervertebral canal and which are not strictly ligaments as (i) their structure more resembles 'bands of fascia' than ligaments proper, and (ii) except for the inferior corporotransverse ligaments, they do not connect two separate bones. However, Giles (1992) showed that some of these structures which traverse the mid-zone of the intervertebral canal, running in the horizontal or vertical planes, are ligaments which contain elastic fibres and small diameter neurovascular structures. Furthermore, in some instances, these ligaments bridge from one bone to another, as confirmed by Church and Buehler (1991) and Giles (1992).

The ligaments within the mid-zone are not constant and are not necessarily present in left and right paired intervertebral canals from a given specimen, raising the possibility that these structures are anomalous variants.

A histological section, cut through the inferior joint recess of the left and right lumbosacral zygapophysial joints respectively, in a 54-year-old male, is shown in Figure 3.20. This shows that particularly large intra-articular synovial folds are located in the lower region of the zygapophysial joint.

Intra-articular synovial folds are also found in the superior joint recesses but are not as large as those found in the inferior joint recesses, as described in Chapter 5.

Detailed anatomy of the lumbar spinal motion segment is presented in the following descriptive Chapters 4–8 and that of the thoracolumbar junction's motion segment is presented in Chapter 12.

References

Amonoo-Kuofi, H.S., El-Badawi, M.G. and Fatani, J.A. (1988a) Ligaments associated with lumbar intervertebral foramina. 1. L1 to L4. *J. Anat.*, **156**, 177–183.

Amonoo-Kuofi, H.S., El-Badawi, M.G., Fatani J.A. *et al.* (1988b) Ligaments associated with lumbar intervertebral foramina. 2. The fifth lumbar level. *J. Anat.*, **159**, 1–10.

Bachop, W. and Hilgendorf, C. (1981a) Transforaminal ligaments of the human lumbar spine. *Anat. Rec.*, **199**, 144.

Bachop, W. and Stern, H. (1981b) Transforaminal ligaments and the straight leg raising test of Lasegue. *Twelfth Annual Biomechanics Conference on the Spine.* Colorado, Biomechanics Laboratory, University of Colorado, Boulder, pp. 281–294.

Bachop, W. and Ro, C.S. (1984) A ligament separating the nerve from the blood vessels at the L5 intervertebral foramen. *The Journal of Bone and Joint Surgery Orthopaedic Transactions*, **8**, 437.

Bogduk, N. and Twomey, L. T. (1991) *Clinical Anatomy of the Lumbar Spine*. Churchill Livingstone, Edinburgh, p. 40.

Brailsford, J.F. (1929) Deformities of the lumbosacral region of the spine. *Br. J. Surg.*, **16**, 562–627.

Bullough, P.G. and Boachie-Adjei, O. (1988) *Atlas of Spinal Diseases*. J.B. Lippincott, Philadelphia, pp. 84–97.

Church, C.P. and Buehler, M.T. (1991) Radiographic evaluation of the corporotransverse ligament at the L5 intervertebral foramen: a cadaveric study. *J. Manipulative Physiol. Ther.*, **14**, 240–248.

DePuky, R. (1935) The physiological oscillation of the length of the body. *Acta Orthop. Scand.*, **6**, 338–347.

Dorwart, R.H. and Genant, H.K. (1983) Anatomy of the lumbosacral spine. *Radiol. Clin. North Am.*, **21**, 201–220.

Epstein, J.A. (1960) Diagnosis and treatment of painful neurological disorders caused by spondylosis of the lumbar spine. *J. Neurosurg.*, **17**, 991–1001.

Giles, L.G.F. (1992) Ligaments traversing the intervertebral canals of the human lower lumbosacral spine. *Neuro-Orthopedics*, **13**, 25–38.

Giles, L.G.F. and Taylor, J.R. (1982) Intra-articular synovial protrusions in the lower lumbar apophyseal joints. *Bulletin of the Hospital for Joint Diseases Orthopaedic Institute*, **12**, 248–255.

Giles, L.G.F., Allen, D.E. and Horne, F. (1991) Thin histological sections prepared from large thick sections : a new technique. *Biotech. Histochem.*, **66**, 273–276.

Hasue, M., Kikuchi, S., Sakuyama, Y. *et al.* (1983) Anatomic study of the interrelation between nerve roots and their surrounding tissues. *Spine*, **8**, 50–58.

Hilton, R.C. (1980) Systematic studies of spinal mobility and Schmorl's nodes. In *The Lumbar Spine and Back Pain* (M.I.V. Jayson, ed.), 2nd edn. Pitman Medical, Kent, pp. 115–134.

Koreska, J., Robertson, D., Mills, R.H. *et al.* (1977) Biomechanics of the lumbar spine and its clinical significance. *Orthop. Clin. North Am.*, **8**, 121–133.

Kraemer, J., Kolditz, D. and Gowin, R. (1985) Water and electrolyte content of human intervertebral discs under variable load. *Spine*, **10**, 69–71.

Keim, H.A. and Kirkaldy-Willis, W.H. (1987) *Clinical Symposia. Low Back Pain*. 39. Ciba-Geigy, New Jersey.

Lewin, T., Moffett, B. and Viidik, A. (1961) The morphology of the lumbar synovial intervertebral arches. *Acta Morphol. Neerlando-Scandinavica*, **4**, 299–319.

Mitchell, G.A.G. (1934) The lumbosacral junction. *J. Bone Joint Surg.*, **16B**, 233–254.

Morris, J.M. (1973) Biomechanics of the spine. *Arch. Surg. (Chicago)*, **107**, 418–423.

Taylor, J.R. and Twomey, L. (1980) Sagittal and horizontal plane movement of the human lumbar vertebral column in cadavers and in the living. *Rheumatol. Rehabil.*, **19**, 223–232.

Tortora, G. J. and Grabowski, S.R. (1993) *Principles of Anatomy and Physiology*, 7th edn. Harper Collins, New York, p. 151.

Tyrrell, A, Reilly, T. and Troup, J.D.G. (1985) Circadian variation in stature and the effects of spinal loading. *Spine*, **10**, 161–164.

White, A.A., III. and Panjabi, M.M. (1978) *Clinical Biomechanics of the Spine*. J.B. Lippincott, Philadelphia.

Wing, P., Tsang, I., Gagnon, F. *et al.* (1992) Diurnal changes in the profile shape and range of motion of the back. *Spine,* **17**, 761–766.

4

Lumbar intervertebral discs

J.R. Taylor and L.G.F. Giles

The anatomy of lumbar intervertebral discs

Disc development

The embryonic vertebral column

The embryonic mesenchymal column is formed as an unsegmented, cylindrical condensation of mesenchyme around the notochord (Taylor and Twomey, 1988). From this primitive, unsegmented connective tissue column, bilateral, segmental processes grow dorsally to encircle the neural tube. The primitive cylindrical column differentiates into alternate light bands and dark bands. Intervertebral discs will develop from the dark bands in this column. The dark bands are relatively slow growing, fibroblastic structures. The rapidly growing light bands will develop into cartilage models of the vertebrae. The more rapid growth of the cartilage models of the vertebral bodies compared to the dark bands contributes to segmental changes in the notochord, which thickens at the centre of each primordial intervertebral disc and gradually thins out and disappears from that part of its course through each vertebral body.

Early disc development

The peripheral cells of each dark band differentiate into fibroblasts which form collagen in a circumferential lamellar arrangement. Centrally, the notochordal segment expands to form the nucleus pulposus (Figure 4.1).

The attenuated part of the notochordal track passing through the centre of each cartilagenous

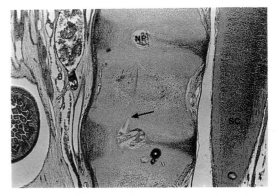

Figure 4.1 A 100 micron median sagittal section showing the lowest two lumbar intervertebral discs in a 20-week fetus. The notochordal segments form the original nucleus pulposus; the mucoid streak (arrow) passes through the cartilage model of the L5 vertebral body, where central cartilage swelling and calcification indicate the appearance of the primary centre of ossification. The anulus fibrosus is already well formed at this stage. NP = nucleus pulposus; SC = spinal cord.

vertebra is known as a mucoid streak. Centres of ossification appear in the centre of each vertebral body, interrupting the mucoid streak and obliterating it from the centre of each vertebra, but the mucoid streak persists in the cartilage plates which cap the cephalic and caudal surfaces of each developing bony vertebral body (Figure 4.2). These cartilage plates are cartilaginous epiphyses of the growing vertebra, but they are also integral parts of the structure of the developing disc (O'Rahilly and Meyer, 1979; Verbout, 1985; Taylor and Twomey, 1988).

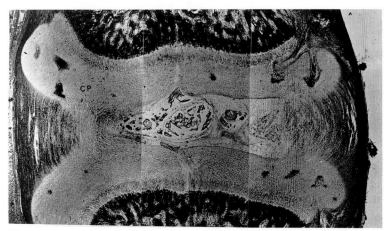

Figure 4.2 A montage of a fetal lumbar intervertebral disc in median sagittal section. The nucleus is now expanding to fill the centre of the disc. The centra are well formed; above and below and the cartilage plates (CP) capping the centra are regions of intersection between the 'cartilaginous epiphyses' of the vertebra and the intervertebral disc. Note the vascular canals in the periphery of the cartilage plates. (Reproduced with permission from Taylor, J.R. and Twomey, L. (1988) Development of the human intervertebral disc. In *Biology of the Intervertebral Disc* (P. Ghosh, ed.), vol l. CRC Press, Boca Raton, Florida, p. 70.)

Disc structure in the fetus

The lamellar structure of the anulus fibrosus, which is typical of the adult disc, is already obvious in the fetal disc (Taylor and Twomey, 1988). The annular lamellae are, from the beginning, continuous with similar lamellae in the cartilage plates, though these cartilage plate lamellae can only be seen by polarized light. The notochordal cells of the nucleus multiply rapidly and produce a proteoglycan-rich mucoid matrix expanding the nucleus pulposus. The continuous lamellae in the anulus and the cartilage plates envelop the rapidly growing nucleus pulposus, the whole structure resembling an elliptical sphere. The notochordal cells of the nucleus also have the capacity to erode the inner aspects of the envelope formed by the anulus and the cartilage plates. The envelope also expands as its lamellae grow in length, to accommodate the growing nucleus pulposus. The continuous envelope around the nucleus, formed by the anulus fibrosus and cartilage plates, is characteristic of the disc at all stages of life.

Disc growth in the infant and child

The rapid expansion of the notochordal nucleus pulposus is the most notable feature of growth in later fetal life and in the infant disc, especially in lumbar discs. The notochordal cells disappear from the nucleus during childhood as the disc grows rapidly in volume and becomes avascular (Taylor, 1974). The fetal and infant disc is a very vascular structure with plentiful blood vessels in its anulus fibrosus and cartilage end-plates, though it normally never has any blood vessels in its nucleus. By the age of 4 years most of these blood vessels have disappeared, leaving only a few small vascular buds projecting from the vertebral marrow into the vertebral aspect of each cartilage plate and a few capillary-like vessels in the outer layers of the anulus fibrosus (Taylor *et al.*, 1992).

This large avascular structure is nourished in later life by diffusion from the vascular buds from the vertebral end-plate and the small blood vessels in the longitudinal ligaments and the most peripheral layers of the anulus (Maroudas *et al.*, 1975). The notochordal cells are unable to survive in an avascular environment and they are replaced during childhood by chondrocytes and fibroblasts, cells better able to survive in the avascular environment (Taylor, 1974).

Water and proteoglycans in the immature disc

The lumbar nucleus of an infant disc is 88% water and the anulus is 80% water (Puschel, 1930). The high water content of this viscous fluid structure is assured by the proteoglycans produced by the notochordal cells and later by chondrocytes which will gradually replace the notochordal cells.

The proteoglycan content of the nucleus and inner anulus remains high as the colonizing cells also produce proteoglycans, in which there is a higher proportion of keratan sulphate, a functional substitute for the originally dominant chondroitin sulphate (Taylor *et al.*, 1992). These cells also produce collagen and the collagen network formed in the

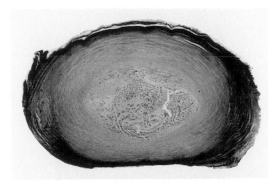

Figure 4.3 A premature infant lumbar intervertebral disc in transverse section. The large notochordal nucleus pulposus occupies the central region, surrounded by the circumferential lamellae of the anulus fibrosus.

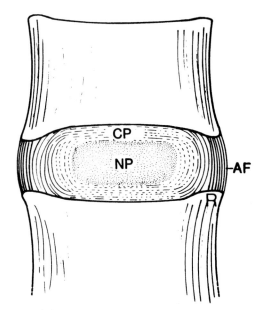

Figure 4.4 A diagram of an adult intervertebral disc in median section. The central nucleus pulposus (NP), rich in proteoglycans, has a sparse population of chondrocytes. The notochordal cells disappeared during maturation. There are two parts of the anulus fibrosus (AF): an outer ligamentous part which attaches to the bony rims (R) of the vertebral bodies, and an inner fibrocartilaginous part which is continuous with the cartilage end-plates (CP) on the surfaces of the vertebrae. The cartilage end-plates and the anulus form a continuous envelope around the nucleus. (Modified from Taylor, J.R. and Twomey, L. T. (1994a) The effects of ageing on the intervertebral discs. In *Grieve's Modern Manual Therapy: The Vertebral Column* (G.D. Boyling, and N. Palastanga, eds.), 2nd ed. Churchill Livingstone, Edinburgh, pp. 177–188.)

nucleus changes it from a viscous fluid to a soft, pulpy, discrete, central mass, which still has a very high water content and behaves as a fluid. As the nucleus matures, in the young adult, it remains soft with a high water content (75–80%) and it continues to behave as a fluid, but its boundaries with the anulus become less distinct. It is central or posterocentral within the disc and occupies about two-thirds of its antero-posterior extent in the mid-sagittal plane (Figure 4.3).

Adult structure

Intervertebral discs from young adults have a broadly similar structure to those of children, with a relatively soft nucleus, rich in proteoglycans, contained by a strong outer fibrous and inner fibrocartilaginous envelope (Taylor, 1990) (Figure 4.4).

However, from the time of appearance of the ring apophyses, at puberty, the outer lamellae of the anulus are anchored in this bony ring, which fuses with the vertebral body at completion of vertebral growth, from 15 to 18 years. The inner lamellae of the young adult anulus fibrosus remain continuous with the lamellar structure of the cartilage plates, forming a complete cartilaginous envelope around the nucleus pulposus. The outer fibrous lamellae of the anulus are almost indistinguishable in structure from the fibrous longitudinal ligaments, but their attachments are different as the fibres of the longitudinal ligaments generally bridge many segments, some inner fibres of the longitudinal ligaments attaching to the vertebral rims at each level. On the other hand, the fibres of the anulus fibrosus only bridge one segment in each case.

Transverse sections of fresh young adult discs show a white glistening appearance with regular concentric annular lamellae. The anterior and lateral parts of the anulus fibrosus are thicker than the posterior part, showing both greater thickness of lamellae and greater numbers of distinguishable lamellae in the antero-lateral anulus fibrosus. The nucleus pulposus is contained under pressure within the anulus and it swells on sectioning, mainly by absorbing more water from the environment.

The nucleus pulposus

The principal changes in the disc on maturation are in the nucleus pulposus. The progressive increase in the collagen content of the nucleus pulposus, begun in childhood, continues in the adult nucleus. At the same time the cell population per unit volume decreases. The more sparse cell population of the adult nucleus, associated with its reduced vascularity, continues to produce proteoglycans; spaces in the bony end plates permit 10% of the vascular spaces of the vertebral marrow to come in contact with the cartilage plates (Maroudas *et al.*, 1975) and the peripheral anulus contains a few small blood vessels. According to Puschel (1930), there is a reduced water content in the young adult nucleus (76%) compared to the newborn disc (88%).

However, normal adult discs still have a high level of hydration, and can absorb more water readily, particularly into the nucleus. Recently cut sections of normal discs buckle due to this rapid absorption of water by the nucleus, even after formalin fixation. Conversely, dehydration of the discs during histological processing inevitably produces some contraction artefact in the nucleus. This artefact characteristically shows horizontal splits near the upper and lower margins of the nucleus, parallel to the adjacent cartilage plates, joined by a vertical split through the centre of the nucleus. This appearance recalls the shape of normal discograms (Taylor, 1990); it may be explained by the distribution of collagen bundles in the nucleus. On high power microscopic examination of a small region of the nucleus pulposus, collagen fibres appear to form a random network, but low power examination of the nucleus as a whole shows that in different parts of the nucleus, bundles of collagen fibres are oriented in preferred directions; in the upper and lower areas of the nucleus, bundles are parallel to the cartilage plates; in the area where the anulus and nucleus merge, loose, poorly formed, lamellar bundles are convex inwards towards the centre of the nucleus; at the centre, a few loosely arranged vertical bundles are seen in the area previously occupied by the 'notochordal debri'. The bilocular 'hamburger' shape of normal discograms is related to the pathways by which the contrast injected into the nucleus spreads most easily between the collagen bundles; this is determined by the orientation of the collagen bundles described.

Our studies in fresh unfixed post-mortem spines show the influence of the turgor in the normal nucleus on lumbar spinal posture. When a normal young adult lumbar spine is hemisected, the nucleus instantly bulges out from its envelope at the cut surface, showing the pressure which the nucleus normally exerts on its constraining envelope. At the time of sectioning, the column both shortens slightly and becomes more lordotic. If the soft, bulging nucleus is compressed back into its cavity the column noticeably lengthens and straightens again. Similarly, in an intact column, when intradiscal pressure is raised by the injection of radio-opaque material for post-mortem discography, lordosis is reduced as intradisc pressure increases and the column straightens (Taylor, unpublished study). Studies of creep i.e. deformation of the disc under load, with prolonged axial loading (Boyd, 1929; Twomey and Taylor, 1991) support the view that, in sustained erect posture, the spine would creep into increased lordosis, whereas with prolonged loading in full flexion, creep may flex the spine beyond the normal end range (Twomey and Taylor, 1982).

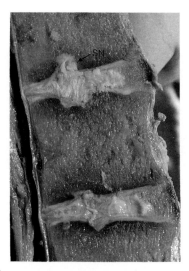

Figure 4.5 An adult vertebral column in sagittal section showing Schmorl's nodes (SN). These protrusions into the vertebral spongiosa occur in adolescence through weak points in the cartilage plates where the notochord originally passed through them. (Reproduced with permission from Taylor, J.R., and Twomey, L. (1988) Development of the human intervertebral disc. In *Biology of the Intervertebral Disc* (P. Ghosh, ed.), Vol l. CRC Press, Boca Raton, Florida, p. 71.)

The nucleus pulposus is separated from the central parts of the vertebral bodies, only by the thin cartilage plates which cap their caudal and cephalic surfaces. At the centres of these, where the notochord originally penetrated the cartilage plates, there are weak points where sudden axial loading of the spine may cause herniation of the young fluid nucleus into the vertebral spongiosa. Such herniations, called Schmorl's nodes (Figure 4.5), appear to occur very commonly in children and adolescents, as they are rarely found in infants and young children but they are seen in 38% of all adults, apparently with little if any adverse effect on the functioning of the intervertebral disc.

The anulus fibrosus

The histology of the adult anulus is similar to that of the child. There are differences between the anterior and posterior parts of the anulus in lumbar discs, related to the lumbar lordosis. Anteriorly, there are more than 20 fairly thick lamellae. The outer lamellae appear entirely fibrous with thick course bundles of fibres which run vertically between the vertebral bony rims. The outer lamellae are loosely fused to the strong anterior longitudinal ligament. The inner lamellae have finer fibres embedded in a densely stained basophilic matrix and they are gently curved with an outward convexity, becoming continuous with the lamellar structure of the 'hyaline' cartilage plates above and below. The lateral anulus resembles the anterior anulus.

The posterior and posterolateral parts of the anulus are much thinner, with 12–15 more closely packed thinner lamellae which are more sharply curved in an outwardly convex U-shaped course. The outer fibres are fused with the thin posterior longitudinal ligament. The outer anular fibres attach to the thinner posterior vertebral rims and the inner fibres are continuous with the cartilage plates.

Blood vessels are frequently seen between the longitudinal ligaments and the anulus, and a few small vessels are usually found within the outer layers of the adult anulus. The inner anulus is not clearly demarcated from the nucleus in the adult disc, and some loose inwardly convex lamellae are usually seen in the transitional area. These are also present in the discs of older children. They cannot be entirely explained on the basis of dehydration contraction artefact. They probably represent an alignment of the collagen bundles in the outer nucleus in response to the mechanical compressive and dynamic forces to which the disc is subjected in weight-bearing and movement.

Thick parasagittal sections of the outer anulus clearly show the alternating direction of the collagen fibres in adjacent lamellae (Figure 4.6); they are arranged such that first, third, and successive layers have parallel fibres while the second, fourth and successive layers have parallel bundles in a direction virtually opposite to that of the fibres in lamellae 1 and 3.

The angle between the crossing fibres of adjacent lamellae (the interstriation angle) is about 50–55° in the lateral anulus of lumbar discs. The angle is less than this in the posterior anulus and may be more than this in the anterior anulus. The complexity of the spiralling concentric lamellae, with the outer layers exchanging fibres with the longitudinal ligaments and some apparent interweaving of fibres in inner lamellae, was said by Walmsley (1953) to 'almost defy description'. However, the elliptical encapsulation of the nucleus by the inner anulus and cartilage plates with the direct bony attachment of the outer anular fibres are essential structural features; the alternating spiral arrangement of the fibres in successive lamellae gives great strength and helps to limit movements, especially rotation (Farfan, 1973; Taylor, 1974; Taylor and Twomey, 1988).

Cartilage plates

At the periphery of each cartilage plate, a ring apophysis appears, fuses with the centrum and forms the hard bony rim of the vertebral end-plate, but the larger central part of each hyaline cartilage plate persists in the adult as part of the envelope of the nucleus (Taylor, 1974; Taylor and Twomey, 1988). In the cartilage plate, the lamellae of the anulus intimately interlock with a persisting part of the cartilage model of the fetal vertebral body. The cartilage plates have a horizontal lamellar arrangement when viewed by polarized light. They are about 1 mm thick and they contribute to the resilience of the mobile segment. They are also important pathways for diffusion of nutrients from the vascular spongiosa into the central parts of the disc, since 10% of each bony vertebral end plate is perforated by small vascular buds which make contact with the cartilage plate. These vascular contacts are more plentiful centrally than peripherally (Maroudas *et al.*, 1975).

Direct neural relations of the disc

The posterior and postero-lateral surfaces of each lumbar disc are directly related to two pairs of spinal nerves (Figure 4.7A and B).

In the intervertebral foramen, the spinal nerves are tucked up under the pedicles, above the level of the disc, but after emerging from the intervertebral foramina, they are in direct contact with the postero-lateral disc surfaces. Within the lateral recesses of the spinal canal, the posterior surface of the same disc is in direct contact with the next pair of spinal nerves, within their root sleeves of spinal arachnoid and dura, as they descend obliquely towards the next pair of

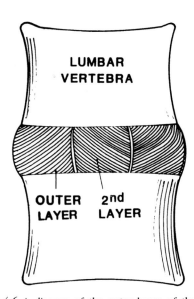

LUMBAR VERTEBRA

OUTER LAYER   **2nd LAYER**

Figure 4.6 A diagram of the outer layers of the anulus fibrosus showing the alternately spiralling arrangement of the fibres in adjacent lamellae. (Reproduced with permission from Taylor, J.R. and Twomey, L.T. (1994a) The effects of ageing on the intervertebral discs. In *Grieve's Modern Manual Therapy: The Vertebral Column* (G. D. Boyling, and N. Palastanga, eds), 2nd edition. Churchill Livingstone, Edinburgh, pp. 177–188.)

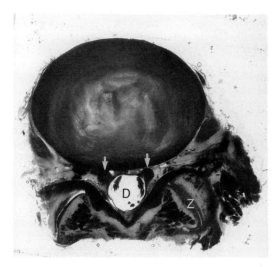

A

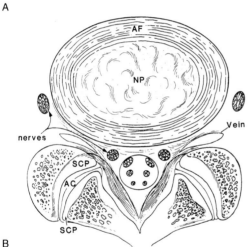

B

Figure 4.7 (A) A transverse section through the L5–S1 disc of a normal adult motion segment, at the level of the lower part of the intervertebral foramen, showing the anulus fibrosus and nucleus pulposus of the disc. On the lateral surface of the anulus, lie the L5 spinal nerves which pass out through the upper parts of the intervertebral foramina. The dural tube (D) occupies the central part of the triangular spinal canal and the S1 nerves lie in the epidural space at the lateral angles (arrows). The zygapophysial joints (Z), postero-lateral to the spinal canal, show articular cartilage supported by a thick subchondral bone plate. The spinous process has been cut off. (Reproduced with permission from Taylor, J.R. and Twomey, L.T. (1994b) Structure and function of lumbar zygapophysial (facet) joints. In *Grieve's Modern Manual Therapy: The Vertebral Column* (G. D. Boyling and N. Palastanga, eds.), 2nd edition. Churchill Livingstone, Edinburgh, pp. 99–108.) (B) A diagram illustrating the anatomy shown in the cadaveric section (7A) A large vein traverses each lower intervertebral foramen; the L5 and S1 nerves are indicated by arrows; AC = articular cartilage; AF = anulus fibrosus; NP = nucleus pulposus; SCP = subchondral bone plate.

intervertebral foramina. On the antero-lateral surface of the disc, the sympathetic chain descends, parallel to the anterior margin of the psoas major muscle, in direct contact with vertebrae and discs (see Figure 14.3); rami communicantes connecting the sympathetic chain to each spinal nerve, pass obliquely across the lateral surfaces of vertebral bodies and intervertebral discs supplying the periosteum and the outer lamellae of the anulus fibrosus (Taylor and Twomey, 1980a) (see Figures 14.12, 17.1 and 17.2B). Other small nerves, arising directly from the spinal nerves or their ventral rami close to the intervertebral foramen, supply the postero-lateral and posterior surfaces of the disc (Taylor and Twomey, 1980a; Bogduk *et al.*, 1981). Those nerves which return into the intervertebral foramina to supply the posterior longitudinal ligament and the posterior anulus are called the sinu-vertebral nerves.

The turgor of the nucleus pulposus

At all stages the nucleus is under tension within its envelope (Nachemson and Elfstrom, 1970), so that it immediately bulges when sectioned at post-mortem. Normal discs from middle aged and old subjects retain this capacity to swell when released from the restraint of the intact anulus.

The capacity of the normal disc to expand by attracting water, due to its rich proteoglycan content, is much greater than its intact, inelastic, outer envelope will allow. An attempt to inject fluid through a needle introduced into the nucleus of a healthy young adult disc is resisted by this intradiscal pressure and the small quantity of fluid which can be injected may subsequently be spontaneously expressed back through the needle into the syringe. As already noted, forceful injection of normal saline into a healthy disc changes the posture of the motion segment which straightens and becomes less lordotic. Conversely, with loss of water and proteoglycans from a degenerate disc, it tends to sag, or creep on axial loadbearing, with greater loss of height than would occur in a healthy young disc.

Nachemson (1965) showed that in healthy discs, the intradiscal pressure varied according to the lumbar posture. Pressure is less in a lordotic posture than in a flexed posture and increased axial loading is reflected by increased intradiscal pressure (Nachemson and Elfstrom, 1970).

In life there is an ever changing equilibrium between the chemical forces in the healthy disc, trying to take in more water and the external mechanical compressive loading, which tends to squeeze water out. On average, we each lose about 1.7 cm of our stature in the course of the day, by axial creep, due to loss of water from our intervertebral discs, most of it in the first few hours after rising, and we recoup it at night when lying down. The water distribution within the disc can also be altered by eccentric loading due to prolonged loading in a fully flexed posture, when water is selectively squeezed out of the anterior part of the disc. Creep in flexion can temporarily alter the normal shape of a lumbar disc (Twomey and Taylor, 1982).

The high proteoglycan and water content of the nucleus pulposus and inner anulus give the disc its elasticity and resilience in weightbearing and movement.

In normal erect posture weightbearing, the fluid nucleus receives the transmitted loading from the vertebra above and redistributes the vertical force equally in all directions, acting as a shock absorber. A normal fresh post-mortem lumbar spine feels quite stiff when it is flexed, extended or laterally flexed, and it will return spontaneously to its resting posture when the deforming force is removed. This is partly due to the elasticity of ligaments like the ligamentum flavum, but also due in large part to the turgor and elasticity of the intervertebral disc (McFadden and Taylor, 1990).

The anulus fibrosus, its attachments and functions

From the fetal stage onwards, two parts can be recognized in the anulus fibrosus: an outer ligamentous part and an inner fibrocartilaginous part. The relatively coarse collagen fibres of the ligamentous, outer anulus attach to the outer margins of the adjacent vertebral bodies. This outer part attaches to the outer rim of the cartilage plate in a child, to the ring apophysis in adolescence and to the vertebral rim in adults, once the bony ring apophysis fuses with the centrum at approximately 18 years. The collagen fibres of the outer anulus have relatively few cells and matrix between them and staining with Alcian Blue reveals a low content of glycosaminoglycans (GAGs) (Taylor *et al.*, 1992).

The fine collagen fibres of the inner anulus are embedded in a plentiful cellular, GAG rich matrix. They are curved with an outward convexity, becoming continuous with the lamellar structure of the cartilage plates above and below, forming a complete elliptical spherical envelope around the nucleus. This arrangement of the inner anulus is seen most clearly in the discs of children but it can still be clearly distinguished in normal adult discs (Taylor, 1974).

The fibres in the whole thickness of the anulus are arranged in circumferential lamellae which spiral between the vertebrae. This arrangement gives the anulus great dynamic strength. The outer anterior lamellae run almost vertically between the vertebrae. This is the thickest part of the disc, and the anulus also has its greatest horizontal thickness here. The fine lamellae of the posterior anulus are, by contrast, sharply curved in a 'U'-shaped form. The posterior region is the thinnest part of the lumbar disc. This wedge shape of the lumbar discs contributes to the

lumbar lordosis, but at the lumbo-sacral level, the body of L5 is also notably wedge-shaped. The posterior margins of the discs, as viewed in transverse section or CT scans are slightly concave where they bound the spinal canal.

The longitudinal ligaments

The anterior anulus is completely covered by the anterior longitudinal ligament, a longitudinal, broad, tough ribbon, whose attachments bridge over many vertebrae, in contrast to the segmental attachments of each anulus. The anterior longitudinal ligament exchanges only a few fibres with each anulus for attachment to each vertebral rim. It is loosely attached to the front of each disc and to the anterior vertebral periosteum, but it may be capable of some slight slip or stretch, in full extension, in contrast to the inelastic, anterior anulus which adapts to movement by change in its curvature. The thinner, posterior longitudinal ligament covers the posterior anulus and is firmly attached to its surface but bridges over each posterior vertebral surface, leaving a space for part of the internal vertebral venous plexus and the basivertebral veins. Its outline is dentate, wide at the discs and narrow where it bridges over each vertebral body.

The arrangement of the anulus in two parts, with their covering ligaments, clearly has functional importance. The outer ligamentous anulus and the anterior and posterior longitudinal ligaments appear designed to bear tensile forces, as in full flexion and extension, and to act as 'check ligaments', preventing excessive movement and the danger of avulsion of the disc from the vertebral body. The anterior structures require greater strength than the posterior anulus and longitudinal ligament as they do not have the additional support given to the posterior structures by the posterior ligamentous complex between the vertebral arches.

'Weight-bearing'

The inner anulus appears designed to cooperate and participate with the enclosed nucleus pulposus in supporting axial loading. First, as the inner anulus and the cartilage plates form a complete, inextensible, envelope around the incompressible, fluid nucleus, this gives the disc a shock absorber function, in response to axial loads. As the anulus and nucleus are capable of changing their shape, this arrangement also enables the disc to act like a strong and rather stiff joint, each disc allowing relatively small movements. The elasticity of the disc, which tends to return it to its resting shape after a movement, also assists the spinal muscles to return the spine to its resting neutral position. In addition to its role as an envelope tightly enclosing the nucleus, the inner anulus, independently of the nucleus, also has the potential to bear axial loads. This is because of the intimate functional relationship of its collagen fibrils with their GAG-rich matrix. Each collagen fibril is closely surrounded and attached to a sheath of proteoglycan macromolecules, which attract and hold water, forming a kind of inflatable cylindrical, collar around each collagen fibril, which tends to straighten it or reduce its curvature (Taylor *et al.*, 1992). Thus, as Markolf and Morris (1974) showed, the disc can still resist axial loads, even when part of its nucleus has been removed.

Movement: the discs and the facets

In general terms, the range of segmental intervertebral movement is proportional to the thickness and compliance of the intervertebral disc and to the slenderness of the column. Measurements of ranges of movements in the lumbar spine as a whole, in both cadavers and living populations suggest that about 50° of sagittal plane movement (flexion plus extension) is the norm, or about 60° in young adult females, who generally have a more slender column than males with more compliant discs (Taylor and Twomey, 1980b). This represents about 10° of movement per motion segment.

However, movement in the spine cannot be discussed without considering the influence of the zygapophysial joint facets. The lumbar zygapophysial joints guide lumbar movements in particular planes and resist, or prevent, movements in other planes, particularly those which would endanger the integrity of the disc (Farfan, 1973; Putz, 1985).

The zygapophysial joints are synovial joints between the superior and inferior articular processes of the laminae (see Chapter 5). Lumbar facets are curved or biplanar in the horizontal plane, but flat in the vertical plane, roughly parallel to the long axis of the lumbar spine. The facet orientation facilitates sagittal plane and coronal plane movements but resists horizontal plane movements (Putz, 1985). The joints have large superior and inferior fat-filled 'polar' recesses to accommodate upward and downward gliding of the facets in flexion, extension and lateral bending. In transverse section or CT scan, two parts can be distinguished in each superior articular process. The larger posterior part is sagittally oriented and the smaller anterior part is almost coronally oriented (Taylor and Twomey, 1986, 1992). These two parts have different functions. The anterior coronal part restrains intersegmental translation in flexion and the posterior part severely restrains axial rotation (Twomey and Taylor, 1983). These functions protect the disc from shearing forces in translation and from overstretch of the fibres of the anulus fibrosus in axial

rotation (Farfan, 1973). As the anular fibres are oriented at approximately 45° to the long axis of the spine, a combination of flexion and axial rotation would have the greatest effect in stretching the posterior fibres of alternate lamellae.

Experiments with single motion segments have shown that true axial rotation is restricted to about 2° in each direction (Farfan, 1973) but studies of the whole lumbar spine suggest a wider range of twisting (Taylor and Twomey, 1980b). Careful observation suggested that this 'more physiologic' movement was partly a coupled movement with lateral bending and flexion accompanying the 'twist' (McFadden and Taylor, 1990). Measurements of facet orientation in the sagittal plane show a very small forward slope of the articular surfaces of the articular processes, making an average angle of 5–8° with the longitudinal axis of the spine.

The protective influence of the facets in resisting translation is of greatest importance at the lumbosacral junction where, as Davis (1961) has shown, in response to the sharply lordotic angle, a much higher proportion of the compressive load is borne by the facets. This is reflected by the increase in the angle formed by the joint plane and the mid-sagittal plane in the lower two superior articular facets compared to higher facets. The load borne by the facets is emphasized by the high frequency of spondylolysis in the arch of L5 in young athletes and the danger to the disc in the absence of this restraint is shown by the effects of spondylolisthesis on the lumbosacral disc.

Ageing of the human intervertebral disc

Decline in stature with ageing is often attributed to reduction in disc height, but osteoporosis is the major cause of loss in stature with ageing (Dent and Watson, 1966). This is due to the increase in vertebral end-plate concavity with ageing and the corresponding ballooning of the disc into the deforming end-plates, as measurement studies of large, unselected, populations, show no evidence of generalized loss in disc height (Twomey and Taylor, 1986). With ageing, disc degeneration is increasingly prevalent but it is not universal and, at least in regard to disc thickness, loss of disc thickness is by no means an inevitable accompaniment of ageing (Twomey and Taylor, 1985).

Measurement studies of cadaveric spines indicate that the average *mid-sagittal* height of most discs is usually maintained during ageing with a tendency to increase, while *peripheral* disc heights tend to decrease (Twomey and Taylor, 1985, 1991).

The functions of the lumbar intervertebral discs are to provide enough strength for stiffness and stability, while giving useful ranges of movement. Considering the high static loading and dynamic forces repeatedly transmitted through the lumbar discs in a lifetime, they maintain these roles well in many elderly people, despite the 'degenerative changes' heralded by the appearance of peripheral osteophytes. The thickest discs are the lower lumbar ones, which are about 12 mm thick. The disc envelope, formed by the anulus and cartilage plates, encloses the nucleus, which continues to behave as a fluid in most older adults, despite the increase in its collagen content and slow age-related changes in its proteoglycan content with reduction in its associated water. The nucleus continues to demonstrate some turgor in older adults; it is still held under tension within its inelastic envelope.

Functional age change: creep and stiffness

The most important age changes in intervertebral discs are biomechanical and functional, rather than obvious structural changes in the gross sense of loss in disc height. The behaviour of a degenerate disc in loadbearing is inconsistent compared to normal discs (Nachemson *et al.*, 1979) and renders the disc less efficient in transmitting loads and maintaining the normal intersegmental stiffness and stability.

The principal, and most consistent, functional changes in the disc with age are a reduction in movement ranges associated with an increase in disc stiffness and an increase in creep in response to loading (Taylor and Twomey, 1980b; Twomey and Taylor, 1982). For instance, the average range of sagittal motion reduces from about 55° in young adults to 40° in the elderly. Creep is greater in the elderly than in young adults, and hysteresis (recovery of initial shape) is slower in the elderly. These functional changes suggest that the disc proteoglycans are less efficient in binding water in older discs than in young discs. The older disc also has a higher collagen content than the young disc (Adams *et al.*, 1977). Thus the old disc is stiffer in its immediate response to muscle forces attempting a normal range of movement, but less stiff in its response to prolonged loading, such as axial loadbearing. Therefore, middle-aged and elderly lumbar columns have a greater tendency to buckle into increased lordosis on prolonged standing, especially if the postural muscle support is inadequate. During creep, fluid and metabolites are expressed from the disc, and in hysteresis they return. The increased response to prolonged loading in the elderly, and the slowing down of recovery, may adversely affect the normal processes of nutrition and predispose to further degenerative change in conditions of prolonged static loading. Such loading could also render the discs of the older spine less resilient, and less able to cope with any sudden demands due to lifting or other strenuous physical activity.

These observations emphasize the importance of healthy muscular activity, producing full ranges of spinal movement, maintenance of strength in lumbar spinal postural muscles, and the avoidance of prolonged loading or overloading of the elderly spine.

Pathology

Disc degeneration

This is not a well defined term. In the literature it is usually synonymous with disc thinning, the presence of circumferential and radial fissures from the nucleus into the anulus, as revealed by discography, and the appearance of marginal osteophytes on plain film radiography (see Figures 4.8A and B, 4.16 and 20.5).

Rolander (1966) described a system of classifying disc age changes, based on their morphological appearance in post-mortem sections. This ranged from normal juvenile discs (grade 0) through the normal age changes of middle age (grade 2) to frank disc degeneration with dessication, thinning and fissuring (grade 3). When Twomey (1981) used this scheme to classify his large range of material of all ages he found that 72% of discs from subjects over 60 years of age were not degenerate, but most remained in grade 2. The commonly accepted view that old discs are dessicated is not quite correct. Puschel's data (1930) showed that most of the water loss in the life history of discs takes place during maturation and the water content of the adult nucleus declines on average by only 6% from young adults to old age. In the same period the GAGs of the disc are said to be generally maintained (Adams *et al.*, 1977). When discs were degenerate (grade 3), the lowest two discs were most frequently affected. These are the discs subjected to the greatest forces, and fissuring of the anulus is seen in L4–5 and L5–S1 with increasing frequency in old age. Trauma, or repeated microtrauma may initially cause circumferential fissures in the anulus leading later to the appearance of radial fissures, most often in the posterolateral regions of the disc (Adams and Hutton, 1985) (Figure 4.8A and B). Disc fissures would provide a possible pathway for nuclear herniation in young or middle-aged adults; in old age, the nucleus pulposus is no longer soft and is too firmly bound by collagen to its surrounding envelope to be able to herniate through the gap, unless very high forces are involved, chemical changes occur in the disc, or the process of herniation is a very slow one. Once again, the discs which most frequently herniate are at L4–5 and L5–S1 (Spangfort, 1972).

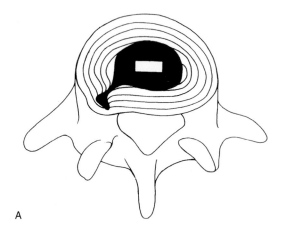

A

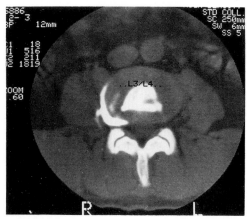

B

Figure 4.8 (A) A diagrammatic representation of a radial fissure penetrating the postero-lateral anulus to its outer third. (Reproduced with permission from Taylor, J.R. and Twomey, L.T. (1994a) The effects of ageing on the intervertebral discs. In *Grieve's Modern Manual Therapy: The Vertebral Column* (G.D. Boyling, and N. Palastanga, eds), 2nd edition. Churchill Livingstone, Edinburgh, pp. 177–188). (B) A discogram of an L3–4 disc, showing the nuclear area outlined by contrast which has also spread via a radial fissure (not seen) to occupy an extensive circumferential fissure on the right side. Contrast is leaking through a fissure into the right lateral surface of the anulus.

Internal disc disruption

Internal disc disruption, as described by Crock (1986), is a much more common degenerative phenomenon, and a much more common cause of low back pain, and/or referred pain to the lower limb, than nuclear herniation with a radiculopathy. This involves both circumferential and radial fissuring of the anulus fibrosus. This fissuring, together with typical pain provocation, can be demonstrated on

discography, and axial discography can also demonstrate clearly the degree of both circumferential and radial fissuring (Figure 4.8B). There is a good correlation between fissuring involving the outer third of the anulus and discogenic pain syndromes (Sachs, 1987). The fissured disc tends, eventually, to become revascularized, by the ingrowth of vessels (see Figures 4.12 and 4.13), often from the vertebral end-plate. According to Vernon-Roberts and Pirie (1977), nerves also grow into the disc with the vessels. Vertical, i.e., intraspongious disc herniations, or Schmorl's nodes (Figure 4.5), are the most common of all disc prolapses, but they are usually a developmental event, probably occurring in childhood or adolescence through a cartilage end-plate weakness left by the notochord. Schmorl's nodes affect 38% of the normal population and Hilton *et al.*, (1976) claimed that these nodes predispose to disc degeneration.

An example of a cartilage end-plate indentation, or weakness, in the superior surface of the first sacral body of a 75-year-old male is shown in Figure 4.9. The lumbosacral intervertebral disc is relatively normal apart from the minor posterior midline herniation. In contrast, the superior end-plate of the fifth lumbar vertebral body shows a small Schmorl's node lesion with calcification surrounding it. The fourth lumbar intervertebral disc shows degenerative changes.

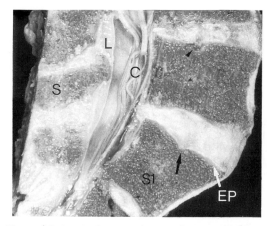

Figure 4.9 A sagittal section showing the lower lumbosacral spine from a 75-year-old male. The L5 intervertebral disc appears to be relatively normal with only slight posterior herniation. The superior surface of the first sacral body (S1) shows cartilage end-plate (EP) indentation or weakness (arrow) in the region where the notochord developed. The superior end-plate of the fifth lumbar vertebral body contains a small Schmorl's node lesion where a vertical, or intraspongious, herniation (arrow head) has occurred with calcification surrounding it. Note the degenerative changes within the L4 intervertebral disc, i.e., thinning with degenerative changes of its nucleus pulposus and anulus fibrosus. C = cauda equina; S = spinous process of L5 vertebra; L = ligamentum flavum.

Instability

Loosening of the motion segment was described by Schmorl and Junghanns (1971), Morgan and King (1957), Crock (1986), Friberg (1987), and Keim and Kirkaldy-Willis (1987) and many others. This is associated with injury or degenerative changes in both the intervertebral disc and the zygapophysial joints (see Figure 20.5). The patient complains of recurrent attacks of low back pain associated with minor stressful incidents and has difficulty in rising to the erect posture from a flexed position. Axial scans often show unilateral subluxed zygapophysial facets, suggesting a rotational strain, as Farfan (1973) and Kirkaldy-Willis (1983) described. A CT axial scan done with the spine in torsion will sometimes demonstrate abnormal zygapophysial facet diastasis during rotation (Kirkaldy-Willis, 1983; McFadden and Taylor, 1990). In the early stages, strengthening of rotary muscle support and control of the lumbar spine may assist in managing the problem, reducing pain, and avoiding surgery. According to Kirkaldy-Willis (1983), the unstable segment tends naturally to stabilize with advancing age.

The age of onset and the rate of progression of intervertebral disc degeneration vary greatly in different individuals, and the role of excessive or chronic stress on the spine can initiate or accelerate disc degeneration (Donohue, 1939). Degradative changes appear in the disc by the second decade and thereafter show variable but relentless progression (Taylor and Ghosh, 1978). Considerable lumbar disc degeneration has been found in most spines of 40 years of age (Schmorl and Junghanns, 1971). In an investigation of ageing and degeneration in lumbar intervertebral discs, Pritzker (1977) found that (a) with ageing, two new cell types appear, that is giant chondrons in discs over 30 years of age and mini-chondrons in association with microfracture of the cartilage end-plate; (b) there were focal histological changes in the cartilage end-plate which appeared to precede histological changes in the nucleus pulposus and anulus fibrosus; and (c) there was generalized thinning, ossification, and disruption of the end-plates; this was seen only in collapsed discs and was indicative of advanced pathological processes.

The major morphological features of the ageing disc, that is, a shrinking in the volume of the nucleus pulposus and a less distinct nucleus pulposus, have been repeatedly asserted (Smith, 1930; Donohue, 1939; Saunders and Inman, 1940; Peacock, 1952; Brown, 1970; Taylor and Akeson, 1971; Bijlsma and Peerboom, 1972) and linked to joint instability.

Progressive desiccation of the nucleus pulposus or injury resulting in the escape of nuclear material is said to allow adjacent vertebrae to approximate each other, leading to bulging of the anulus fibrosus, with lifting of the adjacent periosteum leading to osteophyte formation on the edges of the articulating surfaces of vertebral bodies (McRae, 1977). Also, with advancing age, the hallmarks of spondylosis appear in cases of spinal curvature, first on the concave side of the curvature, with the convex side being relatively spared. On the concave side, disproportionate loading, together with reduced movement can be invoked as responsible for the changes, at least in part (Taylor and Ghosh, 1978).

Intervertebral disc degenerative changes were discussed earlier and details provided elsewhere (Farfan, 1973; Adams and Hutton, 1985; Saal, 1990). However, changes affecting the articular triad are further discussed here, with anatomical and histopathological examples, to emphasize the possible clinical importance of changes which can affect a given spinal level.

Posterolateral intervertebral disc herniation

Early accounts of intervertebral disc herniation were described by Mixter and Barr (1934) and an example of a posterior midline subligamentuous herniation of the second lumbar intervertebral disc, causing compression of the cauda equina, is shown in Figure 4.10. A corresponding parasagittal histological section showing the herniation is depicted in Figure 4.11, which clearly illustrates compression of a root comprising part of the cauda equina.

Posterior herniation of intervertebral disc material, with or without accompanying osteophytic spurs, also frequently causes significant compression of vascular structures within the spinal canal as shown in Figure 4.12.

Blood vessels are frequently seen in degenerating intervertebral discs from elderly cadavers (Figures 4.12 and 4.13) although normal adult intervertebral discs do not possess any blood vessels (Kramer, 1977; Katz *et al.*, 1986; Yasuma *et al.*, 1993).

In some specimens the dural sleeve containing the nerve roots, or nerve root and ganglion, become attached via adhesions to prolapsed intervertebral disc material (Figure 4.14).

Anterolateral intervertebral disc herniation

According to Kramer (1990), increased interest in structural and functional disorders of the spine caused by degenerative change was generated by the mounting incidence of disc-related disorders and the realization that these conditions often affect other organs. Furthermore, emphasis on pathoanatomical alterations led the medical community to neglect functional disturbances which could not be substantiated by morphological findings, with the result that these conditions were then often treated by 'paramedical' practitioners (Kramer, 1990).

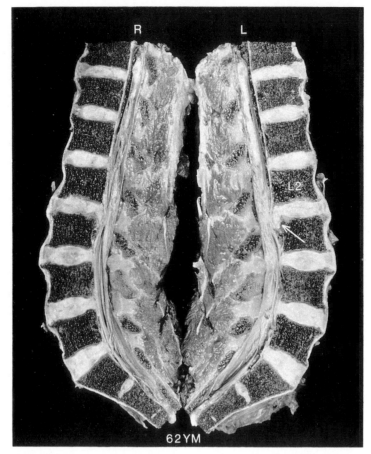

Figure 4.10 Part of a spinal column extending from T11 to S3 is shown bisected in the sagittal plane into left (L) and right (R) halves. The intervertebral discs appear to be relatively normal for a 62-year-old male apart from the large posterior midline subligamentous herniation of the second lumbar intervertebral disc (arrow) which is causing some stenosis with compression of the dural tube and its cauda equina at this level.

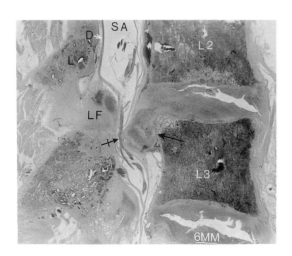

Figure 4.11 Parasagittal compression of the dural tube (D) due to herniation of the L2 intervertebral disc (large arrow) shown in Figure 4.10. Note how in this 200 μm thick histological section a nerve root comprising part of the cauda equina is also compressed (tailed arrow). L = lamina of L2 vertebra; LF = ligamentum flavum; SA = subarachnoid space within the dural tube. (Ehrlich's haematoxylin and light green counterstain.)

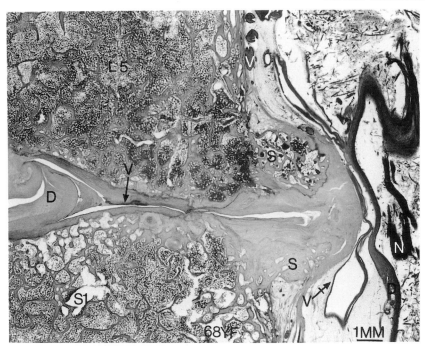

Figure 4.12 A 200 μm thick histological section showing a lumbosacral posterior midline intervertebral disc herniation, with large bilateral osteophytic spurs (S) projecting into the intervertebral canal and causing stenosis of the canal and traction and occlusion of the adjacent vascular structures (V tailed arrow). D = intervertebral disc; L5 = fifth lumbar vertebral body; N = neural structure within the dural tube; S1 = first sacral body; V (arrow) = small blood vessel. (Ehrlich's haematoxylin and light green counterstain.)

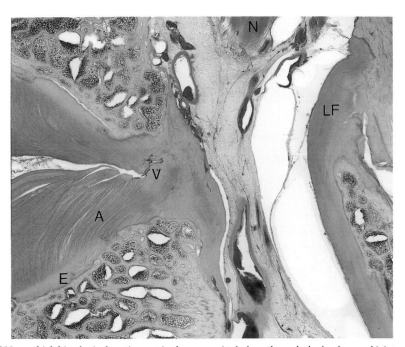

Figure 4.13 A 200 μm thick histological section cut in the parasagittal plane through the lumbosacral joints of an 82-year-old female which shows blood vessels (V) within the posterior region of the anulus fibrosus (A). Note the hyaline articular cartilage of the end-plate (E) and the posterior orientation of the anular fibres in this lumbosacral zygapophysial joint. LF = ligamentum flavum; N = large neural structures within the intervertebral canal. (Ehrlich's haematoxylin and light green counterstain.)

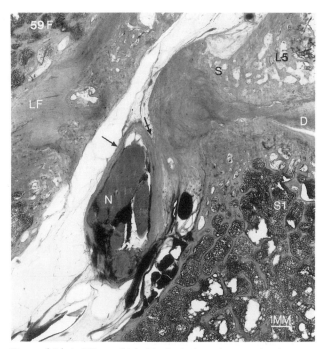

Figure 4.14 A 200 μm thick histological section, cut in the para-sagittal plane through the lumbosacral intervertebral canal of a 59-year-old female which shows an adhesion (tailed arrow) between the dural sleeve (arrow) and the intervertebral disc herniation. D = intervertebral disc; LF = ligamentum flavum; N = neural structures within the dural sleeve (arrow); S = osteophytic spur on the inferior posterolateral margin of the fifth lumbar (L5) vertebral body; S1 = first sacral segment. (Ehrlich's haematoxylin and light green counterstain.)

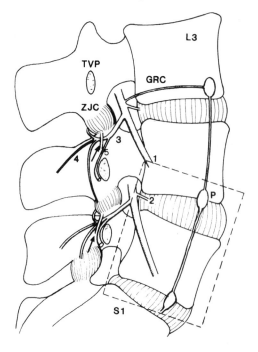

Figure 4.15 Part of the lower lumbosacral spine and its innervation shown schematically (lateral view). 1 = anterior primary ramus of the spinal nerve; 2 = anterior primary ramus branch to the intervertebral disc; 3 = posterior primary ramus of the spinal nerve; 4 = medial branch of the posterior primary ramus with an adjacent zygapophysial joint capsule (articular) branch, and a descending branch to the zygapophysial joint capsule (articular branch) one joint lower; 5 = lateral branch of the posterior primary ramus; GRC = grey ramus communicans; P = paraspinal autonomic ganglion; TVP = transverse process; ZJC = zygapophysial joint capsule; arrow = part of mamillo-accessory ligament. The dashed lines show the approximate region of the L4–S1 vertebral segments retained with some adjacent soft tissues for histological processing and examination. (Modified and reproduced with permission from Giles, L.G.F. (1989) *Anatomical Basis of Low Back Pain*. Williams and Wilkins, Baltimore.)

Intervertebral disc herniation with vertebral body osteophytes which affect the paravertebral autonomic ganglia (Nathan, 1962, 1968, 1987) have been implicated in the vertebrogenic autonomic syndrome by Jinkins *et. al.* (1989) (also see Chapter 17).

This section presents some preliminary morphological findings which show how the paraspinal autonomic nervous system may be subjected to biomechanical (deformation) influences in the region of the paraspinal autonomic ganglia.

Lumbosacral spines were removed at autopsy from three elderly human cadavers aged 73–76 years (mean 74 years) then radiographed in the postero-anterior, lateral, and left and right 45° posterior oblique positions, then cut into blocks of tissues. These blocks comprised parts of the L4–S1 vertebral bodies with some adjacent soft tissues, as dia-

grammatically shown by lateral and superior views, respectively (Figures 4.15 and 4.16), which also show part of the sympathetic chain. The sympathetic chain continues to become closely adherent to the anterior surface of the sacrum, running just medial to the pelvic foramina, to meet on the surface of the coccyx as the ganglion impar (Esses *et al.*, 1991).

Depending upon the position of a section within the block, spines with large osteophytes in the vicinity of paraspinal autonomic nerves and ganglia showed that these structures can be considerably distorted by such osteophytes. The osteoligamentous blocks of tissues removed from the spine were radiographed before being processed and an example of a radiograph from a 73-year-old male shows how large claw osteophytes have developed bilaterally, adjacent to the lateral margins of the L4–5 intervertebral disc (Figure 4.17).

Histological examination of vertebral bodies from L4 to S1 with their adjacent soft tissues, cut in the coronal plane from posterior to anterior, were examined to determine whether lateral vertebral body osteophytosis affected adjacent neural structures. The serial sections included various anatomical

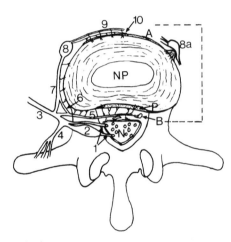

Figure 4.16 Diagram (not to scale) of a superior view of a lumbar vertebra and some of its associated soft tissue structures (see Figure 17.1 for greater detail). A = anterior longitudinal ligament; B = part of Batson's venous (epidural) plexus; N = nerve roots (cauda equina); NP = nucleus pulposus of the intervertebral disc; P = posterior longitudinal ligament; 1 = anterior and posterior spinal roots, respectively, giving rise to a spinal nerve; 2 = spinal ganglion; 3 = anterior primary ramus of the spinal nerve; 4 = posterior primary ramus of the spinal nerve; 5 = sinuvertebral nerve; 6 = autonomic (sympathetic) branch to the sinuvertebral nerve; 7 = grey ramus communicans; 8 = normal paraspinal autonomic ganglion; 8a = paraspinal autonomic ganglion being distorted by an osteophyte projecting from beneath the intervertebral disc; 9 = anterior paraspinal afferent autonomic branch; 10 = anterior paraspinal efferent autonomic branch. The dashed lines show the approximate region of the body with some adjacent soft tissues retained for histological examination.[Modified and redrawn from: Jinkins *et. al.* (1989), Pedersen *et al.* (1956), Edgar and Ghadially (1976), Bogduk (1984).] (Reproduced with permission from Giles, L.G.F. (1992) Paraspinal autonomic ganglion distortion due to vertebral body osteophytosis: a cause of vertebrogenic autonomic syndromes? *J. Manipulative Physiol. Ther.*, **15**, 551–555.)

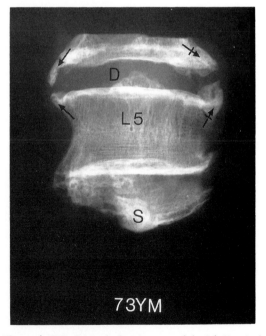

Figure 4.17 Radiograph showing part of the L4–S1 spinal blocks of tissue from a 73-year-old male, with intervertebral disc spaces (D) on each side of the L5 body. S = part of the first sacral segment. Arrows show osteophytes on the left and right sides of the vertebral bodies. (Reproduced with permission from Giles, L.G.F. (1992) Paraspinal autonomic ganglion distortion due to vertebral body osteophytosis: a cause of vertebrogenic autonomic syndromes? *J. Manipulative Physiol. Ther.*, **15**, 551–555.)

structures and part of the corresponding histological anatomy of the L4–5 intervertebral disc and L5 vertebral body shown in Figure 4.16, which shows how a membrane encloses part of the neurovascular structures which are usually in close proximity to the spine (Figure 4.18).

The anulus fibrosus and end-plates are clearly shown on each side of the L4–5 intervertebral disc between the respective vertebral bodies, as are the large osteophytes on these vertebral bodies adjacent to the lateral margins of the disc. On the left of the L4–5 intervertebral disc shown in Figure 4.18, a nerve is being distorted in its course as it passes the lateral osteophytes, and an example of tractioning of the autonomic chain nerves on the right side of the L5–S1 intervertebral joint is seen in Figure 4.19.

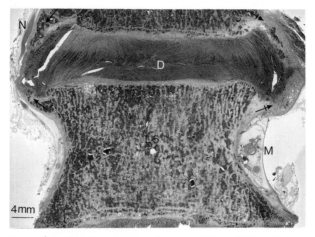

Figure 4.18 Histological section showing a 200 μm thick section cut in the coronal plane through the fifth lumbar vertebral body (L5) with adjacent L4–5 intervertebral disc (D). Note the large osteophytes (arrows) which have developed adjacent to the lateral margins of the L4–5 intervertebral disc bilaterally. A membrane (M) encloses part of the neurovascular structures which are closely related to the spine. On the left side the osteophytes are distorting the nerve (N). There is some unfolding of the innermost anular fibres. (Reproduced with permission from Giles, L.G.F. (1992) Paraspinal autonomic ganglion distortion due to vertebral body osteophytosis: a cause of vertebrogenic autonomic syndromes? *J. Manipulative Physiol. Ther.*, **15**, 551–555.)

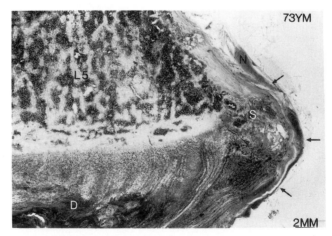

Figure 4.19 The paraspinal autonomic chain on the right side (arrows) is tractioned due to the large osteophyte (S) on the inferior antero-lateral margin of the fifth lumbar (L5) vertebral body. D = intervertebral disc; N = lumbar paraspinal autonomic ganglion.

In some histological sections from the same specimen the claw osteophytes were seen to deform the paraspinal autonomic ganglion (Figure 4.20).

Although numerous authors have documented that radiologically demonstrable but 'asymptomatic' disc disease occurs (Isherwood and Antoun, 1980; Vanharanta *et al.*, 1985), it probably depends on the degree and position of joint osteophytosis as to whether associated paraspinal autonomic tissues are affected. Some authors have suggested that functional disorders of viscera may occur due to vertebral lesions, and Kunert (1965) and Lewit (1985) have attempted to provide a rationale to explain the possible mechanisms involved in any such vertebrogenic symptom complex. However, controlled clinical studies to investigate these hypotheses have not been conducted, so there is, at present, no scientific proof of visceral involvement.

Recent scientific studies have suggested that a relationship may exist between abnormal vascular changes and neural tissue degenerative changes within the intervertebral foramen (Giles and Kaveri, 1990; Giles, 1991; Jayson, 1992; Rydevik, 1992).

A meticulous radiological study was performed by Jinkins *et al.* (1989) to provide an anatomical basis for any possible relationship between lumbar disc extrusion and the vertebrogenic symptom complex, which includes (1) local and referred pain, and (2) autonomic reflex dysfunction, which may be observed as generalized alterations in viscerosomatic tone associated with the autonomic syndrome. Jinkins (1993) also discussed in detail the pathoanatomic basis of somatic and autonomic syndromes originating in the lumbosacral spine and elaborates on these syndromes in Chapter 17.

The vertebrogenic autonomic syndrome could well be associated with lumbar disc degenerative changes with accompanying osteophyte formation causing traction and/or compression of adjacent paraspinal autonomic nerves and ganglia, as has been demonstrated in this histological study. It seems reasonable to postulate that autonomic reflex dysfunction may result from (1) abnormal microvascular circulation in paraspinal autonomic neural structures, and (2) abnormal axoplasmic flow occurring within neural structures affected by osteophytes. These findings may help to explain what has been observed as a clinical impression by chiropractors, osteopaths and medical manipulators that, following spinal manipulation for spinal pain of mechanical origin, some patients report relief from visceral dysfunction, for example in cases of idiopathic 'indigestion'. In addition, other basic science documentation indicates a functional relationship between spinal joints and viscera, as evidenced by the work of Sato (1980, 1992) in which noxious and non-noxious somatic stimuli, at various spinal segmental levels, can reflexly affect visceral organ functions. Clearly, further basic science research is required to shed more light on any possible pathophysiological consequences and mechanisms involved in the vertebrogenic autonomic syndrome.

Intervertebral disc degeneration and its possible effect on zygapophysial joint hyaline articular cartilage and intervertebral canal structures

When the intervertebral disc of the articular triad degenerates, the zygapophysial joints frequently also show degenerative changes. An example of these linked degenerative changes will be shown in this chapter, including plain film radiographs of the specimen used for histological demonstration.

In order to show the clinical relevance of intervertebral disc degeneration and its possible effects on zygapophysial joint hyaline articular cartilage, some important aspects of hyaline articular cartilage are briefly summarized here, although a detailed description of normal and osteoarthritic hyaline articular cartilage is given in Chapter 5.

Normal adult hyaline articular cartilage of the zygapophysial joints (Hadley, 1964; Meachim and Stockwell, 1979; Bullough and Boachie-Adjei, 1988) is considered to be avascular and aneural (Ghadially, 1981; Malemud and Muskowitz, 1981) except at its

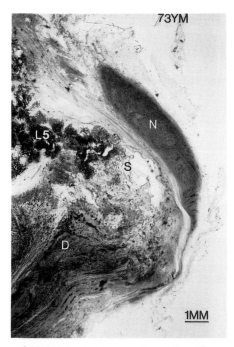

Figure 4.20 A paraspinal autonomic ganglion (N), containing cell bodies, which appears to be tractioned by a large osteophyte (arrow) on the infero-lateral margin of the body of the L5 vertebra. D = intervertebral disc.

periphery (Stockwell, 1979). Cartilage thickness varies in different parts of the same joint (Gardner, 1978) but it is generally thicker at the periphery of concave surfaces and at the centre of convex surfaces (Bullough, 1979), although this does not normally apply to the concave surfaces of zygapophysial joints of the human lumbar spine as the cartilage is thicker at the centre of the concave and convex surfaces (Giles, 1989). The combined thickness of the paired hyaline articular cartilages across the centre of the zygapophysial joints in the lumbar spine is approximately 2–2.4 mm (Fick, 1904; Giles and Taylor, 1984). Hyaline articular cartilage essentially consists of a dense extracellular matrix populated by a sparse, diffuse population of chondrocytes (Woessner *et al.*, 1977). The major components of the matrix are long fibres of collagen, which form an arcade arrangement orientated perpendicular to the subchondral bone plate and arching round to become tangential to the articular cartilage surface (Benninghoff, 1925), and proteoglycans which fill the interstices of this meshwork (see Figure 5.6 A and C).

Just as the physiology of the zygapophysial joints cannot be divorced from consideration of other

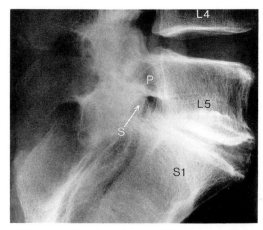

Figure 4.22 Lateral view of the L4 to S1 spinal joints shown in Figure 4.21. Note (1) the spondylosis at L5–S1 with advanced thinning of the intervertebral disc and adjacent osteophyte formation anteriorly and posteriorly, (2) the proximity of the superior articular processes of the sacrum (S) to the adjacent pedicles (P), and (3) narrowing of the intervertebral canal ('foramen') due to the posterolateral osteophytic spur (S) shown in Figure 4.21 to be on the left side of the L5 vertebral body. (Reproduced with permission from Giles, L.G.F. and Kaveri, M.J.P. (1991) Lumbosacral intervertebral disc degeneration revisited: a radiological and histological correlation. *Man. Med.*, **6**, 62–66.)

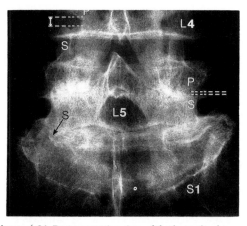

Figure 4.21 Posteroanterior view of the lower lumbosacral spine (L4 to S1 levels) of a 73-year-old male showing a normal intervertebral disc space at L4–5 with relatively normal alignment of the paired articular facet surfaces of the articular processes on the left and right sides of the spine. The relationship of the superior articular processes (S) of the L5 vertebra to the pedicles (P) of the L4 vertebra above, is normal (arrow between dashed lines). The lumbosacral (L5–S1) intervertebral disc space is greatly diminished and there is an osteophytic spur (arrow S) at the inferior posterolateral margin of the L5 vertebral body on the left side. The superior articular processes (S) of the sacrum are in close apposition to the pedicles (P) of the L5 vertebra due to the greatly thinned L5–S1 intervertebral disc, in contrast to the normal superior articular process–pedicle relationship shown at the L4–5 level. (Reproduced with permission from Giles, L.G.F. and Kaveri, M.J.P. (1991) Lumbosacral intervertebral disc degeneration revisited: a radiological and histological correlation. *Man. Med.*, **6**, 62–66.)

elements of the mobile segment, pathological changes of the intervertebral disc may be expected to affect the function of the zygapophysial joints (Farfan, 1973; Kirkaldy-Willis, 1983). Thus, thinning of the intervertebral disc (Figures 4.21 and 4.22), either as a result of a degenerative process or a loss of disc substance, results in approximation of adjacent vertebral bodies, with accompanying subluxation (imbrication, telescoping) of the opposing hyaline articular cartilages of the adjacent zygapophysial joints (Ingelmark, 1959; Hadley, 1964).

Ultimately, osteoarthritic degenerative changes of the zygapophysial joint occur (Figures 4.22–4.24) (Ingelmark, 1959; Farfan, 1977) with encroachment upon the intervertebral canal (Meisel and Bullough, 1984). This segmental instability is also associated with traction spurs (Stokes and Frymoyer, 1987), although the presence of anatomical abnormalities often correlates poorly with the presence of pain (McCarron *et al.*, 1987), probably because of the limitations of clinical imaging systems. However, lumbar intervertebral disc degeneration has a significant association with low back pain (Biering-Sorensen *et al.*, 1988) as is the case with osteoarthritis (Meisel and Bullough, 1984), a ubiquitous, slowly developing articular disease (Swanson and de Groot Swanson, 1985), which is said to be 'primary' when no aetiological factors can be discerned and 'secondary' when there is an identifiable cause (Dick,

1972) such as abnormal wear and tear due to faulty joint mechanics (Mitchell and Cruess, 1977; Bland, 1983; Kerr and Resnick, 1984) which can result from intervertebral disc degeneration.

A histological section of part of the fifth lumbosacral intervertebral disc and part of the left lumbosacral

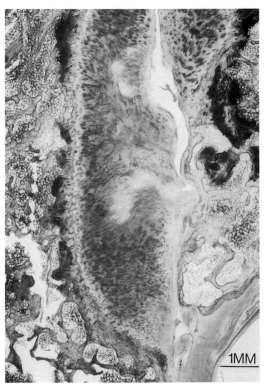

Figure 4.24 Light photomicrograph of the rectangle shown in Figure 4.23 which shows fibrillation and fissuring of the L5 hyaline articular cartilage. (Reproduced with permission from Giles, L.G.F. and Kaveri, M.J.P. (1991) Lumbosacral intervertebral disc degeneration revisited: a radiological and histological correlation. *Man. Med.,* **6,** 62–66.)

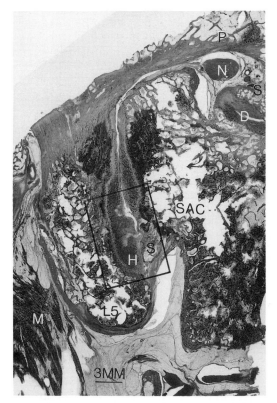

Figure 4.23 A 100 μm thick sagittal section through the left zygapophysial joint and the posterolateral region of the L5–S1 intervertebral disc (D) of a 73-year-old male cadaver. Note the osteophytic spur formation (S), particularly at the inferior posterolateral region of the L5 vertebral body, adjacent to the minor intervertebral disc protrusion, with encroachment upon the intervertebral canal. An osteophytic spur (S) has also developed at the base of the superior articular process (SAC) of the sacrum. Subluxation of hyaline articular cartilage surfaces has resulted in the cartilage on the inferior articular process of the fifth lumbar vertebra (L5) articulating with the boney spur (S) at the base of the superior articular process (SAC) of the sacrum. This has led to fibrillation and deep fissuring within the cartilage. The area enclosed by the rectangle is enlarged for Figures 4.24–4.25. Note the proximity of the superior articular process of the sacrum to the adjacent pedicle (P) of the L4 vertebra which shows some sclerotic changes. (Reproduced with permission from Giles, L.G.F. and Kaveri, M.J.P. (1991) Lumbosacral intervertebral disc degeneration revisited: a radiological and histological correlation. *Man. Med.,* **6,** 62–66.)

zygapophysial joint in Figure 4.21 shows, in Figure 4.23, that intervertebral disc thinning and protrusion can result in (i) osteophytic spur formation adjacent to the intervertebral disc, (ii) subluxation of opposing surfaces of hyaline articular cartilage of the zygapophysial joints, (iii) approximation of the superior articular process of the sacrum to the pedicle of the fifth lumbar vertebra, and (iv) narrowing of the superior to inferior and anteroposterior diameters of the intervertebral canal, which results in diminution in size of the intervertebral canal through which neural and vascular structures pass. Furthermore, subluxation of opposing hyaline articular cartilages can be associated with subsequent degenerative changes within this cartilage, ranging from early fibrillation to fissuring, and finally, to total destruction with eburnation of the subchondral facet surfaces.

Figures 4.23–4.25 show some of these features as seen by light microscopy using transmitted and darkfield techniques, respectively.

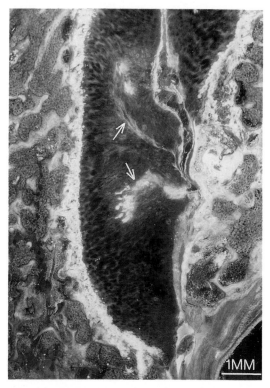

Figure 4.25 Dark field photomicrograph of the rectangle shown in Figure 4.23. Note the additional information recorded, i.e. the deep fissuring of the hyaline articular cartilage (arrows) with clear changes in the appearance of the chondrocytes adjacent to the deep fissures. (Reproduced with permission from Giles, L.G.F. and Kaveri, M.J.P. (1991) Lumbosacral intervertebral disc degeneration revisited: a radiological and histological correlation. *Man. Med.,* **6,** 62–66.)

cartilage where its surface approximates a bony spur; this osteoarthritis represents synovial joint failure (Dieppe and Watt, 1985) and can, in turn, initiate low back pain (Bullough and Boachie-Adjei, 1988). Furthermore, should the large innervated synovial fold, located in the inferomedial joint recess, become pinched, due to zygapophysial joint subluxation, traumatic synovitis could occur with resultant pain (Keim and Kirkaldy-Willis, 1987; Giles, 1989).

This set of radiographs and photomicrographs emphasizes that the interpretation of radiological investigations of low back pain sufferers should take into account the limitation of radiological examinations. Nonetheless, it is emphasized that, in spite of the limitations of radiology, radiographic investigations provide an important and necessary clinical procedure in the differential diagnosis of the low back pain syndrome, which may have a varied pathogenesis and may originate from a variety of anatomical sites (McCarron *et al.,* 1987).

Finally, while degenerative changes affecting the intervertebral disc have frequently been associated with osteoarthritis of the adjacent zygapophysial joints and their hyaline articular cartilage, it is important to note that Ziv *et al.* (1993) found that, even in the young adult, a considerable proportion of fresh post-mortem spines had zygapophysial joint hyaline articular cartilage showing ulceration or severe fibrillation, and that this proportion appeared to remain constant throughout adulthood. Therefore, Ziv *et al.* (1993) suggest that zygapophysial joint hyaline articular cartilage can degenerate early in life, independently of the age-related changes which occur in the intervertebral disc.

Biomechanical implications of intervertebral disc degeneration

Biomechanical studies have shown that, during combined compression and bending loads, the zygapophysial joints carry from 12 to 25% of the total intervertebral load (Bullough and Boachie-Adjei, 1988). However, Adams and Hutton (1983) showed that intervertebral disc narrowing can cause the zygapophysial joints to carry up to 70% of the intervertebral load, dependent on posture and segmental location, within the lumbar spine.

The foregoing case study demonstrates some histological changes which can be associated with advanced thinning of, and minor protrusion of, the intervertebral disc at the lumbosacral joint in a 73-year-old cadaver. The subsequent subluxation of the hyaline articular cartilage surfaces is associated with 'secondary' osteoarthritic changes within the

References

Adams, M.A. and Hutton, W.C. (1983) The mechanical function of the lumbar apophyseal joints. *Spine,* **8,** 327–330.

Adams, M.A. and Hutton, W.C. (1985) Gradual disc prolapse. *Spine,* **10,** 524–531.

Adams, P., Eyre, D.R. and Muir, H. (1977) Biochemical aspects of development and ageing of human lumbar discs. *Rheumatol. Rehabil.,* **16,** 22–29.

Benninghoff, A. (1925) Form und Bau der Gelenk-knorpel in ihren Beziehungen zur Funktion. *Z. Anat. Entwicklungsgesch,* **76,** 43.

Biering-Sorensen, F., Hansen, F.R., Schroll, M. and Runeborg, O. (1988) The relation of spinal X-ray to low-back pain and physical activity among 60-year-old men and women. *N. Engl. J. Med.,* **318,** 291–300.

Bijlsma, F. and Peeraboom, J.W. (1972) The aging pattern of human intervertebral disc. *Gerontology,* **18,** 157–168.

Bland, J.H. (1983) The reversibility of osteoarthritis: a review. *Am. J. Med.,* **74,** 16–26.

Bogduk, N. (1984) The rationale for patterns of neck and back pain. *Patient Management,* **8,** 13–21.

Bogduk, N., Tynan, W. and Wilson, A.S. (1981) The nerve supply to the human lumbar intervertebral discs. *J. Anat.,* **132**, 39-56.

Boyd, E. (1929) The experimental error inherent in measuring the growing human body. *Am. J. Phys. Anthrop.,* **13**, 389-432.

Brown, W.D. (1970) The pathophysiology of disc disease. *Orthop. Clin. North Am.,* **2**, 359-370.

Bullough, P.G. (1979) Pathologic changes associated with the common arthritides and their treatment. *Pathol. Ann.,* **2**, 69-83.

Bullough, P.G. and Boachie-Adjei, O. (1988) *Atlas of Spinal Diseases.* J. B. Lippincott, Philadelphia, pp. 34-41.

Crock, H.V. (1986) Internal disc disruption. *Spine,* **11**, 650-653.

Davis, P.R. (1961) Human lower lumbar vertebrae: some mechanical and osteological considerations. *J. Anat.,* **95**, 337-344.

Dent, C.E. and Watson, L. (1966) Osteoporosis. *Postgrad. Med. J. Suppl.,* **October**, 583-590.

Dick, W.C. (1972) *An Introduction to Clinical Rheumatology.* Churchill Livingstone, London.

Dieppe, P. and Watt, I. (1985) Crystal deposition in osteoarthritis: an opportunistic event? *Clin. Rheum. Dis.,* **11**, 367-391.

Donohue, W.L. (1939) Pathology of the intervertebral disc. *Am. J. Med. Sci.,* **198**, 413-437.

Edgar, M.A. and Ghadially, J.A. (1976) Innervation of the lumbar spine. *Clin. Orthop.,* **115**, 35-41.

Esses, S.I. (1991) Surgical anatomy of the sacrum: a guide for rational screw fixation. *Spine,* **16**, S284-S288.

Farfan, H.F. (1973) *Mechanical Disorders of the Low Back.* Lea and Febiger, Philadelphia.

Farfan, H.F. (1977) A reorientation in the surgical approach to degenerative lumbar intervertebral joint disease. *Orthop. Clin. North Am.,* **8**, 9-21.

Fick, R. (1904) *Handbuch der Anatomie und Mechanik der Gelenke, II.* G.Fischer, Jena, pp. 77-89.

Friberg, O. (1987) Lumbar instability. *Spine,* **12**, 119-129.

Gardner, D.L. (1978) Structure and function of connective tissue and joints. In *Copeman's Textbook of the Rheumatic Diseases* (J.T. Scott, ed.), 5th edition. Churchill Livingstone, London, pp. 78-124.

Ghadially, F.N. (1981) Structure and function of articular cartilage. *Clin. Rheum. Dis.,* **7**, 3-28.

Giles, L.G.F. (1989) *Anatomical Basis of Low Back Pain.* Williams and Wilkins, Baltimore, pp. 12-40, 88.

Giles, L.G.F. (1991) A review and description of some possible causes of low back pain of mechanical origin in *homo sapiens. Proc. Aust. Soc. Hum. Biol.,* **4**, 193-212.

Giles, L.G.F. (1992) Paraspinal autonomic ganglion distortion due to vertebral body osteophytosis: a cause of vertebrogenic autonomic syndromes? *J Manipulative Physiol. Ther.,* **15**, 551-555.

Giles, L.G.F. and Kaveri, M.J.P. (1990) Some osseous and soft tissue causes of human intervertebral canal (foramen) stenosis. *J. Rheumatol.,* **17**, 1474-1481.

Giles, L.G.F. and Kaveri, M.J.P. (1991) Lumbosacral intervertebral disc degeneration revisited: a radiological and histological correlation. *Man. Med.,* **6**, 62-66.

Giles, L.G.F. and Taylor, J.R. (1984) The effect of postural scoliosis on lumbar apophyseal joints. *Scand. J. Rheumatol.,* **13**, 209-220.

Hadley, L.A. (1964) *Anatomico-Roentgenographic Studies of the Spine.* Charles C.Thomas, Springfield, pp. 172-194.

Hilton, R. C., Ball, J. and Benn, R.T. (1976) Vertebral end plate lesions in the dorsolumbar spine. *Ann. Rheum. Dis.,* **35**, 127-132.

Ingelmark, B.E. (1959) Function of and pathological changes in the spinal joints. *Acta Anat.,* **38**, 12-60.

Isherwood, I. and Antoun, N.M. (1980) CT scanning in the assessment of lumbar spine problems. In *The Lumbar Spine and Back Pain* (M.I.V. Jayson, ed.), 2nd edition. Pitman Medical, Kent, pp. 247-264.

Jayson, M.I.V. (1992) The role of vascular damage and fibrosis in the pathogenesis of nerve root damage. *Clin. Orthop. Rel. Res.,* **279**, 40-48.

Jinkins, J.R. (1993) The pathoanatomic basis of somatic and autonomic syndromes originating in the lumbosacral spine. *Neuroimaging Clin North Am,* **3**, 443-463,

Jinkins, J.R., Whittemore, A.R. and Bradley, W.G. (1989) The anatomic basis of vertebrogenic pain and the autonomic syndrome associated with lumbar disk extrusion. *Am. J. Neuroradiol.,* **10**, 219-232.

Katz, M.M., Hargens, A.R., Garfin, S.R. (1986) Intervertebral disc nutrition. Diffusion versus convection. *Clin. Orthop. Rel. Res.,* **210**, 243-245.

Keim, H.A. and Kirkaldy-Willis, W.H. (1987) Low back pain. *Clinical Symposia* 39, Ciba-Geigy Corp., New Jersey.

Kerr, R. and Resnick, D. (1984) Degenerative diseases of the spine. *Aust. Radiol.,* **28**, 319-329.

Kirkaldy-Willis, W.H. (1983) The pathology and pathogenesis of low back pain. In *Managing Low Back Pain* (W.H. Kirkaldy-Willis, ed.). Churchill Livingstone, New York, pp. 23-43.

Kramer, J. (1977) Pressure dependent fluid shifts in the intervertebral disc. *Orthop. Clin. North Am.,* **8**, 211-216.

Kramer, J. (1990) *Intervertebral Disk Diseases: Causes, Diagnosis, Treatment and Prophylaxis,* 2nd edition. Georg Thieme Verlag, Stuttgart, New York, p. 1.

Kunert, W. (1965) Functional disorders of internal organs due to vertebral lesions. *Ciba Symposium,* **13**, 85-96.

Lewit, K. (1985) *Introduction. Manipulative Therapy in Rehabilitation of the Motor System.* Butterworths, London, pp. 1-9.

Malemud, C.J. and Moskowitz, R.W. (1981) Physiology of articular cartilage. *Clin. Rheum. Dis.,* **7**, 29-55.

Markolf, K.L. and Morris, J.M. (1974) The structural components of the intervertebral disc. *J. Bone Joint Surg.,* **56A**, 675-687.

Maroudas, A., Stockwell, R.A., Nachemson, A. and Urban, J. (1975) Factors in the nutrition of the human intervertebral disc. *J. Anat.,* **120**, 113-130.

McCarron, R.F., Wimpee, M.W., Hudkins, P.G. and Laros, G.S. (1987) The inflammatory effect of nucleus pulposus. A possible element in the pathogenesis of low back pain. *Spine,* **10**, 445-451.

McFadden, K.D. and Taylor, J.R. (1990) End-plate lesions of the lumbar spine. *Spine,* **14**, 867-869.

McRae, D.L. (1977) Radiology of the lumbar spinal canal. In *Lumbar Spondylosis. Diagnosis, Management and Surgical Treatment* (P.R. Weinstein, G. Ehni and C.B. Wilson, eds), Year Book Medical Publishers, Chicago, pp. 92-114.

Meachim, G. and Stockwell, R.A. (1979) The matrix. In *Adult Articular Cartilage* (M.A.R. Freeman, ed.), 2nd edition. Pitman Medical, Kent, pp. 1-68.

Meisel, A.D. and Bullough, P.G. (1984) *Atlas of Osteoarthritis.* Lea and Febiger, Philadelphia, pp. 8.1-8.20.

Mitchell, N.S. and Cruess, R.H. (1977) Classification of degenerative arthritis. *Can. Med. Assoc. J.,* **117**, 763-765.

Mixter, W.J. and Barr, J.S. (1934) Rupture of the intervertebral disc with involvement of the spinal canal. *N. Engl. J. Med.,* **211**, 210-215.

Morgan, F.P. and King, T. (1957) Primary instability of lumbar vertebrae as a common cause of low back pain. *J. Bone Joint Surg.,* **39B**, 6-22.

Nachemson, A.L. (1965) The effect of forward leaning on lumbar intradiscal pressure. *Acta Orthop. Scand.,* **35**, 314.

Nachemson, A.L. and Elfstrom, G. (1970) Intradiscal dynamic pressure measurements in lumbar discs. *Scand. J. Rehabil. Med.,* **Suppl.**, 1.

Nachemson, A.L., Schultz, A.B. and Berkson, M.H. (1979) Mechanical properties of human lumbar spine motion segments. *Spine,* **4**, 1-8.

Nathan, H. (1962) Osteophytes of the vertebral column. *J. Bone Joint Surg.,* **44A**, 243-268.

Nathan, H. (1968) Compression of the sympathetic trunk by osteophytes of the vertebral column in the abdomen: an anatomical study with pathological and clinical considerations. *Surgery,* **63**, 609-625.

Nathan, H. (1987) Osteophytes of the spine compressing the sympathetic trunk and splanchnic nerves in the thorax. *Spine,* **12**, 527-532.

O'Rahilly, R. and Meyer, D.B. (1979) The timing and sequence of events in the development of the human vertebral column during the embryonic period proper. *Anat. Embryol.,* **157**, 167-176.

Peacock, A. (1952) Observations on the postnatal structure of the intervertebral disc in man. *J. Anat.,* **86**, 162-178.

Pedersen, H.E., Blunck, C.F.J. and Gardner, E. (1956) The anatomy of lumbo-sacral posterior rami and meningeal branches of spinal nerves (sinu-vertebral nerves) with an experimental study of their function. *J. Bone Joint Surg.,* **38A**, 377-391.

Pritzker, K.P.H. (1977) Aging and degeneration in the lumbar intervertebral disc. *Orthop. Clin. North Am.,* **8**, 65-77.

Puschel, J. (1930) Der Wassergehalt normaler und degenerierter Zwischenbandscheiben. *Beitr. Path. Anat.,* **84**, 123-130.

Putz, R. (1985) The functional morphology of the superior articular processes of the lumbar vertebra. *J. Anat.,* **143**, 181-187.

Rolander, S.D. (1966) Motion of the lumbar spine with special reference to the stabilising effect of posterior fusion. *Acta Orthop. Scand.,* **Suppl.**, 90.

Rydevik, B.L. (1992) The effects of compression on the physiology of nerve roots. *J. Manipulative Physiol. Ther.,* **15**, 62-66.

Saal, J.A. (1990) Intervertebral disc herniation: advances in nonoperative treatment. *Phys. Med. Rehabil.,* **4**, 175-190.

Sachs, B.L. (1987) Dallas discogram description – a new classification of CT/discography in low back disorders. *Spine,* **12**, 287-294.

Sato, A. (1980) Physiological studies of the somatoautonomic reflexes. In *Modern Developments in the Principles and Practice of Chiropractic* (S. Haldeman, ed.), Appleton-Century-Crofts, New York, pp. 93-105.

Sato, A. (1992) The reflex effects of spinal somatic nerve stimulation on visceral function. *J. Manipulative Physiol. Ther.,* **15**, 57-61.

Saunders, J.B. and Inman, T. (1940) Pathology of the intervertebral disk. *Arch. Surg.,* **40**, 389-416.

Schmorl, G. and Junghanns, H. (1971) *The Human Spine in Health and Disease,* 2nd American edition. Grune and Stratton, New York, p. 211.

Smith, N. (1930) The intervertebral discs. *Br. J. Surg.,* **18**, 358-375.

Spangfort, E.V. (1972) The lumbar disc herniation. *Acta Orthop. Scand.,* **142** (Suppl), 1-80.

Stockwell, R.A. (1979) *Biology of Cartilage Cells.* Cambridge University Press, Cambridge, p. 1.

Stokes, I.A.F. and Frymoyer, J.W. (1987) Segmental motion instability. *Spine,* **12**, 760-764.

Swanson, A.B. and de Groot Swanson, G. (1985) Osteoarthritis of the hand. *Clin. Rheum. Dis.,* **11**, 393-420.

Taylor, J.R. (1974) *Growth and Development of Human Intervertebral Discs.* PhD Thesis, University of Edinburgh.

Taylor, J.R. (1990) The development and structure of lumbar intervertebral discs. *Man. Med.,* **5**, 43-47.

Taylor, J.R., Scott, J.E., Bosworth, T.R. and Cribb, A.M. (1992) Human intervertebral disc acid glycosaminoglycans. *J. Anat.,* **180**, 137-141.

Taylor, J.R. and Twomey, L.T. (1980a) Innervation of lumbar intervertebral discs. *N. Z. J. Physio.,* **8**, 36-37.

Taylor, J.R. and Twomey, L.T. (1980b) Sagittal and horizontal plane movement of the human lumbar spine in cadavers and in the living. *Rheumatol. Rehabil.,* **19**, 223-232.

Taylor, J.R. and Twomey, L.T. (1986) Age changes in lumbar zygapophysial joints: observations on structure and function. *Spine,* **11**, 739-745.

Taylor, J.R. and Twomey, L.T. (1988) Development of the human intervertebral disc. In *Biology of the Intervertebral Disc,* (P. Ghosh, ed.), vol. 1. CRC Press, Boca Raton, Florida, pp. 39-82.

Taylor, J.R. and Twomey, L.T. (1992) Structure and function of lumbar zygapophysial joints: a review. *J. Orthop. Med.,* **14**, 71-78.

Taylor, J.R. and Twomey, L.T. (1994a) The effects of ageing on the intervertebral discs. In *Grieve's Modern Manual Therapy: The Vertebral Column* (G. D. Boyling, and N. Palastanga, eds.), 2nd edition. Churchill Livingstone, Edinburgh, pp. 177-188.

Taylor, J.R. and Twomey, L.T. (1994b) Structure and function of lumbar zygapophysial (facet) joints. In *Grieve's Modern Manual Therapy: The Vertebral Column* (G.D. Boyling, and N. Palastanga, eds), 2nd edition. Churchill Livingstone, Edinburgh, pp. 99-108.

Taylor, T.K.F. and Akeson, W.H. (1971) Intervertebral disc prolapse. A review of morphologic and biochemic knowledge concerning the nature of prolapse. *Clin. Orthop.,* **76**, 54-79.

Taylor, T.K.F. and Gosh, P. (1978) Ageing and the intervertebral disc. Ageing in Australia. Australian Association of Gerontology. In *Proceedings of the Satellite Conference of the 11th Congress of the International Association of Gerontology* (J.W. Donald, A.V. Everett and P.J. Wheele, eds). Pot Still Press, Sydney, pp. 113-115.

Twomey, L.T. (1981) *Age Changes in the Human Lumbar Vertebral Column.* PhD thesis, University of Western Australia.

Twomey, L.T. and Taylor, J.R. (1982) Flexion creep deformation and hysteresis in the lumbar column. *Spine,* **7**, 116-122.

Twomey, L.T. and Taylor, J.R. (1983) A quantitative study of the role of the posterior vertebral elements in sagittal movement of the lumbar vertebral column. *Arch. Phys. Med. Rehab.,* **64**, 322-325.

Twomey, L.T. and Taylor, J.R. (1985) Age changes in lumbar intervertebral discs. *J. Anat.* **143**, 233-234.

Twomey, L.T. and Taylor, J.R. (1986) Bone density and structure in lumbar vertebrae. In *Modern Manual Therapy: The Vertebral Column,* (G. Grieve, ed.), Churchill Livingstone,Edinburgh, pp. 121-128.

Twomey, L.T., and Taylor, J.R. (1991) Age-related changes in the lumbar spine and spinal rehabilitation. *CRC Crit. Rev. Phys. Rehabil. Med.,* **2**, 153-169.

Vanharanta, H., Korpi, J., Heliovaara, J. and Troup, J.D.G. (1985) Radiographic measurements of lumbar spinal canal size and their relation to back mobility. *Spine,* **10**, 461-466.

Verbout, A.J. (1985) The development of the vertebral column. In *Advances in Anatomy, Embryology and Cell Biology* (F. Beck, W. Hild and R. Ortmann, eds.) vol. 90. Springer Verlag, Berlin.

Vernon-Roberts, B. and Pirie, C.J. (1977) Degenerative changes in the IV discs of the lumbar spine and their sequelae. *Rhematol. Rehab.,* **16**, 13-21.

Walmsley, R. (1953) The development and growth of the intervertebral disc. *Edin. Med. J.,* **60**, 341-364.

Woessner, F.F., Sapolsky, A.I., Nagase, H. and Howell, D.S. (1977) Role of proteolytic enzymes in cartilage matrix breakdown in osteoarthritis. *Arthritis Rheum.,* **20**, 116-123.

Yasuma, T., Arai, K. and Yamauchi, Y. (1993) The histology of lumbar intervertebral disc herniation: the significance of small blood vessels in the extruded tissue. *Spine,* **18**, 1761-1765.

Ziv, I., Maroudas, C., Robin, G. and Maroudas, A. (1993) Human facet cartilage: swelling and some physicochemical characteristics as a function of age. *Spine,* **18**, 136-146.

5

Zygapophysial (facet) joints

L.G.F. Giles

Anatomy

The lumbar zygapophysial (facet, interlaminar) synovial joints lie posterolateral to the lumbar spinal canal
and posterior to the intervertebral canals (foramina)
(Baddeley, 1976). The lumbar articular processes and
zygapophysial joints, originally oriented in the coronal plane, assume their final form and orientation
during childhood (Lutz, 1967). These joints are
approximately sagittally oriented in the upper lumbar
spine, rotating toward the coronal plane at the
lumbosacral junction (Pheasant, 1975; Park, 1980)
(Figure 5.1).

The lumbar zygapophysial joints are biplanar, with
the major posterior parts of the joint approximated to
the sagittal plane (Taylor and Twomey, 1986). There is
a wide range of variability of the lumbosacral joint
planes in the horizontal plane, and asymmetry
(tropism) in the joint planes comparing left and right
sides is common (Cihak, 1970) (Figure 5.2).

Tropism, especially if it is marked, is currently a
subject of intense interest because it has the potential
markedly to alter the biomechanics of lumbar spinal
movements and precipitate early degenerative changes either in the joint or adjacent intervertebral discs,
abnormalities that may contribute to back pain (Tulsi
and Hermanis, 1993).

A relationship exists between the orientation of
the zygapophysial joints and the orientation of their
related laminae, for example, at L5–S1 the zygapophysial joints and the laminae are more coronally
orientated (van Schaik *et al.*, 1985). The superior
articular processes project upward, curving dorsally
and laterally from the junction of the pedicle and
upper margin of the lamina, and have a smooth
concave cartilaginous articular surface averaging 10
× 18 mm in adults (Weinstein *et al.*, 1977) (Figure
5.3).

On the posterior aspect of the base of the superior
articular process, extending posteriorly, is a protuber-
ance of variable size called the mamillary process
(Rauschning, 1983), and at the base of the transverse
process, posteriorly, is a small accessory process
(Farfan, 1973; Gardner *et al.*, 1975). Between the
mamillary and accessory processes a fibrous band,
called the mamillo-accessory ligament (Bogduk, 1981;
Francois *et al.*, 1985), usually bridges over a groove of
variable depth forming a tunnel about 6 mm long
(Bradley, 1974). This ligament is occasionally ossified,
rather than being fibrous (Bogduk, 1981), and can
then be seen on radiographs (Koehler and Zimmer,
1968). This tunnel transmits the medial branch of the
posterior primary ramus as it descends from the
intervertebral canal immediately above (Bogduk *et al.*,
1982), as well as small blood vessels, to the posterior
paraspinal muscles (Farfan, 1973). The medial branch
of the posterior primary ramus and its associated
structures are discussed in detail in Chapter 14.

The zygapophysial joint is a synovial joint which is
formed by the convex laterally facing inferior articular process of the upper vertebra, and the concave
medially facing superior articular process of the
lower vertebra (Hadley, 1961; Koreska *et al.*, 1977;
Taylor and Twomey, 1986). It is a true diarthrodial
joint, complete with a joint capsule (Figure 5.4) and
synovial lining (Keim and Kirkaldy-Willis, 1987).

The joint cavity is normally potential rather than
real because it contains only a very small volume of
synovial fluid (Moore, 1992) and the capacity of the
lumbar zygapophysial joints is only 1–2 ml (El-Khoury
and Renfrew, 1991). Parts of the lumbar zygapophysial joint synovial folds project into the joint, from
above and below, but particularly from the larger
inferior recess (Giles and Taylor, 1984, 1985; Giles,
1989). The normal appearance of L4–5 and L5–S1
zygapophysial joint superior and inferior recesses
during arthrography shows that the inferior recesses

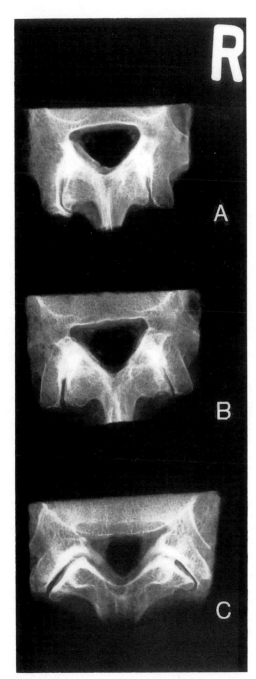

Figure 5.1 Superior to inferior radiographic images of the L3–S1 zygapophysial joints. Note that the horizontal plane of the L3–4 zygapophysial joint (A) is more sagittal than that of the L5–S1 zygapophysial joint (C). B = L4–5 zygapophysial joint.

132 SPECIMENS (264 ARTICULAR FACETS)

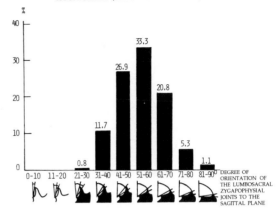

Figure 5.2 The variability of lumbosacral joint planes. (Modified from Cihak, R. (1970) Variations of lumbosacral joints and their morphogenesis. *Acta Universitatis Carolinae Medica*, **16**, 145–165.) (Reproduced with permission from Giles, L.G.F. (1989) *Anatomical Basis of Low Back Pain*. Williams and Wilkins, Baltimore.)

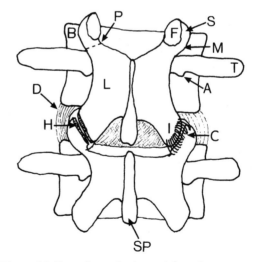

Figure 5.3 Two adjacent lumbar vertebrae. A = accessory process; B = body of vertebra; C = capsule (fibrous portion); D = intervertebral disc of the intervertebral joint (an amphiarthrodial joint); F = facet of superior articular process; H = hyaline articular cartilage of the zygapophysial synovial joint (a diarthrodial joint); I = inferior articular process; L = lamina; M = mamillary process; P = pars interarticularis; S = superior articular process; SP = spinous process; T = transverse process.

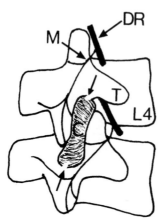

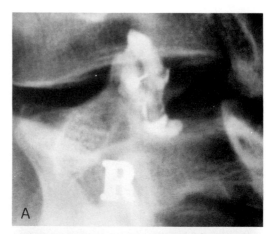

Figure 5.4 Large recesses are present within each extremity of the zygapophysial joint capsule; these recesses contain synovial lined adipose tissue which communicates with extracapsular adipose tissue through a small foramen within the capsule at approximately the pole of each capsule (arrows). L4 = body of 4th lumbar vertebra; T = transverse process; C = capsule of joint; DR = dorsal ramus (posterior primary ramus); M = medial branch of posterior primary ramus. (Modified from Dory, M.A. (1981) Arthography of the lumbar facet joints. *Radiology* **140**, 23–27.)

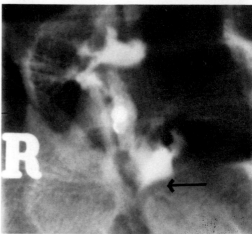

are larger, and that the inferior recess is larger at L5–S1 than at L4–5; the contrast medium can appear well below the level of the lumbosacral joint capsule (Giles, 1984) due to contrast medium passing into the extracapsular recess (Figure 5.5).

Each *superior articular recess* lies directly above the cranial end of the joint space. It is bounded posteriorly by the dorsal leaf of the intertransverse ligament, medially by the lateral surface of the vertebral lamina, and ventrally by the lateral part of the ligamentum flavum, which protrudes slightly beyond the lamina at this point (Lewin *et al.*, 1961). The ligamentum flavum does not completely separate the recess from the intervertebral canal and the adipose tissue in the recess becomes continuous with that around the spinal nerve in the intervertebral canal (Tondury, 1940; Lewin *et al.*, 1961).

Each *inferior articular recess* lies caudal and anteromedial to the tip of the inferior articular process, where its location is identified by a conspicuous bony fossa on the posterior surface of the adjacent lamina of the lower vertebra (Lewin *et al.*, 1961). The lateral boundary of this fossa is formed by a ridge of bone which runs from the lamina to the base of the superior articular process; the inferior recess of the lumbosacral joint is marked by a similar but larger fossa on the posterior aspect of the sacrum (Lewin *et al.*, 1961).

According to Tondury (1940) and Dorr (1958), the function of the adipose tissue in the recesses is to cushion and moderate the load on the joint process.

Figure 5.5 Normal oblique zygapophysial joint arthrograms of a 21-year-old male. Note the well delineated superior and inferior joint recesses of the L4–5 joint capsule (A) and the apparent 'leakage' (arrows) of contrast medium well below the margin of the L5–S1 joint capsule (B) due to contrast medium passing into the extracapsular recess (see Figure 18.1). (Reproduced with permission from Giles, L.G.F. (1984) Lumbar apophyseal joint arthrography. *J. Manipulative Physiol. Ther.*, **7**, 21–24.)

However, Lewin *et al.* (1961) disagree because the adipose tissue extends through the joint capsule, thus becoming an ideal, easily displaceable space filler which facilitates, rather than restricting, movement of the joint processes, the articular processes of which can move 5–7 mm on each other in the sagittal plane. The adipose tissue which extends inside the joint capsule is covered with synovial lining cells which lubricate the joint (Lewin *et al.*, 1961; Giles, 1989) (see Figure 5.15).

Furthermore, the combination of synovial and adipose tissue is characteristically seen in those parts of joints where the loading is minimal (Lewin *et al.*, 1961).

Function

The function of the lumbar zygapophysial joints is to guide and restrain movement between vertebrae and to protect the discs from shear forces, excessive flexion, and axial rotation (Adams and Hutton, 1983; Putz, 1985; Taylor and Twomey, 1986). The transfer of biomechanical forces from one zygapophysial joint facet to the adjacent facet occurs via particular areas in flexion and extension loadings, e.g. on the superior articular surface, the contact area moves from the upper tip in maximum flexion to the lower margin in extension, while on the inferior articular facet, the contact area moves from the upper and central areas in maximum flexion to the lower tip in extension (Shirazi-Adl and Drouin, 1987).

According to Hakim and King (1976), who used an intervertebral load cell (a transducer (Prasad *et al.*, 1973) inserted into the inferior portion of a cadaveric lumbar vertebral body to deduce facet loads), normal lumbar facets may carry up to 40% of the incumbent body weight. Using a similar method, Yang and King (1984) found that normal facets carry up to 25% of the incumbent body weight. Using cadaveric lumbar spines on a hydraulic servo-controlled testing machine, which gave outputs of applied force against deformation, Hutton and Adams (1980) found that an average of 16% of the axial load is carried by the facets. It is difficult to account for the large discrepancy between these estimates obtained by different investigators. In cadaveric osteoarthritic joints, facet loading may increase to as high as 47% of the total axial load (Yang and King, 1984). According to Gregersen and Lucas (1967), the lumbar facets are orientated so as to restrict axial rotation of the lumbar vertebral column to less than 9 degrees, and the facets and the disc both play major roles in resisting axial torsion movements (Farfan, 1983; Tencer and Mayer, 1983). The restraints to movement at each joint are of two types: *passive restraint* (due to the articular facet orientation and resistance in joint capsules, the adjacent ligaments, and the intervertebral disc), and *active restraint* (provided by muscular contraction) (Smeathers and Biggs, 1980). The principal plane of movement in the lumbosacral spine is flexion–extension (Weinstein *et al.*, 1977).

Hyaline articular cartilage

Hyaline articular cartilage is a highly specialized form of connective tissue which lines sliding joint surfaces (Walmsley, 1972; Rhodin, 1974; Mankin, 1975; Bullough, 1979), including those of the zygapophysial joints (Bland, 1987; Giles, 1987). According to Ziv *et al.* (1993), at the L4–5 level it is approximately 1.45 mm (SD 0.27 mm) thick at the

centre of the concave (superior) zygapophysial joint facet, and 1.12 mm (SD 0.25 mm) at the centre of the convex (inferior) zygapophysial joint facet. However, some authors have found the combined thickness of the paired hyaline articular cartilages across the centre of the joints in the lumbar spine to be approximately 2–2.4 mm (Fick, 1904; Giles and Taylor, 1984). Its chemical content and cell density vary in different parts of the same joint and at different depths within the tissue (Stockwell, 1979). Also, using cadaveric spines, Tobias *et al.* (1992) found that zygapophysial joint facet cartilage is underhydrated *in situ*, perhaps reflecting the permanent presence of stresses *in vivo* on some part of the zygapophysial joints, the position of the loaded site changing with time. Its histologic zones (Edwards and Chrisman, 1979; Meachim and Stockwell, 1979; Junqueira *et al.*, 1986; Giles, 1992a) are shown in Figure 5.6.

Some authors describe hyaline articular cartilage as consisting of three ill-defined zones, i.e. superficial zone (with small flattened or oval chondrocytes, and fine fibres arranged tangentially to the surface), middle zone (with chondrocytes arranged in columns perpendicular to the surface with decussating fibres), and deep zone (with small chondrocytes in calcified cartilage lying adjacent to bone) (Benninghoff, 1939; Collins, 1949; Barnett *et al.*, 1961; Ghadially *et al.*, 1965; Ghadially and Roy, 1969; Ham and Cormick, 1979). Hence, according to Ham and Cormick (1979), synovial joint articular cartilage is unique in that the surface it presents to articulate with its opposing articular cartilage is that of naked cartilage matrix. However, the ultrastructure of adult articular cartilage has been described in a number of human and animal studies (Cameron and Robinson, 1958; Davies *et al.*, 1962; Collins *et al.*, 1965; Meachim, 1967; Roy and Meachim, 1968; Ruttner and Spycher, 1968; Weiss *et al.*, 1968; Meachim and Roy, 1969; Stofft and Graf, 1983) and some reference is made in the literature to a chondrosynovial membrane which is only a few tenths of a micron thick (Wolf, 1969) and which Wolf (1969, 1972, 1975) refers to as being of cartilaginous origin which may be torn off the articular surface 'like a sheet of paper'. According to Wolf (1975), the uppermost layer of amorphous substance forms the actual smooth 'glide' surface of articular cartilage and can be distinguished from the undersurface layer of thin collagenous fibrils which smoothly pass with their fibrillar structure into the cartilaginous tissue beneath the membrane. Davies *et al.* (1962) described a narrow surface lamina, devoid of fibres, appearing to correspond to the lamina splendens, while Weiss *et al.* (1968) concluded that the lamina was fibrous. Using phase contrast illumination to microscopically examine human adult fresh and cadaveric cartilage, MacConaill (1951) showed a thin bright line at the surface

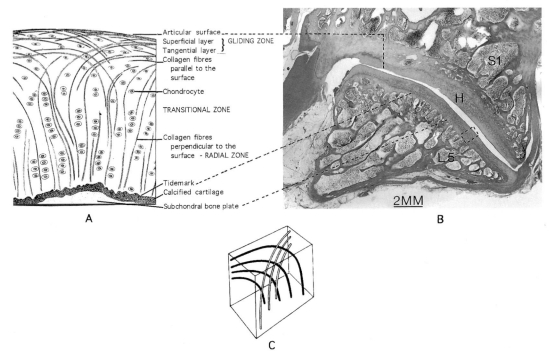

Figure 5.6 (B) A 100 μm thick section cut in the horizontal plane through the right lumbosacral zygapophysial joint of a 69-year-old female. The articular facet of the superior articular process (S1) of the sacrum and the inferior articular process (L5) of the fifth lumbar vertebra, are lined with hyaline articular cartilage (H). The rectangle on the L5 inferior articular process is approximately represented in (A) (magnified) which shows the histological zones of hyaline articular cartilage. The deeper chondrocytes are more spherical and are arranged in approximately vertical rows, whereas the superficial chondrocytes are flattened and are randomly located. Collagen fibres in the deeper zones are perpendicular to the cartilage surface, then they become parallel to the surface in the more superficial zones as shown in the schematic diagram (C). (Adapted from Junqueira, L.C., Carneiro, J. and Long, J.A. (1986) *Basic Histology*, 5th edition. Lange Medical Publications, California, pp. 201–203.)

of articular cartilage which was not visible by ordinary light illumination; it was so conspicuous that it merited the name of lamina splendens. However, according to Aspden and Hukins (1979), the so-called lamina splendens described by MacConaill (1951) is an artefact of phase contrast microscopy due to a Fresnel diffraction pattern on the edge of a section of cartilage, while Sokoloff (1969) suggested that MacConaill's bright line was a 'halo' resulting from phase contrast microscopy.

However, Giles (1992a) reported a narrow acellular surface lamina on the hyaline articular cartilage in some 'normal' human lower lumbar zygapophysial joints. In specimens showing relatively normal zygapophysial joints for the age group of 46–78 years (mean 60 years; 9M:11F) a narrow surface lamina was seen in 20 out of 80 joints (25%), as shown in Figures 5.7A and B which include low and high power transmitted light photomicrographs. In some instances there appeared to be continuity of the surface lamina up to the adjacent synovial folds.

Figure 5.7 (A) A transmitted light photomicrograph of a section cut in the horizontal plane, at a thickness of 200 μm, from the left lumbosacral zygapophysial joint of a 67-year-old female which shows relatively normal hyaline articular cartilage (H) on the facet surfaces bordering the joint 'cavity'. The cartilage surfaces show minor focal fibrillation at the centre of the joint with minor tinctorial changes along the length of the cartilage indicating minor changes in the chondrocytes and cartilage matrix. IAP = inferior articular process of the L5 vertebra; SAP = superior articular process of the sacrum. A narrow surface lamina of acellular tissue is seen (arrows) which appears to extend to the adjacent fibrous synovial fold (S) adjoining to the inner surface of the ligamentum flavum (L). Ehrlich's haematoxylin stain with light green counterstain.(Reproduced with permission from Giles, L.G.F. (1992a) The surface lamina of the articular cartilage of human zygapophysial joints. *Anat. Rec.*, **233**, 350–356.) (B) A higher magnification of the adjacent cartilage surfaces showing the narrow surface lamina and the adjoining fibrous synovial fold (S) seen in Figure 4.4A. (Reproduced with permission from Giles, L.G.F. (1992a) The surface lamina of the articular cartilage of human zygapophysial joints. *Anat. Rec.*, **233**, 350–356.)

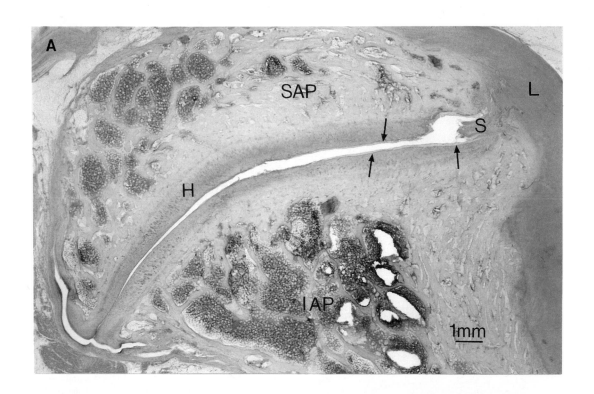

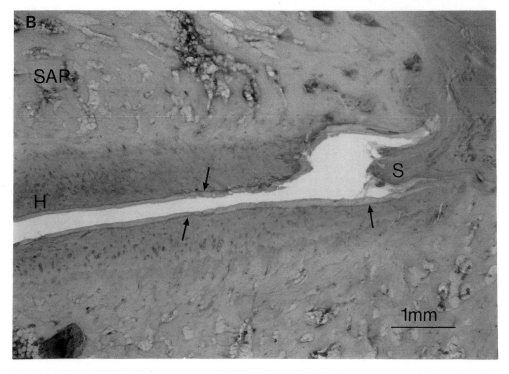

Using the same histological and photographic techniques for osteoarthritic joints, the narrow surface lamina was not found in joints showing advanced osteoarthritic changes. The hyaline articular cartilage changes associated with osteoarthritic changes are discussed later in this chapter.

Joint capsule and synovial folds

Lumbar zygapophysial joint capsules differ from those of other synovial joints in having a quite unique capsular structure anteromedially, the ligamentum flavum, while posterolaterally having a typical fibrous capsule (Keller, 1953; Hirsch *et al.*, 1963; Reilly *et al.*, 1978) (Figure 5.8). A detailed description of the joint capsule and its inferior recess *in situ* in dissected cadavers, and in histological sections prepared from cadavers, as well as an example of a fresh (surgical) specimen, has been recorded elsewhere (Giles, 1989).

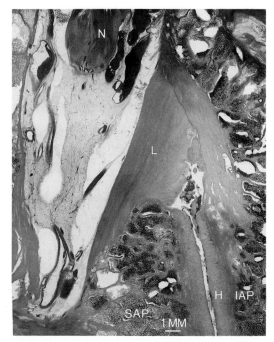

Figure 5.9 A 200 mm thick histological section cut in the parasagittal plane through the superior articular recess of the L4–5 zygapophysial joint of a 69-year-old female showing how the superior articular recess of the joint is 'closed' by the ligamentum flavum (L) in this particular section. H = hyaline articular cartilage; N = large neural structures within the intervertebral canal; SAP = superior articular process of L5 vertebra; IAP = inferior articular process of L4 vertebra. Ehrlich's haematoxylin and light green counterstain.

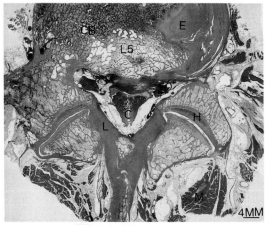

Figure 5.8 A 200 μm thick histological section cut slightly obliquely in the horizontal plane through the fifth lumbar vertebra of a 56-year-old male. C = cauda equina; CB = cancellous bone of the vertebral body; E = end-plate cartilage; H = hyaline articular cartilage; I = interspinous ligament; L = ligamentum flavum; L5 = fifth lumbar vertebral body; M = muscle; S = spinous process. Ehrlich's haematoxylin and light green counterstain.

Ligamentum flavum

The ligamenta flava are a series of interlaminar ligaments (Figures 5.8 and 5.9) located within the spinal canal (Dommisse, 1975; Levine, 1979), covering most of the dorsal bony wall of the spinal canal (Rolander, 1966; Twomey, 1981).

The fibre direction is said to be essentially perpendicular in the medial interlaminar portion and slightly oblique in the capsular portion (Naffziger *et al.*, 1938; Ramsey, 1966). The anteromedial border of each ligament passes around the joint, skirts the posterior edge of the intervertebral foramen (Brown, 1938) and forms its roof (Ramsey, 1966). The medial part of each ligament is thicker and unites the laminae, while the lateral thinner portion surrounds the joints and blends with their fibrous capsules (Epstein, 1976).

Microscopically, the ligamenta flava consist of elastic connective tissue fibres (80%) with collagen fibres (20%) interspersed among the elastic fibres (Ramsey, 1966; Kirkaldy-Willis *et al.*, 1984). The elastic fibres measure about 1 μm in diameter and consist of fine, parallel fibres, without striations, when viewed by transmission electron microscopy (Barnett *et al.*, 1961). The adult ligamentum flavum is quite cell-poor, and the basic cell appears to be the spindle-shaped fibrocyte (Ramsey, 1966).

Where the laminae fuse to form the spinous process (Williams and Warwick, 1980), the ligamenta flava meet the membranous interspinous ligament posteriorly (Horwitz, 1939; Heylings, 1978; Reilly *et al.*, 1978; Fairbank and O'Brien, 1980; Williams and Warwick, 1980) (Figure 5.8). However, small midline intervals are present in the ligamenta flava for the passage of vessels (Williams and Warwick, 1980; Giles, 1989) (Figure 5.10) although Brown (1938), Ramsey (1966), Kapandji (1974), Lee and Atkinson (1978), and Ellis and Feldman (1979) thought the posterior margins of the ligamenta flava fused completely in the midline. Figure 5.10 shows that the posterior margins of the ligamenta flava do not completely fuse in the midline except for a very short distance adjacent to the junction of the laminae and spinous process of the vertebra above and below a given mobile segment.

In ventroflexion of the lumbar spine, the ligamenta flava are stretched, while in lordosis, the fibres of the ligamenta flava become slack, and the cross-sectional thickness of the ligaments increases (Breig, 1960). These ligaments act, to some degree, as check ligaments in preventing hyperflexion, their elasticity serving to re-establish and maintain normal posture after flexion and rest (Weinstein *et al.*, 1977). However, according to Rolander (1966) and Twomey (1981), the posterior ligaments play only a minor role in limiting ventroflexion and their main function is to maintain the posterolateral wall of the spinal column smooth in all postures of the spine. This main function of providing a smooth covering for the posterior part of the spinal canal appears to be correct as the ligamenta flava extend into the sacral canal, as shown in Figure 5.11, where there is no movement between bony structures.

The ligamentum flavum not only has the structure and function of a ligament, but also acts as a capsule on the ventral surface of the lumbar zygapophysial joint and as an elastic band keeping the spinal nerves free from compression when passing through the intervertebral canal during movements in the lumbar spine (Hirsch *et al.*, 1963).

Numerous measurement studies of the ligamentum flavum thickness variously report them as 2–10 mm thick (Horwitz, 1939; Dockerty and Love, 1940; Herzog, 1950; Ramsey, 1966; Schmorl and Junghanns, 1971; Crawford, 1978; Reilly *et al.*, 1978; Moir, 1980; Giles, 1982; Giles and Taylor, 1984; Parkin and Harrison, 1985). The variation would depend, in part, on where the measurements were made (Giles and Taylor, 1984). According to Horwitz (1939), they are thickest at the L4–5 and L5–S1 levels and their height varies from 1.0 to 2.0 cm (Herzog, 1950).

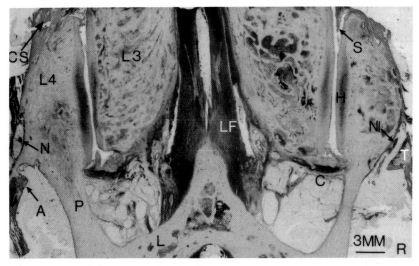

Figure 5.10 A histological section cut in the coronal plane as shown by the line on Figure 14.5, from a 36-year-old woman. The histological section is slightly oblique as the mamillo-accessory ligament is clearly seen enclosing the medial branch of the posterior primary ramus (N) on the left of the specimen, whereas on the right side the medial branch of the posterior primary ramus (N1) is seen coursing behind part of the transverse process (T). A = accessory process; C = fibrous capsule inferiorly meshing with the ligamentum flavum (LF). The ligamenta flava join at the junction of the laminae. CS = fibrous capsule superiorly; H = hyaline articular cartilage on the superior articular process of the L4 vertebra forming part of the zygapophysial joint; L = lamina of the L4 vertebra; P = pars interarticularis of the L4 vertebra; S = synovial fold projecting into the joint from the superior recess. Ehrlich's haematoxylin and light green counterstain. (Reproduced with permission from Giles, L.G.F. (1991a) The relationship between the medial branch of the lumbar posterior primary ramus and the mamillo-accessory ligament. *J. Manipulative Physiol. Ther.*, **14**, 189–192.)

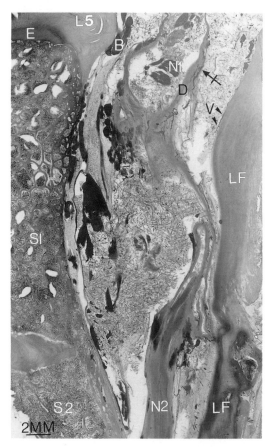

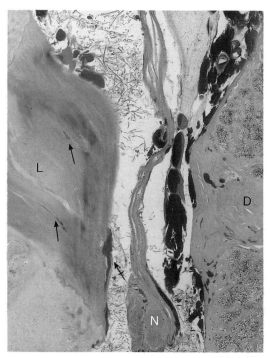

Figure 5.11 A 200 μm thick histological section cut in the sagittal plane through the first and second sacral segments (S1, S2) from an 82-year-old female. Note how the ligamentum flavum (LF) lines the posterior wall of the sacral canal. Small blood vessels (V) supply the ligamentum flavum. B = blood vessels of Batson's venous plexus; D = dural sleeve showing its abundant vascular supply (tailed arrow); L5 = fifth lumbar intervertebral disc with its hyaline articular cartilage end-plate (E); N1 = nerve root trunks within the dural sleeve; N2 = nerve root trunks at the lower end of the cauda equina. Ehrlich's haematoxylin and light green counterstain.

Figure 5.12 A 200 μm thick histological section cut in the parasagittal plane through the ligamentum flavum (L) and the intervertebral disc (D) at the lumbosacral level. Note the small blood vessels (arrows) within the ligamentum flavum. There is also a vascular supply to the surface of the ligamentum flavum (tailed arrow). N = large neural structures within the entrance zone of the intervertebral canal. Some blood vessels are seen within the intervertebral disc. Ehrlich's haematoxylin and light green counterstain.

Blood supply of the ligamentum flavum

The posterior artery of the vertebral canal supplies the ligamenta flava and the vertebral arch via their anterior surfaces (Rickenbacher *et al.*, 1985). The ligamentum flavum is described as having only a few irregularly dispersed blood vessels which are said to be capillaries and other small, thin-walled blood vessels (Ramsey, 1966), and this is confirmed in histological studies (Figures 5.11–5.13).

However, using horizontal section views from the lower part of zygapophysial joints (Figure 5.13), bilateral vascular channels are found passing into the ligamentum flavum, a short distance anterior to the joints. These bilateral vascular channels are a constant finding and seem to confirm Dorr's (1958) opinion that these vascular channels supply the adjacent part of the zygapophysial joint.

Thus the ligamentum flavum is not as poorly vascularized as suggested by Herzog (1950). No lymphatics were observed in the body of the ligamentum flavum confirming the findings of Dockerty and Love (1940) and Ramsey (1966).

Structure and function of synovial folds

Synovial folds

Synovial folds consist of a synovial lining layer with a subsynovial layer. The earliest appearance of a fold of synovial membrane in zygapophysial joints is when the articular gap appears at the onset of ossification

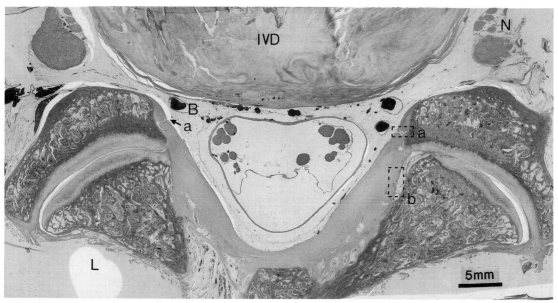

Figure 5.13 A section cut in the horizontal from the lower region of the lumbosacral zygapophysial joints of a 54-year-old male cadaver. B = Batson's venous plexus; IVD = intervertebral disc; N = spinal ganglion with nerve roots; rectangles show: bilateral vascular channels (a) and blood vessels in the ligamentum flavum adjacent to an intra-articular synovial fold (b); L = left side of specimen. Ehrlich's haematoxylin stain with light green counterstain. (Reproduced with permission from Giles, L.G.F. (1989) *Anatomical Basis of Low Back Pain*. Williams and Wilkins, Baltimore.)

of the vertebral arches (in fetuses of 70 mm crown–rump length) and a synovial fold is noted at the medial side of the joint, developing from a richly vascular interarticular mesenchyme (Tondury, 1972).

Intra-articular synovial folds, which consist of various shapes and sizes, and have numerous small blood vessels in fibrous connective tissue and adipose tissue, are described in all the zygapophysial joints (Schmincke and Santo, 1932; Tondury, 1940, 1972; Keller, 1953, 1959; Dorr, 1958, 1962; Hadley, 1961, 1964; De Marchi, 1963; Penning and Tondury, 1963; Kos, 1969; Schmorl and Junghanns, 1971; Tondury, 1972; Benini, 1979; Putz, 1981; Giles and Taylor, 1982; Rickenbacher *et al.*, 1985; Giles, 1986a; Agur, 1991; Moore, 1992). In addition to the synovial folds, intra-articular 'mesenchymatous' menisci are also described, extending ventrally and dorsally into the zygapophysial joints from the capsule (Lewin, 1968; Schmorl and Junghanns, 1971).

There is some controversy on the subject and nomenclature of 'synovial folds' (Giles and Taylor, 1987a,b) and 'meniscoid' structures (Bogduk and Twomey, 1991) in zygapophysial joints. According to Lewin *et al.* (1961), true mesenchymal intra-articular menisci are present in the zygapophysial joints, and Engel and Bogduk (1980, 1982) refer to semi-lunar fibrous structures which remotely resemble menisci. However, according to Tondury (1972), there are no true menisci in zygapophysial joints, which supports

the earlier study by Barnett *et al.* (1961) who found true menisci or discs only in the knee, temporomandibular, sternoclavicular, wrist, and acromioclavicular joints in humans.

Some of the confusion arises from variations in the histology of synovial folds themselves, which may relate to their different functions. Areolar synovium is apparently adapted for greater movement, while fibrous synovium is generally seen in areas most subject to strain (Schumacher, 1975) and may be the result of mechanical nipping of areolar synovium. The free irregular margins of the synovial folds may be quite long and thin (Hadley, 1964) and frequently project between the articulating surfaces and are often fibrous at their tips (Giles and Taylor, 1982; Jee, 1983; Kirkaldy-Willis, 1984; Giles, 1989) or even 'fibro-cartilaginous' (Tondury, 1972; Kos and Wolf, 1972). Keller (1959) could not find any cartilaginous metaplasia in the intra-articular synovial fold inclusions of intervertebral joints; however, he agreed that they may become fibrous as a result of being nipped within the joint.

Three types of intra-articular structures were identified by Engel and Bogduk (1982) when they examined human lumbar zygapophysial joints, excluding the lumbosacral joints, i.e. *adipose tissue pads* and *fibroadipose meniscoids* (both located at the superior and inferior poles of the joint), and connective tissue rims (located posteriorly and anteriorly).

Synovial membrane

The synovial membrane, which lines synovial folds, is one of the characteristic features of synovial joints (Walmsley, 1972). It is a complex lining tissue (Simkin, 1979; Simkin and Nilson, 1981) which is necessary to maintain the normal function of the synovial joint; it is the conduit for the exchange of nutrients and waste between blood and the joint tissues, and its cells synthesize and secrete the proteins and proteoglycans necessary for normal joint lubrication (Hasselbacher, 1981). The synovial membrane has three principal functions: (a) secretion of synovial fluid hyaluronate, (b) phagocytosis due to the phagocytic capacity of the 'A' cells involved in the clearing of waste materials, and (c) regulation of the movement of solutes, electrolytes, and proteins (Paget and Bullough, 1980).

The synovial membrane lines not only the inner surface of the fibrous articular capsule but also those intracapsular parts of the bone which are not covered by articular cartilage, and it extends around fat pads which fill joint recesses (Collins, 1949; Barnett *et al.*, 1961; Dieppe and Calvert, 1983). There is no distinct basal membrane between the synovial lining membrane and the subsynovial tissue (Efskind, 1941; Hasselbacher, 1981; Dieppe and Calvert, 1983).

According to Barnett *et al.* (1961), the synovial membrane of synovial joints overlaps the non-articular margins of the cartilage, becomes gradually thinner, then terminates without a clear line of demarcation. This overlapping part of the synovial membrane contains the 'circulus articuli vasculosus', i.e., a fringe of looped vascular anastomoses. It is considerably more vascular than the fibrous periarticular structures supporting the joint, such as the capsule, ligaments, and tendons (Liew and Dick, 1981).

The synovial membrane usually consists of two parts: (a) a lining layer bounding the joint space referred to as the *synovial lining* or the synovial intima (predominantly cellular with an abundant blood supply), and (b) a supportive or backing layer which should be called the subintima but is usually referred to as the *subsynovial layer* or subsynovial tissue (formed of loose fibrous connective tissue rich in blood vessels, lymphatics, and adipose tissue in varying proportions) (Davies, 1950; Ghadially and Roy, 1969; Paget and Bullough, 1980).

Synovial lining (intimal) layer

The surface of the synovial membrane is smooth, moist, and glistening, with small villi and fringe-like folds (Ghadially and Roy, 1969; Paget and Bullough, 1980; Giles and Taylor, 1982) (Figure 5.14) which increase the surface area of the synovial membrane.

The cells of the synovial lining layer, which are secreting fibroblasts, form an intricate meshwork

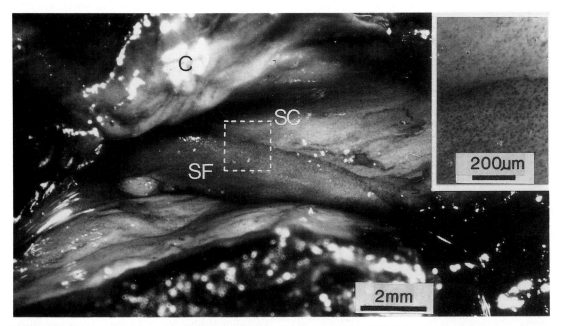

Figure 5.14 Fresh adolescent specimen (15-year-old female; L2–3 zygapophysial joint) showing a fat-filled intra-articular synovial fold projecting from the posterior capsule into the joint cavity. The insert shows minute villi on the synovial fold and on the synovial lining of the joint cavity. C = joint capsule reflected; SC = synovial 'cavity'; SF = synovial fold (immersed in 0.01% methylene blue). (Reproduced with permission from Giles, L.G.F. and Taylor, J.R. (1982) Intra-articular synovial protrusions in the lower lumbar apophyseal joints. *Bull. Hosp. J. Dis. Orthop. Inst.*, **42**, 248–255.)

between the joint cavity and the underlying capillary bed (Barland *et al.*, 1962; Rhodin, 1974; Wassilev, 1981). The synovial cells do not form a continuous compact layer like true epithelium (Ghadially and Roy, 1969); rather they form a layer which varies in depth, or they may be absent, leaving minute gaps in the synovial lining layer (Hadler, 1981; Giles, 1989) (Figure 5.15).

The significance of the extensive blood supply of the synovial folds will be discussed in relation to low back pain later in this chapter

Electron microscopy studies of the synovial lining layer which is formed by one to three layers of cells of two types, i.e. A and B cells, have been described in detail elsewhere (Schumacher, 1975; Junqueira *et al.*, 1986).

Subsynovial (subintimal) layer

The structure of the subsynovial layer varies in different parts of the same joint (Ghadially and Roy, 1969); it can be fibrous, fibroareolar, areolar, or areolar–adipose (Castor, 1960). It is a loose fibrous connective tissue found in the synovial folds and is rich in blood vessels, lymphatics, and adipose tissue (Shaw and Martin, 1962; Rhodin, 1974), and the adipose cells form compact lobules, surrounded by vascular fibroelastic septa which impart firmness, deformability, and elastic recoil during joint movement (Williams and Warwick, 1980). Sometimes it contains organized laminae of collagen and elastin fibres running parallel to the synovial lining surface (Davies, 1950). In addition to fibroblasts and lipocytes, the subsynovial tissue also contains macrophages (Ghadially and Roy, 1969) and mast cells (Shaw and Martin, 1962; Ghadially and Roy, 1969).

Compared with the synovial lining, the richly vascular *subsynovial tissue* has received scant attention from electron microscopists apart from the studies by Ghadially and Roy (1969), Giles *et al.* (1986), and Giles and Taylor (1987a) which showed two common types of subsynovial tissue, i.e. fibrous (characterized by innumerable bundles of collagen fibres), and fatty (made up of lipocytes interspersed with small amounts of fibrous tissue).

Appearance of synovial folds in histological sections

Cadaveric zygapophysial joints cut in the horizontal plane, are shown in Figures 5.16 and 5.17. Figure 5.16 shows a section from the upper half of each lumbosacral joint and Figure 5.17 shows a slightly oblique section from the lower end of each lumbosacral joint including the inferior joint recess. In Figure 5.17 the right side of the section is lower than the left side, as shown by the ala of the sacrum on the right side, whereas the intervertebral canal is seen on the left side. As previously mentioned, it can be seen how the ligamentum flavum forms a thick medial capsule at both spinal levels. By contrast, the posterolateral part of the joint is closed by a thin lax fibrous capsule. The inferior joint recess is enclosed by the ligamentum flavum medially and by fibrous capsular material posteriorly.

In the region of the lumbosacral zygapophysial joint inferior recess (Figure 5.17), a large fat-filled synovial fold projects forwards (arrow) into the medial aspect of each joint. The synovial fold consists of *white* adipose tissue, i.e. a single droplet of lipid occupies most of the volume of the cell – these fat cells are unilocular, which distinguishes them from

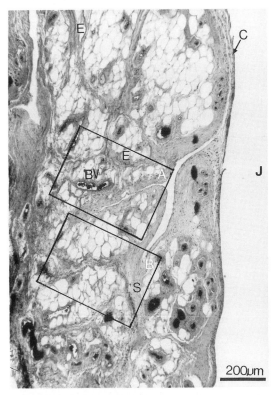

Figure 5.15 This 30 μm thick section shows part of a synovial fold from the lumbosacral zygapophysial joint of a 45-year-old female. Note the irregularly spaced synovial lining cells (C) in the synovial lining (intimal) layer. BV = blood vessels containing blood cells; J = joint cavity; S = interlocular fibrous septum in the subsynovial (subintimal) layer. There is a rich blood supply and the unilocular fat cells indicate that synovial folds consist of white adipose tissue in adults. The rectangles A and B highlight some areas where elastic fibres run in various directions in the subsynovial tissue within interlocular fibrous septa. (Modified Schofield's silver impregnation and Verhoeff's haematoxylin counterstain.) (Reproduced with permission from Giles, L.G.F. (1988) Human lumbar zygapophysial joint inferior recess synovial folds: a light microscope examination. *Anat. Rec.*, **220**, 117–124. Copyright AR Liss, New York.)

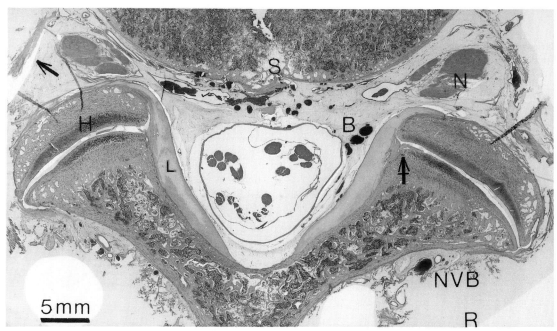

Figure 5.16 A 100 μm thick horizontal section from the upper half of the lumbosacral zygapophysial joint of a 54-year-old male. B = Batson's venous plexus; H = hyaline articular cartilage on the sacral superior articular process; L = ligamentum flavum; N = spinal ganglion with anterior and posterior nerve roots; NVB = neurovascular bundle; R = right side; S = sacrum. Tailed arrow shows a fibrous intra-articular synovial lined fold projecting from the ligamentum flavum into the upper one-third of the right zygapophysial joint and arrow shows part of a transforaminal ligament. Ehrlich's haematoxylin stain with light green counter stain. (Reproduced with permission from Giles, L.G.F. (1987) Lumbosacral zygapophysial joint tropism and its effect on hyaline cartilage. *Clin. Biomech.*, **2**, 2–6. Copyright John Wright, London.)

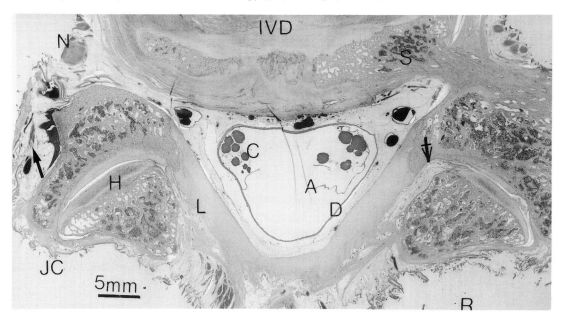

Figure 5.17 A 100 μm thick horizontal section of the lumbosacral zygapophysial joints at the level of the inferior joint recesses, from a 54-year-old male (the plane of section is slightly oblique). A = arachnoid membrane; C = cauda equina; D = dura mater; H = hyaline articular cartilage; IVD = intervertebral disc; JC = posterolateral fibrous capsule; L = ligamentum flavum; N = spinal ganglion; R = right side; S = sacrum; SP = base of trimmed off spinous process. The intra-articular synovial fold is shown by the tailed arrow. A neurovascular bundle is shown by the arrow. Ehrlich's haematoxylin stain with light green counterstain. Reproduced with permission from Giles, L.G.F. and Taylor, J.R. (1982) Intra-articular synovial protrusions in the lower lumbar apophyseal joints. *Bull. Hosp. J. Dis. Orthop. Inst.*, **42**(2), 248–255.)

brown adipose tissue, which contains multiple small droplets of lipid of varying size and which is, therefore, multilocular (Bloom and Fawcett, 1975). The synovial folds would be expected to contain white adipose tissue since brown adipose tissue disappears from most sites in humans after the first decade of life (Ross and Reith, 1985).

Multifidus muscle

The multifidus muscle covers the posterior joint capsule and the joint recesses (Lewin *et al.*, 1961; Hirsch *et al.*, 1963; Lewin, 1964; Bogduk, 1979). A tendon of the multifidus muscle is clearly applied to the fibrous capsule as it crosses the joint to attach to the mamillary process and to the posterior aspect of the joint capsule (Barnett *et al.*, 1961; Cyron and Hutton, 1981; Adams and Hutton, 1983; Taylor and Twomey, 1986). Deep to the multifidus muscle there may be some adipose tissue which extends into the inferior recess of the joints (Hirsch *et al.*, 1963; Giles, 1989).

The multifidus muscle consists of a number of fleshy and tendinous fasciculi which fill the groove beside the spines of the vertebrae from the sacrum to the axis; they are best developed in the lumbosacral region (Williams and Warwick, 1980). Fasciculi are attached inferiorly to the back of the fourth sacral level, the posterior sacroiliac ligament, and lumbar mamillary processes; they pass obliquely upwards and medially to an upper attachment to the whole length of the spinous process of a vertebra two or three segments above; the fasciculi vary in length, with the deepest fasciculi connecting contiguous vertebrae (Quiring and Warfel, 1960; Williams and Warwick, 1980). Some fibres merge with the fibrous capsule of the zygapophysial joint, thus keeping the capsule taut and free from impingement between the hyaline articular cartilages (Lewin *et al.*, 1961) under normal circumstances.

The deeper tendinous sheet of the multifidus muscle forms the posterior boundary of the extra-capsular part of the inferior recess adipose pads. According to Lewin *et al.* (1961) and Taylor and Twomey (1986), because the multifidus muscle has some control over the tension within the fibrous capsule, it must affect the potential spaces of the intra- and extracapsular recesses and their adipose pads as the zygapophysial joint goes through various ranges of movement.

Blood supply of the synovial folds

My findings support those of Lewin *et al.* (1961) and Kos (1969) that the blood supply to the synovial fold is by means of arteries which pass through the multifidus muscle, i.e. branches of the posterior spinal branch, to enter the extracapsular recess. The

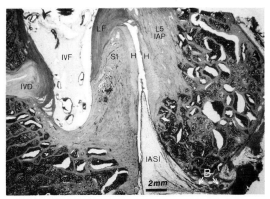

Figure 5.18 Large highly vascular intra-articular synovial fold with a small fibrotic tip, within the inferior recess of the lumbosacral zygapophysial joint from a 56-year-old male. The cartilage on the sacral superior process appears to have become moulded adjacent to the fibrotic tip of the synovial fold, presumably due to pressure on the fibrotic tip. B = blood vessels; H = hyaline articular cartilage; IASI = intra-articular synovial fold; IVD = intervertebral disc of the lumbosacral joint; IVF = intervertebral foramen of the lumbosacral joint; LF = ligamentum flavum; L5 IAP = L5 inferior articular process; S1 = superior articular process of the sacrum. Ehrlich's haematoxylin stain with light green counterstain. (Reproduced with permission from Giles, L.G.F. (1988) Human lumbar zygapophysial joint inferior recess synovial folds. A light microscope examination. *Anat. Rec.,* **220**, 117–124. Copyright AR Liss, New York.)

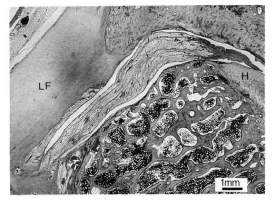

Figure 5.19 A large intra-articular synovial fold showing the extensive blood supply of a lumbosacral synovial fold from a 54-year-old male. Note the fibrotic tip of the synovial fold where it has been pinched between the hyaline articular cartilage surfaces. H = hyaline articular cartilage; LF = ligamentum flavum (Ehrlich's haematoxylin stain with light green counterstain). (Reproduced with permission from Giles, L.G.F. and Taylor, J.R. (1982) Intra-articular synovial protrusions in the lower lumbar apophyseal joints. *Bull. Hosp. J. Dis. Orthop. Inst.,* **42**, 248–255.)

blood vessels then supply and ramify within the synovial folds. Two examples to show the possible extent of intra-articular synovial folds, with their blood supply, extending between the zygapophysial joint hyaline articular cartilages are shown in Figures 5.18 (sagittal plane) and Figure 5.19 (horizontal plane).

Synovial fluid

The synovial fluid (or synovia) is a viscous, pale yellow, clear fluid which consists of a dialysate of plasma, to which hyaluronate protein has been added as a result of secretion of the synovial lining cells (Paget and Bullough, 1980). Nutrients flow through the synovial fluid to reach the articular cartilage, the source of the synovial fluid and its nutrients being the capillary bed surrounding the joint cavity and the capillaries occurring in the synovial membrane (Knight and Levick, 1983).

Only a film of synovial fluid separates the moving surfaces in joints, and the intra-articular cavity is primarily a potential space, containing so little free fluid (less than 1 ml in small joints), that none can be recovered from small joints by needle aspiration (Simkin, 1979; Paget and Bullough, 1980). The synovial fluid acts not only as a lubricant but also as an adhesive which helps to hold the articular cartilages in close apposition (Semlak and Ferguson, 1970; Simkin, 1979).

Pathology

Articular process degenerative changes

As mentioned in Chapter 4, mechanical stresses affecting the articular triad can result in the superior and inferior articular processes showing degenerative osteophytosis.

An example of osteophytic changes affecting the lateral and medial margins of the articular processes is shown in Figure 5.20, where the lateral margin of the superior articular process, and the medial margin of the inferior articular process, show osteophytic changes; osteoarthritic fibrillation changes affecting the hyaline articular cartilage on the facets of both articular processes is also noted.

Zygapophysial joint osteoarthritic changes

Zygapophysial joint hyaline articular cartilage changes associated with ageing are different from those occurring in osteoarthritis (degenerative joint disease). Ageing results in thinning but not in the diffuse

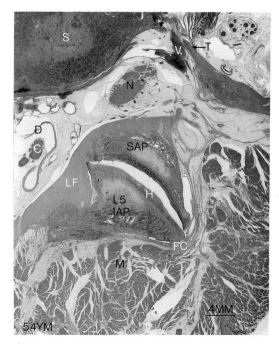

Figure 5.20 A 100 μm thick section cut in the horizontal plane through the middle of the right lumbosacral zygapophysial joint of a 54-year-old male. C = cauda equina nerve root trunks; D = dural membrane; FC = fibrous capsule; H = hyaline articular cartilage; L5IAP = inferior articular process of fifth lumbar vertebra; LF = ligamentum flavum; M = muscle; N = neural complex within the intervertebral canal; S = sacrum; SAP = superior articular process; T = part of a transforaminal ligament; V = blood vessel. Ehrlich's haematoxylin and light green counterstain.

evidence of degradation and repair which is characteristic of osteoarthritis (Ferguson, 1975). With advancing years, the water content of hyaline articular cartilage is reduced, whereas in osteoarthritis, it is normal or increased (Dick, 1972). In adults the hyaline articular cartilage often develops areas of disintegration and erosion (Meachim, 1969), and Ziv *et al.* (1993) found from a study of fresh post-mortem spines that zygapophysial joint hyaline articular cartilage degenerates early in life, leading to back pain which is unrelated to the age-related changes occurring in the adjacent intervertebral disc.

In some specimens, early osteoarthritic changes, such as tinctorial variations (a staining variation (Giles, 1986b) presumed to be due to changes in cartilage matrix) may precede early fibrillation and the narrow surface layer of acellular tissue may also be seen by transmitted light and darkfield microscopy to show early fibrillation of its margin (Figures 5.21 A and B).

In specimens showing advanced osteoarthritic changes in zygapophysial joints the acellular layer is not present when examined by transmitted light and darkfield microscopy (Figure 5.22 A and B).

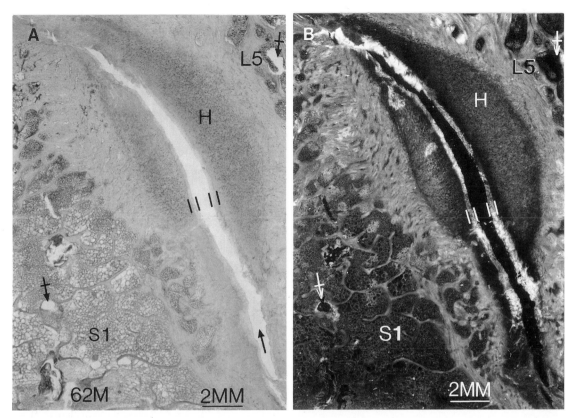

Figure 5.21 (A) A transmitted light photomicrograph showing a section cut in the parasagittal plane through the lumbosacral zygapophysial joint of a 62-year-old male. Note that the acellular surface layer of the hyaline articular cartilage (H) on the inferior articular process of the fifth lumbar (L5) vertebra and the superior articular process of the sacrum (S1) show early osteoarthritic changes and that there are tinctorial changes in the cellular region of the cartilages. A part of the narrow strip of acellular surface layer is shown between the paired parallel lines (II) on each surface. The joint 'space' is shown by an arrow. Some artefact spaces, where small pieces of bone marrow have been lost during processing, are shown by tailed arrows. Ehrlich's haematoxylin stain with light green counterstain. (B) A darkfield photomicrograph of the specimen shown in Figure 5.21A. Note the dramatically enhanced narrow strip of acellular surface layer between the paired parallel lines (II). (Reproduced with permission from Giles, L.G.F. (1992a) The surface lamina of the articular cartilage of human zygapophysial joints. *Anat. Rec.*, **233**, 350–356. Copyright Wiley-Liss Inc.)

It should be noted that with darkfield microscopy of 'normal' to early osteoarthritic joint cartilage surfaces (Figures 5.21B) the narrow strip of acellular lamina of the cartilage bounding the joint space is enhanced. As would be expected, there is no acellular lamina in joints with advanced osteoarthrosis (Figure 5.22B). Also, areas of tissue adjacent to artefact spaces (caused by loss of small parts of tissue during processing (for example Figure 5.21 B), do not show corresponding areas of enhancement. Therefore, the acellular layer does exist in joints not exhibiting advanced degenerative changes and it is not an artefact (Giles, 1992a). The thickness of the acellular layer can vary from 20 to 200 μm along the surface of the cartilage, and from one specimen to another, and appears to be unrelated to age or sex.

This study illustrates the existence of an acellular layer, or lamina splendens, lining the surface of some

lower lumbar zygapophysial joint facet cartilages in middle-aged human cadavers which exhibit 'normal' joints, or only early osteoarthritic changes for this age group. This appears to support the findings of MacConaill (1951), Davies *et al.* (1962), and Weiss *et al.* (1968), who reported a narrow surface lamina on articular cartilage. Perhaps an explanation of the fact that the narrow lamina is not seen in all 'normal' joints relates to technical difficulties involved in decalcifying and generally processing large blocks of osteoligamentous tissues for several months before sectioning can commence. Once advanced osteoarthrosis is present, the layer of acellular tissue is no longer recognizable and, in such specimens, no 'white' line is seen on the osteoarthritic cartilage surface by darkfield microscopy, nor is there any enhancement of the cut edge of any other joint structures. This, and the fact that an acellular layer

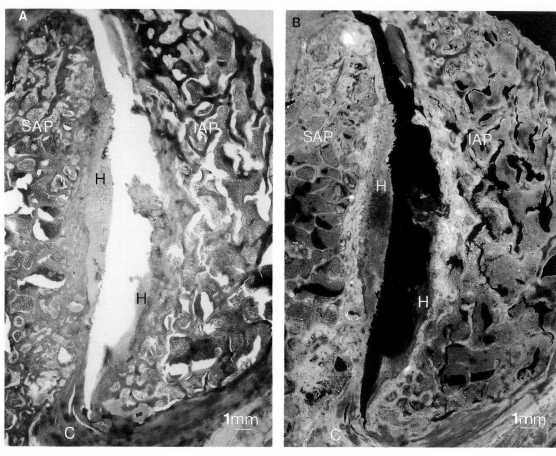

Figure 5.22 (A) A transmitted light photomicrograph of a 200 μm thick section cut in the parasagittal plane through the lumbosacral zygapophysial joint of a 78-year-old male. There is advanced fibrillation and loss of the hyaline articular cartilage (H) on the facets of the superior articular process of the sacrum (SAP) and the inferior articular process (IAP) of the fifth lumbar vertebra, respectively. The fibrous capsule (C) is seen at the inferior margin of the joint. (B) A darkfield photomicrograph of the specimen shown in Figure 5.22A shows no surface lamina. Importantly, there is no evidence of significant light artefacts along the cut edges of the residual osteoarthritic cartilages, or any other parts of the joint, which could simulate a surface lamina. (Reproduced with permission from Giles, L. G. F. (1992a) The surface lamina of the articular cartilage of human zygapophysial joints. *Anat. Rec.,* **233**, 350–356. Copyright Wiley-Liss Inc.)

can be seen on normal light illumination, indicates that the lamina splendens is not an artefact. However, the possible physiological significance of this acellular tissue will not be speculated upon in this text.

Pathoanatomical studies and clinical significance of lumbosacral zygapophysial (facet) joints – the facet syndrome

Jackson (1992) believes the diagnosis of facet syndrome is not a reliable clinical diagnosis. However, when patients present with local tenderness in the low back, muscle spasm, and low back pain referred to the back of the thigh, the mid-calf, or to the ankle they are considered to have the facet syndrome (Kirkaldy-Willis, 1983; Kirkaldy-Willis and Cassidy, 1984). Furthermore when alleviation of this pain is achieved by injection into the joint of local anaesthetic, with or without steroid suspension, under fluoroscopic control (Mooney and Robertson, 1976; Kirkaldy-Willis and Tchang, 1983; Aprill, 1986), this diagnosis is supported (Destouet *et al.*, 1982; Lewinnik and Warfield, 1986).

Because not all cases respond to injection within the zygapophysial joint, it is possible that pain could also result from mechanical irritation of soft tissue structures outside the joint which are adjacent to osteophytes on degenerative zygapophysial joints

(Giles and Kaveri, 1990; Giles, 1992b). Such degenerative margins of the joint (Altman and Dean, 1989), can lead to lumbar spinal stenosis, which may involve the intervertebral canal and/or the spinal canal (Kirkaldy-Willis and McIvor, 1976).

Radiologically demonstrable osteophytic degenerative changes in the spine do not normally regress, whereas symptoms of low back pain with referred pain to the leg can vary, with remissions and exacerbations, so there is a poor correlation between the severity of radiographic changes and back pain (Stockwell, 1985). This may be due to the possible multifactorial causes of mechanical back pain that can affect a given level of the spine.

The effect of joint dysfunction on associated soft tissue structures, with possible venous stasis and nerve ischaemia (Giles, 1973, Sunderland, 1980; Hoyland *et al.*, 1989; Giles and Kaveri, 1990), and soft tissue entrapment (Kos and Wolf, 1972; Giles and Taylor, 1987b; Giles, 1991b) has been postulated as a potential mechanism for causing back pain of mechanical origin which cannot be shown on imaging procedures which only give a shadow of the truth, as previously mentioned.

The following large cross-sectional area histological section viewed by low magnification light microscopy show soft tissue structures associated with zygapophysial joints which may be compromised due to joint dysfunction but which cannot be seen on imaging. The sections provide good detail of the relationship between various spinal structures but limited information on histopathological changes and no direct relationship with pain.

Apart from some degree of posterolateral intervertebral disc protrusion (17% at L4–5 and 50% at L5–S1) and one minor central posterior bulge at the lumbosacral level, several soft tissue structures which could theoretically be involved in low back pain of mechanical origin were histologically identified as (a) the large intra-articular synovial folds of the zygapophysial joints, (b) joint capsule fibrous tissues which become attached by adhesions to the adjacent hyaline articular cartilage, (c) distorted and tractioned blood vessels within the intervertebral canal foramen, (d) neural structures which become attached by adhesions to densely fibrotic intra-articular synovial folds, and (e) stenosis of the intervertebral canal foramen due to hypertrophy of the ligamentum flavum with, or without, adjacent posterolateral intervertebral disc herniation.

A highly vascular intra-articular synovial fold with a fibrotic tip projecting between the osteoarthritic hyaline articular cartilage surfaces, indicating that this tip was probably 'nipped' during life, is shown within the right lumbosacral joint of a 74-year-old male in Figure 5.23

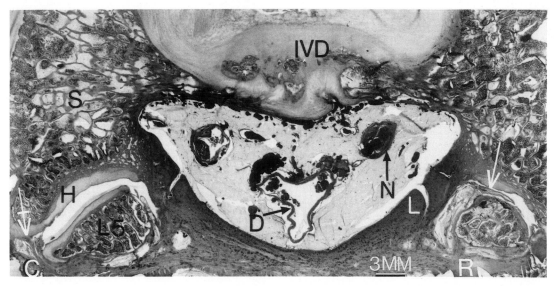

Figure 5.23 A 100 µm thick section cut in the horizontal plane from the lower one-third of the lumbosacral zygapophysial joints of a 74-year-old male cadaver. The right (R) zygapophysial joint shows a large highly vascular intra-articular synovial fold (arrow) with a fibrotic tip, projecting between osteoarthritic hyaline articular cartilage surfaces. The tip is probably fibrotic due to 'nipping' of the synovial fold between the joint surfaces during life. C = fibrous capsule, some fibres of which have become attached to the surface of the hyaline articular cartilage (H) on the sacral facet (tailed arrow) between the articulating surfaces; D = dural sac containing the cauda equina; IVD = a small midline bulge of the intervertebral disc; L = ligamentum flavum with vascular channel; L5 = inferior articular process of the fifth lumbar vertebra; N = nerve roots in the dural sleeve; S = sacral ala. (Reproduced with permission from Giles, L.G.F. (1991b) A review and description of some possible causes of low back pain of mechanical origin in *homo sapiens. Proc. Aust. Soc. Hum. Biol.*, **4**, 193–212.)

Kos and Wolf (1972) described vascular 'menisci' in zygapophysial joints and claimed that they are well innervated, although they did not present any histologic evidence of innervation. They advance the theory that these may become entrapped between articular surfaces causing the syndrome of 'vertebral block'. The entrapment of 'meniscoid inclusions' may mechanically interfere with movement (Lewit, 1968), leading to pain and muscle spasm (Giles and Taylor, 1982). Zukschwerdt *et al.* (1955), Bourdillon (1973), Giles and Taylor (1987a,b), and Giles and Harvey (1987) have also implicated synovial fold inclusions in some cases of low back pain due to the impingement of the articular surfaces on synovial tissue. Kraft and Levinthal (1951), Tondury (1972), and Kirkaldy-Willis (1984) believe impingement is accompanied by oedema, synovitis, and then distension of the capsule; this causes nerve root irritation (Harmon, 1966). According to Bogduk and Jull (1985), meniscus entrapment as an explanation for the pathologic basis for acute locked back is inconsistent with the clinical features of acute back pain, because (a) fibrous inclusions 'do not project into the joint space', and (b) there is the possibility of 'cleavage' of the adipose type of inclusion when traction is applied to it. However, following the histologic examination of numerous zygapophysial joint synovial folds in serial sections, it is the opinion of this author that by far the majority of innervated synovial folds do project into inferior and superior joint recesses and remain intact and do not undergo cleavage.

Figure 5.23 also shows adhesions between the posterolateral part of the left fibrous capsule and the surface of the hyaline articular cartilage on the superior articular process of the sacrum. The adhesions have caused part of the fibrous capsule to be drawn between the articular surfaces of the hyaline articular cartilage. This could be nipped between joint surfaces, causing pain.

Figure 5.24 shows how a blood vessel can be deformed and tractioned by an osteophytic spur projecting into the intervertebral canal (foramen) from the superior articular process of the fifth lumbar vertebra of a 79-year-old male. This figure also shows a large densely fibrotic intra-articular synovial lined fold, arising from the joint's fibrous capsule–ligamentum flavum junction superiorly, and projecting between the osteoarthritic hyaline articular cartilage surfaces.

An example of a highly vascular connective tissue adhesion between a densely fibrotic intra-articular synovial fold, in the superior articular recess of a lumbosacral zygapophysial joint, and the adjacent neural complex, in an 82-year-old female, is shown in Figure 5.25.

Clearly, it is not possible to correlate these histopathological findings in cadavers with the facet syndrome. However, the vascular synovial folds in the zygapophysial joints have been shown to contain

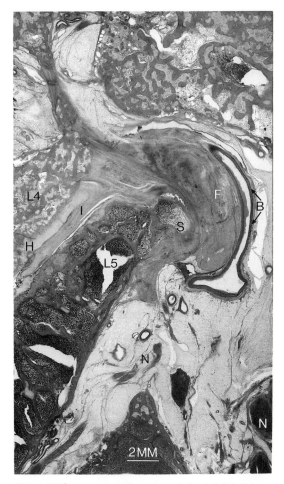

Figure 5.24 A parasagittal section of the left L4–5 intervertebral canal (foramen) from a 79-year-old male. Note how a blood vessel (B) can be deformed and tractioned by an osteophytic spur (S) projecting from the superior articular process of the L5 vertebra and how the blood vessel conforms to the contour of the osteoarthritic joint as it passes around the margin of the joint and its capsule. F = fibrous joint capsule–ligamentum flavum junction; H = hyaline articular cartilage (osteoarthritic); I = fibrous intra-articular synovial lined fold arising from the fibrous joint capsule–ligamentum flavum junction superiorly; L4 = part of the inferior articular process of the L4 vertebra; L5 = part of the superior articular process of the L5 vertebra; N = neural structures within the intervertebral canal foramen. (Reproduced with permission from Giles, L.G.F. (1991b) A review and description of some possible causes of low back pain of mechanical origin in *homo sapiens. Proc. Aust. Soc. Hum. Biol.*, 4, 193–212.)

both paravascular and non-paravascular nerve fibres of small (nociceptive) diameter (Giles and Taylor, 1987b; Gronblad *et al.*, 1991a), as well as small diameter substance P positive profiles (nerves) (Giles and Harvey, 1987; Gronblad *et al.*, 1991b). Substance

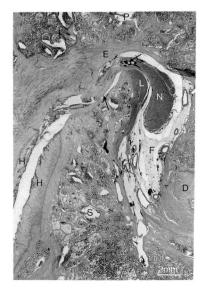

Figure 5.25 A parasagittal section of the left lumbosacral intervertebral canal foramen from an 82-year-old female showing how the neural complex (N) and a dense fibrous intra-articular synovial fold (arrow) have become attached to each other via a highly vascular connective tissue adhesion (tailed arrow). D = intervertebral disc; E = eburnation of the inferior aspect of the pedicle (P) of the L5 vertebra; F = intervertebral canal (foramen); H = hyaline articular cartilage (arthritic); L = ligamentum flavum on the superior articular process of the sacrum (S). (Reproduced with permission from Giles, L.G.F. (1991b) A review and description of some possible causes of low back pain of mechanical origin in *homo sapiens. Proc. Aust. Soc. Hum. Biol.,* **4**, 193–212.)

P is thought to be involved in nociception (Jessell and Iversen, 1977; Marx, 1979; Cuello *et al.*, 1982; Henry, 1982; Rossell, 1982; Salt *et al.*, 1982; Liesi *et al.*, 1983; Korkala *et al.*, 1985), so it is possible that, should the synovial folds become 'nipped' and cause traumatic synovitis (Kirkaldy-Willis, 1984), this could result in low back pain, with or without referred pain to the leg, and muscle spasm. As previously mentioned, such pain can be alleviated by injecting local anaesthetic, with or without steroid suspension, into the joints under fluoroscopic control, supporting this etiology (Mooney and Robertson, 1976; Carrera, 1979; Destouet *et al.*, 1982; Kirkaldy-Willis and Tchang, 1983; Aprill, 1986; Lewinnik and Warfield, 1986).

When adhesions occur between the fibrous capsule and the surface of the hyaline articular cartilage, it is possible that some spinal movements could result in low back pain, as the fibrous joint capsule contains small diameter nociceptive (free ending) nerve fibres (Ikari, 1954; Pedersen *et al.*, 1956; Hirsch *et al.*, 1963; Hadley, 1964; Reilly *et al.*, 1978) and Substance P positive profiles (Giles and Harvey, 1987; El-Body *et*

al., 1988). These nociceptors may be activated as a result of (i) traction of the fibrous joint capsule against the cartilage surface during lumbar flexion or some rotational movements, or (ii) pinching of parts of the fibrous joint capsule between the hyaline articular cartilage surfaces, for example during lumbar extension.

Where blood vessels are vulnerable to compression and or traction distortion, as shown in Figures 5.19, 5.24 and 5.25, back pain may well occur due to mechanical irritation of the innervated blood vessels, or possibly as a result of venous stasis (Giles, 1973; Sunderland, 1980; Hoyland *et al.*, 1989; Giles and Kaveri, 1990; Jayson, 1992). Vascular stasis could cause ischaemia of the related neural structures with accumulation of metabolic waste products (such as lactic acid), pain, epineurial, perineurial and intraneural fibrosis, with neural dysfunction, and degeneration as postulated in Figure 5.26.

Pain of vascular origin is a well known clinical phenomenon (Kuntz, 1953), and may be perceived centrally via the sinuvertebral nerves which supply these vessels with autonomic and somatic sensory fibres (Hovelacque, 1925). Where adhesions occur between zygapophysial joint structures, such as fibrotic synovial folds and the associated neural complex (Figure 5.25), the neural complex could be compromised due to traction of its neural and microvascular structures, resulting in pain. Pinching

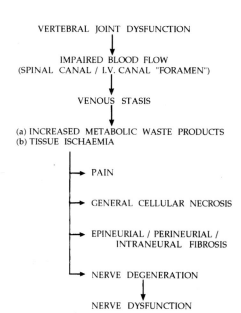

Figure 5.26 An hypothesis for vertebral joint dysfunction possibly causing pain and nerve dysfunction. (Reproduced with permission from Giles, L.G.F. (1991b) A review and description of some possible causes of low back pain of mechanical origin in *homo sapiens. Proc. Aust. Soc. Hum. Biol.,* **4**, 193–212.)

between bony surfaces across the highly vascular connective tissue adhesion could also result in pain of vascular origin.

If disruption occurs to the periradicular and radicular microvasculature due to intervertebral canal foramen stenosis caused by encroachment by zygapophysial joint or intervertebral disc structures, this also raises the question of whether low back pain of mechanical origin could be due to vascular stasis.

These preliminary descriptive findings suggest how some anatomical structures, which are not demonstrable by various imaging procedures, may contribute to zygapophysial joint dysfunction and the facet syndrome. Such dysfunction could conceivably result in low back pain of mechanical origin which is often relieved by appropriate spinal manipulation (Sandoz, 1976; Farfan, 1980; Keim and Kirkaldy-Willis, 1987; Kirkaldy-Willis, 1988; Meade *et al.*, 1990).

References

Adams, M.A. and Hutton, W.C. (1983) The mechanical function of the lumbar apophyseal joints. *Spine*, **8**, 327-330.

Agur, A.M.R. (1991) *Grant's Atlas of Anatomy*, 9th edition. Williams and Wilkins, Baltimore.

Altman, R.D. and Dean, D. (1989) Pain in osteoarthritis - introduction and overview. *Semin. Arthr. Rheum.*, **18**, 1-3.

Aprill, C. (1986) Lumbar facet joint arthrography and injection in the evaluation of painful disorders of the low back (abstract). Presented at a meeting of the International Society for the Study of the Lumbar Spine, Dallas.

Aspden, R.M. and Hukins, D.W.L. (1979) The lamina splendens of articular cartilage is an artefact of phase contrast microscopy. *Proc. R. Soc. Lond.*, **B206**, 109-113.

Baddeley, H. (1976) Radiology of lumbar spinal stenosis. In *The Lumbar Spine and Back Pain* (M. Jayson, ed.), Sector Publishing, London, pp. 151-172.

Barland, P., Novikoff, A.B. and Hamerman, D. (1962) Electron microscopy of the human synovial membrane. *J. Cell Biol.*, **14**, 207-220.

Barnett, C.H., Davies, D.V. and MacConaill, M.A. (1961) *Synovial Joints: Their Structure and Mechanics*. Longmans, London, pp. 24, 47, 48, 50.

Benini, A. (1979) Das Kleine Gelenk der Lendenwirbelsaule. *Fortschr. Med.*, **97**, 2103-2106.

Benninghoff, A. (1939) *Lehrbuch der Anatomie des Menschen*, Band I. Munich, Lehmann JF, Verlag.

Bland, J.H. (1987) *Disorders of the Cervical Spine: Diagnosis and Medical Management*. WB Saunders, Philadelphia, p. 65.

Bloom, W. and Fawcett, D.W. (1975) *A Textbook of Histology*. WB Saunders, Philadelphia, pp. 196-208.

Bogduk, N. (1979) The lumbar zygapophysial joints. *Proceedings of Low Back Pain Symposium, Manipulative Therapists Association of Australia*, Sydney, Australia, pp. 32-40.

Bogduk, N. (1981) The lumbar mamillo-accessory ligament: its anatomical and neurological significance. *Spine*, **6**, 162-167.

Bogduk, N. and Jull, G. (1985) The theoretical pathology of acute locked back: a basis for manipulation. *Man. Med.*, **1**, 78-82.

Bogduk, N. and Twomey, L.T. (1991) *Clinical Anatomy of the Lumbar Spine*, 2nd edition. Churchill Livingstone, Edinburgh.

Bogduk, N., Wilson, A.S. and Tynan, W. (1982) The lumbar dorsal rami. *J. Anat.*, **134**, 383-397.

Bourdillon, J.F. (1973) *Spinal Manipulation*, 2nd edition. William Heinemann Medical Books, London, pp. 22-23.

Bradley, K.C. (1974) The anatomy of backache. *Aust. N. Z. J. Surg.*, **44**, 227-232.

Breig, A. (1960) *Biomechanics of the Central Nervous System*. Almqvist and Wiksell, Stockholm.

Brown, H.A. (1938) Enlargement of the ligamentum flavum. *J. Bone Joint Surg.*, **20**, 325-338.

Bullough, P.G. (1979) Pathologic changes associated with the common arthritides and their treatment. *Pathol. Ann.*, **2**, 69-83.

Cameron, D.A. and Robinson, R.A. (1958) Electron microscopy of epiphyseal and articular cartilage matrix in the femur of the newborn infant. *J. Bone Joint Surg.*, **40A**, 163.

Carrera, G.F. (1979) Lumbar facet arthrography and injection in low back pain. *Wisc. Med. J.*, **78**, 35-37.

Castor, C.W. (1960) The microscopic structure of normal human synovial tissue. *Arthritis Rheum.*, **3**, 140.

Cihak, R. (1970) Variations of lumbosacral joints and their morphogenesis. *Acta Universitatis Carolinae Medica*, **16**, 5-165.

Collins, D.H. (1949) *The Pathology of Articular and Spinal Diseases*. Edward Arnold, London.

Collins, D.H., Ghadially, F.N. and Meachim, G. (1965) Intracellular lipids of cartilage. *Ann. Rheum. Dis.*, **24**, 123.

Crawford, J.S. (1978) *Principles and Practice of Obstetric Anaesthesia*, 4th edition. Blackwell Scientific Publications, Oxford, p. 170.

Cuello, A.C., Priestley, J.V. and Milstein, C. (1982) Immunocytochemistry with internally labelled monoclonal antibodies. *Proc. Natl Acad. Sci. USA*, **79**, 665-670.

Cyron, B.M. and Hutton, W.C. (1981) The tensile strength of the capsular ligaments of the apophyseal joints. *J. Anat.*, **132**, 145-150.

Davies, D.V. (1950) Structure and function of synovial membrane. *Br. Med. J.*, **1**, 92-95.

Davies, D.V., Barnett, C.H., Cochrane, W. and Palfrey, A.J (1962) Electron microscopy of articular cartilage in the young adult rabbit. *Ann. Rheum. Dis.*, **21**, 11-22.

DeMarchi, F. G. (1963) Le articolazioni intervertebrali Studio anatomo-istologica. *Clin. Orthop.*, **15**, 26-33.

Destouet, J.M., Gilula, L.A., Murphy, W.A. and Monsess, B. (1982) Lumbar facet joint injection: indication, technique, clinical correlation and preliminary results. *Radiology*, **5**, 321-325.

Dick, W.C. (1972) *An Introduction to Clinical Rheumatology*. Churchill Livingstone, London, p. 24.

Dieppe, P. and Calvert, P. (1983) *Crystals and Joint Disease*. Chapman and Hall, London, p. 14.

Dockerty, M.B. and Love, J.G. (1940) Thickening and fibrosis (so-called hypertrophy) of the ligamentum flavum: pathological study of fifty cases. *Proc. Staff Meet. Mayo Clin.*, **15**, 161-166.

Dommisse, G.F. (1975) Morphological aspects of the lumbar spine and lumbo-sacral region. *Orthop. Clin. North Am.*, **6**, 163-175.

Dorr, W. (1958) Uber die Anatomie der Wirbelgelenke. *Arch. Orthop. Unfall. Chir.*, **50**, 222-243.

Dorr, W. (1962) Nochmals zu den Menisci in der Wirbelbo-gengelenken. *Z. Orthop.*, **96**, 457-461.

Dory, M.A. (1981) Arthrography of the lumbar facet joints. *Radiology*, **140**, 23-27.

Edwards, C.C. and Chrisman, O.D. (1979) Articular cartilage. In *The Scientific Basis of Orthopaedics* (J.A. Albright and R.A. Brand, eds). Appleton-Century-Crofts, New York, pp 315-347.

Efskind, I. (1941) Anatomy and physiology of the joint capsule. *Acta Orthop. Scand.*, **12**, 214-260.

El-Bohy, A., Cavanaugh, J.M., Getchell, M.L. *et al.* (1988) Localization of substance P and neurofilament immuno-reactive fibres in the lumbar facet joint capsule and supraspinous ligament of the rabbit. *Brain Res.*, **460**, 379-382.

El-Khoury, G.Y. and Renfrew, D.L. (1991) Percutaneous procedures for the diagnosis and treatment of lower back pain: diskography, facet-joint injection and epidural injection. *AJR*, **157**, 685-691.

Ellis, H. and Feldman, S. (1979) *Anatomy for Anaesthetists*, 3rd edition. Blackwell Scientific Publications,Oxford, pp. 138-143.

Engel, R.M. and Bogduk, N. (1980) The menisci of the lumbar zygapophysial joints. Presented at the annual conference of the *Anatomical Society of Australia and New Zealand*, University of Sydney, Sydney, Australia.

Engel, R.M. and Bogduk, N. (1982) The menisci of the lumbar zygapophysial joints. *J. Anat.*, **135**, 795-809.

Epstein, B. (1976) *The Spine. A Radiological Text and Atlas*, 4th edition. Lea and Febiger, Philadelphia, p. 42.

Fairbank, J.C.T. and O'Brien, J.P. (1980) The abdominal cavity and thoraco-lumbar fascia as a stabiliser of the lumbar spine in patients with low back pain. In *Engineering Aspects of the Spine*. Mechanical Engineering Publications, London, pp. 83-88.

Farfan, H.F. (1973) *Mechanical Disorders of the Low Back*. Lea and Febiger, Philadelphia, pp. 5, 21.

Farfan, H.F. (1980) The scientific basis of manipulative procedures. *Clin. Rheum. Dis.*, **6**, 159-178.

Farfan, H.F. (1983) Biomechanics of the lumbar spine. In *Managing Low Back Pain* (W.H. Kirkaldy-Willis, ed.), Churchill Livingstone, New York, pp. 9-21.

Ferguson, A.B. (1975) The pathology of degenerative arthri-tis. In *Surgical Management of Degenerative Arthritis of the Lower Limbs* (R.L. Cruess and N.S. Mitchell, eds). Lea and Febiger, Philadelphia, pp. 3-9.

Fick, R. (1904) *Handbuch der Anatomie und Mechanik der Gelenke*. II. G.Fischer, Jena, pp. 77-89.

Francois, R.J., Bywaters, E.G.L. and Aufdermaur, M. (1985) Illustrated glossary for spinal anatomy. *Rheumatol. Int.*, **5**, 241-245.

Gardner, E., Gray, D.J. and O'Rahilly, R. (1975) *Anatomy and Regional Study of Human Structure*, 4th edition. W.B. Saunders, Philadelphia.

Ghadially, F.N. and Roy, S. (1969) *Ultrastructure of Synovial Joints in Health and Disease*. Butterworths,London, pp. 1-48.

Ghadially, F.N., Meachim, G. and Collins, D.H. (1965) Extra-cellular lipid in the matrix of human articular cartilage. *Ann. Rheum. Dis.*, **24**, 136.

Giles, L.G.F. (1973) Spinal fixation and viscera. *J. Clin. Chiroprac. Arch.*, **3**, 4-165.

Giles, L.G.F. (1982) *Leg Length Inequality with Postural Scoliosis: Its Effect On Lumbar Apophyseal Joints*. M.Sc. thesis, Department of Anatomy and Human Biology, The University of Western Australia, Perth.

Giles, L.G.F. (1984) Lumbar apophyseal joint arthrography. *J. Manipuative Physiol. Ther.*, **7**, 21-24.

Giles, L.G.F. (1986a) Lumbo-sacral and cervical zygapophy-sial joint inclusions. *Man. Med.*, **2**, 89-92.

Giles, L.G.F. (1986b) Pressure related changes in human lumbo-sacral zygapophysial joint articular cartilage. *J. Rheumatol.*, **13**, 1093-1095.

Giles, L.G.F. (1987) Lumbo-sacral zygapophysial joint tro-pism and its effect on hyaline cartilage. *Clin. Biomech.*, **2**, 2-6.

Giles, L.G.F. (1988) Human lumbar zygapophysial joint inferior recess synovial folds: a light microscope examina-tion. *Anat. Rec.*, **220**, 117-124.

Giles, L.G.F. (1989) *Anatomical Basis of Low Back Pain*. Williams and Wilkins, Baltimore.

Giles, L.G.F. (1991a) The relationship between the medial branch of the lumbar posterior primary ramus and the mamillo-accessory ligament. *J. Manipulative Physiol. Ther.*, **14**, 189-192.

Giles, L.G.F. (1991b) A review and description of some possible causes of low back pain of mechanical origin in *homo sapiens*. *Proc. Aust. Soc. Hum. Biol.*, **4**, 193-212.

Giles, L.G.F. (1992a) The surface lamina of the articular cartilage of human zygapophysial joints. *Anat. Rec.*, **233**, 250-356.

Giles, L.G.F. (1992b) Pathoanatomic studies and clinical significance of lumbosacral zygapophysial (facet) joints. *J. Manipulative Physiol. Ther.*, **15**, 36-40.

Giles, L.G.F. and Harvey, A.R. (1987) Immunohistochemical demonstration of nociceptors in the capsule and synovial folds of human zygapophysial joints. *Br. J. Rheumatol.*, **26**, 362-364.

Giles, L.G.F. and Kaveri, M.J.P. (1990) Some osseous and soft tissue causes of human intervertebral canal (foramen) stenosis. *J. Rheumatol.*, **17**, 1474-1481.

Giles, L.G.F. and Taylor, J.R. (1982) Intra-articular synovial protrusions in the lower lumbar apophyseal joints. *Bull. Hosp. J. Dis. Orthop. Inst.*, **42**, 248-255.

Giles, L.G.F. and Taylor, J.R. (1984) The effect of postural scoliosis on lumbar apophyseal joints. *Scand. J. Rheuma-tol.*, **13**, 209-220.

Giles, L.G.F. and Taylor, J.R. (1985) Osteoarthrosis in human cadaveric lumbo-sacral zygapophysial joints. *J. Manip-ulative Physiol. Ther.*, **8**, 239-243.

Giles, L.G.F. and Taylor, J.R. (1987a) Innervation of human lumbar zygapophysial joint synovial folds. *Acta Orthop. Scand.*, **58**, 43-46.

Giles, L.G.F. and Taylor, J.R. (1987b) Human zygapophysial joint capsule and synovial fold innervation. *Br. J. Rheuma-tol.*, **26**, 93-98.

Giles, L.G.F., Taylor, J.R. and Cockson, A. (1986) Human zygapophysial joint synovial folds. *Acta Anat.*, **126**, 110-114.

Gregersen, G.G. and Lucas, D.B. (1967) An in vivo study of axial rotation of the human thoracolumbar spine. *J. Bone Joint Surg.*, **49A**, 247.

Gronblad, M., Weinstein, J.N. and Santavirta, S. (1991a) Immunohistochemical observations on spinal tissue innervation. *Acta Orthop. Scand.*, **62**, 614-622.

Gronblad, M., Korkala, O., Konttinen, Y.T. *et al.* (1991b) Silver impregnation and immunohistochemical study of nerves in lumbar facet joint plical tissue. *Spine,* **16**, 34–38.

Hadler, N.M. (1981) The biology of the extracellular space. *Clin. Rheum. Dis.,* **7**, 71–97.

Hadley, L.A. (1961) Anatomico-roentgenographic studies of the posterior spinal articulations. *Am. J. Roentgenol.,* **86**, 270–276.

Hadley, L.A. (1964) *Anatomico-Roentgenographic Studies of the Spine.* Charles C. Thomas, Springfield, IL, pp. 179, 186, 189, 190.

Hakim, N.S. and King, A.I. (1976) Static and dynamic articular facet loads. In *Proceedings, 20th Stapp Car Crash Conference*, pp. 609–637.

Ham, A.W. and Cormack, D.H. (1979) *Histology*, 8th edition. J.B. Lippincott, Philadelphia, pp. 476, 642.

Harmon, P.H. (1966) Congenital and acquired anatomic variations, including degenerative changes of the lower lumbar spine: role in production of painful back and lower extremity syndromes. *Clin. Orthop.,* **44**, 171–186.

Hasselbacher, P. (1981) Structure of the synovial membrane. *Clin. Rheum. Dis.,* **7**, 57–69.

Henry, J.L. (1982) Relation of substance P to pain transmission: neurophysiological evidence. In *Substance P in the nervous system* (R. Porter and M. O'Connor, eds). Ciba Foundation Symposium, Pitman Co, London, pp. 206–224.

Herzog, W. (1950) Morphologie und pathologie des ligamentum flavum. *Frankfurter Zeitschrift fur Pathologie,* **61**, 250–267.

Heylings, D.J.A. (1978) Supraspinous and interspinous ligaments of the human lumbar spine. *J. Anat.,* **125**, 127–131.

Hirsch, C., Ingelmark, B.E. and Miller, M. (1963) The anatomical basis for low back pain. *Acta Orthop. Scand.,* **33**, 1–17.

Horwitz, T. (1939) Lesions of the intervertebral disc and ligamentum flavum of the lumbar vertebrae: anatomic study of 75 human cadavers. *Surgery,* **6**, 410–425.

Hovelacque, A. (1925) Le nerf sinuvertebral. *Ann. d'Anat. Pathol.,* **5**, 435–443.

Hoyland, J.A., Freemont, A.J. and Jayson, M.I.V. (1989) Intervertebral foramen venous obstruction. A cause of periradicular fibrosis? *Spine,* **5**, 558–568.

Hutton, W.C. and Adams, M.A. (1980) The forces acting on the neural arch and their relevance to low back pain. In *Engineering Aspects of the Spine*. Mechanical Engineering Publications, London, pp. 49–55.

Ikari, C. (1954) A study of the mechanism of low back pain. The neurohistological examination of the disease. *J. Bone Joint Surg.,* **36A**, 1272–1281.

Jackson, R.P. (1992) The facet syndrome. Myth or reality? *Clin. Orthop. Rel. Res.,* **279**, 110–121.

Jayson, M.I.V. (1992) The role of vascular damage and fibrosis in the pathogenesis of nerve root damage. *Clin. Orthop. Rel. Res.,* **279**, 40–48.

Jee, W.S.S. (1983) The skeletal tissues. In *Histology: Cell and Tissue Biology* (L. Weiss, ed.), 5th edition. Macmillan, New York, p. 254.

Jessell, T.M. and Iversen, L.L. (1977) Opiate analgesics inhibit substance P release from rat trigeminal nucleus. *Nature (Lond),* **268**, 549–551.

Junqueira, L.C., Carneiro, J. and Long, J.A. (1986) *Basic Histology*, 5th edition. Appleton-Century-Crofts, Norwalk, Connecticut, pp. 201–303.

Kapandji, I.A. (1974) The physiology of the joints. *The Trunk and the Vertebral Column*. Vol 3. Churchill Livingstone, Edinburgh, p. 78.

Keim, H.A. and Kirkaldy-Willis, W.H. (1987) Low back pain. *Clin. Symp.,* **39**, 1987.

Keller, G. (1953) Die Bedeutung der Veranderungen an den kleinen Wirbelgelenken als Ursache des lokalen Ruckenschmerzes. *Z. Orthop.,* **83**, 517–547.

Keller, G. (1959) Die Arthrose der Wirbelgelenke in ihrer Beziehung zum Ruckenschmerz. *Zeitschrift fur Orthopadie,* **91**, 538–550.

Kirkaldy-Willis, W.H. (1983) The pathology and pathogenesis of low back pain. In *Managing Low Back Pain* (W.H. Kirkaldy-Willis, ed.). Churchill Livingstone, New York, pp. 23–43.

Kirkaldy-Willis, W.H. (1984) The relationship of structural pathology to the nerve root. *Spine,* **9**, 49–52.

Kirkaldy-Willis, W.H. (1988) A comprehensive outline of treatment. In *Managing Low Back Pain* (W.H. Kirkaldy-Willis, ed.), 2nd edition. Churchill Livingstone, New York, pp 247–264.

Kirkaldy-Willis, W.H. and Cassidy, J.D. (1984) Toward a more precise diagnosis of low back pain. In *Spine Update, 1984. Perspectives in Radiology, Orthopaedic Surgery and Neurosurgery* (H.K. Genant, ed.), Radiology Research and Education Foundation, San Francisco, pp. 5–16.

Kirkaldy-Willis, W.H. and McIvor, G.W.D. (1976) Lumbar spinal stenosis – editorial comment. *Clin. Orthop. Rel. Res.,* **115**, 2–3.

Kirkaldy-Willis, W.H. and Tchang, S. (1983) Diagnosis. In *Managing Low Back Pain* (W.H. Kirkaldy-Willis, ed.), Churchill Livingstone, New York, pp. 109–127.

Kirkaldy-Willis, W.H., Heithoff, K.B., Tchang, S. *et al.* (1984) Lumbar spondylosis and stenosis: correlation of pathological anatomy with high resolution computed tomographic scanning. In *Computed Tomography of the Spine* (M.J.D. Post, ed.). Williams and Wilkins, Baltimore, pp. 495–505.

Knight, A.D. and Levick, J. (1983) The density and distribution of capillaries around a synovial cavity. *Q. J. Exp. Physiol.,* **68**, 629–644.

Koehler, A. and Zimmer, E.A. (1968) *Borderlands of the Normal and Early Pathologic Skeletal Radiology*, 3rd edition. Translated and edited by S.P. Wilk. Grune and Stratton, New York.

Koreska, J., Robertson, D., Mills, R.H. *et al.* (1977) Biomechanics of the lumbar spine and its clinical significance. *Orthop. Clin. North Am.,* **8**, 121–133.

Korkala, D., Gronblad, M., Liesi, P. and Karaharju, E. (1985) Immunohistochemical demonstration of nociceptors in the ligamentous structures of the lumbar spine. *Spine,* **10**: 156–157.

Kos, J. (1969) Contribution a l'etude de l'anatomie et de la vascularisation des articulations intervertebrales. *Bull. Assoc. Anat. Berlin,* **142**, 1.088–1.105.

Kos, J. and Wolf, J. (1972) Les menisques intervertebraux et leur role possible dans les blocages vetebraux. *Ann. Med. Phys.,* **15**, 203–217.

Kraft, G.L. and Levinthal, D.H. (1951) Facet synovial impingement: a new concept in the etiology of lumbar vertebral derangement. *Surg. Gynecol. Obstet.,* **93**, 439–443.

Kuntz, A. (1953) *The Anatomic Nervous System*. Lea and Febiger, Philadelphia, pp. 157, 161.

Lee, J.A. and Atkinson, R.S. (eds) (1978) *Sir Robert Mackintosh's Lumbar Puncture and Spinal Analgesia, Intradural and Extradural*, 4th edition. Churchill Livingstone, Edinburgh, pp 24-70.

Levine, D.B. (1979) The painful low back. In *Arthritis and Allied Conditions* (D.J. McCarthy, ed.), 9th edition. Lea and Febiger, Philadelphia, pp 1044-1079.

Lewin, T. (1964) Osteoarthritis in lumbar synovial joints. *Acta Orthop. Scand. Suppl.*, **73**, 1-111.

Lewin, T. (1968) Anatomical variations in lumbosacral synovial joints with particular reference to subluxation. *Acta Anat.*, **71**, 229-248.

Lewin, T., Moffett, B. and Viidik, A. (1961) The morphology of the lumbar synovial intervertebral arches. *Acta Morphol. Neerlando-Scand.*, **4**: 299-319.

Lewinnik, G.E. and Warfield, C.A. (1986) Facet joint degeneration as a cause of low back pain. *Clin. Orthop.*, **213**, 216-222.

Lewit, K. (1968) Beitrag zur reversiblen Gelenksblockierung. *Zeitschr. Orthop.*, **105**, 150.

Liesi, P., Gronblad, M., Korkala, O. *et al.* (1983) Substance P: neuropiptide involved in low back pain. *Lancet*, **1**, 1328-1329.

Liew, M. and Dick, W.C. (1981) The anatomy and physiology of blood flow in a diarthrodial joint. *Clin. Rheum. Dis.*, **7**, 131-148.

Lutz, G. (1967) Die Entwicklung der kleinen Wirbelgelenke. *Z. Orthop.*, **104**, 19-28.

MacConaill, M.A. (1951) The movements of bones and joints (a) The mechanical structure of articulating cartilage. *J. Bone Joint Surg.*, **33B**, 251-257.

Mankin, H.J. (1975) Localization of tritiated thymedine in articular cartilage of rabbits. III. Mature articular cartilage. *J. Bone Joint Surg.*, **45A**, 529.

Marx, J.L. (1979) Brain peptides: is substance P a transmitter of pain signals? *Science*, **205**, 886-889.

Meachim, G. (1967) The histology and ultrastructure of cartilage. In *Proceedings of a Workshop on Cartilage: Degradation and Repair* (C.A.L. Bassett, ed.). National Research Council, Washington, p. 3.

Meachim, G. (1969) Age changes in articular cartilage. *Clin. Orthop.*, **64**, 33-44.

Meachim, G. and Roy, S. (1969) Surface ultrastructure of mature adult, human articular cartilage. *J. Bone Joint Surg.*, **51B**, 521-539.

Meachim, G. and Stockwell, R.A. (1979) The matrix. In *Adult Articular Cartilage* (M.A.R. Freeman, ed.), 2nd edition. Pitman Medical, Kent, pp 1-68.

Meade, T.W., Dyer, S., Brown, W. *et al.* (1990) Low back pain of mechanical origin: randomised comparison of chiropractic and hospital outpatient treatment. *Br. Med. J.*, **300**, 31-37.

Moir, D.D. (1980) *Obstetric Anaesthesia and Analgesia*, 2nd edition. Bailliére Tindall, London, p. 192.

Mooney, V. and Robertson, J. (1976) The facet syndrome. *Clin. Orthop.*, **115**, 9-156.

Moore, K.L. (1992) *Clinically Oriented Anatomy*, 3rd edition. Williams and Wilkins, Baltimore.

Naffziger, H.C., Inman, V. and Saunders, J.B. (1938) Lesions of the intervertebral disc and ligamenta flava. *Surg. Gynecol. Obstet.*, **66**, 288-299.

Paget, S. and Bullough, P.G. (1980) Synovium and synovial fluid. In *Scientific Foundations of Orthopaedics and Traumatology*. (R. Owen, J. Goodfellow and P. Bullough, eds). William Heinemann Medical Books, London, pp. 18-22.

Park, W.M. (1980) The place of radiology in the investigation of low back pain. *Clin. Rheum. Dis.*, **6**, 93-132.

Parkin, I.G. and Harrison, G.R. (1985) The topographical anatomy of the lumbar epidural space. *J. Anat.*, **141**, 211-217.

Pedersen, H.E., Blunck, C.F.J. and Gardner, E. (1956) The anatomy of lumbosacral posterior rami and meningeal branches of spinal nerves (sinu-vertebral nerves) with an experimental study of their function. *J. Bone Joint Surg.*, **38A**, 377-391.

Penning, L. and Tondury, B. (1963) Entstehung Bau und Funktion der meniscoiden Strukturen in den Halswirbelgelenken. *Z. Orthop.*, **98**, 1-14.

Pheasant, H.C. (1975) Sources of failure in laminectomies. *Orthop. Clin. North Am.*, **6**, 319-329.

Prasad, P., King, I., Denton, R.A. and Begeman, P.C. (1973) Intervertebral force transducer. In *Proceedings of the 10th International Conference of Medical Biological Engineers*, Dresden, p. 137.

Putz, R. (1981) Funktionelle Anatomie der Wirbelgelenke. In *Normale und Pathologische Anatomie*, Vol. 43. Georg Thieme Verlag, Stuttgart, pp. 31, 32.

Putz, R. (1985) The functional morphology of the superior articular processes of the lumbar vertebrae. *J. Anat.*, **143**, 181-187.

Quiring, D.P. and Warfel, J.W. (1960) *The Head, Neck and Trunk: Muscles and Motor Points*. Henry Kimpton, London, p. 57.

Ramsey, R.H. (1966) The anatomy of the ligamenta flava. *Clin. Orthop.*, **44**, 129-140.

Rauschning, W. (1983) Computed tomography and cryomicrotomy of lumbar spine specimens. *Spine*, **8**, 170-180.

Reilly, J., Yong-Hing, K., MacKay, R.W. and Kirkaldy-Willis, W.H. (1978) Pathological anatomy of the lumbar spine. In *Disorders of the Lumbar Spine* (S.J. Helfet and D.M. Gruebel, eds). J.B. Lippincott, Philadelphia, pp. 26-50.

Rhodin, J.A.G. (1974) *Histology: A Text and Atlas*. Oxford University Press, London, pp. 200, 340-362.

Rickenbacher, J., Landolt, A.M. and Theiler, K. (1985) *Applied Anatomy*. Springer-Verlag, Berlin, pp. 30, 31.

Rolander, S.D. (1966) Motion of the lumbar spine with special reference to the stabilising effect of posterior fusion. *Acta Orthop. Scand. Suppl.* 90.

Ross, M.H. and Reith, E.J. (1985) *Histology: A Text and Atlas*. Harper and Row, New York, pp. 114-120.

Rossell, S. (1982) Discussion. In *Substance P in the Nervous System*. Ciba Foundation Symposium 91, Pitman, London, p. 219.

Roy, S. and Meachim, G. (1968) Chondrocyte ultrastructure in adult human articular cartilage. *Ann. Rheum. Dis.*, **27**, 544.

Ruttner, J.R. and Spycher, M.A. (1968) Electron microscopic investigations on aging and osteoarthritic human cartilage. *Pathol. Microbiol.*, **31**, 14.

Salt, T.E., Crozier, C.S. and Hill, R.G. (1982) The effects of capsaicin pre-treatment on the responses of single neurones to sensory stimuli in the trigeminal nucleus caudalis of the rat: evidence against a role for substance P as the neurotransmitter serving termal nociception. *Neuroscience*, **7**, 11.

Sandoz, R. (1976) Some physical mechanisms and effects of spinal adjustments. *Ann. Swiss Chiropract. Assoc.*, **6**, 91-141.

Schmincke, A. and Santo, E. (1932) Zur normalen und pathologischen anatomie der halswirbelsaule. *Zbl. Allg. Path. Path. Anat.*, **55**, 369-372.

Schmorl, G. and Junghanns, H. (1971) *The Human Spine in*

Health and Disease, 2nd edition. Grune and Stratton, New York, pp. 23, 28, 188, 211.

Schumacher, H.R. (1975) Ultrastructure of the synovial membrane. *Ann. Clin. Lab. Sci.*, **5**, 489-498.

Semlak, K. and Ferguson, A.B. (1970) Joint stability maintained by atmospheric pressure. *Clin. Orthop.*, **68**, 294-300.

Shaw, N.E. and Martin, B.F. (1962) Histological and histochemical studies on mammalian knee joint tissues. *J. Anat.*, **96**, 359.

Shirazi-Adl, A. and Drouin, G. (1987) Load-bearing role of facets in a lumbar segment under sagittal plane loading. *J. Biomech.*, **20**, 601-613.

Simkin, P.A. (1979) Synovial physiology. In *Arthritis and Allied Conditions*, (D.J. McCarthy, ed.), 9th edition. Lea and Febiger, Philadelphia, pp. 167-178.

Simkin, P.A. and Nilson, K.L. (1981) Trans-synovial exchange of large and small molecules. *Clin. Rheum. Dis.*, **7**, 99-129.

Smeathers, J.E. and Biggs, W.D. (1980) Mechanics of the spinal column. In *Engineering Aspects of the Spine*. Mechanical Engineering Publications, London, pp. 103-109.

Sokoloff, L. (1969) *The Biology of Degenerative Joint Disease*. University Press, Chicago, p. 38.

Stockwell, R.A. (1979) *Biology of Cartilage Cells*. Cambridge University Press, Cambridge, p. 1.

Stockwell, R.A. (1985) *A Pre-Clinical View of Osteoarthritis*. A Sir John Struthers Lecture. Teviot Place, The Medical School, Edinburgh.

Stofft, E. and Graf, J. (1983) Scanning electron microscopic study of hyaline cartilage. *Acta Anat.*, **16**, 114-125.

Sunderland, S. (1980) The anatomy of the intervertebral foramen and the mechanisms of compression and stretch of nerve roots. In *Modern Developments in the Principles and Practice of Chiropractic* (S. Haldeman, ed.). Appleton-Century-Crofts, New York, p. 45-64.

Taylor, J.R. and Twomey, L. (1986) Age changes in lumbar zygapophysial joints: observations on structure and function. *Spine*, **11**, 739-745.

Tencer, A.F. and Mayer, T.G. (1983) Soft tissue strain and facet face interaction in the lumbar intervertebral joint. II: Calculated results and comparison with experimental data. *J. Biomech. Eng.*, **105**, 210-215.

Tobias, D., Ziv, I. and Maroudas, A. (1992) Human facet cartilage: swelling and some physico-chemical characteristics as a function of age. *Spine*, **17**, 694-700.

Tondury, G. (1940) Beitrag zur Kenntniss der kleinen Wirbelgelenke. *Z. Anat. Entw. Gesch.*, **110**, 568-575.

Tondury, G. (1972) Anatomie fonctionelle des petites articulations de rachis. *Ann. Med. Phys.*, **15**, 173-191.

Tulsi, R.S. and Hermanis, G.M. (1993) A study of the angle of inclination and facet curvature of superior lumbar zygapophysial joints. *Spine*, **18**, 1311-1317.

Twomey, L.T. (1981) *Age Changes in the Human Lumbar Vertebral Column*. Ph.D. thesis. Department of Anatomy and Human Biology, University of Western Australia, Perth.

Van Schaik, J.P.J., Verbiest, H. and van Schaik, F.D.J. (1985) The orientation of laminae and facet joints in the lower lumbar spine. *Spine*, **10**, 59-63.

Walmsley, R. (1972) Joints. In *Cunningham's Textbook of Anatomy* (G.J. Romanes, ed.), 11th edition. Oxford University Press, London, p. 211.

Wassilev, W. (1981) Funktionelle struktur der synovialmembran. *Verh. Anat. Ges.*, **75**, 221-234.

Weinstein, P.R., Ehni, G. and Wilson, C.B. (1977) Clinical features of lumbar spondylosis and stenosis. In *Lumbar Sprondylosis: Diagnosis, Management and Surgical Treatment* (P.R. Weinstein, G. Ehni and C.B. Wilson, eds). Year Book Medical Publishers, Chicago, pp. 115-133.

Weiss, C., Rosenberg, L. and Helfet, A.J. (1968) An ultrastructural study of normal, young adult, human articular cartilage. *J. Bone Joint Surg.*, **50A**, 663-674.

Williams, P.L. and Warwick, T. (1980) *Gray's Anatomy*, 36th edition. Churchill Livingstone, London, pp. 271, 427, 445, 545.

Wolf, J. (1969) Chondrosynovial membrane serving as joint cavity lining with a sliding and barrier function. *Fol. Morphol.*, **17**, 291-308.

Wolf, J. (1975a) Les ménisques intervertébraux et leur rôle possible dans les blocages vertébraux. *Ann. Méd. Phys.*, **15**, 204-218.

Wolf, J. (1975b) Function of chondral membrane on surface of articular cartilage from point of view of its mechanical resistance. *Fol. Morphol.*, **23**, 77-87.

Yang, K.H. and King, A.I. (1984) Mechanism of facet load transmission as a hypothesis for low back pain. *Spine*, **9**, 559-565.

Ziv, I., Maroudas, C., Robin, G. and Maroudas, A. (1993) Human facet cartilage: swelling and some physicochemical characteristics as a function of age. *Spine*, **18**, 136-146.

Zukschwerdt, L., Emminger, E., Biedermann, F. and Zettel, H. (1955) *Wirbelgelenk und Bandscheibe*. Stuttgart.

6

Spinal and intervertebral canals

L.G.F. Giles

Anatomy

Spinal canal

In cross section, the lumbar spinal canal usually approximates a triangular outline (Figures 3.13 and 3.15), but it can become trefoil in shape because incurved laminae and/or superior facets may encroach upon it (McRae, 1977). According to Eisenstein (1980), a trefoil configuration is a common non-pathologic condition, usually of the fifth lumbar vertebral canal, and is not necessarily dependent on or related to increasing age, osteophytosis, or spinal stenosis. However, Keim and Kirkaldy-Willis (1987) point out that the formation of osteophytes around the periphery of the vertebral body of zygapophysial joints may narrow the central or lateral neural canals, causing stenosis, which may produce pressure or tension on adjacent nerves inducing the nerve root entrapment syndrome. The spinal canal encloses the spinal dural tube and its contents, the conus medullaris, cauda equina, and their blood vessels, bathed in cerebrospinal fluid (CSF) (McRae, 1977). The extradural 'space' is filled by varying amounts of fat, areolar tissue, and blood vessels (McRae, 1977), including the valveless extradural veins (Batson, 1957; Shapiro, 1975). Hasue *et al.* (1983) also described an epidural membrane, interposed between the dura and ligamentum flavum, as being continuous with an epiradicular sheath around the nerve roots and Wiltse *et al.* (1993) recently reported a detailed study which re-investigated the contents of the spinal canal, including the fibrovascular membrane (Fick, 1904) and Hofmann's (1898) ligaments.

The lumbar spinal canal lateral width increases steadily from L1 (23.7 ± 0.92 mm) to L5 (27.1 ± 0.88 mm), with an average transverse diameter of

25 mm (Dommisse, 1975). The spinal canal antero-posterior depth decreases from L1 (19.0 ± 0.67 mm) to L3 (17.5 ± 0.53 mm) then increases from L3 to L5 (19.7 ± 0.49 mm) (Panjabi *et al.*, 1992). While the cross-sectional area decreases from L1 (320 ± 18.10 mm²) to L2 (281 ± 15.38 mm²), it is approximately constant from L2 to L4, then increases at L5 (330 ± 21.2 mm²) (Panjabi *et al.*, 1992).

Intervertebral canal

The intervertebral canal (intervertebral foramen, lateral canal, nerve root tunnel, radicular canal, root canal, interpedicular canal) is clinically a very important structure, which exits from the spinal canal via the lateral recess (Dorwart and Genant, 1983). Therefore, it is described in considerable detail in this chapter.

Over the years, standard anatomical textbooks such as *Gray's Anatomy* (Williams and Warwick, 1980), *Cunningham's Textbood of Anatomy* (Romanes, 1981), *A Colour Atlas of Human Anatomy* (McMinn and Hutchings, 1977), and *Clinically Oriented Anatomy* (Moore, 1992) have used the term 'intervertebral foramina' to describe both the osseous nerve root canals and their medial and lateral 'openings'. However, Dommisse (1975) correctly suggests that the term 'foramen' should only be used to describe the inner and outer boundaries of intervertebral canals. The term 'intervertebral canal' is used in this text since it appears to be a more accurate description of the structure which can be quite long, particularly at the lumbosacral level.

The first detailed histological study of the human intervertebral canal was reported by Swanberg (1915a,b) and various subsequent studies have been documented by several authors (Oppenheimer, 1937;

Larmon, 1944; Magnuson, 1944; Crelin, 1973; Dorwart and Genant, 1983; Yeager, 1986; Rauschning, 1987; Twomey and Taylor, 1988; Peretti *et al.*, 1989; Giles and Kaveri, 1990; Giles, 1992; Jayson, 1992). Within the intervertebral canal are found important neural structures originating from the spinal cord as small anterior and posterior *rootlets* which converge caudally to form a common *nerve root trunk*, the posterior root of which has a spinal ganglion, beyond which the anterior and posterior roots mix and form a *spinal nerve* (Figure 6.1).

The relatively large spinal nerve roots and ganglion pass obliquely through each of these lumbar osteoligamentous intervertebral canals (Figures 6.1 and 6.2), which have a *medial* and *lateral* foramen (Dommisse, 1975), as does the relatively small neural structure, the recurrent meningeal nerve (Von Luschka, 1850)

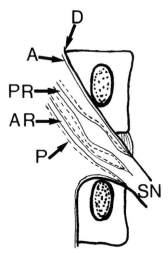

Figure 6.2 Diagram showing an enlargement of the interpedicular zone of a lumbar intervertebral canal, referred to in Figure 6.1, with its adjacent relatively large neural structures, the anterior root (AR), the posterior root (PR) with its spinal ganglion, and the spinal nerve (SN). The nerve roots and the spinal ganglion are bathed within the cerebrospinal fluid as far as the intervertebral foramen. The dura mater (D) and arachnoid mater (A) of the dural sac extend as the dural sleeve as far as the spinal nerve. The dura mater blends with the epineurium of the spinal nerve. The subdural space is a potential space containing a film of serous fluid whereas the subarachnoid space is well defined and contains the cerebrospinal fluid. Note the proximity of the dural sleeve and some neural structures to the cephalad pedicle. (Modified and reproduced with permission from Giles, L.G.F. (1994) A histologicigal investigation of human lower lumbar intervertebral canal (foramen) dimensions. *J. Manipulative Physiol. Ther.*, **17**, 4–14.

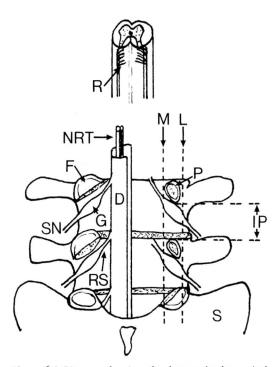

Figure 6.1 Diagram showing the human lumbar spinal canal, the medial (M) and lateral (L) borders of the intervertebral canal, and the remains of the pedicles on the right side (P) from which the vertebral arches have been removed. Anterior and posterior rootlets (R) leave the spinal cord then converge to form anterior and posterior nerve root trunks (NRT), the posterior root of which has a spinal ganglion (G), beyond which the anterior and posterior roots join to form a spinal nerve (SN). D = dura with arachnoid lining; F = facet (partly resected) of superior articular process; IP = interpedicular zone of the intervertebral canal; RS = root sleeve; S = sacrum. (Reproduced with permission from Giles, L.G.F. (1994) A histological investigation of human lower lumbar intervertebral canal (foramen) dimensions. *J. Manipulative Physiol. Ther.*, **17**, 4–14.

which is present at all vertebral levels (Kimmel, 1961a,b) and contains autonomic and somatic sensory fibres (Allbrook, 1974).

The oblique course of the intervertebral canals is approximately 18.5 mm long at the L4–5 level and 22.7 mm long at the lumbosacral (L5–S1) level in males and females of 60 years and over (Twomey and Taylor, 1988), although the pedicle width in the horizontal plane ranges from 8.7 to 12.0 mm at L4, and from 8.4 to 14.7 mm at L5 (Berry *et al.*, 1987; Scoles *et al.*, 1988). For clinical purposes, the intervertebral canal is considered to have three zones (Lee *et al.*, 1988), each with its own characteristic shape and contents (Figure 6.3).

The intervertebral canal starts in the spinal canal at the point where the nerve root sheath comes off the dural sac and ends where the spinal nerve emerges from the intervertebral canal laterally (Kirkaldy-Willis and McIvor, 1976), i.e. at the area surrounding the intervertebral foramen proper (Rauschning, 1987). Therefore the *spinal nerve* does not pass through the length of the intervertebral canal.

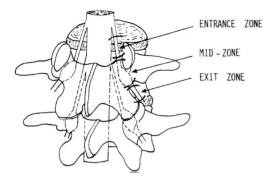

ENTRANCE ZONE

MID - ZONE

EXIT ZONE

Figure 6.3 The three zones of the intervertebral canal of the lumbar spine are shown by the brackets. (Reproduced with permission from Giles, L.G.F. (1992) Ligaments traversing the intervertebral canals of the human lower lumbosacral spine. *Neuro-Orthopedics*, **13**, 25–38.)

The intervertebral canal's clinically important three zones are: the *entrance zone* (lateral recess area), the *mid-zone* (sublamina blind zone) and the *exit zone* (near the intervertebral 'foramen' (Lee, 1988; Lee *et al.*, 1988)) (Figure 6.3).

Large diameter neural structures, such as the dorsal root ganglion and the nerve root, contained in the intervertebral canal zones are (1) the lumbar nerve root, covered by dura mater and bathed in CSF in the *entrance zone*, (2) the dorsal root ganglion and ventral motor nerve root (funiculus) covered by a fibrous connective tissue extension of the dura mater, bathed in CSF, in the *mid-zone*, and (3) the lumbar peripheral (spinal) nerve, which is covered by perineurium, in the *exit zone* (Lee *et al.*, 1988). The relatively small diameter neural structure contained in the intervertebral canal, the sinuvertebral nerve, arises from the anterior primary ramus and the gray ramus communicans (von Luschka, 1850; Bogduk, 1980), re-enters the intervertebral canal (von Luschka, 1850; Hovelacque, 1925) before dividing into terminal branches which supply the walls of extradural veins (Hovelacque, 1925), the posterior longitudinal ligament (Spurling and Bradford, 1939), bone on the posterior aspects of vertebral bodies, the adjacent outer layer of the anulus fibrosus (Hovelacque, 1925) and the flaval ligaments (Roofe, 1970; Wyke, 1970). The sinuvertebral nerve is discussed in greater detail in Chapter 14.

According to Peretti *et al.* (1989), the spinal nerve root and ganglion lie immediately below the pedicle of the subjacent vertebra, although Williams and Warwick (1980), Haughton and Williams (1982), Rydevik *et al.* (1984) and Van der Linden (1984) describe the spinal ganglion as lying within the central or lateral portion of the intervertebral canal, and Hasue *et al.* (1989) classify the L5 and S1 spinal ganglia as being (a) intraspinal, in which more than

half the ganglion lies in the spinal canal, (b) intraforaminal, or (c) extraforaminal, in which most of the ganglion lies outside the intervertebral canal.

The spinal nerve roots do not have the same amounts of protective connective tissue sheaths as the more peripheral nerves (Rydevik, 1992), which has led to the suggestion that the spinal nerve roots are more susceptible to mechanical deformation from spinal degenerative disorders than are peripheral nerves (Rydevik *et al.*, 1984). According to Crelin (1982), the 'spacious lumbar intervertebral foramen' contains a combination of delicate, loose areolar and fatty tissue which fills the space between the bony margins and the dural sheath. Also passing through the intervertebral canal are small blood vessels, nerves (Crelin, 1982) and lymphatics (Rauschning, 1987).

The average superior-to-inferior diameter of the interpedicular zone of the intervertebral canals is 19 mm (L4–L5 level), and 12 mm (L5–S1 level), respectively, while its average anteroposterior diameter is 7 mm (Magnuson, 1944) from the vertebral body to the ligamentum flavum at both the L4–L5 and L5–S1 levels. The average anteroposterior diameter of the ganglion at both levels is also 7 mm (Magnuson, 1944), or only a fraction of a millimeter less (Larmon, 1944). Postural changes result in variation of the size of this opening (Breig, 1960) which, according to Epstein (1960), is estimated to be normally five to six times as large as the transverse area of the nerve passing through it in the lumbar region, allowing for a generous reserve cushion (Dommisse, 1974; Sunderland, 1975). The cross-sectional area of the intervertebral canal increases from L1–L2 to L4–L5 but at L5–S1 it is smaller than the rest, even though the L5 spinal nerve is the largest lumbar nerve (Hasue *et al.*, 1983) and is approximately equal in size to the first sacral nerve (Swanberg, 1915a).

Crelin (1973) removed the areolar tissue surrounding the *spinal nerves* emerging from the *lateral* borders of the intervertebral canals in order to expose these *lateral* borders of the canal, then used gross mechanical stress studies (extreme flexion, extension and lateral bending) on three infant and three adult (35–76 year) human spines to examine and measure this artificially induced spatial relationship between *spinal nerves* and the adjacent *lateral* borders of the intervertebral canals; the method of measurement was not described. It is misleading to draw conclusions about the possible effect on more remote neural function when only the relationship between *spinal nerves* and the size of their intervertebral canal's *lateral* border dimension is examined, while completely ignoring the far more anatomically and clinically important *interpedicular zone* of the intervertebral canal relationship with its related neural structures. Therefore, a histological study was specifically undertaken by

Giles (1994) to measure accurately the cross-sectional area of the important *interpedicular zone* of intervertebral canals, i.e. between their *medial* and *lateral* borders (Dommisse, 1975), and their related large neural structures at the L4–L5 and L5–S1 levels in nine lumbosacral spines using blocks of osteoligamentous tissue (Figures 6.4 and 6.5) for histological processing.

The mounted histological sections (Figure 6.5) were used to locate the medial and lateral openings of the intervertebral canal and for histological and measurement studies (Giles, 1994).

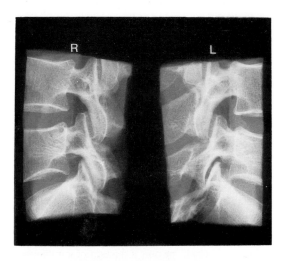

Figure 6.4 These osteoligamentous blocks of tissue show the paired left (L) and right (R) anatomical regions retained for histological processing. (Reproduced with permission from Giles, L.G.F. (1992) A histological investigation of human lower lumbar intervertebral canal (foramen) dimensions.) (Reproduced with permission from Giles, L.G.F. (1992) Ligaments traversing the intervertebral canals of the human lower lumbosacral spine. *Neuro-Orthopedics*, **13**, 25–38.)

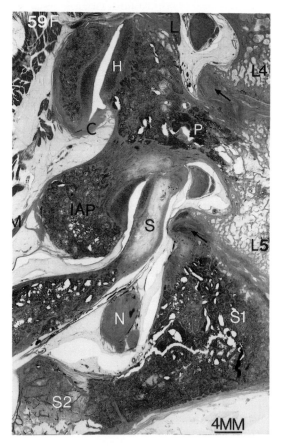

Figure 6.5 A 200 μm thick histological section cut in the parasagittal plane which shows parts of the fourth lumbar (L4) to first sacral (S1) spinal segments of a 59-year-old female. The large neural structures, i.e. the nerve roots and ganglion (N), which float in the cerebrospinal fluid, are shown within the L4–L5 and L5–S1 intervertebral canals and within the sacral canal. Posterolateral intervertebral disc herniations (arrows) with thinning of the L4 and L5 intervertebral discs is demonstrated; this has resulted in approximation of the vertebral bodies and imbrication (subluxation) of the opposing facets with their hyaline articular cartilages (H). The zygapophysial joint imbrication appears to have caused some tractioning of the L4–L5 joint capsule (C) inferiorly and 'buckling' of the ligamentum flavum at the L5–S1 level. This 'buckling', together with early osteophytosis of the superior articular process (S) of the sacrum, has caused deformation and unilateral compression of the adjacent neural structure. IAP = inferior articular process of L5 vertebra; L = ligamentum flavum; M = multifidus muscle tendon; P = pedicle of L5 vertebra; Ehrlich's haematoxylin and light green counterstain. (Modified and reproduced with permission from Giles, L.G.F. (1994) A histological investigation of human lower lumbar intervertebral canal (foramen) dimensions. *J. Manipulative Physiol. Ther.*, **17**, 4–14)

Visual comparison of the L4-L5 and L5-S1 intervertebral discs to estimate any degree of intervertebral disc thinning showed that there was only thinning of 75% at one L4-L5 and two L5-S1 intervertebral discs out of the nine spines examined. From the nine spines bisected in the median plane, 18 L4-L5 and 18 L5-S1 left and right intervertebral canals were examined in the parasagittal plane providing information on a total of 36 intervertebral canal interpedicular zones.

Neural and vascular structures were found to be deformed within some intervertebral canals and an example of a deformed neural structure at the lumbosacral level is shown in Figure 6.5. Due to posterolateral herniation and thinning of the L4-L5 and lumbosacral intervertebral discs in this 59-year-old female, there is a subluxation of the L4-L5 and L5-S1 facet surfaces. At L5-S1 this has caused buckling of the ligamentum flavum, resulting in an indentation of the adjacent large neural structure.

The measurement study (Giles, 1994) was clinically important as it showed:

(i) the mean *cross-sectional area ratio* of the interpedicular zone of the intervertebral canal to large neural structures, for the L4-L5 level (left and right sides combined) ranges from 22.9 (SD 6.7) to 30.8 (SD 4.4)%, and for the L5-S1 level from 24.9 (SD 5.3) to 31.1 (SD 5.3)%, i.e. the intervertebral canal is 3.3 (SD 0.5) to 4.8 (SD 1.7) times larger than that of the large neural structures at the L4-L5 level, and 3.3 (SD 0.6)-4.2 (SD 0.8) at the L5-S1 level.

(ii) The mean *height* of the interpedicular zone of the intervertebral canal ranges from 15.3 (SD 1.8) to 21.7 (SD 2.5) mm at L4-L5, and from 12.2 (SD 1.5) to 20.1 (SD 2.9) mm at L5-S1.

(iii) The mean *width* of the interpedicular zone of the intervertebral canal from the ligamentum flavum to the vertebral body ranges from 8.0 (SD 1.1) to 12.3 (SD 1.8) mm at L4-L5, and from 8.6 (SD 1.2) to 13.6 (SD 2.4) mm at L5-S1.

(iv) The mean minimum distance between the large neural structure(s) and the boundary of the interpedicular zone ranges from 0.4 (SD 0.4) to 0.8 (SD 0.9) mm at the L4-L5 level, and from 0.4 (SD 0.4) to 0.6 (SD 0.3) mm at the L5-S1 level, and

(v) The *average length* of the interpedicular zone of the intervertebral canal, based on the number of 200 μm thick histological sections spanning the zone of the canals examined, ranges from 8.2 to 10.2 mm at L4-L5, and from 8.2 to 12.2 mm at L5-S1.

It is unfortunate that in Crelin's (1973) study of three infant and three adult cadavers, which were not radiographed, he did not refer to the earlier and not insignificant adult postmortem studies by Larmon

(1944) and Magnuson (1944), and to Swanberg's (1915a,b) histological examination of a 5-month-old infant's right seventh thoracic intervertebral canal. Larmon's (1944) study of ten unselected human lumbosacral spines, obtained at autopsy, found that '1: comparing the average size of the fourth and fifth lumbar nerves (which measured a fraction of a millimetre less than 7 mm) to the average anteroposterior diameter of the foramina, which measured 7 mm, one is impressed by the intimate relationship of the nerve to the foramen, and 2: moderate swelling of the capsular ligamentum flavum can cause compression of the nerve in the foramen'. Magnuson (1944) confirmed that 'any swelling or inflammation around the foramen could narrow the canal sufficiently to cause pressure upon the nerve root'. As Swanberg (1915a) noted, the size of the intervertebral canal as compared to the nerves is dependent upon the part of the nerves within the intervertebral canal. Nonetheless, Crelin (1973) concluded from his biomechanical studies that (a) there was 'never less than 4 mm of space surrounding the lumbar nerves' in adults, (b) 'under all conditions, a relatively large amount of space surrounded the nerves in the foramina', and (c) 'any reduction in the size of the intervertebral foramina during the application of torsional force was insignificant in relation to the spinal nerves passing through the foramina'. However, Crelin's (1973) conclusions were based only on his examination of the relatively insignificant *lateral border* of the exposed (dissected) intervertebral canals and their emerging spinal nerves.

The histological study by Giles (1994) demonstrates that, between the *medial* and *lateral* borders of the interpedicular zone of the intervertebral canal, its horizontal length ranges from 8.2 to 10.2 mm at L4-L5 and from 8.2 to 12.2 mm at L5-S1, which is in agreement with the findings of Berry *et al.* (1987) and Scoles *et al.* (1988) for pedicle width, although pedicle width can be greater at both the fourth and fifth lumbar levels according to Krag *et al.* (1986, 1988), Zindrick *et al.* (1987) and Panjabi *et al.* (1992) with a maximum width of 14.1 mm at L4 and 18.6 mm at L5 (Panjabi *et al.*, 1992). The ratio of the mean cross-sectional area of the large neural structure(s) to that of the interpedicular zone of the intervertebral canal ranges from 22.9 to 30.8% at the L4-L5 level, and 24.9-31.1% at the L5-S1 level. This can also be expressed in terms of the cross-sectional area of the interpedicular zone of the intervertebral canal being approximately only 3.3-4.8 times larger than the large neural structures at the L4-L5 level and 3.3-4.2 times larger than the large neural structures at the L5-S1 level, which results in a less generous reserve cushion than that suggested by Epstein (1960), Crelin (1973), Dommisse (1975) and Sunderland (1974).

The original histological technique used by Giles and Taylor (1983) to study large blocks of spinal osteoligamentous tissues showed that there was an overall shrinkage factor of 8.6% between osseous structures seen on X-ray images of the unprocessed blocks and these same osseous structures as seen on mounted histological sections. Shrinkage for individual soft tissue structures was not determined, but it would be reasonable to expect it to be at least as much as for osseous structures. Bearing this in mind, the figures shown in the present study would most likely represent the minimum space occupied by the soft tissue structures within the mainly osseous interpedicular zone of the intervertebral canal.

Clinical implications

At the L4–L5 spinal level, the minimum distance between the neural structures and the boundary of the *interpedicular zone* of the intervertebral canal ranges from 0.4 (SD 0.4) to 0.8 (SD 0.9) mm. At the L5–S1 level, this distance ranges from 0.4 (SD 0.4) to 0.6 (SD 0.3) mm. In view of this, Crelin's (1973) finding that there was never less than 4 mm of space surrounding the lumbar 'nerves' in adults at the *lateral* border of the foramen of the intervertebral canal, which lead to his statement that 'under all conditions, a relatively large amount of space surrounds the nerves in the foramina', is meaningless as a basis for considering the possible physiological and or pathophysiological functions of spinal nerves beyond the intervertebral canal as he did not examine the important interpedicular zone. Furthermore, documented evidence by Peretti *et al.* (1989), describing lumbar and the first sacral roots as lying immediately below the subjacent pedicle, raises serious concerns about the conclusions of Crelin's (1973) study.

When the interpedicular zone space is further diminished by (i) intervertebral disc herniation, with or without accompanying osteophytosis of the adjacent vertebral body or of the adjacent part of the zygapophysial joint facet (Isherwood and Antoun, 1980; Giles and Kaveri 1990), (ii) transforaminal ligaments (Chapter 7), or (iii) 'buckling' or hypertrophy of the ligamentum flavum (Rothman and Simeone, 1975), it is quite conceivable that direct pressure upon neural structures will occur within the interpedicular zone of the intervertebral canal. Such deformation and unilateral compression of neural structures has been demonstrated in this chapter (Figure 6.5) and in other publications (Giles and Kaveri, 1990). The foregoing clearly shows that it is wrong to draw conclusions on 'spinal nerves passing through the foramina' when the *nerve roots* and the *spinal ganglion* within the important interpedicular zone of the intervertebral canal, upon whose normal function the *spinal nerves* depend for *their* normal physiological function, are not studied.

As the findings of Larmon (1944), Magnuson (1944) and Giles (1994) indicate that nerve roots and the spinal ganglion do not necessarily have a generous protective reserve cushion within the important interpedicular zone of the intervertebral canal, their respective nerve roots and spinal ganglia may well be subjected to mechanical deformation and compression. This could induce a sequence of events including impairment of nerve root blood flow and oxygen supply, and increased microvascular permeability. This could lead to intraneural oedema formation with blockage of axonal transport, which may lead to long-term alterations in nerve function (Rydevik *et al.*, 1990; Rydevik, 1992). Mechanical deformation and compression of the dural sleeve and its contents may also lead to interference with the normal movement of CSF around the nerve roots and the spinal ganglion. Furthermore, compressive irritation of the nociceptive receptor system embedded in the dural sleeves surrounding the lower spinal nerve roots may arise, especially should there be intervertebral disc and/or osteophytic projection into the intervertebral canals (Wyke, 1982).

It seems perfectly reasonable to discount as irrelevant the conclusion made in Crelin's (1973) paper that 'the exertion of pressure on a spinal nerve does not occur' as he only dissected then examined spinal nerves emerging from the *lateral* foramen of the intervertebral canal and he did not examine the important structures within the interpedicular zone of the intervertebral canal which unite to form the spinal nerve which, after all, does not function in isolation.

It is obvious from Giles' (1994) histological investigation of neural structures within the important interpedicular zone of the intervertebral canal that neural and associated vascular structures may well be compromised due to vertebral joint subluxation. This may result in chronic compression, of yet undetermined magnitude, upon neural and vascular structures within the confines of the anatomically and clinically important interpedicular zone of the intervertebral canal. The clinical significance of such compression is yet to be determined. However, nerve fibres in spinal nerve roots, as well as in peripheral nerves, are dependent upon a continuous supply of oxygen and other nutrients in order to maintain proper function; interference with the nutritional supply to nervous tissue from chronic compression lesions such as spinal stenosis can lead to deterioration of nerve function (Rydevik *et al.*, 1990) (see Chapter 16).

Because of the clinical importance of the structures passing through the three zones of the intervertebral canal, further details of the clinical anatomy of this canal follow, with some emphasis on the possible effects of stenosis upon the neurovascular structures.

Pathology

Stenosis

Spinal stenosis may result from developmental or acquired lesions or a combination of both; it may be symmetrical or asymmetrical, central or lateral, and may be due to soft tissue changes, such as intervertebral disc herniation, fibrous scar, ligamentum flavum hypertrophy (see Figure 13.11) tumour, or bony changes (Bullough and Boachie-Adjei, 1988). According to Dorwart *et al.* (1983), stenosing lesions of the spine can have three anatomic sites, i.e. central canal, subarticular canal and the intervertebral canal.

Patients with lumbar central canal stenosis (see Figure 4.1) may present with a variety of clinical symptoms including back pain, radiculopathy, and neurogenic claudication (Herzog *et al.*, 1991).

Much attention has been paid to the causes of vertebral canal stenosis in humans but relatively little has been documented with regard to intervertebral canal stenosis. This is an important clinical issue because, as the dural sleeve ends at the outer opening of the intervertebral canal, a false 'normal' myelogram is possible when a space occupying lesion occurs beyond the subarachnoid space. Also, if stenosis affects only vascular structures, compression of these structures cannot be noted during myelography, so venous stasis may be overlooked.

It is well known that degenerative changes in the intervertebral discs are always accompanied by osteophyte formation on the margins of the vertebral bodies and remodelling changes in the zygapophysial joints (Vernon-Roberts and Price, 1977; Kirkaldy-Willis *et al.*, 1984), and there is usually a direct relationship between the degree of disc degeneration, vertebral body marginal osteophyte formation, and zygapophysial joint changes (Vernon-Roberts and Price, 1977). These degenerative changes can lead to lumbar spinal stenosis, which may involve the spinal canal and/or the intervertebral canal (Kirkaldy-Willis and McIvor, 1976). In this chapter, emphasis is placed on intervertebral canal stenosis.

Intervertebral canal zones

The most common causes of stenosis in the three zones are (a) in the *entrance zone*, hypertrophic osteoarthritis of the zygapophysial joint (particularly of the superior articular process), while other causes are developmental variations of the zygapophysial joints, and the pedicle (if short), or an osteophytic ridge or bulging anulus anterior to the nerve root, (b) in the *mid-zone*, osteophyte formation under the pars interarticularis where the ligamentum flavum is attached, and fibrocartilaginous or bursal tissue hypertrophy at a spondylolytic defect, and (c) in the

exit zone, hypertrophic osteoarthritic changes of the zygapophysial joints, with facet subluxation (imbrication, telescoping), and osteophytic ridge formation along the superior margin of the disc (Lee *et al.*, 1988). The osteoarthritic changes of zygapophysial joints are characterized by defects or abnormalities of articular cartilage with related changes in the subchondral bone, bony margins of the joint, surrounding capsule, synovium, and para-articular structures (Altman and Dean, 1989), and the L4–L5 and L5–S1 spinal levels are most frequently involved in zygapophysial joint and intervertebral disc degenerative changes (McRae, 1977; Bullough and Boachie-Adjei, 1988).

Herniated intervertebral discs or osteophytes which cause nerve root compression have long been implicated in low back pain and sciatica (Mixter and Barr, 1934; Coventry *et al.*, 1945; Bullough and Boachie-Adjei, 1988), although there is a poor correlation between the severity of radiographic changes and back pain (Stockwell, 1985). Furthermore, osteophytic degenerative changes do not regress, whereas symptoms of low back pain and sciatica can vary, with remissions and exacerbations.

Therefore, a cadaveric study was undertaken to investigate some causes of intervertebral canal stenosis due to encroachment by bony and soft tissue structures, with the following findings.

Some degree of osteophytosis involving the intervertebral joints of all the cadavers was found on various radiographic views. Histological investigation of these lumbosacral spines showed that six out of 12 (50%) lumbosacral intervertebral joints showed unilateral posterolateral contained (i.e. non-sequestrated) intervertebral disc herniation, varying from minor (i.e. with no pressure on neural or vascular structures) to large (i.e. causing deformation of neural and vascular structures due to the herniation projecting up to 5 mm into the intervertebral canal).

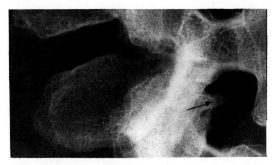

Figure 6.6 A lateral radiographic view of the L5–S1 intervertebral canal in a 71-year-old female. Note the relatively normal thickness of the intervertebral disc, and the large osteophyte (arrow) causing intervertebral canal stenosis. (Reproduced with permission from Giles, L.G.F. and Kaveri, M.J.P. (1990) Some osseous and soft tissue causes of human intervertebral canal (foramen) stenosis. *J. Rheumatol.*, **17**, 1474–1481.)

In this study, *contained herniation* refers to nuclear material which has not escaped from the confines of the anular fibres. In each case, the herniation was found to be at the posterolateral region of the disc and no midline posterior herniations were found. Two out of 12 (17%) minor contained unilateral posterolateral intervertebral disc herniations were found at the L4–L5 level. Various shapes and sizes of osteophytes involved 24 of the 48 zygapophysial joints examined histologically and some of the osteophytes were large enough to be recorded radiographically as causing considerable stenosis of the intervertebral canal. An example of a large osteophyte projecting from the superior articular process of the sacrum into the adjacent intervertebral canal in a 71-year-old female is shown in Figure 6.6. A further radiographic example is shown for an 83-year-old female (Figure 6.7) with associated histopathological findings (Figure 6.8).

In Figure 6.7, there is approximately 40% thinning of the lumbosacral intervertebral disc with intervertebral canal stenosis caused by subluxation of the zygapophysial joint facet surfaces and osteophytosis (arrow) at the superior margin of the sacral articular facets. On the anteroposterior radiograph of this specimen, some vertebral body posterolateral osteophytosis was noted on the left side, and this was found to be associated with a minor contained intervertebral disc herniation upon histological investigation, as demonstrated in Figure 6.8 which is a parasagittal histological section through the left lumbosacral zygapophysial joint showing an osteophyte at the superior margin of the sacral facet. Note how this osteophyte, together with the minor contained intervertebral disc herniation and its adjacent osteophyte, have a 'pincer' effect across the centre of the intervertebral canal, resulting in stenosis of the anteroposterior diameter of this part of the canal and disruption of the dorsal root ganglion and the spinal nerves with their associated blood vessels.

The L5–S1 zygapophysial joint shows advanced osteoarthritic changes, with fibrillation and loss of hyaline articular cartilage on the superior articular process of the sacrum, with almost complete loss of the cartilage on the inferior articular process of the fifth lumbar vertebra. Sclerosis is evident in both subchondral surfaces of the facets.

When a posterolateral intervertebral disc herniation occurs, varying degrees of intervertebral canal

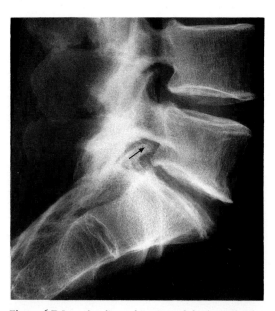

Figure 6.7 Lateral radiographic view of the lower lumbosacral spine of an 83-year-old female. Approximately 40% thinning of the lumbosacral intervertebral disc is noted with anterior osteophytosis, and stenosis of the intervertebral canal due to subluxation of the L5–S1 zygapophysial joint facet surfaces and osteophytic enlargement of the sacral articular facets (arrow). (Reproduced with permission from Giles, L.G.F. and Kaveri, M.J.P. (1990) Some osseous and soft tissue causes of human intervertebral canal (foramen) stenosis. *J. Rheumatol.*, **17**, 1474–1481.)

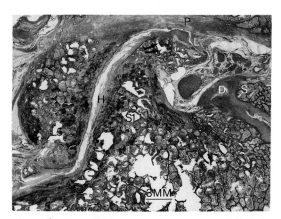

Figure 6.8 A parasagittal section (cut at a thickness of 100 μm) through the left lumbosacral intervertebral canal of an 83-year-old female, at the posterolateral region of the intervertebral disc, and the zygapophysial joint, of the specimen in Figure 6.7. D = a minor, 3 mm long, contained posterolateral herniation of the intervertebral disc with adjacent osteophytic spur (S) which, in conjunction with the large 5 mm long osteophytic spur (arrows) at the superior margin of the superior articular process, cause stenosis of the intervertebral canal and deformation of the motor and sensory nerves with their associated blood vessels. H = osteoarthritic hyaline articular cartilage on the superior articular process of the first sacral segment (S1); L5 = inferior articular process of L5; L = ligamentum flavum; P = pedicle of L5 vertebra. Ehrlich's haematoxylin and light green counterstain. (Reproduced with permission from Giles, L.G.F. and Kaveri, M.J.P. (1990) Some osseous and soft tissue causes of human intervertebral canal (foramen) stenosis. *J. Rheumatol.*, **17**, 1474–1481.)

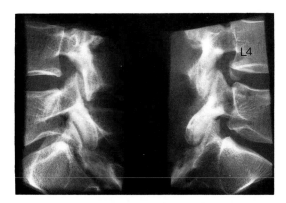

Figure 6.9 Radiograph showing the left and right sides of a sagittally bisected lower lumbosacral spine of a 45-year-old male. Note the osteophytic spur at the posterolateral inferior margin of the L4 vertebral body and the calcification inside the margin of the intervertebral disc space.

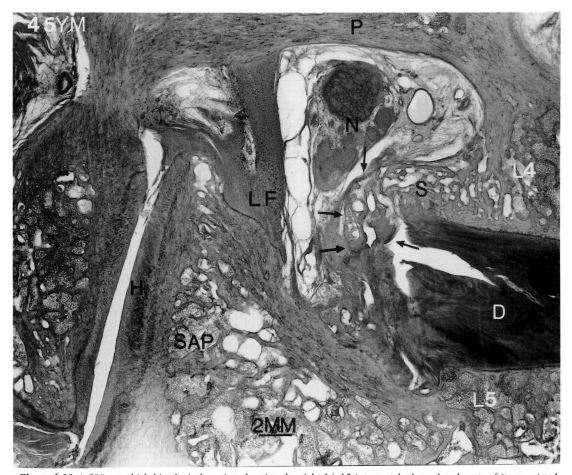

Figure 6.10 A 200 µm thick histological section showing the right L4–L5 intervertebral canal and parts of its associated intervertebral disc (D) and zygapophysial joint. H = hyaline articular cartilage of the fifth lumbar superior articular process (SAP); LF = ligamentum flavum; N = large neural structures; P = pedicle. Note the intervertebral disc degenerative changes and the associated large osteophytic spur (S) projecting (arrows) into the intervertebral canal which causes stenosis of this canal (Ehrlich's haematoxylin and light green counterstain).

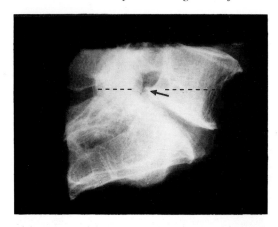

Figure 6.11 There is advanced thinning of the lumbosacral intervertebral disc with discogenic spondylosis (67-year-old female). The arrow indicates an osteophyte which appears to project posteriorly into the lumbosacral intervertebral canal. The dotted line shows the approximate level of the histological section shown in Figure 6.12.

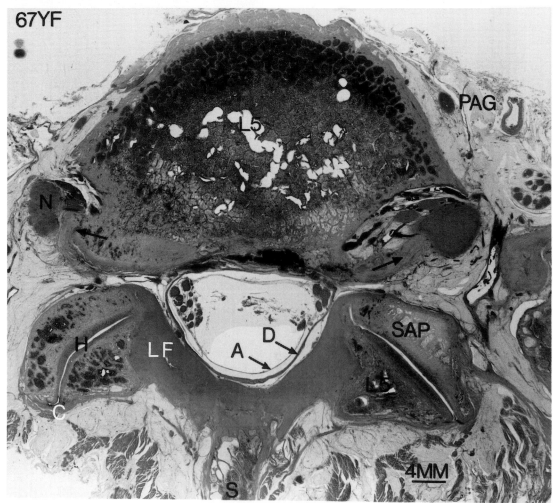

Figure 6.12 A 200 μm thick histological section cut in the horizontal plane through the lumbosacral joint of the 67-year-old female whose radiograph is shown in Figure 6.11. Large bilateral osteophytes project (arrows) towards the exit zone of the left and right intervertebral canals and deform the associated fifth lumbar large neural structures (N). A = arachnoid membrane; C = fibrous joint capsule; D = dural membrane; H = hyaline articular cartilage on facet surfaces; L5 = fifth lumbar vertebral body; LF = ligamentum flavum; PAG = paravertebral autonomic ganglion; S = spinous process; SAP = superior articular process of the sacrum.

stenosis can occur. For example, the radiograph of the lower lumbosacral spine of a 45-year-old male, which has been bisected in the median plane, shows degenerative osteophytosis involving the right L4–L5 intervertebral canal (Figure 6.9). This causes some stenosis of the intervertebral canal which is more fully appreciated on the corresponding histological section (Figure 6.10).

It is important to recognize that, in particular, plain film radiographs provide only a shadow of the truth. As an example of this, note the numerous histopathological degenerative changes seen in Figure 6.8, some of which could not be observed from the radiograph (Figure 6.7). A further example of this important clinical fact is noted in the radiographic examination of a lumbosacral spine from a 67-year-old female which showed osteophytosis (best seen on the lateral view (Figure 6.11) involving the posterior inferior margin of the fifth lumbar vertebra as part of generalized discogenic spondylosis of the lumbosacral intervertebral joint.

The histological appearance of the fifth lumbar vertebra, at the approximate level shown in Figure 6.11 is shown in Figure 6.12. This figure shows that the fifth lumbar spinal ganglia are being deformed by large bilateral osteophytes which project more laterally than posteriorly into the exit zones of the intervertebral canals bilaterally. This was not obvious from the plain film radiographs due to the superimposition of various osseous structures.

Thus, any planned treatment procedure must take into account the fact that degenerative changes seen as a result of various imaging procedures may be accompanied by far more significant soft tissue pathology due to the degenerative process.

The extraforaminal course of spinal nerves and their relationship to both hard and soft tissues are not always appreciated (Olsewski *et al.*, 1991) but should be borne in mind as a large posterolateral herniation of the lumbosacral intervertebral disc can project towards the ala of the sacrum, i.e. beyond the exit zone of the intervertebral canal, and can compromise the neural structures contributing to the sacral plexus. Such an example in a 78-year-old male is shown in Figure 6.13.

Also, the 'far out syndrome' can be due to impingement of the fifth lumbar spinal nerve between the sacral ala and the transverse process of the fifth lumbar vertebra (Wiltse *et al.*, 1993). Furthermore, large osteophytes on the inferior border of the fifth lumbar vertebra, coupled with 'tightness' of the lumbosacral ligament, often cause entrapment and compression of the L5 spinal nerve against the sacral ala (Nathan *et al.*, 1982) as the nerve passes through the osteofibrotic tunnel formed between the lumbosacral ligament and the sacrum.

In a study of cadavers (60–98 years age), Olsewski *et al.* (1991) examined the anterior primary rami of fifth lumbar nerves which were believed to be

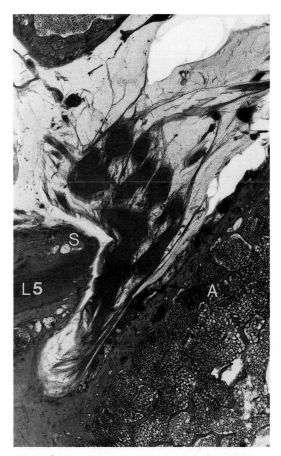

Figure 6.13 A 200 μm thick parasagittal section cut through the lumbosacral intervertebral disc (L5) and the adjacent sacral ala (A) of a 78-year-old male. Note the large osteophytic spurs (S) accompanying the intervertebral disc herniation and how this 'complex' deforms part of the neural structures contributing to the sacral plexus (Ehrlich's haematoxylin and light green counterstain).

trapped (11 out of 102) by lumbosacral ligaments. They found histological evidence of chronic compression as suggested by perineurial and endoneurial fibrosis, peripheral thinning of myelin sheaths, or subjective evidence of a shift in fibre diameter to a population of smaller size fibres in three of the 11 nerves judged to be compressed.

An example of a large posterolateral contained intervertebral disc herniation, which has caused considerable stenosis of the lumbosacral intervertebral canal in a 74-year-old male, is shown in Figure 6.14. In this example, the large contained nucleus pulposus herniation has resulted in only relatively slight deformation of the neural complex which is located in the upper half of the intervertebral canal. However, the blood vessels have been confined to a narrow region in the lower half of the

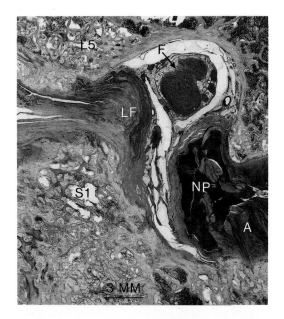

Figure 6.14 The large posterolateral contained intervertebral disc herniation shown in this parasagittal section from the left intervertebral canal of a 74-year-old male, projects 5 mm into the lower half of the intervertebral canal, below the neural complex, causing advanced stenosis of the canal. A = anulus fibrosus; LF = ligamentum flavum; L5 = fifth lumbar vertebra; NP = contained herniated nucleus pulposus; S1 = sacral superior articular process. There appears to be some disruption and congestion of the blood vessels in the lower half of the intervertebral canal opposite the contained herniation, and there is evidence of minor focal epineurial fibrosis (F) of the neural complex, particularly on the opposite side to that adjacent to the herniation. (Ehrlich's haematoxylin and light green counterstain.) (Reproduced with permission from Giles, L.G.F. and Kaveri, M.J.P. (1990) Some osseous and soft tissue causes of human intervertebral canal (foramen) stenosis. *J. Rheumatol.*, **17**, 1474–1481.)

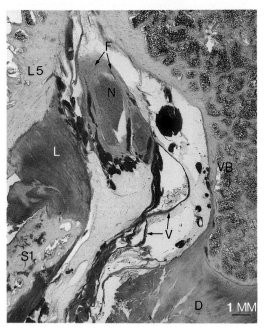

Figure 6.15 A parasagittal 100 μm thick histological section across the L5–S1 intervertebral canal in a 71-year-old male cadaver with a relatively normal lumbosacral intervertebral disc. Note the large very dilated thin walled vein (V) and the numerous adjacent congested blood vessels in the intervertebral canal, particularly in the vicinity of the neural complex (N) which occupies a relatively small cross-sectional area of the intervertebral canal in comparison to the total cross-sectional area occupied by blood vessels. The blood vessels appear to be congested with thrombus formation, although this must be considered as speculative when examining cadaveric material, particularly at a section thickness of 100 μm. There is marked perineurial fibrosis (F) of the neural complex. It is interesting to note that the perineurial fibrosis is not related to intervertebral disc herniation or to an osteophyte. D = intervertebral disc; L = ligamentum flavum; L5 = inferior articular process of the fifth lumbar vertebra; S1 = superior articular process of the sacrum; VB = posterolateral border of the fifth vertebral body. (Reproduced with permission from Giles, L.G.F. and Kaveri, M.J.P. (1990) Some osseous and soft tissue causes of human intervertebral canal (foramen) stenosis. *J. Rheumatol.*, **17**, 1474–1481.)

intervertebral canal by the herniation and there is a loss of the normally clearly defined outlines of the blood vessels in this area, suggesting congestion of these vessels. There is evidence of focal epineurial fibrosis affecting the neural complex, mainly on the opposite side to that adjacent to the herniation.

An example to show how extensive the blood supply can be within the intervertebral canal of a 71-year-old male is shown in Figure 6.15. The large,

dilated, thin walled vein and the blood vessels adjacent to the neural complex occupy a large area of the intervertebral canal and there is marked perineurial fibrosis of the neural complex, a finding which has also been noted by Jayson (1992) in cadavers.

Figure 6.16 shows a further example of how stenosis, caused by a posterolateral contained intervertebral disc herniation, with adjacent osteophytic

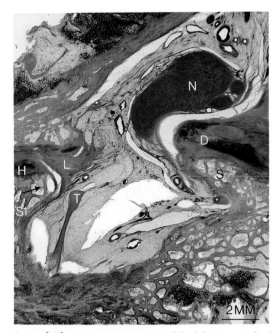

Figure 6.16 A parasagittal section of the left intervertebral canal of a 73-year-old male. D = posterolateral contained intervertebral disc herniation projecting 5 mm into the intervertebral canal, with an adjacent osteophytic spur (S) projecting from the junction between the lumbosacral disc and the sacrum; H = hyaline articular cartilage on the superior articular process of the sacrum (S1) which has developed a minor osteophytic spur (arrow); L = ligamentum flavum; T = part of a transforaminal ligament; N = nerve complex, including the dorsal root ganglion, which has been markedly deformed by the intervertebral disc herniation (D), resulting in some epineurial fibrosis. (Ehrlich's haematoxylin and light green counterstain.) (Reproduced with permission from Giles, L.G.F. and Kaveri, M.J.P. (1990) Some osseous and soft tissue causes of human intervertebral canal (foramen) stenosis. *J. Rheumatol.*, **17**, 1474–1481.)

spurs, can markedly deform the neural structures and blood vessels in the intervertebral canal of a 73-year-old male, resulting in possible slight epineural fibrosis associated with the posterior root ganglion.

Advanced zygapophysial joint osteophytosis can result in considerable stenosis of the intervertebral canal, as shown in Figure 6.17 where a large osteophyte has formed at the superior margin of the articular process of the first sacral segment and this articulates with the inferior surface of the pedicle above, where 'fibrocartilaginous' bumpers have developed between the osteophyte and the pedicle. The contours of the blood vessels adjacent to the osteophyte indicate that some of the vessels within the intervertebral canal are deformed by the osteophyte in this 71-year-old male.

In summary, intervertebral canals are defined superiorly and inferiorly by the pedicles of adjacent vertebral arches, posteriorly by the articular processes and the ligamentum flavum, and anteriorly by the vertebral bodies and the intervertebral disc (Rickenbacher *et al.*, 1985). The neural structures passing through the intervertebral canal are surrounded by adipose tissue which has numerous blood vessels coursing through it. The anatomy of the neural structure(s) passing through a given region of the intervertebral canal depends upon whether the entrance zone, mid-zone, or exit zone is being considered.

In this chapter all intervertebral canal photomicrographs showing the canal in its vertical dimension represent parasagittal histological sections at the junction between the *mid-* and *exit zones*. It can be seen that, although the sinuvertebral nerve has not been demonstrated at the magnification used, in some specimens the large neural complex occupies the superior region of the intervertebral canal, for example (Figures 6.5, 6.10 and 6.14), which is its usual location in the lumbar spine (Hadley, 1964). In some instances, contrary to the findings of Hoyland *et al.* (1989), the large neural structures can occupy the inferior region, as illustrated in Figure 6.8. In some cases, large neural stuctures can be deformed by contained intervertebral disc herniation and osteophytes. The neural complex can be considerably distorted when it is subjected to a 'pincer' like force between an osteophytic spur on the superior articular process and a contained intervertebral disc herniation with an adjacent osteophyte, particularly when the neural complex passes through the lower region of the intervertebral canal (Figure 6.8).

According to Pedowitz *et al.* (1992), nerve root compression, for example with disc herniation causing spinal stenosis, may induce a variety of symptoms in terms of sensory deficit, motor weakness, and pain. Nervi nervorum located on the dorsal root ganglion, as well as the peripheral nerves, are mechanically sensitive nociceptors, so the epineurium of the posterior root ganglion may be directly activated by compression or mechanical stimulation of these nociceptors (Weinstein, 1991). It is reasonable to assume that, when this degree of neural distortion occurs, associated vascular and microvascular structures may likewise be distorted. There is also evidence of frequent distortion of the numerous vascular structures by contained intervertebral disc herniation, or by zygapophysial joint osteophytosis, in the lower lumbar spine. This raises the question of whether low back pain, with or without sciatica, can arise as a result of venous stasis causing ischaemia of the neural structures, followed by perineurial and intraneurial fibrosis, neural dysfunction, and degeneration, as hypothesized in Chapter 5 (Figure 5.26). This seems a logical possibility in view of the evidence

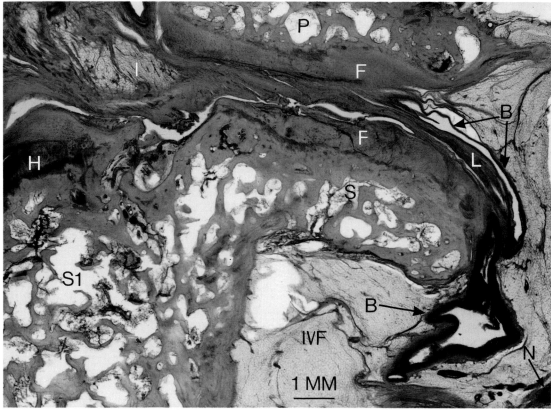

Figure 6.17 A parasagittal section through a large osteophytic spur (S) at the L5–S1 zygapophysial joint of a 71-year-old male. The superior margin of the articular process of the first sacral segment (S1) has developed a large osteophyte which protrudes 6 mm into the intervertebral canal. A bumper 'fibrocartilage' (F) has developed between the osteophyte and the adjacent pedicle (P) of the fifth lumbar vertebra which has also developed similar bumper 'fibrocartilage' (F). The blood vessels (B) adjacent to the osteophyte appear to conform largely to the contour of the osteophyte, indicating that they are being deformed and perhaps tractioned by it. H = hyaline articular cartilage on the superior articular process of S1; I = part of an intra-articular synovial fold; IVF = part of the intervertebral canal; N = part of a nerve within the intervertebral canal. The ligamentum flavum (L) has been disrupted and distorted by the large osteophyte. (Reproduced with permission from Giles, L.G.F. and Kaveri, M.J.P. (1990) Some osseous and soft tissue causes of human intervertebral canal (foramen) stenosis. *J. Rheumatol.*, **17**, 1474–1481.)

provided which tends to show epineurial and peri-neurial fibrosis (Figures 6.14 and 6.15) related to pressure distortion of neural and vascular structures. Even at the thickness of these histological sections there is evidence of perineurial and epineural fibrosis and this is not necessarily related to direct pressure by an intervertebral disc herniation or an osteophyte.

The effects of acute compression on intraneural blood flow (Olmarker *et al.*, 1989a, 1991), nerve root vascular permeability (Olmarker *et al.*, 1989b), and solute transport to nerve roots (Olmarker *et al.*, 1990) has been well documented *in vivo* porcine cauda equina graded unilateral posterior compres-sion experiments, and Rydevik *et al.* (1991) and Pedowitz *et al.* (1992) suggest that a pressure threshold of 50–75 mm mercury can cause a neu-rophysiological deficit due to 2 or 4 hours of acute nerve root compression.

As venous stasis may occur within the inter-vertebral canal, it would appear that patients suffer-ing from idiopathic low back pain should be encour-aged to remain active in order to promote better circulation around the neural structures within the intervertebral canal. When sitting, such patients may well obtain some relief by using a rocking chair to promote circulation.

While the results of cadaveric studies are spec-ulative regarding the possibility of low back pain, with or without sciatica, being caused by spinal nerve ischaemia and fibrosis, there is no doubt that ischaemia can be a cause of pain in other regions of the body (Guyton, 1986), and mechanical de-formation and compression may cause injury and dysfunction due to the resulting local tissue ischaemia (Pedowitz *et al.*, 1992). Naturally occurring biologic substances have been implicated by Sicuteri *et al.* (1974) as producing pain in vascular disorders, including bradykinin, 5-hydroxytryptamine, potassium, and adenosine triphosphate which are grouped under the term 'vaso-neuroactive substances'. As previously noted, according to Kuntz (1953), pain of vascular origin is a well recognized clinical phenomenon, although the nature of the stimuli required to produce such pain is not fully understood, nor is the way in which signals related to tissue damage are transmitted to the central nervous system (Dubner and Hargreaves, 1989).

References

Allbrook, D. (1974) The intervertebral disc. In *Low Back Pain: Proceedings of a Conference on Low Back Pain* (L.T. Twomey, ed.). Institute of Technology, Western Australia, pp. 14–19.

Altman, R.D. and Dean, D. (1989) Pain in osteoarthritis – introduction and overview. *Semin. Arthr. Rheum.* **18**, 1–3.

Batson, O.V. (1957) The vertebral vein system. *Am. J. Roentgenol.*, **78**, 195–212.

Berry, J.L., Moran, J.M., Berg, W.S. and Steffee, A.D. (1987). A morphometric study of human lumbar and selected thoracic vertebrae. *Spine* **13**, 362–367.

Bogduk, N. (1980). The anatomy and physiology of lumbar back disability. *Bulletin of the Post-Grad Committee in Medicine*, University of Sydney, pp 2–17.

Breig, A. (1960) *Biomechanics of the Central Nervous System*. Almqvist and Wiksell, Stockholm.

Bullough, P.G. and Boachie-Adjei, O. (1988). *Atlas of Spinal Diseases*. J.B. Lippincott Philadelphia, pp. 84–97.

Coventry, M.B., Ghormley, R.K. and Kernohan, J.W. (1945) The intervertebral disc: its microscopic anatomy and pathology. Part II. Changes in the intervertebral disc concomitant with age. *J. Bone Joint Surg.* **27A**, 233–252.

Crelin, E.S. (1973) A scientific test of the chiropractic theory. *Am. Sci.*, **61**, 574–580.

Crelin, E.S. (1982). Functional anatomy of the lumbosacral spine: In S.L. Gordon, A.A. White, (eds): *American Academy of Orthopaedic Surgeons Symposium on Idiopathic Low Back Pain.* CV Mosby, St Louis, pp. 59–77.

Dommisse, G.F. (1975) Morphological aspects of the lumbar spine and lumbo-sacral region. *Ortho. Clin. North Am.* **6**, 163–175.

Dorwart, R.H. and Genant, H.K. (1983) Anatomy of the lumbosacral spine. *Radiol. Clin. North Am.* **21**, 201–220.

Dorwart, R.H., Vogler, J.B. and Helms, C.A. (1983) Spinal stenosis. *Radiol. Clin. North Am.* **21**, 301–325.

Dubner, R. and Hargreaves, K.M. (1989) The neurobiology of pain and its modulation. *Clin. J. Pain* **5** (Suppl 2), S1–6.

Eisenstein, S. (1980) The trefoil configuration of the lumbar vertebral canal. *J. Bone Joint Surg.* **62B**, 73–77.

Epstein, J.A. (1960) Diagnosis and treatment of painful neurological disorders caused by spondylosis of the lumbar spine. *J. Neurosurg*, **17**, 991–1001.

Fick, R. (1904). *Anatome und Mechanik der Gelenke*. Jena Verlag Von Gustav Fischer, p. 81.

Giles, L.G.F. (1993) A histological investigation of human lower lumbar intervertebral canal (foramen) dimensions. *J. Manip. Physiol. Ther.*, **15**, 551–555.

Giles, L.G.F. (1992) Ligaments traversing the intervertebral canals of the human lower lumbosacral spine. *Neuro-Orthopedics*, **13**, 25–38.

Giles, L.G.F. and Kaveri, M.J.P. (1990) Some osseous and soft tissue causes of human intervertebral canal (foramen) stenosis. *J. Rheumatol*, **17**, 1474–1481.

Giles, L.G.F. and Taylor, J.R. (1983) Histological preparation of large specimens. *Stain Technol.*, **58**, 45–49.

Guyton, A.C. (1986) *Textbook of Medical Physiology.*, 7th edn. W.B. Saunders, Philadelphia, pp. 320, 345, 598.

Hadley, L.A. (1964) *Anatomico-Roentgenographic Studies of the Spine*, Charles C. Thomas, Springfield, Illinois. pp. 172–194.

Hasue, M., Kikuchi, S., Sakuyama, Y. and Ito T. (1983) Anatomic study of the interrelation between nerve roots and their surrounding tissues. *Spine* **8**, 50–58.

Hasue, M., Kunogi, J., Konno, S. and Kikuchi, S. (1989) Classification by position of dorsal root ganglia in the lumbosacral region. *Spine*, **14**, 1261–1264.

Haughton, V.M. and Williams, A.L. (1982) *Computed Tomography of the Spine*. C.V. Mosby, St Louis p. 88.

Herzog, R.J., Kaiser, J.A., Saal, J.A. and Saal, J.S. (1991) The importance of posterior epidural fat pad in lumbar central canal stenosis. *Spine*, **16**, S227–S233.

Hofmann, M. (1898) Die befestigung der dura mater im wirbelcanal. *Arch F. Anat. Physiol. (Anat Abt)* 403.

Hovelacque, A. (1925). Le nerf sinuvertebral. *Ann. d'Anat. Path.*, **5**, 435–443.

Hoyland, J.A., Freemont, A.J. and Jayson, M.I.V. (1989) Intervertebral foramen venous obstruction. A cause of periradicular fibrosis? *Spine*, **14**, 558–568.

Isherwood, I. and Antoun, N.M. (1980) CT scanning in the assessment of lumbar spine problems. In *The Lumbar Spine and Back Pain*. (M.I.V. Jayson (ed.) Edn 2. Kent, Pitman Medical, pp. 247–264.

Jayson, M.I.V. (1992) The role of vascular damage and fibrosis in the pathogenesis of nerve root damage. *Clin. Orthop. Rel. Res*, **279**, 40–48.

Keim, H.A. and Kirkaldy-Wills, W.H. (1987) Low back pain. *Clin. Symp.*, 39.

Kimmel, D.L. (1961a) Innervation of spinal dura mater and dura mater of the posterior cranial fossa. *Neurology*, **11**, 800–109.

Kimmel, D.L. (1961b) The nerves of the cranial dura mater and their significance in dural headaches and referred pain. *Chicago Medical School Quarterly*, **22**, 16–26.

Kirkaldy-Willis, W.H., Heithoff, KB., Tchang, S., Bowen, C.V.A., Cassidy, J.D. and Shannon, R. (1984) Lumbar spondylosis and stenosis. Correlation of pathological anatomy with high resolution computed tomographic scanning. In Post MJD (ed): *Computed Tomography of the Spine*. Baltimore: Williams & Wilkins, pp 495–505.

Kirkaldy-Willis, W.H. and McIvor, G.W.D. (1976) Lumbar spinal stenosis – editorial comment. *Clin. Orthop. Rel. Res.*, **115**, 2–3.

Krag, M.H., Beynonn, B.D. and Pope, M.H., *et al.* (1986) An internal fixator for posterior application to short segments of the thoracic, lumbar or lumbosacral spine: design and testing. *Clin. Orthop.*, **203**, 75–98.

Krag, M.H., Weaver, D.L., Beynnon, B.D. and Haugh, L.D. (1988) Morphometry of the thoracic and lumbar spine related to transpedicular screw placement for surgical spinal fixation. *Spine*, **13**, 27-32.

Kuntz, A. (1953). *The Autonomic Nervous System*. Lea and Febiger, Philadelphia, pp. 157, 161.

Larmon, W.A. (1944) An anatomic study of the lumbosacral region in relation to low back pain and sciatica. *Ann. Surg.*, **119**, 892-896.

Lee, C.K. (1988) Office management of low back pain. *Orthop. Clin. North Am.*, **19**, 797-804.

Lee, C.K. Rauschning, W. and Glenn, W. (1988) Lateral lumbar spinal canal stenosis: classification, pathologic anatomy and surgical decompression. *Spine*, **13**, 313-320.

Magnuson, P.G. (1944) Differential diagnosis of causes of pain in the lower back accompanied by sciatic pain. *Ann. Surg.*, **179**, 878.

McMinn, R.H.M. and Hutchings, R.T. (1977) *A Colour Atlas of Human Anatomy*. Wolf Medical Publications, London. p 90.

McRae, D.L. (1977). Radiology of the lumbar spinal canal. In *Lumbar Spondylosis. Diagnosis. Management and Surgical Treatment* P.R. Weinstein, G Ehni, C.B. Wilson (eds): Chicago, Year Book Medical Publishers, pp 92-114.

Mixter, W.J. and Barr, J.S. (1934) Rupture of the intervertebral disc with involvement of the spinal canal. *N. Engl. J. Med.*, **211**, 210-215.

Moore, K.L. (1992), *Clinically Oriented Anatomy*, 3rd edn. Williams & Wilkins, Baltimore.

Nathan, H., Weizenbluth, M. and Halperin, N. (1982) The lumbosacral ligament with special emphasis on the 'lumbosacral tunnel' and the entrapment of the 5th lumbar nerve. *Int. Orthop.*, **6**, 197-202.

Olmarker, K., Rydevik, B., Holm, S. and Bagge, U. (1989a) Effects of experimental graded compression on blood flow in spinal nerve roots: a vital microscopic study on the porcine cauda equina. *J. Orthop. Res.*, **7**, 817-823.

Olmarker, K., Rydevik, B. and Holm, S. (1989b) Edema formation in spinal nerve roots induced by experimental, graded compression: an experimental study on the pig cauda equina with special reference to differences in effects between rapid and slow onset of compression. *Spine*, **14**, 569-573.

Olsewski, J.M., Simmons, E.H., Kallen, F.C. and Mendel, F.C. (1991) Evidence from cadavers suggestive of entrapment of fifth lumbar spinal nerves by lumbosacral ligaments. *Spine*, **16**, 336-347.

Olmarker, K., Rydevik, B., Hansson, T. and Holm, S. (1990) Compression-induced changes of the nutritional supply to the porcine cauda equina. *J. Spinal Disord.*, **3**, 25-29.

Olmarker, K., Holm, S., Rosenqvist, A.-L. and Rydevik, B. (1991) Experimental nerve root compression: a model of acute, graded compression of the porcine cauda equina and an analysis of neural and vascular anatomy. *Spine*, **16**, 61-69.

Oppenheimer, A. (1937) Diseases affecting the intervertebral foramina. *Radiology*, **28**, 582-591.

Panjabi, M.M., Goel, V.K., Oxland, T. *et al.* (1992) Human lumbar vertebrae. Quantitative three-dimensional anatomy. *Spine*, **17**, 299-306.

Pedowitz, R.A., Garfin, S.R., Massie, J.B. *et al.* (1992) Effects of magnitude and duration of compression on spinal nerve root conduction. *Spine*, **17**, 194-199.

Peretti de, F., Micalef, J.P., Bourgeon, A. *et al.* (1989) Biomechanics of the lumbar spinal nerve roots and the first sacral root within the intervertebral foramina. *Surg. Radiol. Anat.*, **11**, 221-225.

Rauschning, W. (1987) Normal and pathologic anatomy of the lumbar root canals. *Spine*, **12**, 1008-1019.

Romanes, C.J. (1981) *Cunningham's Textbook of Anatomy*, 12th edn. Oxford University Press, Oxford, pp. 207-257.

Roofe, P.G. (1940) Innervation of anulus fibrosus and posterior longitudinal ligament. *Arch. Neurol. Psychiatry*, **44**, 100-103.

Rothman, R.H. and Simeone, F.A. (1975) *The Spine*. Vol 1. W.B. Saunders Company, Philadelphia, p. 407.

Rydevik, B.L. (1992). The effects of compression on the physiology of nerve roots. *J. Manip. Physiol. Ther.* 1, 62-66.

Rydevik, B., Brown, M.D. and Lundborg, G. (1984) Pathoanatomy and pathophysiology of nerve root compression. *Spine*, **9**, 7-15.

Rydevik, B., Holm, S., Brown, M.D. and Lundborg, G. (1990) Diffusion from the cerebrospinal fluid as a nutritional pathway for spinal nerve roots. *Acta Physiol. Scand.* **138**, 247-248.

Rydevik, B.L., Pedowitz, R.A. and Hargens, A.R., *et al.* (1991) Effects of acute, graded compression on spinal nerve root function and structure: an experimental study of the pig cauda equina. *Spine*, **16**, 487-493.

Scoles, P.V., Linton, A.E., Latimer, B., Levy, M.E. and Digiovanni, B.F. (1988) Vertebral body and posterior element morphology. The normal spine in middle life. *Spine*, **13**, 1082-1086.

Shapiro, R. (1975) *Myelography*, 3rd ed. Year Book Medical Publishers, Chicago. pp. 77-94.

Sicuteri, F., Franchi, G., Anselm, B. and Del Bianco, P.L. (1974) Headache and cardiac pain. Physiopathologic and therapeutic perspectives. In Bonica JJ, Procacci P, Pagni CA (eds): *Recent Advances on Pain: Pathophysiology and Clinical Aspects*. Springfield, IL, Charles C. Thomas, pp 82-104.

Spurling, R.G. and Bradford, F.K. (1939) Neurologic aspects of herniated nucleus pulposus. *JAMA*, **113**, 2019-2022.

Stockwell, R.A. (1985) A Pre-clinical view of osteoarthritis. A Sir John Struthers Lecture. The Medical School, Edinburgh.

Sunderland, S. (1974) Mechanisms of cervical root avulsion in injuries of the neck and shoulder. *J. Neurosurg.*, **51**, 705-714.

Swanberg, H. (1915a) *The Intervertebral Foramina in Man*. Scientific Publishing Co, Illinois.

Swanberg, H. (1915b) The intervertebral foramina in man. *Med. Rec.*, Jan 30th, 176-180.

Twomey, L. and Taylor, J. (1988). Age changes in the lumbar spinal and intervertebral canals. *Paraplegia*, **26**, 238-249.

Vanderlinden, R.G. (1984) Subarticular entrapment of the dorsal root ganglion as a cause of sciatic pain. *Spine*, **9**, 19-22.

Vernon-Roberts, B. and Pirie, C.J. (1977) Degenerative changes in the intervertebral discs of the lumbar spine and their sequelae. *Rheumatol Rehab.*, **16**, 13-21.

von Luschka, H. (1850) *Die Nerven des Menschlichen Wirbelkanales*. Tubingen, Laupp and Siebeck.

Weinstein, J.N. (1991) Anatomy and neurophysiologic mechanisms of spinal pain. In *The Adult Spine: Principles and*

Practice (J.W. Frymoyer ed.). Raven Press, NY. pp. 593–610.

Williams, P.L. and Warwick, T. (1980). *Gray's Anatomy*, 36th edn. London, Churchill Livingstone.

Wiltse, L.L., Fonseca, A.S., Amster, J. *et al*. (1993) Relationship of the dura, Hofmann's ligaments, Batson's plexus and a fibrovascular membrane lying on the posterior surface of the vertebral bodies and attaching to the deep layer of the posterior longitudinal ligament. *Spine*, **18**, 1030–1043.

Wyke, B.D. (1982) Receptor systems in lumbosacral tissues in relation to the production of low back pain. In *American Academy of Orthopaedic Surgeons Symposium on Idiopathic Low Back Pain* (A.A. White, S.L. Gordon, eds). CV Mosby St Louis, 1982, pp 97–107.

Wyke, B.D. (1970). The neurological basis of thoracic spinal pain. *Rheumatol. Phys. Med.*, **110**, 356–367.

Yeager, V.L. (1986). Anatomy of the lumbar vertebral column. *Semin. Neurol.*, **6**, 341–349.

Zindrick, M.R., Wiltse, L.L. and Doornik, A. et al. (1987) Analysis of morphometric characteristics of the thoracic and lumbar pedicles. *Spine*, **12**, 160–166.

7

Ligaments related to the intervertebral canal and foramen

Harold S. Amonoo-Kuofi and Mohammed G. Y. El-Badawi

Introduction

Such is the complexity of low back pain that the management could fall squarely within the domain of the physician, rheumatologist, neurologist, neurosurgeon, orthopaedic surgeon, gynaecologist, general practitioner, physiotherapist, osteopath, chiropractor, and quite often the psychiatrist. Low back pain affects 50–80% of the population (White and Gordon, 1982). Spondylogenic back pain accounts for a large proportion of cases seen in practice. In the majority of patients with back pain, it is not possible to make a firm diagnosis of the cause of the pain (Roland and Morris, 1983).

Pain is always an expression of a disturbance of neurological function (Wyke, 1987). A precise understanding of the neurological mechanisms involved in its production is therefore an important prerequisite to a rational, ordered approach to management. Understanding of the mechanisms depends on availability of accurate anatomical, physiological and pathological information in sufficient detail. This chapter attempts to bring together some relevant contemporary anatomical, neuroanatomical and clinical data on the structural and functional interaction between the lumbar spinal nerve (within its sheath) and its surroundings as it traverses the intervertebral canal and foramen. It is hoped that this information will contribute to informed assessment of low back pain patients and thus facilitate the choice of clinical management strategies.

The lumbar spinal nerve emerges from the lumbar thecal sac, ensheathed in a dural sleeve (Figure 7.1), and runs in an osteoligamentous tunnel in the lateral recess of the vertebral canal, inferomedial to the pedicle of the vertebra. This tunnel, orientated obliquely caudad and laterally, is known as the lumbar spinal nerve root canal (Crock, 1981) or intervertebral canal (Lee *et al.*, 1988). It has a funnel-shaped entrance zone, lateral to the dura and a somewhat oval exit foramen laterally, known as the intervertebral foramen. The topography, subdivisions and contents of

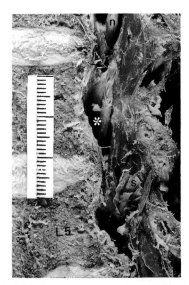

Figure 7.1 Median sagittal section through the lower lumbar region, showing the entrance zones of the intervertebral canals. p = posterior longitudinal ligament; f = ligamentum flavum. The lateral edge of the ligamentum flavum is closely related to the nerve, n. White asterisk * = entrance zone of the L4 level. Note the fine nerve roots (of L4) surrounded by the sheath. s = dural sleeve of L5 spinal nerve. The nerve (n) occupies a spacious opening superior to the horizontal mid-transforaminal ligament (☆). The ligament does not appear to be encroaching on the neural space. The opening for the veins (→) are separated from the nerve by the ligament. Scale: small divisions = mm.

this canal have been dealt with in detail in Chapter 6. Only a brief mention will be made of the aspects of its morphology that are directly relevant to the subject of this chapter. The posterior longitudinal ligament, which is placed in the midline on the dorsal surface of the vertebral bodies, sends lateral extensions at the level of the intervertebral discs to contribute to the formation of the anterior wall of the intervertebral canal (Figures 7.1 and 7.2). The posterior wall of the canal is formed by the lamina (pars interarticularis) of the vertebra and the lateral part of the ligamentum flavum and anterior surface to the zygapophysial joint. The outlet of the intervertebral canal, the foraminal exit zone (Rauschning, 1987), is the intervertebral foramen (see Chapter 6). It is bounded superiorly by

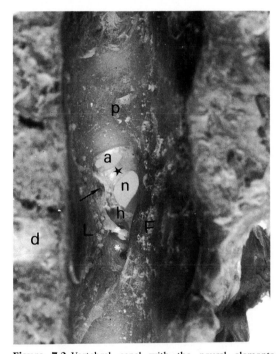

Figure 7.2 Vertebral canal with the neural elements removed to show the internal aspect of the intervertebral canal at L1. F = ligamentum flavum. The upper part of its free, lateral border forms the posterior boundary of the mid-zone while the lower part of the border is closely related to the venous foramina. L = lateral extensions of the posterior longitudinal ligament forming part of the anterior wall of the mid-zone. p = inferomedial surface of the right pedicle of L1 vertebra. The oblique superior transforaminal ligament (☆) separates the opening of the nerve (n) from the arterial opening (a). The anterior end of the ligament inserts on the posterior border of the deep anterior intraforaminal ligament which forms the posterior boundary of the opening for the sinuvertebral nerve (→). h = horizontal mid-transforaminal ligament. The oblique inferior transforaminal ligament is represented by two bands (*, white asterisks). Note two venous openings in the lower part of the exit zone. d = the L1/L2 intervertebral disc.

the inferior vertebral notch of the vertebra above and inferiorly by the superior vertebral notch of the vertebra below. The anterior boundary is formed by the posterolateral surfaces of the contiguous vertebrae separated by the intervertebral disc, while the posterior boundary is formed by the lateral free edge of the ligamentum flavum placed anterior to the zygapophysial joint and the anterior surface of the superior articular process of the vertebra below. The area immediately beyond the outlet of the intervertebral foramen has been described as the postcanal zone (Rauschning, 1987). The foramen contains the neural complex (root sleeve, dorsal root ganglion and the nerve trunk), spinal branches of the lumbar segmental artery, the recurrent meningeal (sinuvertebral) nerve, proximal or pedicle veins, distal or disc veins and a plug of fat. The nerve root complex occupies 30–50% of the cross-sectional area of the foramen (Sunderland, 1980). Most of the contents are pain sensitive and would give rise to pain when subjected to compression.

The lumbar spine is highly mobile. It is involved in most movements of the body. During certain movements, e.g. lateral flexion, the size of the foramen may be reduced markedly because of the presence of the two movable joints forming part of the boundary (Brieg, 1960; Maurice-Williams, 1981). Furthermore, the neural complex slides to and fro continually in a piston-like manner during movements of the limbs and trunk (Sunderland, 1980). The L5 root may move out of its foramen by between 2 mm and 6 mm. The proximal lumbar roots move less (Maurice-Williams, 1981). The displacement of the individual foraminal structures (especially the neural complex) would be multidirectional, i.e. varying combinations of anteroposterior, cephalocaudal and to and fro sliding displacements, depending on the complexity of limb and trunk movements. Normal daily activities that involve movement of the trunk do not give rise to pain. This means that the foraminal contents have adequate room and are protected from compression or encroachment during posture and movement.

The mechanism by which this protection is ensured is not fully known. It is widely accepted that the fat plug that obturates the foramen is largely contributory. Other structures within the intervertebral canal, and at the foraminal exit zone, have been suggested as playing various roles. These include Hoffmann ligaments (Hoffmann 1898; Luyendijk *et al.*, 1966; Rauschning, 1987; Wiltse *et al.*, 1993), the dural pouch formed by the emerging nerve roots (Sunderland, 1974, 1980), condensations of fascial tissue attaching the nerve root to the pedicles (Sunderland, 1974; Hayashi *et al.*, 1977; Spencer *et al.*, 1983; Rauschning, 1987; Kubo *et al.*, 1994), and internal and external foraminal ligaments traversing the exit zone (Nathan *et al.*, 1982; Amonoo-Kuofi *et al.*, 1988a,b; Giles, 1992; Nowicki and Haughton, 1992a; Transfeldt *et al.*, 1993).

In this chapter, the topography of the ligaments related to the intervertebral canal will be described with emphasis on the ligaments traversing the exit zone. The role that these ligaments could play in the causation of back pain will be discussed.

Classification of the ligaments of the intervertebral canal

Various connective tissue structures and ligaments are connected or related to the neural complex as it passes through the intervertebral canal. Some of these ligaments form parts of the walls of the intervertebral canal while others traverse the exit zone. Pathological changes in any of these ligaments could predispose to structural or functional changes that could produce back pain.

These ligaments may be classified into three broad categories according to their location within the intervertebral canal:

1. Ligaments of the entrance zone
   - Posterior longitudinal ligament
   - Hoffmann ligament
   - Peridural membrane
2. Ligaments of the mid-zone
   - Fascial condensations attaching the nerve root sleeve to the pedicles
   - Ligamentum flavum
3. Ligaments of the exit zone (intervertebral foramen)
   - Internal ligaments
   - Transforaminal ligaments
   - External ligaments
4. Ligament of the post-canal zone
   - Lumbar cribriform fascia

Topography of the ligaments of the intervertebral canal

Ligaments of the entrance zone

Often referred to as the lateral recess, this infundibular space houses the dural root sleeve and the enclosed nerve roots.

Posterior longitudinal ligament

The posterior longitudinal ligament will be described in Chapter 9 and has been labelled in Figures 3.5 and 3.11. Only a brief mention will be made here to highlight its role in the protection of the neural complex. The main part of the posterior longitudinal ligament is related to the dorsal surface of the vertebral bodies in the midline, i.e. in the anterior wall of the vertebral canal. It is adherent to the intervertebral discs and the adjacent margins of the vertebral bodies. In between attachments to the intervertebral discs, the ligament is separated from the posterior surfaces of the vertebral bodies by the basivertebral veins and the venous channels connecting them to the anterior internal vertebral venous plexus. At the level of the intervertebral discs, the posterior longitudinal ligament gives lateral extensions which may form a large part of the ventral boundary of the intervertebral canal and the exit foramen (Figures 7.1 and 7.2). Histologically, it is made up of dense connective tissue (type I collagen) arranged in layers. Within its layers it contains some of the venous channels that are part of the extradural venous (Batson's) plexus.

In 2–3% of the population, the lumbar portion of the posterior longitudinal ligament may become ossified (Wennekes *et al.*, 1985; Bitar *et al.*, 1987; Terayama *et al.*, 1987; Albisinni *et al.*, 1988; Lee *et al.*, 1990; Ermachenko *et al.*, 1992). The condition is generally asymptomatic but, in some individuals, it can contribute to stenosis of the intervertebral canal, thereby causing a myelopathy or mimicking intermittent neurogenic claudication seen in nerve root vascular impairment (Wennekes *et al.*, 1985; Ermachenko *et al.*, 1992). There is a significant association between ossification of the posterior longitudinal ligament and ossification of the ligamentum flavum (Tezuka *et al.*, 1976; Ikata *et al.*, 1977; Otani *et al.*, 1986; Terayama *et al.*, 1987; Lee *et al.*, 1990; Brown *et al.*, 1991).

Hoffmann ligaments

These are bands of connective tissue that segmentally attach the thecal sac to the anterior wall of the vertebral canal and the superficial layer of the posterior longitudinal ligament. They were first described by Hoffmann in 1898. Their existence has been confirmed by Luyendijk *et al.* (1966), Sunderland (1974, 1980), Hayashi *et al.* (1977), Brieg (1978), Hasue *et al.* (1983), Spencer *et al.* (1983), Rauschning (1987), Wiltse *et al.* (1993). The ligaments are bilateral and vary from narrow thread-like bands to broad bands which may meet in the midline. They are stronger and broader in the proximal segments (about 1 cm wide at L2) and become thinner at lower levels, and thread-like at L5. They may be absent at the first sacral level. The fibres pass cranially from the anterior surface of the dural sheath to attach to the posterior longitudinal ligament immediately proximal to the point where the latter ligament blends with the anulus fibrosus. The dural attachment may extend laterally to the anterior aspect of the dural sleeve of the nerve root within the entrance zone of the intervertebral canal (Spencer *et al.*, 1983). These ligaments prevent the neural complex from moving posteriorly when a disc bulges against it from the anterior aspect. This could produce pain (radicular pain) even though there is plenty of room for the nerve in the bony canal posteriorly. The lateral extensions of the dural attachment could also help in preventing excessive traction on the nerve roots.

Peridural membrane

This is a connective tissue sheath that lines the vertebral canal (Fick, 1904; Schmorl and Junghanns, 1959; Dommisse, 1975, 1979; Hayashi *et al.*, 1977; Kikuchi, 1982; Schellinger *et al.*, 1990; Wiltse *et al.*, 1993). Originally described as the membranous lining of the vertebral canal, it was Dommisse (1979) who introduced the term 'peridural membrane'. The membrane serves as the periosteum of the vertebral canal. It does not cross the disc space. The extradural plexus of veins (Batson's plexus) is sandwiched between this membrane and the posterior longitudinal ligament which lies superficial to it. Posteriorly, the peridural membrane lines the laminae while laterally it is loosely attached to the medial and caudal border of the pedicle. It can be peeled off easily with the thumbnail through gloves (Wiltse *et al.*, 1993). In the lateral parts of the vertebral canal, as the dura gives tubular extensions to surround the emerging spinal nerve roots, the peridural membrane gives extensions, which together with the lateral extensions of the posterior longitudinal ligament, form a lining for the lateral part of the bony canal and the entrance zone of the intervertebral canal. This membrane and ligament form a thick membranous sheath around the dural sleeve. This sheath has been described by Kikuchi (1982) as the epiradicular sheath, and by Wiltse *et al.* (1993) as the circumneural sheath. Circumneural sheath is probably a more accurate description, since the sheath extends laterally to cover the dorsal root ganglion and the proximal segment of the spinal nerve trunk. The tissue forming the circumneural sheath may be implicated in pathological conditions associated with fibrosis and narrowing at the entry zone of the intervertebral canal.

Ligaments of the mid-zone

This is an obliquely orientated cylindrical space, inferomedial to the pedicle. The dorsal root ganglion lies within this zone together with arteries, veins and sinuvertebral nerves. The ligamentum flavum is posterior to the ganglion in this part of the intervertebral canal.

Fascial condensations attaching the nerve root sleeve to the pedicles

Ligaments 'anchoring' the exiting nerve root sheath to the medial surface of the pedicle above, and to the lateral surface of the pedicle below, have been described by Sunderland (1974), Hayashi *et al.* (1977), Spencer *et al.* (1983), Rauschning (1987) and Kubo *et al.* (1994). These ligaments are thought to be condensations in the fascial tissue surrounding the root sleeve. In meticulous microdissections of the cervical vertebral canal, Kubo *et al.* (1994) suggested that 'ligamentous anchors' found anteriorly in the mid-zone were derived from the superficial layer of the posterior longitudinal ligament. More work is still needed to ascertain whether these fascial condensations are different from the sheath derived from the peridural membrane. These anchors are believed to protect the nerve root from avulsion injury (Kubo *et al.*, 1994). Kinking of the nerve root (Macnab, 1971; Hasue, 1983) may be due to caudad traction on the nerve root by these ligamentous anchors, following descent of the pedicle, as in isolated disc resorption. Inflammation involving the fascial condensations could also produce pain.

Ligamentum flavum

The ligamentum flavum is mentioned here in so far as it forms the posterior boundary of the intervertebral canal. It is related to both the entrance and midzones. Its morphology is described in Chapter 9 and has been labelled in several figures, e. g. Figures 3.5, 3.9, 3.14, 3.20, 6.14 and 6.15.

The ligamentum flavum is a broad, predominantly elastic ligament. It is attached superiorly to the anterior surface of the lower border of the lamina. The fibres run nearly vertically downwards to gain attachment to the posterior surface of the upper border of the subjacent lamina. The lateral half of the ligament may incline slightly obliquely, downwards and laterally. Posteromedially, the edges of the right and left ligaments may be partially united in the midline, leaving only small intervals for the passage of veins. Anterolaterally, the ligament has a free border (Figures 7.1 and 7.2). The posterior surface of this border fuses with the anterior aspect of the capsule of the zygapophysial joint. The ligament is interposed between the exiting nerve root sheath and the zygapophysial joint, forming the posterior wall of the mid-zone (Figure 7.1). Its lower part is also related to the large veins emerging from the venous foramina at the inferior angle of the exit zone (Figure 7.2). The horizontal mid-transforaminal ligaments (Figure 3.16) and the inferior corporotransverse ligaments (Figure 3.15) are closely related to the lateral edge of the ligament (Giles, 1992). Histologically, the ligamentum flavum of young adults is made up of 80% elastic fibres and 20% type I collagen fibres (Yong Hing *et al.*, 1976). With ageing, there is an increase in the relative amount of fibrous tissue (Yong Hing *et al.*, 1976, Panjabi *et al.*, 1987).

The ligamentum flavum may be subject to hypertrophy (Beamer *et al.*, 1993) or calcification (Towne and Reichert, 1931; Moiel *et al.*, 1967; Otani *et al.*,

1986; Nakamura *et al.*, 1990; Brown *et al.*, 1991; Baba *et al.*, 1993; Kashiwagi *et al.*, 1993). Localized mechanical stresses affecting the ligament (Otani *et al.*, 1986) and age-related changes (Kashiwagi, 1993) have been suggested as probable aetiological factors. Hypertrophy or ossification alone do not necessarily cause neurologic symptoms unless other factors coexist (Omojola *et al.*, 1982; Kudo *et al.*, 1983). These changes could nevertheless cause narrowing of the anteroposterior diameter of the intervertebral canal which, in turn, could produce pressure on the foraminal contents (Moiel *et al.*, 1967; Verbiest, 1975; Baba *et al.*, 1993). Intermittent claudication is a common presentation in symptomatic cases (Verbiest, 1975; Baba *et al.*, 1993), but the condition may progress to radiculopathy and, eventually, to myelopathy (Moiel *et al.*, 1967; Tezuka *et al.*, 1976; Ikata *et al.*, 1977; Guo-Xiang *et al.*, 1988).

Ligaments of the exit zone (intervertebral foramen)

The exit zone is a shallow anular opening bounded by the lateral borders of the pedicles and the lateral edge of the ligamentum flavum (Rauschning, 1987). This corresponds to the intervertebral foramen (Nomina Anatomica, 1983).

Most descriptions of the intervertebral foramina often leave the reader with the impression that the lumbar intervertebral foramina are large oval openings devoid of any ligamentous partitions (Crelin, 1982; Williams *et al.*, 1989; Parke, 1992). This impression is reinforced by the appearance of these foramina on plain radiographs. Normal ligamentous tissue is radiolucent, and therefore cannot be imaged by conventional plain film radiography. Constraints in the modern curricula of anatomy courses do not permit detailed dissection of the lumbar intervertebral foramina. This limitation is compounded by the fact that, in the preferred posterior approach to the lumbar spine, the surgeon does not get a good opportunity to explore the parts of the intervertebral foramina that are anterior to the exiting ventral root. It is within reason, therefore, that earlier reports of the presence of ligaments traversing the intervertebral foramina have not engendered much inquiry. It is pertinent, however, to give a brief history of the work that has been done on this important aspect of the morphology of the lumbar spine.

Historical gleanings

In a quest for factors that could produce compression or irritation of the spinal nerves in the intervertebral foramina, Larmon (1944) dissected ten unpreserved autopsy lumbar spines. In three cases he noted that 'a ligament connected the transverse process of the fifth with the body of the fifth and the first sacral vertebrae.

This ligament lay directly over the intervertebral foramen at the exit of the fifth lumbar nerve'. He added that evidence of compression could not be demonstrated in two cases, although the ligament bound the nerve firmly to the body of the first sacral vertebra in all three cases. Golub and Silverman (1969), in an attempt to extend Larmon's (1944) report, dissected ten spines obtained at autopsy in the fresh state. Their subjects were selected to exclude cases with disorders of the spine or sciatica. They found 'a total of forty-seven anomalous transforaminal ligaments of various types' in nine of the ten spines dissected. The ligaments were random in pattern and distribution, but were found at each of the five lumbar levels. The ligament at the fifth lumbar level was present in all nine spines. Right and left sides of some spines showed symmetrical ligaments, while others differed. The ligaments were easily distinguishable from the overlying fibrous covering because they were strong, unyielding structures of varied width and thickness, ranging from 2 to 5 mm. In one specimen, the corporotransverse ligament at the fifth lumbar level was completely ossified. Golub and Silverman (1969) classified the ligaments into five major types, namely: corporotransverse superior, corporotransverse inferior, superior transforaminal, mid-transforaminal, and inferior transforaminal ligaments. They concluded that there was no evidence to suggest that the ligaments were acquired structures, although they might sometimes be involved in nerve root entrapment syndromes. These findings were confirmed by Bachop and Hilgendorf (1981) and Bachop and Ro (1984), who added that the ligaments could be flat, wide and flexible, or rod-like and rigid. Both forms could coexist in any individual spine. Nathan *et al.* (1982) added to the reports on the fifth lumbar level by showing that a lumbosacral ligament, extending from the transverse process and body of the fifth lumbar vertebra to attach to the ala of the sacrum, formed an osteofibrotic tunnel for the fifth lumbar nerve and vessels that accompanied it. They dissected 42 specimens. The ligament was present in all cases but the size, thickness, shape and attachments were variable. The ligament was found to cause entrapment and compression of the nerve in some cases but they did not give the incidence. No mention was made of the corporotransverse ligament described by earlier reports. Mamillo-accessory ligaments associated with the dorsal rami were described by Bogduk (1981) and confirmed by Ro and Bachop (1984). Inspite of the clarifications brought by these studies, the question of whether these structures were true ligaments or not remains unresolved. None of the studies appeared to have looked at the reasons why the ligaments were found at some levels and not others. Amonoo-Kuofi *et al.* (1988a,b) dissected the lumbosacral spines of 12 adult cadavers and one fetal spine, which were carefully selected to exclude diseases or anomalies of the vertebral column. They showed, for the first time, that all lumbar intervertebral foramina were crossed by ligaments which subdivided the openings into smaller compartments for the protection of the structures passing through. The ligaments were better developed in some subjects than in others. The morphology of the ligaments at the lumbosacral junction were distinctly different from those of the upper lumbar levels. A classification based on their attachments was suggested. This will be adopted in the ensuing description. The finding of ligaments in the lumbar intervertebral foramina of the fetal specimen corroborated the suggestion of Golub and Silverman (1969) that these structures were not only integral parts of the lumbar spine but were also present at birth. These observations were strengthened by the results of a sectional anatomical study reported by Nowicki and Haughton (1992a). They sectioned the lumbar spines of 15 cadavers and found that fibrous ligaments were present in every lumbar intervertebral foramen. They described six different types of ligaments. The morphology of some of the ligaments appeared to differ somewhat from those described by previous workers. At the time of their study, Nowicki and Haughton (1992a) were unaware of the earlier report of Amonoo-Kuofi *et al.* (1988a,b). This fact enhanced the significance of their corroborative information. Radiological studies by Church and Buehler (1991) and Nowicki and Haughton (1992b) brought evidence to show that computerized axial tomographic and magnetic resonance imaging techniques could be modified to image these ligaments under experimental conditions. Giles (1992) carried out a histological study of the fourth and fifth lumbar intervertebral canals and confirmed the presence of ligaments in the mid-zones of these two levels. He stressed that there was no evidence of compression of the large nerves and blood vessels by these ligaments in his study. His report was the first to show that the transforaminal ligaments contained blood vessels and nerves.

Topography of the ligaments of the exit zone

The ligaments traversing the exit zones of the upper four lumbar levels differ from those of the fifth lumbar foramen. They will therefore be described separately, beginning with the foramina of the upper four lumbar levels.

Ligaments traversing the foramina of the upper four lumbar segments

Internal ligament

The oblique inferior transforaminal ligament

This is a tough, flat ligament measuring between 3 and 5 mm in width. It is located in the lower parts of the upper four intervertebral foramina. It arises from the posterolateral surface of the intervertebral disc and passes obliquely downwards and posteriorly to gain attachment to the lower part of the anterior surface of the superior articular facet (Figure 7.3). It crosses the lateral free border of the ligamentum flavum. The ligament bridges over the superior vertebral notch to convert it into a foramen which, in all spines, was seen to transmit a large vein. In some spines, the ligament was represented by multiple smaller bands thus giving rise to many smaller foramina, all of which transmitted veins (Figure 7.2). This ligament was described by Nowicki and Haughton (1992a) as a variant of their type 2 ligament.

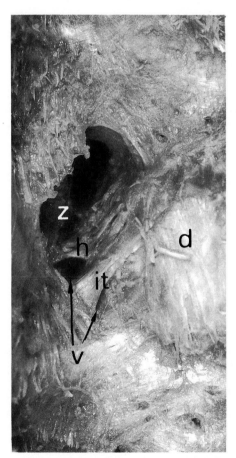

Figure 7.3 Photograph of the L4 intervertebral foramen with the external ligaments removed to show the lower intraforaminal ligaments. h = horizontal mid-transforaminal ligament; it = oblique inferior transforaminal ligament; z = anterior surface of the capsule of the zygapophysial joint; d = intervertebral disc between L4 and L5 vertebrae; v = venous compartments. (Reproduced with permission from Amonoo-Kuofi, H.S., El-Badawi, M.G. and Fatani, J.A. (1988a) Ligaments associated with lumbar intervertebral foramina. 1.L1 to L4. *J. Anat.*, **156**,177-183.)

Intraforaminal ligaments

These ligaments are attached to the margins of the intervertebral foramen. There are three types of intraforaminal ligaments:

(a) Oblique superior transforaminal ligament
(b) Deep anterior intraforaminal ligament
(c) Horizontal mid-transforaminal ligament

Oblique superior transforaminal ligament

This is a strong flat band measuring 1.5–2 mm. It is attached superiorly to the inferior border of the posterior end of the pedicle. The ligament passes obliquely downwards and forwards to attach to the posterolateral surface of the body of the vertebra above the level of the intervertebral disc (Figure 7.4). In some individuals, the lower attachment was to the posterior border of the deep anterior intraforaminal ligament (Figure 7.2). The ligament bridges the upper part of the inferior vertebral notch to form a vascular foramen. The main spinal branch of the lumbar segmental artery was seen passing through this foramen to enter the vertebral canal. The ligament was represented by two bands in some spines, thus creating two foramina, both of which transmitted arteries (see Figure 7.5). A similar ligament was illustrated by Golub and Silverman (1969) but they did not differentiate it from their corporotransverse superior ligament.

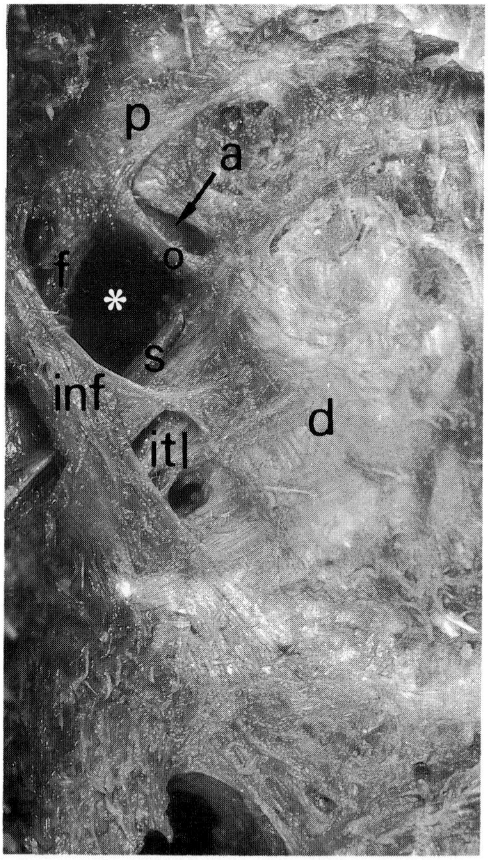

Figure 7.4 Photograph of the L3 intervertebral foramen showing the external ligaments. In this subject, ligaments were highly developed and mostly flattened. o = oblique superior transforaminal ligament; p = root of the right pedicle of L3 vertebra; d = intervertebral disc between L3 and L4 vertebrae; inf = inferior corporotransverse ligament of L3 level; s = superior corporotransverse ligament of L4 level; * = opening for the nerve trunk; a = arterial opening; f = lateral edge of ligamentum flavum; itl = oblique inferior transforaminal ligament. (Reproduced with permission from Amonoo-Kuofi, H.S., El-Badawi, M.G. and Fatani, J.A. (1988a) Ligaments associated with lumbar intervertebral foramina. 1.L1 to L4. *J. Anat.*, **156**, 177–183.)

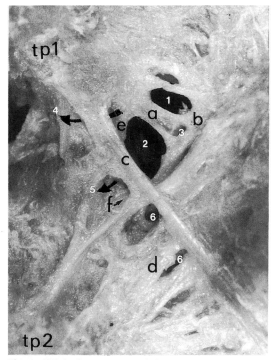

Figure 7.5 A close-up view of the right L1 intervertebral foramen showing the compartments of the lumbar intervertebral foramen. a = oblique superior transforaminal ligament; b = deep anterior intraforaminal ligament; c = inferior corporotransverse ligament of L1; d = superior corporotransverse ligament of L2; e = ligamentum flavum; f = horizontal mid-transforaminal ligament; tp1 and tp2 = transverse processes of L1 and L2 vertebrae respectively. For explanation of the numbered openings, refer to Figure 7.6. (Reproduced with permission from Amonoo-Kuofi, H.S., El-Badawi, M.G. and Fatani, J.A. (1988a) Ligaments associated with lumbar intervertebral foramina. 1.L1 to L4. *J. Anat.*, **156**, 177–183.)

Deep anterior intraforaminal ligament

This is a vertically orientated ligament located in the anterior part of the exit zone.

It is the smallest of the ligaments of the intervertebral foramen. It is attached superiorly to the lower border of the root of the pedicle. The ligament passes vertically downwards to gain attachment to the lower part of the posterior surface of the vertebral body at the junction with the intervertebral disc (Figure 7.2). As mentioned previously, the posterior edge of this ligament gave attachment to the oblique superior transforaminal ligament in some specimens. The osteofibrous foramen formed by this ligament transmitted the sinuvertebral nerve and a small artery.

Horizontal mid-transforaminal ligament

This is a strong ligament, placed horizontally at the junction between the upper two-thirds and the lower one-third of the intervertebral foramen. It is attached posteriorly to the anterior surface of the upper part of the superior articular facet. Anteriorly, the ligament is attached to the posterior part of the intervertebral disc and the adjacent part of the upper border of the vertebral body (Figures 7.1, 7.2 and 7.3). Its width ranges from 0.5 mm to 2 mm. The superior surface of the ligament forms a gutter that serves as the bed for the exiting spinal nerve. This ligament was described as the inferior transforaminal ligament by Golub and Silverman (1969) and by Nowicki and Haughton (1992a) as a variant of the type 2 ligament. Giles (1992) demonstrated it histologically and showed that it contained blood vessels and nerves. Owing to its thickness, the medial part of the ligament was seen in parasagittal sections of the mid-zone (Giles, 1992).

External ligaments

These ligaments are related to the outer surface of the intervertebral foramen. In dissections, they appear to radiate from the anterior surface of the root of the transverse process in three discrete bands, namely ascending, transverse and descending, of which the transverse band passes horizontally to the waist of the vertebra without crossing an intervertebral foramen (Figure 7.5). Because of their attachments to the transverse process as well as to the vertebral body, they are classified as the corporotransverse ligaments. These were the most variable ligaments in terms of thickness, appearance and in position.

Superior corporotransverse ligament

This ligament arises from the upper border of the root of the transverse process. It may vary from a strong rounded ligament to a broad, flat one. It passes obliquely, superiorly and anteriorly, crossing the lower part of the exit foramen below the spinal nerve, to insert into the posterolateral aspect of the lower border of the vertebra above and the adjacent part of the intervertebral disc (Figures 7.4 and 7.5). It is *transarticular* and therefore it is expected that lateral flexion of the lumbar spine will cause changes in tension within the ligament. This ligament corresponds to the inferior corporotransverse ligament described by Golub and Silverman (1969).

Inferior corporotransverse ligament

This ligament arises from the lower border of the root of the transverse process. It forms a rounded or flat structure, with a width ranging from 1 mm to 3.5 mm. It passes obliquely, downwards and anteriorly, crossing superficial to the superior corporotransverse ligament of the vertebra below (Figures 7.4 and 7.5). It inserts into the posterolateral aspect of the upper border of the vertebra below and the adjacent part of the intervertebral disc. The ligament is inferomedial to the exiting spinal nerve. The medial surface of the proximal part of this ligament is closely related to the lateral border of the ligamentum flavum and the horizontal mid-transforaminal ligament (Figures 7.2, 7.4 and 7.5). The ligament forms the posteroinferior boundary of the neural foramen (see below). Like the superior corporotransverse ligament, this ligament is also *transarticular* and therefore is expected to exhibit variations in tension during lateral flexion.

Compartments of the exit foramina of the upper four lumbar segments

The arrangement of the internal, intra- and external foraminal ligaments is such that the exit foramen is partitioned into neural, arterial and venous openings (Figures 7.4, 7.5 and 7.6). Owing to the differences in the mobility and consistency of the individual foraminal contents, this arrangement is beneficial considering the fact that the lumbar spine is constantly in motion.

The opening for the spinal nerve is centrally placed. The nerve is the most mobile structure within the foramen and its central location ensures that it stays clear of the bony walls of the opening. It glides on the grooved smooth superior surface of the horizontal mid-transforaminal ligament, which also ensures that it is kept clear of the inferior pedicle and the vulnerable veins interposed between the pedicle and the nerve. The *transarticular* attachments of the superior and inferior corporotransverse ligaments, which contribute to the antero-inferior and postero-inferior boundaries of the neural foramen, respectively, enable the size of the neural opening to alter during movement.

The vascular foramina surround the neural foramen. The vessels are relatively non-mobile and by

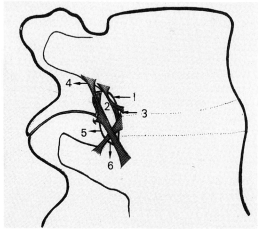

Figure 7.6 Schematic diagram showing the attachments of the ligaments of the external aspect of the lumbar intervertebral foramen, and their contribution towards the partitioning of the foramen. Based on Figures 7.4 and 7.5. 1 = compartment for the spinal artery; 2 = compartment for the ventral ramus of the spinal nerve; 3 = compartment for the recurrent meningeal nerve – this compartment also transmits a small branch of the segmental artery; 4 and 5 = tunnels transmitting the medial and lateral divisions of the dorsal primary ramus respectively, and accompanying vessels; 6 = compartment for veins (often multiple). [Reproduced with permission from Amonoo-Kuofi, H.S.,El-Badawi, M.G. and Fatani, J.A. (1988a) Ligaments associated with lumbar intervertebral foramina. 1.L1 to L4. *J. Anat.*, **156**, 177–183.]

keeping them close to the margins of the foramen, they can be plastered to the walls of the intervertebral canal. The branches of the arteries can, therefore, course to their destinations along the walls, without having to cross the intervertebral canal space. Similarly, the veins coming from the epidural plexus continue along the walls to exit through the venous openings, without crossing any space in the canal. The nerve root sleeve is free to slide to and fro within the intervertebral canal without endangering any vascular structures. The neural (radicular) branches of the spinal vessels join the nerve outside the foramen, and accompany the nerve through the neural opening. Therefore, they are protected by the circumneural sheath.

Ligaments traversing the fifth lumbar exit zone

The fifth lumbar intervertebral foramen is located in a region of structural and functional transition. The highly mobile lumbar spine, articulating with the immobile sacrum, makes the mechanical conditions at this junction different from the upper four lumbar levels (Amonoo-Kuofi *et al.*, 1988b). The spinal nerve trunk and its ventral and dorsal rami not only cross the junction but are also closely related to two mobile

joints – the ventral ramus to the intervertebral joint and the dorsal ramus to the zygapophysial joint (Amonoo-Kuofi *et al.*, 1988, 1991). The series of bends that the nerve turns through, as it runs towards the pelvic cavity, are such that, if it were not protected, it would bowstring anteriorly during flexion of the lumbosacral junction (Amonoo-Kuofi *et al.*, 1988b, 1991; Smith *et al.*, 1993). This would result in compression of the nerve against the inferior surface of the L5 transverse process, which overhangs the intervertebral foramen, and consequently produce pain. The presence of ligaments, and their arrangement, however, prevents this from happening (Nathan *et al.*, 1982; Amonoo-Kuofi *et al.*, 1988b; Transfeldt *et al.*, 1993).

Four ligaments have been identified as playing important roles in the mechanism by which the fifth lumbar spinal nerve and its two rami are protected from the effects of movement at the lumbosacral junction. These are:

1. The lumbosacral ligament
2. The lumbosacral hood
3. The L5 corporotransverse ligament
4. The mamillo-transverso-accessory ligament

The lumbosacral ligament

This is more of a vertebropelvic ligament than a juxtaforaminal ligament. Although it is described in most standard texts of anatomy, some aspects of its morphology, that are not fully described, were uncovered in our dissections. The ligament is included here for two reasons. First of all, it bears important relationships to both the ventral and dorsal rami of the fifth lumbar spinal nerve. Secondly, it gives attachment to the lumbosacral hood and the mamillo-transverso-accessory ligament.

This ligament bridges the interval between the antero-inferior border of the fifth lumbar transverse process and the upper surface of the ala of the sacrum. Its attachment to the sacrum is to the ridge that corresponds to the transverse process element of the ala of sacrum (Figures 7.7, 7.8 and 7.10). The upper part of the ligament, immediately subjacent to the transverse process, is thickened to form a rounded cord which continues laterally to reinforce the iliolumbar ligament (Figures 7.7, 7.8 and 7.10). The lumbosacral ligament has a free, crescentic medial border, that stops short of the lateral surface of the body of the fifth lumbar vertebra. The fibres in this free border are vertically orientated, unlike the rest of the ligament which has horizontally orientated fibres (Figures 7.8 and 7.9a). This border forms the lateral boundary of an opening through which the ventral ramus of the fifth lumbar spinal nerve emerges to descend into the pelvis (Figure 7.8). The medial boundary of the opening is formed by the lateral surface of the lumbosacral intervertebral disc

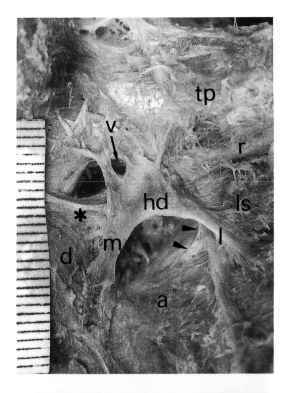

Figure 7.7 Ventral view of the fifth lumbar intervertebral foramen. The blood vessels and nerves have been removed to show the anterior ligaments *in situ*. tp = transverse process of the fifth lumbar vertebra; ls = lumbosacral ligament; a = upper surface of the ala of sacrum; d = intervertebral disc between fifth lumbar and first sacral vertebrae; r = thickened upper part of the lumbosacral ligament forming a rounded cord; hd = lumbosacral hood; * = corporotransverse ligament passing deep to the lumbosacral hood to insert on the intervertebral disc. m = medial limb of the lumbosacral hood; l = lateral limb of lumbosacral hood; arrow head = crescentic, medial border of the lumbosacral ligament; v = opening for the descending branches of the fourth lumbar segmental vessels to the fifth lumbar. Scale = mm. (Reproduced with permission from Amonoo-Kuofi, H.S., El-Badawi, M.G., Fatani, J.A. and Butt, M.M. (1988b) Ligaments associated with lumbar intervertebral foramina. 2. The fifth lumbar level. *J. Anat.*, **159**, 1-10.)

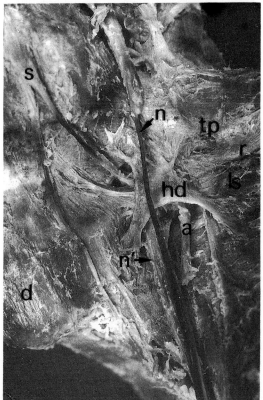

Figure 7.8 Photograph of the lumbosacral junction dissected to show the fifth lumbar intervertebral foramen and the related structures on the left side of an adult specimen. d = lumbosacral intervertebral disc (and sacral promontory); tp = transverse process of L5; s = ganglion of sympathetic chain giving a grey ramus communicans to L5; n = communicating branch from L4 ventral ramus to L5 ventral ramus (n′); a = branch of iliolumbar artery to the fifth lumbar foramen; hd = lumbosacral hood; ls = lumbosacral ligament; r = thickened upper part of the lumbosacral ligament.

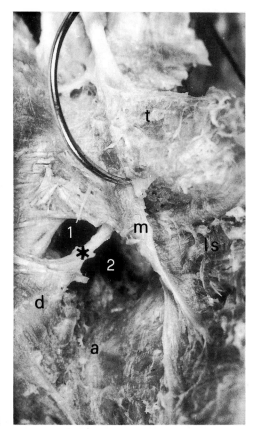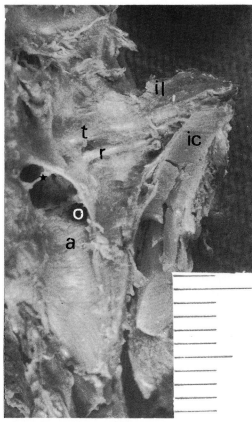

A   B

Figure 7.9 (A). Photograph of the ventral aspect of the L5/S1 exit zone on the left side showing the corporotransverse ligament (*). The medial limb of the lumbosacral hood (m) has been partially reflected laterally to expose this strong band. Note that the inferomedial attachment of the corporotransverse ligament includes the intervertebral disc (d); t = transverse process of the fifth lumbar vertebra; ls = lumbosacral ligament; a = ala of sacrum; 1 = superomedial opening; 2 = inferolateral opening. (B). Photograph of the ventral view of the lumbosacral junction of a fetus showing the exit zone of the left fifth lumbar intervertebral canal. t = transverse process of the fifth lumbar vertebra; il = iliolumbar ligament; r = thickened upper part of the lumbosacral ligament; ic = cartilaginous iliac crest; a = medial part of the ala of sacrum; o = opening for the medial division of the dorsal primary ramus inferior to the transverse (anterior) part of the mamillo-transverso-accessory ligament; *, = corporotransverse ligament. Scale, small divisions = mm. (Reproduced with permission from Amonoo-Kuofi, H.S., El-Badawi, M.G., Fatani, J.A. and Butt, M.M. (1988b) Ligaments associated with lumbar intervertebral foramina. 2. The fifth lumbar level. *J. Anat.*, **159**, 1-10.)

and adjacent part of the body of the fifth lumbar vertebra. The superior boundary of the opening is formed by the medial part of the inferior border of the transverse process, while the inferior boundary is formed by the medial part of the ala of sacrum (Figure 7.9). The opening so defined lies in the same vertical plane as the ventral sacral foramina.

The lumbosacral hood

This is a tent-like ligament that forms a roof over the ventral ramus, and its accompanying vessels, as they course over the smooth upper surface of the ala of sacrum (Amonoo-Kuofi *et al.*, 1988b). Superiorly, it is attached to the anteroinferior edge of the transverse

process of the fifth lumbar vertebra. There is usually an opening or two in the attachment for the passage of intersegmental vessels – mainly pedicular veins draining into the ascending lumbar vein (Figure 7.7). Laterally, the hood is attached to the anterior surface of the lumbosacral ligament. It has two crescentic, free borders – one medial and one inferior. The inferior border arches over the ventral ramus and the lumbar branches of the iliolumbar vessels (Figure 7.8). It gains attachment to the intervertebral disc and sacrum, respectively, by two limbs – one medial and one lateral. The medial limb is attached to the lateral aspect of the lumbosacral intervertebral disc and the adjacent part of the first sacral vertebra. The lateral limb is attached to the lower part of the anterior

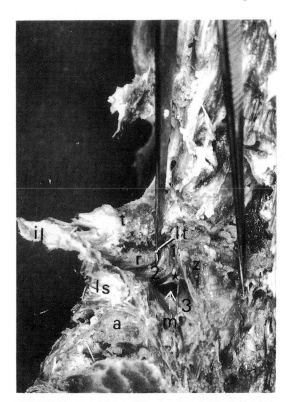

Figure 7.10 Dorsal view of the junction between the fifth lumbar and first sacral vertebrae on the left side of an adult specimen. t = posterior surface of the transverse process of the fifth lumbar vertebra; z = L5/S1 zygapophysial joint; a = ala of the sacrum; ls = lumbosacral ligament; r = thickened upper part of the lumbosacral ligament; il = iliolumbar ligament; ★ mamillo-transverso-accessory ligament (1 = superior attachment, 2 = anterior attachment, 3 = posterior attachment); lt = opening for the lateral division of the L5 dorsal ramus. The thick part of the lumbosacral ligament has reduced this opening to a narrow slit within which the nerve can easily be entrapped. m = opening for the medial division of the dorsal ramus. (Reproduced with permission from Amonoo-Kuofi, H.S., El-Badawi, M.G., Fatani, J.A. and Butt, M.M. (1988b) Ligaments associated with lumbar intervertebral foramina. 2. The fifth lumbar level. *J. Anat.*, **159**, 1–10.)

surface of the lumbosacral ligament and the adjacent part of the anterior surface of the ala of the sacrum. The presence of the lumbosacral hood was confirmed by Giles (1992).

Because of its attachments to the fifth lumbar transverse process and the body, as well as the ala, of the sacrum, the lumbosacral hood is, functionally, a *transarticular* ligament. Therefore, during flexion of the hip, as in straight leg raising, when the nerve rises toward the roof of the tunnel (Maurice-Williams, 1981; Smith *et al.*, 1993), the tension in the ligament will also be reduced as the distal and proximal attachments are approximated.

The grey ramus communicans from the sympathetic trunk to the fifth lumbar spinal nerve, enters the lumbosacral atrium (Amonoo-Kuofi *et al.*, 1988b) by passing through an opening, bounded laterally by the upper part of the medial border of the lumbosacral hood. The medial and inferior boundaries of this opening are formed by the root of the transverse process and the medial end of the corporotransverse ligament, respectively (Figure 7.7). The 'lumbosacral' ligament, described by Nathan *et al.* (1982) was similar to this ligament, except that the medial part of their ligament was attached along the whole of its length to the side of the fifth lumbar vertebra. The lumbosacral hood may vary in size, shape or thickness in different individuals (Nathan *et al.*, 1982; Amonoo-Kuofi *et al.*, 1988b). It was present in fetal specimens dissected by our group. The ligament forms the roof of an osteofibrous tunnel, through which the ventral ramus and its accompanying vessels, embedded in a dense plug of fat, pass to reach the pelvic cavity. The descending branch of the fourth lumbar spinal nerve, coming to join the fifth lumbar ventral ramus (to form the lumbosacral trunk), passes superficial to the hood (Figure 7.8).

The L5 corporotransverse ligament

The L5 corporotransverse ligament is a strong, cord-like ligament measuring 2–5 mm in diameter. Proximally, it is attached to the medial part of the accessory process of the fifth lumbar vertebra. From this attachment, it passes obliquely downwards, forwards and medially, across the lateral surface of the fifth lumbar intervertebral foramen, to gain insertion into the lateral surface of the lower part of the fifth lumbar vertebral body and the adjacent part of the lumbosacral disc (Amonoo-Kuofi *et al.*, 1988b; Amonoo-Kuofi *et al.*, 1991). This ligament lies under cover of the lumbosacral hood. Its inferior attachment is often deep to the medial limb of the hood (Figures 7.7 and 7.9a). In fetal specimens, it is a thin, thread-like, but nevertheless strong, structure (Figure 7.9b). As it crosses the intervertebral foramen, the ligament divides the foramen into a smaller superomedial and a larger inferolateral compartment. The superomedial opening transmits the grey ramus communicans from the sympathetic trunk to the fifth lumbar nerve. The inferolateral opening transmits the spinal nerve trunk medially, the venous plexus laterally, and the spinal branch of the lumbar division of the iliolumbar artery between them (see Figure 7.8). The orientation of the corporotransverse ligament causes the nerve to slide laterally as it rises towards the transverse process during flexion of the hip (Amonoo-Kuofi *et al.*, 1988b; Amonoo-Kuofi *et al.*, 1991). This ensures that the moving nerve is kept clear of the lateral surface of the vertebral body. Owing to its attachment to the intervertebral disc, the ligament will slacken during hip flexion (as the nerve rises towards it) and, therefore, minimize the possibility of impingement. The vessels are not at risk of compression by the nerve because, during hip flexion, the nerve initially rises towards the transverse process before sliding laterally (Maurice-Williams, 1981; Smith *et al.*, 1993). There is no evidence to suggest that the vessels move to the same extent as the nerve during flexion and extension of the hip.

The corporotransverse ligament was reported by Larmon (1944), Golub and Silverman (1969), Macnab (1971), Bachop and Hilgendorf (1981), Bachop and Ro (1984), Janse and Bachop (1985) and Church and Buehler (1991) but their accounts of the topography and attachments of the ligament appeared to be incomplete.

The mamillo-transverso-accessory ligament

This is a strong, flattened, tripartite ligament which, though not related to the fifth lumbar intervertebral foramen, deserves mention because of its important relationship to the two divisions of the dorsal ramus of the fifth lumbar spinal nerve. The potential for entrapment of the branches of the dorsal ramus by this ligament appears to be greater than that of the ventral ramus by its related ligament.

The ligament has the shape of an inverted Y (Amonoo-Kuofi *et al.*, 1988b). The stem of the Y is attached to the posterior part of the accessory process of the fifth lumbar vertebra. As the ligament is followed inferiorly, it bifurcates into anterior and posterior limbs. The posterior limb descends anterolateral to the L5/S1 zygapophysial joint to gain insertion into the upper border of the superior articular facet of the sacrum. It may be adherent to the anteromedial part of the capsule of the zygapophysial joint (Figure 7.10). This part of the ligament is, clearly, an accessory ligament of the L5/S1 zygapophysial joint. The anterior limb of the ligament runs horizontally forwards to gain attachment to the posterior surface of the lumbosacral ligament. It defines two openings, superior and inferior (Amonoo-Kuofi *et al.*, 1988b, 1991). The superior opening is a triangular, often slit-like, space bounded anterosuperiorly by the posterior surface of the lumbosacral ligament, posteriorly by the stem of the mamillotransverso-accessory ligament, and posteroinferiorly by the anterior limb of the ligament. It transmits the lateral division of the dorsal ramus. The inferior opening is more spacious. Superiorly, it is bounded by the anterior limb of the ligament, and anteriorly by the lower part of the lumbosacral ligament. The posterior boundary is formed by the posterior limb of the ligament, and the inferior boundary by the upper surface of the ala of sacrum. It gives passage to the medial division of the dorsal ramus. This ligament is, probably, the most inaccessible of the ligaments associated with the lumbar intervertebral foramina. The narrowness of the slit for the lateral division of

the dorsal ramus means that there is a greater risk of entrapment of that nerve than there is of the medial division or of the ventral ramus. It should be considered in the differential diagnosis of low back pain localized at the level of the posterolateral part of the iliac crest.

Ligament of the postcanal zone

Lumbar cribriform fascia

This fascia has been described as a fibrous sheet that overlies the foraminal exit (Golub and Silverman, 1969; Bogduk and Twomey, 1987; Rauschning, 1987; Paz-Fumagalli and Haughton, 1993). It is a sagittally orientated fascia that separates the overlying psoas major muscle from the intervertebral foramen. The exact nature of this fascia is not very clear. Bogduk and Twomey (1987) described it as the ventral leaflet of the intertransverse ligament. The histological account by Rauschning (1987) suggests that it is the anterior layer of the thoracolumbar fascia. Anteriorly, it is attached to the posterolateral aspect of the vertebral body, the lateral parts of the anterior longitudinal ligament, and the intervertebral disc. Posteriorly, it is attached to the transverse and articular processes. At all levels, the cranial part of the fascia is thicker, while the caudal part is thinner and more delicate. All accounts agree that the fascia is more difficult to visualize and demonstrate at the L5/S1 level. The middle and caudal thirds of the fascia are penetrated by vessels and nerves. We noted, in our dissections, that on removal of the psoas major muscle, there was a fascial condensation, deep to the muscle, but it did not form a sheet that could be peeled off as one layer. It had to be removed by dissection. Deep to the fascia, opposite each intervertebral foramen, there was a complex array of arteries, veins and communicating nerves (Figure 7.11A). Sandwiched between these and the foraminal exit, there was a plexus, or polygonal ring, of veins, that completely obscured the view of the foramen (Figure 7.11B). These juxtaforaminal venous rings received tributaries from the intervertebral foramina and were connected by longitudinal intersegmental veins to form the ascending lumbar vein. The intervertebral foramina, and the ligaments associated with them are, therefore, separated from the lumbar cribriform fascia and the overlying psoas major muscle, by this rich plexus of veins.

Histological studies of ligaments associated with the intervertebral foramina

The ligaments associated with the intervertebral foramina are not easily accessible by dissection. Because of this, some workers have resorted to sectional anatomic techniques in attempts to study

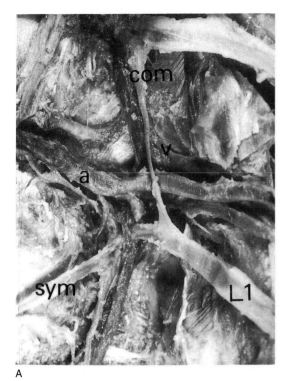
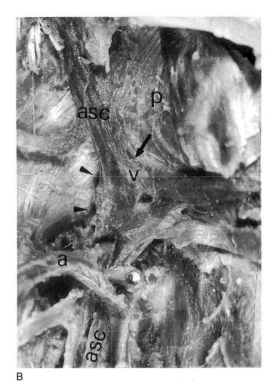

A   B

Figure 7.11 (A). Photograph showing the superficial relations of the left L1 intervertebral foramen. The segmental artery (a) is seen coursing dorsally, across the upper part of the foramen, accompanied by its vein. The spinal branch of the artery and other smaller branches are also seen entering the foramen. Note the plexus of veins (v) sandwiched between the intervertebral foramen and the dorsal continuation of the segmental artery. L1 = ventral ramus of the first lumbar spinal nerve receiving a communicating branch (com) from T12 nerve; sym = sympathetic ramus. (B). The segmental artery, a, and the ventral ramus have been reflected ventrally to show the underlying venous network. The somewhat polygonal ring of veins (v) receives tributaries from the postvertebral region. It also communicates with similar rings at the other lumbar levels through the ascending lumbar vein (asc). Tributaries enter the deep surface of the ring from the intervertebral canal; p, pedicle of L1; →, upper border of the intervertebral foramen; arrow head = anterior margin of the foramen. [Reproduced with permission from Amonoo-Kuofi, H.S., (El-Badawi, M.G. and Fatani, J.A. (1988a). Ligaments associated with lumbar intervertebral foramina. 1.L1 to L4. *J. Anat.*, **156**, 177-183.)

them. These studies have confirmed the presence of ligaments traversing the foramina (Rauschning, 1987; Giles, 1992; Nowicki and Haughton, 1992a), although sections have not given detailed information on the exact topography of the ligaments. One limitation of this technique is that no single orthogonal plane of section gives a clear picture of the three-dimensional relationships of the ligaments. Reconstruction techniques are needed to make sectional studies more informative. Histological studies, on the other hand, give valuable information needed to answer some of the questions that have been raised on the nature of these ligaments.

Giles *et al.* (1991) developed a technique whereby ligaments identified by sectional anatomic study of thick sections could be removed and re-embedded for histological study. This enabled detailed microscopic studies of these structures to

be carried out (see Chapter 3). Giles (1992) studied 26 blocks of L4/L5 and 26 blocks of L5/S1 intervertebral canals cut from 13 bisected spines by parasagittal sections. Another set of 32 blocks of L5/S1 intervertebral canals, cut from 16 spines, were also cut horizontally for histological study. The depth of ligaments within the exit zones of the L4/L5 and the L5/S1 intervertebral canals was calculated by viewing serial sections of known thicknesses to see in which section the first, and last, fibres of the ligament were noted. The length and width of the ligaments were measured using a calibrated scale and a known magnification of a Wild photomacroscope. In 16 out of 26 (61%) sagittally cut L4/L5 intervertebral canals and in 25 of the 58 (43%) sagittally and horizontally cut L5/S1 intervertebral canals, he was able to confirm the presence of ligaments. He stressed that the ligaments did not compromise the large neural structures. At the L4/L5 level the length of the horizontal (mid-transforaminal) ligament in parasagittal sections ranged from 3.1 to 9.8 mm (with a mean of 5.7 mm). Its width ranged from 0.4 mm to 1.9 mm (with a mean of 1.1 mm). The ligament was placed at a depth of 1.0–3.0 mm (mean 1. 8 mm) from the outer margin of the intervertebral foramen. Morphometric study of the ligament at the L5/S1 level showed that its dimensions and depth were similar to the ligament at L4/L5 level. Measurements of the ligaments in horizontal sections confirmed gross anatomic observations that the ligaments varied markedly in the extent to which they were developed in different individuals.

Thin sections of the horizontal mid-transforaminal ligament showed it was made, mainly, of regularly arranged collagenous fibres, with some elastic fibres interspersed among the collagenous fibres (Giles, 1992). Blood vessels and nerves were seen within the ligament. The presence of a myelinated nerve within the ligament was beautifully illustrated. Rhalmi *et al.* (1993) have demonstrated that in all specimens of spinal ligamentous tissue they studied, blood vessels and collagenous fibres were associated with abundant neurofilament-protein-immunoreactive nerve fibres. These fibres tended to end as free nerve endings. The technique offers an additional tool for studying the detailed innervation of foraminal ligaments.

Radiological studies of the ligaments traversing the lumbar intervertebral foramina

Hitherto, plain lateral radiographs of the lumbar spine have not demonstrated the ligaments of the intervertebral foramina because the normal, unossified or uncalcified, foraminal ligament cannot be visualized by either plain film radiography or conventional linear tomography. In studies of the corporotransverse ligament at the L5 intervertebral foramen, Church and Buehler (1991) showed that the superior soft tissue imaging capabilities of computerized tomography enabled the corporotransverse ligament to be well demonstrated under experimental conditions in cadaveric material. Their observations have been confirmed and extended by Nowicki and Haughton (1992b) who studied 114 neural foramina at 57 spinal levels by axial and parasagittal computerized tomography (CT) and 27 neural foramina by magnetic resonance (MR) imaging. The supraspinal, and paraspinal muscles of their specimens were completely removed by sharp dissection before imaging. They were able to visualize ligaments at all five lumbar levels by computerized tomography. The attenuation coefficients of the ligaments were similar

to those of the intervertebral disc and the ligamentum flavum. In the parasagittal CT images most of the bands were found in the lateral aspects of the neural foramina. They stressed that the accuracy of CT in depicting the foraminal ligaments depended on the size and shape of the ligaments, and the imaging plane used. Axial MR images also showed bilateral ligaments at all lumbar levels. The origins of the ligaments from the posterolateral margins of the intervertebral discs, or vertebral body, and insertions into the superior articular process, transverse process, or pedicles, could be easily identified. Parasagittal MR images showed the ligaments to be linear or curvilinear. Their evidence did not suggest that the ligaments caused entrapment of the neural or vascular structures. The ligaments had a signal intensity lower than that of the adjacent fat. The signal intensity was similar to those of the intervertebral disc and the ligamentum flavum. Nowicki and Haughton (1992b) clarified, however, that the CT and MR imaging techniques employed in this cadaveric study cannot be used for imaging patients. Further work was needed to develop the technique for use in clinical imaging.

Role of the foraminal ligaments in the production of low back pain

The weight of morphological, histological and clinical evidence suggests that these ligaments are normal structures which play a role in the function of the lumbar spine. Nevertheless, like other normal structures in the body, they are subject to structural variations or pathological change. Under these altered conditions they may either produce pain, or predispose to pain.

There are two main mechanisms by which foraminal ligaments can contribute to low back pain. These are:

1. Inflammatory: activation of fine, non-myelinated pain endings as a result of local tissue distortion or release of chemical irritants following inflammation.
2. Mechanical: direct pressure on the neural complex giving rise to severe pain and paraesthesiae along the distribution of the nerve.

Inflammatory

Foraminal ligaments, like other fibrous tissue elsewhere, may become inflamed. The vasodilatation and oedema that accompany the inflammatory reaction will cause an increase in tissue pressure. The effect of this will be the distortion of the various components of the ligaments (i.e. blood vessels, neural elements and fibres). The walls of blood vessels, and the surrounding fat, are known to have free nerve endings and plexuses of non-myelinated nerves within them (Wyke, 1970, 1977, 1987; Maurice-Williams, 1981; Rhalmi *et al.*, 1993). Distortion of these endings will give rise to pain. Furthermore, oedematous ligaments could exert pressure on neighbouring vessels. The venous structures are especially sensitive to pressure (Hoyland *et al.*, 1989).

The chemical irritants released by the inflamed tissue are also known to activate the nociceptive endings (Rydevik *et al.*, 1984; Jayson, 1987). Pain arising as a result of inflammation of the ligaments will usually be localized, except when the swelling is severe enough to cause pressure either on the neural complex or on its vessels; in this case, vascular impairment could cause nerve fibre dysfunction and consequently produce radicular symptoms (Rydevik *et al.*, 1984; Watanabe and Parke, 1986; Parke, 1991). Pain arising from acute inflammation will resolve once the inflammation is treated. However, if the inflammation persists, then fibrosis, and possible contracture, of the ligaments could result in encroachment on foraminal contents, making the pain intractable.

Mechanical

Foraminal ligaments may exert pressure on the neural complex in one of the following ways, namely:

(a) Periradicular fibrosis
(b) Malposition of the ligaments – congenital and acquired
(c) Ossification of foraminal ligaments
(d) Anomalies of the nerve trunks, e.g. conjoint nerve roots
(e) Entrapment of the dorsal root ganglion

Periradicular fibrosis

As discussed previously, the neural complex is surrounded by a fibrous sheath and fascial condensations. These may be involved in inflammatory processes. A history of viral or bacterial meningitis, or invasive procedures (e.g. myelography, spinal or epidural anaesthesia, laminectomy), or ischaemic pain may be antecedent. Post-inflammatory fibrosis of the connective tissue around the neural complex and spinal cord could result in (i) damage of the nerve or nerve roots (Jayson, 1987), or (ii) interruption of its arterial supply or venous drainage (Watanabe and Parke, 1986; Hoyland *et al.*, 1989). Chronic pressure resulting from the fibrosis will not only activate nociceptive endings (especially in the dorsal root ganglion), but will also lead to intraneural ischaemia. This will aggravate intra- and extraneural fibrosis

(Rydevik *et al.*, 1984; Jayson, 1987) and produce chronic back pain associated with demyelination or axonal degeneration.

Malposition of the ligaments

Transforaminal ligaments are subject to marked variation (Larmon, 1944; Golub and Silverman, 1969; Bachop and Ro, 1985; Janse *et al.*, 1985; Amonoo-Kuofi *et al.*, 1988a; Amonoo-Kuofi *et al.*, 1988b) If the ligament is placed in such a way as to encroach severely on the neural foramen, the resultant narrowing of the neural foramen may cause entrapment of the nerve (Magnusson, 1944; Golub and Silverman, 1969; Macnab, 1977; Nathan *et al.*, 1982; Bachop *et al.*, 1985). This would lead to pressure on the nerve and its blood supply. The pain in such cases would mimic the pain produced by a prolapsed intervertebral disc associated with nerve root compression.

Variation or malpositioning of the foraminal ligaments could be congenital since these structures are normal components of the spine, but the onset of pain could be delayed till adolescence or adulthood, i.e. when the ligaments mature. Normally, the vertebral column and its associated structures continue to undergo regeneration and remodelling throughout life (Oda *et al.*, 1988). Peak changes take place in the third decade of life (Humzah and Soames, 1988; Amonoo-Kuofi, 1991, 1992, 1995). It has been shown from biomechanical studies that the strength of the spine (and presumably the extent of maturation attained by its associated ligaments) is determined, partly, by the amount of physical activity undertaken (Porter *et al.*, 1989). It is, therefore, possible that pressure symptoms due to a maldeveloped foraminal ligament could be delayed until the ligaments mature. Strong and physically active individuals who are genetically predisposed, would have a higher risk of developing symptoms in the third decade of life, if not earlier.

Acquired malpositioning of foraminal ligaments, due to reduction or loss of intervertebral disc height, could affect ligaments that are *transarticular*, i.e. the superior and inferior corporotransverse ligaments of the upper lumbar levels, the L5 corporotransverse ligament, and the lumbosacral hood. Reduction or loss of intervertebral disc space, could result from isolated disc resorption (Crock, 1970; Venner and Crock, 1981), age-related changes (Vernon-Roberts and Pirie, 1977; Twomey and Taylor, 1985; Amonoo-Kuofi, 1991) or disc surgery. Descent of the vertebra can cause changes in the position of the *transarticular* ligaments. At the upper four lumbar levels, the corporotransverse ligaments form the boundaries of the neural foramen. The integrity of the intervertebral disc ensures that the neural opening alters its shape during movement to accommodate the nerve. This function will be impaired when the disc space is compromised. At the fifth lumbar level, the ventral ramus is at increased risk of entrapment and compression because it passes between the L5 corporotransverse ligament and the ala of sacrum. Isolated disc resorption is most common at the L5–S1 junction. Venner and Crock (1981) demonstrated that, in this condition, the symptoms were similar to those of prolapsed disc, although the cause of the nerve root compression was not clear.

Ossification of the foraminal ligaments

This appears to be a rarer cause of encroachment and entrapment of the contents of the intervertebral foramen. Nevertheless, it should be considered in the differential diagnosis. The only reported case of ossification of a transforaminal ligament was brought by Golub and Silverman (1969). The ossified ligament was the right corporotransverse ligament at the lumbosacral level. The nerve root emerged below the ossified ligament. During flexion of the hip, the nerve would not only glide under the ossified ligament, but it would also be exposed to the risk of entrapment. Pain could result from attrition or entrapment.

Vascular impairment from ossified ligaments is less likely, since the relationship between ossified ligaments and vessels would remain unchanged during movement.

Conjoint nerve roots

The space in the neural foramen is normally adequate for the segmental nerve (Amonoo-Kuofi *et al.*, 1988a,b). Anatomical variations have been described in which contiguous nerve roots may be conjoined intrathecally (Ethelberg and Riishede, 1952; Postacchini *et al.*, 1982; Hasue *et al.*, 1983; Kadish and Simmons, 1984; Hasue *et al.*, 1989; Philips and Park, 1993). The incidence of conjoint roots is estimated to be between 4% and 14% (Kadish and Simmons, 1984). The conjoined nerve roots either separated just before leaving the vertebral canal or they remained conjoined and left the vertebral canal, through one neural foramen (Hasue *et al.*, 1983; Kadish and Simmons, 1984). If this happens, the exiting conjoint nerve root would be disproportionately larger than the space available. This would result in compression of the nerve with radicular symptoms.

Entrapment of the dorsal root ganglion

The dorsal root ganglia are exquisitely sensitive to mechanical pressure. Evidence suggests that they are an important anatomic factor in the pathophysiology of pain (Cohen *et al.*, 1990). Compression of these structures, unlike mechanical pressure in other parts of the spinal nerve root, induces prolonged electrical activity (Howe *et al.*, 1977; Rydevik *et al.*, 1984; Cohen *et al.*, 1990) (see Chapter 16). Their size and

anatomical location may, therefore, have relevance in the differential diagnosis of lumbosacral pain disorders (Cohen *et al.*, 1990). Hasue *et al.* (1989) showed that in 8.4% of 144 subjects they studied, the dorsal root ganglion at the L5 level was extraforaminal. Since the diameter of the ganglion is normally greater than that of the ventral root (Cohen *et al.*, 1990), the likelihood of entrapment and compression by the corporotransverse ligament was high. Saal *et al.* (1988) suggested that chronic pressure on the dorsal root ganglion would lead to an increase in the release of the pain neurotransmitter, substance P, from the dorsal root ganglion. This would be passed to the point of entry of the dorsal root in the spinal cord. The result of this would be an increased sensitivity of the dorsal root ganglion and the nerve root to any stimulus, whether painful or not.

References

Albisinni, U., Chianura, G., Merlini, L. *et al.* (1988) Ossificazione del legamento longitudinale posteriore del rachide lombare. *Radiol. Med. Torino*, **75**, 482–485.

Amonoo-Kuofi, H.S. (1991) Morphometric changes in the heights and anteroposterior diameters of the lumbar intervertebral discs with age. *J. Anat.*, **175**, 159–168.

Amonoo-Kuofi, H.S. (1992) Changes in the lumbosacral angle, sacral inclination and the curvature of the lumbosacral spine during aging. *Acta Anat.*, **145**, 373–377.

Amonoo-Kuofi, H.S. (1995) Age related variations in the horizontal and vertical diameters of the pedicles of the lumbar spine. *J. Anat.*, **186**, 321–328.

Amonoo-Kuofi, H.S., El-Badawi, M.G. and Fatani, J.A. (1988a) Ligaments associated with lumbar intervertebral foramina. 1. L1 to L4. *J. Anat.*, **156**, 177–183.

Amonoo-Kuofi, H.S., El-Badawi, M.G., Fatani, J.A. and Butt, M.M. (1988b) Ligaments associated with lumbar intervertebral foramina. 2. The fifth lumbar level. *J. Anat.*, **159**, 1–10.

Amonoo-Kuofi, H.S., El-Badawi, M.G., Fatani, J.A. and Butt, M.M. (1991) Extraspinal course of the fifth lumbar spinal nerve: an update of its topographical relationships. *Clin. Anat.*, **4**, 1–9.

Baba, H., Komita, T., Maesawa, Y. and Imura, S. (1993) Intermittent claudication of the spinal cord due to ossification of the ligamentum flavum. A report of two cases. *International Orthopaedics (SICOT)*, **17**, 169–172.

Bachop, W. and Hilgendorf, C. (1981) Transforaminal ligaments of the human lumbar spine. *Anat. Rec.*, **199**, 14A.

Bachop, W. and Ro, C.S. (1984) A ligament separating the nerve from the blood vessels at the L5 intervertebral foramen. *Orthop. Transac. Int. Soc. Stud. Lumbar Spine*, **8**, 437.

Bachop, W. and Ro, C.S. (1985) Location of the dorsal ramus, ventral ramus and gray ramus communicans of the L5 spinal nerve relative to a transforaminal ligament at the L5 intervertebral foramen and diagnostic implications thereof. *Anat. Rec.*, **211**, 359.

Beamer, Y.B., Garner, J.T. and Shelden, C.H. (1973) Hypertrophied ligamentum flavum. Clinical and surgical significance. *Arch. Surg.*, **106**, 289-292.

Bitar, E., Mohasseb, G., Tabbara, W. *et al.* (1987) A propos de l'ossification du ligament longitudinal posterieur du rachis lombaire. *Rev. Rheum. Mal. Osteoartic.*, **54**, 789-793.

Bogduk, N. (1981) The lumbar mamillo-accessory ligament. Its anatomical and neurosurgical significance. *Spine*, **6**, 162-167.

Bogduk, N. and Long, D.M. (1979) The anatomy of the so-called 'articular nerves' and their relationship to facet denervation in the treatment of low back pain. *J. Neurosurg.*, **51**, 172-177.

Bogduk, N. and Twomey, L.T. (1987) *Clinical Anatomy of the Lumbar Spine*. Churchill Livingstone, London, p. 40.

Brieg, A. (1960) *Biomechanics of the Central Nervous System*. Almqvist and Wiksell, Stockholm.

Brieg, A. (1978) *Adverse Mechanical Tension in the Central Nervous System*. John Wiley and Sons, New York.

Brown, T.R., Quinn, S.F. and D'Agostino, A.N. (1991) Deposition of calcium pyrophosphate dihydrate crystals in the ligamentum flavum: evaluation with MR imaging and CT. *Radiology*, **178**, 871-873.

Church, C.P. and Buehler, M.T. (1991) Radiographic evaluation of the corporotransverse ligament at the L5 intervertebral foramen: a cadaveric study. *J Manipulative Physiol. Ther.*, **14**, 240-248.

Cohen, M.S., Wall, E.J., Brown, R.A. *et al.*, (1990) Cauda equina anatomy II: Extrathecal nerve roots and dorsal root ganglia. *Spine*, **15**, 1248-1251.

Crelin, E.S. (1982) Functional anatomy of the lumbosacral spine. In *Symposium on Idiopathic low back pain. Miami Fla. December, 1980.* (A.A. White and S.L. Gordon, eds). C.V.Mosby, St Louis. pp. 59-77.

Crock, H.V. (1970) A reappraisal of intervertebral disc lesions. *Med. J. Aust.*, **1**, 983-989.

Crock, H.V. (1981) Normal and pathological anatomy of the lumbar spinal nerve root canals. *J. Bone Joint Surg.*, **63B**, 487-490.

Dommisse, G. (1975) Morphological aspects of the lumbar spine and lumbosacral region. *Orthop.Clin. North Am.*, **6**, 163-175.

Ermachenko, B.A., Makarov, A.I. and Leikin, I.B. (1992) Ossifikatsiia zadnei prodol'noi sviazki. *Vestn. Rentgenol. Radiol.*, **2**, 30-34.

Ethelberg, S. and Riishede, J. (1952) Malformation of lumbar spinal roots and sheaths in the causation of low back ache and sciatica. *J. Bone Joint Surg.*, **34B**, 442-446.

Fick, R. (1904) *Anatomie und Mechanik der Gelenke.* Verlag von Gustav Fischer, p. 81.

Giles, L.G.F. (1992) Ligaments traversing the intervertebral canals of the human lower lumbosacral spine. *Neuro-Orthop.*, **13**, 25-38.

Giles, L.G.F., Allen, D.E. and Horne, F. (1991) Thin histological sections prepared from large thick sections: a new technique. *Biotechnic and Histochemistry*, **66**, 273-291.

Golub B.S. and Silverman, B.(1969) Transforaminal ligaments of the lumbar spine. *J. Bone Joint Surg.*, **51A**, 947-956.

Guo-Xiang, J., Wei-Dong, X. and Ai-Hao, W. (1988) Spinal stenosis with meralgia paraesthetica. *J. Bone Joint Surg.*, **70B**, 272-273.

Hasue, M., Kikuchi, S., Sakuyama, Y. and Ito, T. (1983) Anatomic study of the interrelation between lumbosacral nerve roots and their surrounding tissues. *Spine*, **8**, 50-58.

Hasue, M., Kunogi J., Konno, S., Kikuchi, S. (1989) Classification by position of dorsal root ganglia in the lumbodorsal region. *Spine*, **14**, 1261-1264.

Hayashi, K., Yabuki, T., Kurokawa, T. *et al.* (1977) The anterior and the posterior longitudinal ligaments of the lower cervical spine. *J. Anat.*, 633-636.

Hoffmann, M. (1898) Die befestigung der dura mater im wirbelcanal. *Arch. F. Anat. Physio.(Anat. Abt.)*, 403.

Howe, J.F., Loeser, J.D. and Calvin, W.H. (1977) Mechano-sensitivity of dorsal root ganglia and chronically injured axons: a physiological basis for the radicular pain of nerve root compression. *Pain*, **3**, 25-41.

Hoyland, J.A., Freemont, A.J. and Jayson, M.I.V. (1989) Intervertebral foramen venous obstruction. A cause of periradicular fibrosis? *Spine*, **14**, 558-568.

Humzah, M.D. and Soames, R.W. (1988) Human intervertebral disc: structure and function. *Anat. Rec.*, **220**, 337-356.

Ikata, T. and Onomura, T. (1977) General conception of ossification of ligamenta flava. *Clin. Orthop. Surg. (Jpn.)*, **12**, 322-324.

Janse, J., Ro, C-S. and Bachop, W. (1985) Clinical implications of a transforaminal ligament at the L5 intervertebral foramen. Paper presented at the *International Anatomical Congress*, London, August, 1985.

Jayson, M.I.V. (1987) Chronic inflammation and fibrosis in back pain syndromes. In *The Lumbar Spine and Back Pain* (M.I.V. Jayson, ed.)., Churchill Livingstone, London, pp. 411-418.

Kadish, L.J. and Simmons, E.H. (1984) Anomalies of the lumbosacral nerve roots. An anatomical investigation and myelographic study. *J. Bone Joint Surg.*, **66B**, 411-416.

Kashiwagi, K. (1993) Histological changes of the lumbar ligamentum flavum with age. *Nippon-Seikeigeka Gakkai-Zasshi*, **67**, 221-229.

Kikuchi, S. (1982) Anatomical and experimental studies of nerve root infiltration. *J. Japan Orthop. Assoc.*, **56**, 605-614.

Kubo, Y., Waga, S., Kojima, T. *et al.* (1994) Microsurgical anatomy of the lower cervical spine and cord. *Neurosurgery*, **34**, 895-902.

Kudo, S., Ono, M. and Russell, W.J. (1983) Ossification of thoracic ligamenta flava. *AJR*, **141**, 117-121.

Larmon, W. A. (1944) An anatomical study of the lumbosacral region in relation to low back pain and sciatica. *Annals of Surgery*, **119**, 892-896.

Lee, C.K., Rauschning, W. and Glenn, W. (1988) Lateral lumbar spinal canal stenosis: classification, pathologic anatomy and surgical decompression. *Spine*, **13**, 313-320.

Lee, T., Chacha, P.B. and Khoo, J. (1990) Ossification of posterior longitudinal ligament of the cervical spine in non-Japanese Asians. *Surg. Neurol.*, **35**, 40-44.

Luyendijk, W. and van Voorthuisen, A.E. (1966) Contrast examination of the spinal epidural space. *Acta Radiol. Diagn. (Stockh.)*, **5**, 1051-1066.

Macnab, I. (1971) Negative disc exploration - an analysis of the causes of nerve root involvement in sixty eight patients. *J. Bone Joint Surg.*, **53A**, 891-907.

Macnab, I. (1977) *Backache*. Williams and Wilkins, Baltimore, pp. 53-56, 97-102.

Magnusson, P.B. (1944) Differential diagnosis of causes of pain in the lower back accompanied by sciatic pain. *Ann. Surg.*, **119**, 878–891.

Maurice-Williams, R. S. (1981) *Spinal Degenerative Disease.* John Wright, London, pp. 15–25, 181–209.

Moiel, R.H., Ehni, G. and Anderson, M.S. (1967) Nodule of the ligamentum flavum as a cause of nerve root compression. *J. Neurosurg.*, **27**, 456–458.

Nakamura, T., Hashimoto, N., Maeda, Y. *et al.* (1990) Degeneration and ossification of the yellow ligament in unstable spine. *J. Spinal Disord.*, **3**, 288–292.

Nathan, H., Weizenbluth, M. and Halperin, N. (1982) The lumbosacral ligament (LSL) with special emphasis on the lumbosacral tunnel and the entrapment of the 5th lumbar nerve. *International Orthopaedics (SICOT)*, **6**, 197–202.

Nomina Anatomica (1983) Fifth edition. Incorporating *Nomina Histologica* (2nd edn) and *Nomina Embryologica* (2nd edn). Williams and Wilkins, Baltimore.

Nowicki, B.H. and Haughton,V.M. (1992a) Ligaments of the lumbar neural foramina: a sectional anatomic study. *Clin. Anat.*, **5**, 126–135.

Nowicki, B.H. and Haughton, V.M. (1992b) Neural foraminal ligaments of the lumbar spine: appearance at CT and MR imaging. *Radiology*, **183**, 257–264.

Oda, J., Tanaka, H. and Tsuzuki, N. (1988) Intervertebral disc changes with aging human cervical vertebra. Neonate to 80 years. *Spine*, **13**, 1205–1211.

Omojola, M.F., Cardoso, E.R., Fox, A.J. *et al.* (1982) Thoracic myelopathy secondary to ossified ligamentum flavum. *J. Neurosurg.*, **56**, 448–450.

Otani, K., Aihara, T., Tanaka, A. and Shibasaki, K. (1986) Ossification of the ligamentum flavum of the thoracic spine in adult kyphosis. *International Orthopaedics (SICOT)*, **10**, 135–139.

Panjabi, M.M., Hult, J.E. and White, A.A. (1987) Biomechanical studies in cadaveric spines. In *The Lumbar Spine and Back Pain* (M.I.V. Jayson, ed.)., Churchill Livingstone, London, pp. 161–176.

Parke, W.W. (1991) The significance of venous return impairment in ischaemic radiculopathy and myelopathy. *Orthop. Clin. North Am.*, **22**, 213–221.

Parke, W.W. (1992) Applied anatomy of the spine. In *The Spine*, Vol.1.(R.A. Rothman and F.A. Simeone, eds). W.B. Saunders, Philadelphia, pp. 35–87.

Paz-Fumagalli, R. and Haughton, V.M. (1993) Lumbar cribriform fascia: appearance at freezing microtomy and MR imaging. *Radiology*, **187**, 241–243.

Philips, L.H. and Park, T.S. (1993) The frequency of intradural conjoined lumbosacral dorsal nerve roots found during selective dorsal rhizotomy. *Neurosurgery*, **33**, 88–91.

Porter, R.W., Adams, M.A. and Hutton, W.C. (1989) Physical activity and the strength of the lumbar spine. *Spine*, **14**, 201–203.

Postacchini, F., Urso, S. and Ferro, L. (1982) Lumbosacral nerve root anomalies. *J. Bone Joint Surg.*, **64A**, 721–729.

Rauschning, W. (1987) Normal and pathologic anatomy of the lumbar root canals. *Spine*, **12**, 1008–1019.

Rhalmi, S., Yahia, L.H., Newman, N. and Isler, M. (1993) Immunohistochemical study of nerves in lumbar spine ligaments. *Spine*, **18**, 264–267.

Ro, C-S. and Bachop, W. (1984) Topographic anatomy of the dorsal ramus of the lumbar level spinal nerve. *Anat. Rec.*, **208**, 148A.

Roland, M and Morris, R. (1983) A study of the natural history of low back pain. Part II. Development of guidelines for trials of treatment in primary care. *Spine*, **8**, 145–150.

Rydevik, B., Brown, M.D. and Lundborg, G. (1984) Pathoanatomy and pathophysiology of nerve root compression. *Spine*, **9**, 7–15.

Saal, J.A., Dillingham, M.F., Gamburd, R.S. and Fanton, G.S. (1988) The pseudoradicular syndrome: lower extremity peripheral nerve entrapment masquerading as lumbar radiculopathy. *Spine*, **13**, 79–83.

Schellinger, D., Manz, H., Vidic, B. *et al.* (1990) Disc fragment migration. *Radiology*, **175**, 831–836.

Schmorl, G. and Junghanns, H. (1971) *The Spine in Health and Disease* (Translation). Grune and Stratton, New York, pp. 35–39.

Smith, S.A., Massie, J.B., Chesnut, R. and Garfin, S.R. (1993) Straight leg raising. Anatomical effects on the spinal nerve root without and with fusion. *Spine*, **18**, 992–999.

Spencer, D.L., Irwin, G.S. and Miller, J.A.A. (1983) Anatomy and significance of fixation of the lumbosacral nerve roots in sciatica. *Spine*, **8**, 672–679.

Sunderland, S. (1974) Meningeal-neural relations in the intervertebral foramen. *J. Neurosurg.*, **40**, 756–763.

Sunderland, S. (1980) The anatomy of the intervertebral foramen and the mechanisms of compression and stretch of nerve roots: In *Modern Developments in the Principles and Practice of Chiropractic* (S. Haldeman, ed.). Appleton-Century-Croft, Norwalk, pp. 45–64.

Terayama, K., Ohtsuka, K., Merlini, L. *et al.* (1987) Ossification of the spinal ligament. A radiographic re-evaluation in Bologna, Italy. *Nippon Seikeigeka Gakkai Zasshi.*, **61**, 1373–1378.

Tezuka, A., Yonezawa, M. and Hasegawa, H. (1976) Report of cases with ossification of posterior longitudinal ligament. *Clin. Orthop. Surg. (Jpn.)*, **11**, 1142–1147.

Towne, E.B. and Reichert, F.L. (1931) Compression of the lumbosacral roots of the spinal cord by thickened ligamenta flava. *Ann. Surg.*, **94**, 327–336.

Transfeldt, E.E., Robertson, D. and Bradford, D.S. (1993) Ligaments of the lumbosacral spine and their role in possible extraforaminal spinal nerve entrapment and tethering. *J. Spinal Disord.*, **6**, 507–512.

Twomey, L. and Taylor, J. (1985) Age changes in lumbar intervertebral discs. *Acta Orthop. Scand.*, **56**, 496–499.

Venner, R.M. and Crock, H.V. (1981) Clinical studies of isolated disc resorption in the lumbar spine. *J. Bone Joint Surg.*, **63B**, 491–494.

Verbiest, H. (1975) Pathomorphologic aspects of developmental lumbar stenosis. *Orthop. Clin. North Am.*, **6**, 177–196.

Vernon-Roberts, B. and Pirie, C. (1977) Degenerative changes in the intervertebral discs of the lumbar spine and their sequelae. *Rheum. Rehab.*, **16**, 13–21.

Watanabe R. and Parke, W.W. (1986) Vascular and neural pathology of lumbosacral spinal stenosis. *J. Neurosurg.*, **64**, 64–70.

Wennekes, M.J., Anten, H.W. and Korten, J.J. (1985) Ossification of the posterior longitudinal ligament. *Clin. Neurol. Neurosurg.*, **87**, 297–302.

White, A.A. and Gordon, S.L. (1982) Synopsis: workshop on idiopathic low back pain. *Spine*, **7**, 141–149.

Williams, P.L., Warwick, R., Dyson, M. and Bannister, L.H. (1989) *Gray's Anatomy.* 37th edn. Churchill Livingstone, London, p.1334.

Wiltse, L.L., Fonseca, A.S., Amster, J. *et al.* (1993) Relationship of the dura, Hofmann's ligaments, Batson's plexus and a fibrovascular membrane lying on the posterior surface of the vertebral bodies and attaching to the deep layer of the posterior longitudinal ligament. An anatomical, radiological and clinical study. *Spine,* **18**, 1030-1043.

Wyke, B.D. (1970) The neurological basis of thoracic spinal pain. *Rheumatol. Phys. Med.*, **10**, 356-367.

Wyke, B.D. (1977) Neurological mechanisms of spinal pain. In: *Patologia de la Columna Vertebral.* (S. Hernández Conesa and J. Seiquer, eds). Ferrer Internacional, Murcia, p. 45.

Wyke, B.D. (1987) The neurology of low back pain. In: *The Lumbar Spine and Back Pain* (M.I.V. Jayson, ed.), 3rd edn. Churchill Livingstone, London, pp. 56-99.

Yong-Hing, K., Reilly, J. and Kirkaldy-Willis, W.H. (1976) The ligamentum flavum. *Spine,* **1**, 226-234.

8

Blood supply of lumbosacral vertebrae, spinal cord, nerve roots and ganglia

Hidezo Yoshizawa and Henry Vernon Crock

Arterial supply of the lumbosacral spine

The lumbosacral spine is nourished by lumbar segmental arteries which arise in pairs from the posterior wall of the abdominal aorta and from the median sacral artery which arises from the back of the aorta just above its bifurcation and by branches from both iliac arteries (Figure 8.1). Lumbar segmental arteries pass laterally on each side remaining closely applied to the centre of the fronts and sides of the vertebral bodies until they reach the intervertebral foramina. In this part of their course the lumbar segmental arteries give off branches to the lumbar vertebral bodies (Figure 8.1).

Each lumbar segmental artery gives off sets of branches in relation to the vertebral body. The first of these are short centrum branches which penetrate vascular foramina at regular intervals, subjacent to the segmental artery. The second are the longer ascending and descending branches which form dense networks on the fronts and sides of the vertebral bodies (Figure 8.2). Their terminal branches penetrate the bone in the area adjacent to each vertebral end-plate while other branches form fine vertical networks on the surface of the anterior longitudinal ligament and discs.

At the level of the intervertebral foramina, but just outside them, each segmental artery divides into three major branches, 1) anterior (abdominal wall) branches, 2) intermediate (spinal canal) branches, and 3) posterior branches (Figure 8.3).

Anterior (abdominal wall) branches

They lie medial to and then behind the psoas muscles anterior to the lumbar plexus. Neural branches

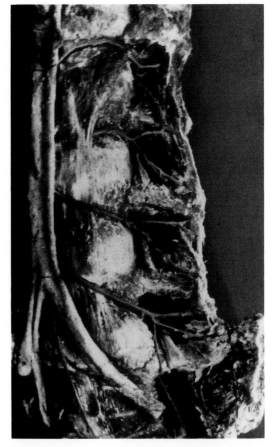

Figure 8.1 Origin and distribution of lumbar segmental arteries. (Reproduced with permission from Crock, H.V. and Yoshizawa, H. (1977). *The Blood Supply of the Vertebral Column and Spinal Cord in Man*. New York, Springer-Verlag.)

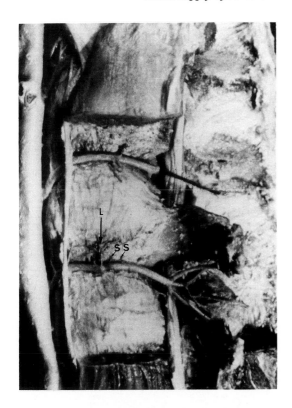

Figure 8.2 Short centrum branches (S) and a longer ascending branch (L) of lumbar segmental arteries. (Reproduced with permission from Crock, H.V. and Yoshizawa, H. (1976). The blood supply of the lumbar vertebral column. *Clin. Orthop.*, **115**, 6–21.)

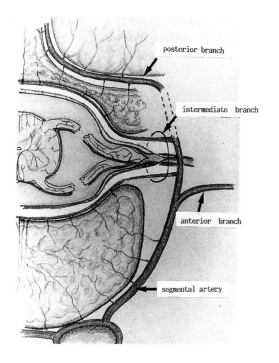

Figure 8.3 A schematic drawing of three major branches of the lumbar segmental artery: 1) anterior (abdominal wall) branch; 2) intermediate (spinal canal) branch; 3) posterior branch.

descend with each lumbar nerve. The abdominal wall branches pass laterally across the quadratus lumborum, piercing the posterior aponeurosis of the transversus abdominis, to pass forwards between this and the internal oblique muscle.

Intermediate (spinal canal) branches

The intermediate branch divides into three subdivisions in the intervertebral foramen, (a) anterior spinal canal branches, (b) nervous system branches, and (c) posterior spinal canal branches.

Almost immediately on entering the spinal canal, the anterior spinal canal branch bifurcates into an ascending and descending branch, the latter being closely related to the superior border of the pedicle of the lower vertebra at the interspace. Each ascending limb crosses the disc in its outer one third as it passes upwards to join the descending branch from the segmental lumbar artery above it, thus forming an arcade system on the anterior wall of the spinal canal.

The convexities of the right and left-sided arches are close together in the centre of each vertebral body (Figure 8.4).

The calibre of posterior spinal canal branches is marginally smaller than the corresponding anterior spinal canal branches. They too are disposed in an arcuate pattern, though their branches form a more closely woven network on the anterior surfaces of the laminae and ligamenta flava, from which vessels penetrate each lamina. Usually a well marked central artery penetrates the base of the spinous process to run backwards towards its tip. Unlike the main branches of the anterior arcuate system, those forming the posterior spinal arcuate system run a tortuous course (Figure 8.5).

Nervous system branches include vessels nourishing the dura mater and radicular vessels accompanying the nerve root towards the spinal cord.

The dorsal root ganglion is nourished by an independent branch.

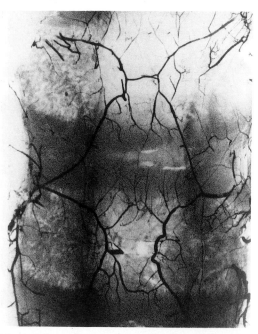

Figure 8.4 Distribution of anterior spinal branches of the lumbar segmental arteries on the anterior surface the spinal canal. (Reproduced with permission from Crock, H.V. and Yoshizawa, H. (1977) *The Blood Supply of the Vertebral Column and Spinal Cord in Man*. New York, Springer-Verlag.)

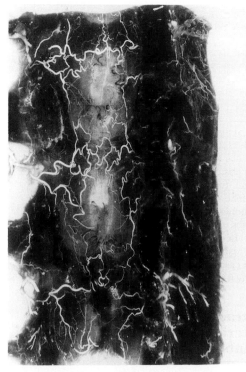

Figure 8.5 Distribution of posterior spinal branches of the lumbar segmental arteries on the posterior surface of the spinal canal. (Reproduced with permission from Crock, H.V. and Yoshizawa, H. (1977) *The Blood Supply of the Vertebral Column and Spinal Cord in Man*. New York, Springer-Verlag.)

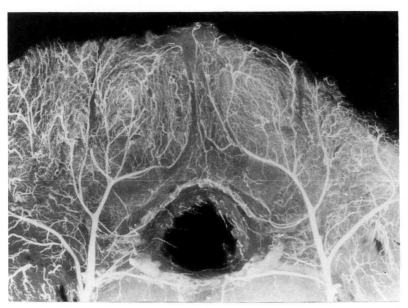

Figure 8.6 Posterior branches of the lumbar segmental artery. (Reproduced with permission from Crock, H.V. and Yoshizawa, H. (1976) The blood supply of the lumbar vertebral column. *Clin. Orthop.*, **115**, 6–21.)

Posterior branches

These dorsal vessels cross each pars interarticularis and pass backwards in contact with the outer surface of the laminae. They enter the sacrospinalis muscles and course medially and backwards, being applied closely to the middle of each spinous process, on the surface of which they form an open meshed plexus. The density of branches in the paraspinal muscles is such as to obscure the underlying simple design of the vascular arcades. Beautiful arterial arches form around the posterior vertebral (zygapophysial) joints, from which tributaries penetrate the outer surfaces of the laminae and the joints themselves. As these dorsal branches pass medially towards the spinous processes, they give off vertical branches which ascend and descend in the substance of the paraspinal (sacrospinalis) muscles. From the plexuses on the outer aspect of the laminae and the spinous processes, many fine arteries penetrate the bones (Figure 8.6).

Intraosseous distribution of arteries and veins in the lumbosacral spine

The centrum of the vertebral body is penetrated radially in the horizontal plane by small arteries derived from the abdominal portions of the lumbar arteries anterolaterally, and posteriorly by somewhat larger arteries derived from the arcuate branches of the anterior spinal canal division of the lumbar segmental arteries. An arterial grid is formed then in the centre of the vertebral body (Figure 8.7A), from which vertical branches ascend and descend in slightly tortuous paths toward respective vertebral end-plates, forming a brush border of arterioles which pass vertically into capillary beds in the vertebral end-plate.

In coronal (Figure 8.7B) and sagittal sections (Figure 8.7C), contributions from the ascending and descending branches of the lumbar arteries and analogous branches from the anterior spinal canal arcuate arteries to the vertebral bodies can be seen; these, too, have their entry points orientated circumferentially around the vertebral bodies. However, as the branches which enter the anterolateral aspects of the body penetrate to the interior, their main stems form triangular wedge-shaped patterns viewed in both the coronal and sagittal planes, with apices near the junctions of the lateral and middle thirds, or anterior and middle thirds, of the vertebral body. From the sloping sides of these triangles, vertical branches turn upwards or downwards towards the vertebral end-plate areas (Figure 8.7C).

A study of these intraosseous patterns in three dimensions suggests that the arterial grid in the centrum is concerned ultimately with the blood supply of the central third of the vertebral body and its respective central vertebral end-plates. The remaining segments of the vertebral end-plates are supplied anterolaterally by the vertical branches arising from the triangular water-shed described above, and poste-

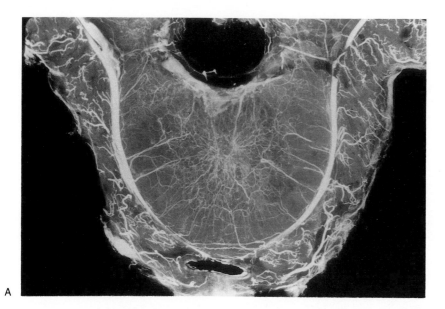

A

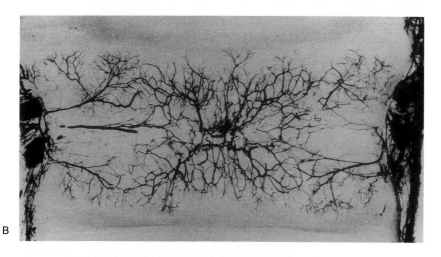

B

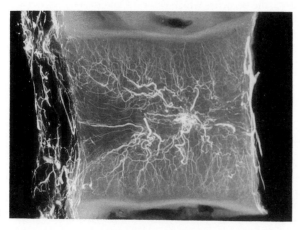

C

Figure 8.7 (A) Transverse, (B) coronal and (C) sagittal sections of the lumbar vertebral body, showing intrinsic arterial distribution. (Reproduced with permission from Crock, H.V. and Yoshizawa, H. (1976) The blood supply of the lumbar vertebral column. *Clin. Orthop.*, **115**, 6–21. Reproduced with permission from Crock, H.V. and Yoshizawa, H. (1977). *The Blood Supply of the Vertebral Column and Spinal Cord in Man*. New York, Springer-Verlag.)

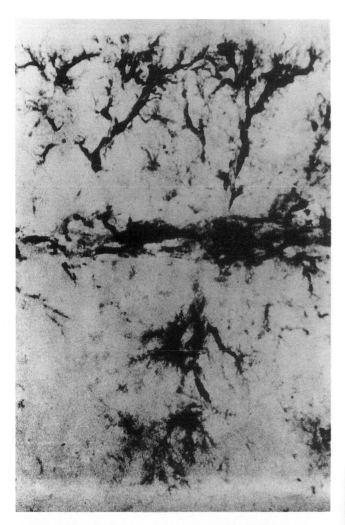

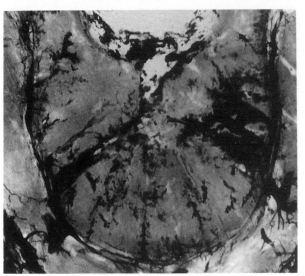

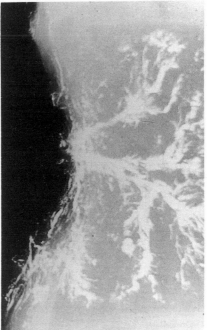

Figure 8.8 Central coronal (top), lateral coronal (bottom right) and transverse (bottom left) sections of lumbar vertebral bodies showing intrinsic venous distribution. (Reproduced with permission from Crock, H.V. and Yoshizawa, H. (1977). *The Blood Supply of the Vertebral Column and Spinal Cord in Man*. New York, Springer-Verlag. Reproduced with permission from Crock, H.V. and Yoshizawa, H. (1976) The blood supply of the lumbar vertebral column. *Clin. Orthop.*, **115**, 6–21.)

riorly by the ascending and descending branches of the arcuate arteries on the anterior wall of the spinal canal.

Basi-vertebral veins

The basi-vertebral system of veins is orientated horizontally in the centrum. It is arranged in the middle of the vertebral body along with the radiate arteries, forming a large scale venous grid into which the vertical veins of the vertebral body flow from above and below. The basi-vertebral veins converge posteriorly to drain into the anterior internal vertebral venous plexus, sometimes as a single vein, sometimes as two separate tributaries. Anteriorly, they join the external vertebral venous plexus, of which the lumbar veins are intrinsic components.

The main vertical venous channels are of large calibre and run gently tortuous courses. They are formed by the confluence of numbers of equally large branches which enter the main stems obliquely, and at regular intervals, along their courses and around the circumferences. Individual branches themselves are

formed of the union of innumerable short fine radicles (Figure 8.8).

In the region of the vertebral body adjacent to the vertebral end-plate, large venous channels are found orientated horizontally and running parallel to the end-plate area when viewed in sagittal or coronal sections. This large venous channel (horizontal subarticular collecting vein) is built up in the central area of the vertebral body by large calibre tributaries of the vertical veins of the centrum, which turn abruptly from their vertical courses to run horizontally, some passing anteriorly, others posteriorly, and still others laterally. In the posterior part of the vertebral body some of the tributaries from this horizontally orientated network run directly into the anterior internal vertebral venous plexus. Anteriorly and around the circumference of the vertebral body, tributaries of veins, draining directly into the external vertebral venous plexus, also contribute to the formation of the horizontal subarticular collecting vein system (Figure 8.9).

At the vertebral end-plate level, there is another vascular network of smaller calibre, orientated horizontally, which we have named the subchondral post-capillary venous network of the vertebral bodies.

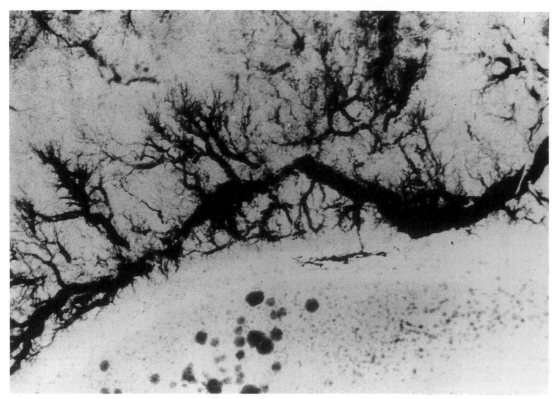

Figure 8.9 A sagittal section through the fifth lumbar vertebral body showing the horizontal subarticular collecting vein system of the vertebral body draining the subchondral post-capillary venous network. (Reproduced with permission from Crock, H.V. and Yoshizawa, H. (1976) The blood supply of the lumbar vertebral column. *Clin. Orthop.*, **115**, 6–21.)

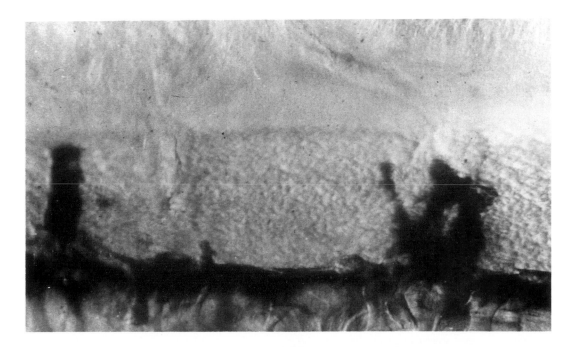

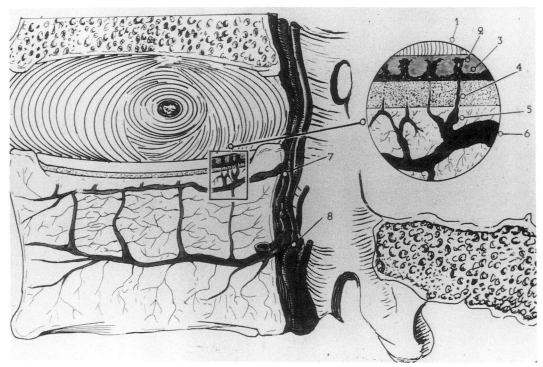

Figure 8.10 Vascular buds in the bone disc junction draining into the subchondral post-capillary venous network. 1. Intervertebral disc. 2. Capillary bed in vertebral end-plate cartilage. 3. Subchondral post-capillary venous network on the vertebral end-plate. 4. Vertebral end-plate perforated by short vertical venous tributaries. 5. Vertical tributary from the subchondral post-capillary venous network, draining to the horizontal subarticular collecting vein. 6. Horizontal subarticular collecting vein. 7. Horizontal subarticular collecting vein joining the anterior internal vertebral venous plexus. 8. Basivertebral vein joining the anterior internal vertebral venous plexus. (Reproduced with permission from Crock, H.V. and Yoshizawa, H. (1976) The blood supply of the lumbar vertebral column. *Clin. Orthop.*, **115**, 6–21.)

Short vertical tributaries from this network drain into the horizontal subarticular collecting vein system. This subchondral post-capillary venous network receives tributaries at right angles to its plane of orientation from the vascular buds in the bone-disc junction (Figure 8.10).

Venous drainage of the lumbosacral spine

The venous blood from the lumbosacral spine drains into the external and internal vertebral venous plexuses.

The external vertebral venous plexus is subject to many variations in the arrangements of its tributaries. Described in simplest terms, its main posterior branches form large veins which relate themselves to the sides of the spinous processes and course forward across the laminae on each side toward the intervertebral foramina. They coalesce outside the foramina with emerging intervertebral veins (Figure 8.11). Here, they are joined also by anteriorly directed veins which drain the body wall, the confluence forming segmental veins related to the sides of the vertebral bodies. In the lumbar region they are known as the lumbar veins, corresponding to the named arteries in this region, but are connected by a variable series of longitudinally directed channels, the ascending lumbar veins and the lumbar azygos veins.

The lower lumbar veins drain into the inferior vena cava (Figure 8.12), while the azygos systems in the chest drain into the superior vena cava and left brachiocephalic veins. From a functional point of view, these are important anastomoses between the external vertebral venous system and certain visceral veins such as the pelvic plexus and the renal veins.

The internal vertebral venous plexus extends from the region of the sphenoidal clivus within the skull, where it anastomoses with the sinuses at the base of the skull, to the sacral region below. It is in two parts, the anterior internal vertebral venous plexus and the posterior internal vertebral venous plexus. Batson (1940) described the importance of its continuity with the prostatic plexus and noted its large capacity. When intra-abdominal pressure is high, venous blood from the pelvic plexus passes upward in the internal vertebral venous system. Likewise, when the jugular veins are obstructed, blood leaves the skull via this plexus.

Both the anterior and posterior internal vertebral venous plexuses are arranged in an arcuate pattern overlying the sharply defined arterial arcades (Figure 8.13). The plexuses surround emerging nerve roots at the level of the intervertebral foramina and, just outside them, fuse with the segmental veins of the external vertebral venous plexus.

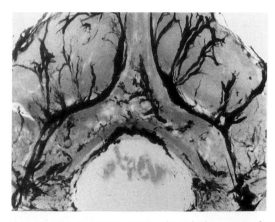

Figure 8.11 A transverse section through the centre of a lumbar spinous process and lamina showing the distribution of the posterior branches of the lumbar vein system. (Reproduced with permission from Crock, H.V. and Yoshizawa, H. (1976) The blood supply of the lumbar vertebral column. *Clin. Orthop.*, **115**, 6–21.)

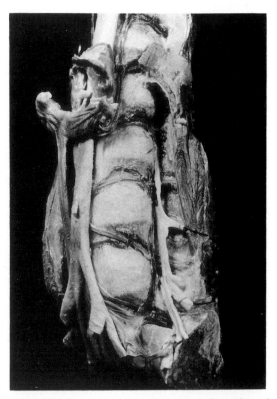

Figure 8.12 The external venous plexus on the surface of the lumbosacral spine. (Reproduced with permission from Crock, H.V. and Yoshizawa, H. (1977) *The Blood Supply of the Vertebral Column and Spinal Cord in Man*. New York, Springer-Verlag.)

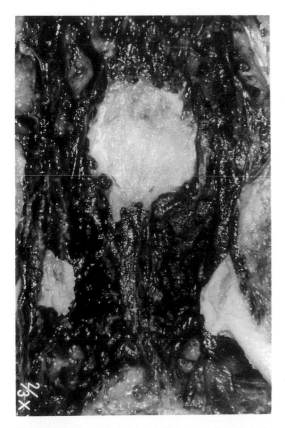

Figure 8.13 The anterior internal venous plexus on the anterior surface of the lumbar spinal canal. (Reproduced with permission from Crock, H.V. and Yoshizawa, H. (1977) *The Blood Supply of the Vertebral Column and Spinal Cord in Man*. New York, Springer-Verlag.)

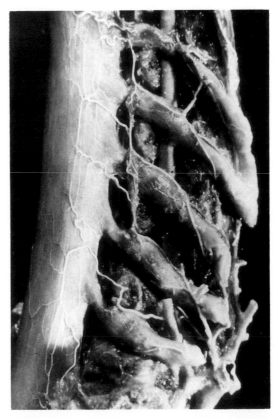

Figure 8.14 The arterial plexus of the back of the cervical dura mater. (Reproduced with permission from Crock, H.V. and Yoshizawa, H. (1977) *The Blood Supply of the Vertebral Column and Spinal Cord in Man*. New York, Springer-Verlag.)

Blood supply of meninges

The vessels on the dural sac are very fine and usually not easily seen in life. They are, nonetheless, arranged in regular patterns. Just inside the spinal canal, fine branches from the segmental artery bifurcate to form a longitudinally orientated channel in the epidural space. From this channel, midway between adjacent nerve roots, main stem branches pass on to the side of the dural sac, running transversely backward toward the midline where they anastomose with corresponding arteries from the other side. These unnamed segmental arteries are joined into an open plexus on the side, and posterior surfaces of the dural sac by an irregular number of longitudinal branches (Figure 8.14). A similar pattern is found on the anterior surface of the dural sac, based on meningeal branches from the nerve root arteries.

Blood supply of the spinal cord

The spinal cord, covered with the meninges, lies in the spinal canal below the measure of the upper line of the atlas. The cranial side of the spinal cord leads to the medulla oblongata in the foramen magnum. The location of the bottom of the spinal cord, that is, the conus medullaris, differs from child to adult. To be more exact, during fetal life, as the spine matures, the tip of the conus gradually moves cephalad.

It proceeds up to as high as the third lumbar vertebra at birth, and continues to go upward during development up to the height of the upper part of the lumbar vertebra, until maturity. The filum terminale, which is a cord without nerve function, tethers the conus. The cervical and lumbar segments of the spinal cord supply the extremities. They are described as the cervical (C3–T2 spinal level) and lumbar enlargements (T10–T12 spinal level), respectively.

Anterior nerve root filaments, that is, *centrifugal motor neurons*, which come out of the anterior horn of the spinal cord, and posterior nerve root filaments, that is, *centripetal sensory neurons*, which go into the posterior horn of the spinal cord, come out of the spinal cord with a certain vertical width to each other, and become one as a spinal nerve in the intervertebral foramen, and then move on distally. The nerve root inside the spinal canal, as it goes down, runs downward, leaning towards the outside as it's target, the intervertebral foramen, moves downward. Thus, lumbosacral nerve roots in the most caudal part run down almost vertically to the applicable intervertebral foramen. Inside the lumbar thecal sac, many anterior and posterior nerve roots are bundled together, resembling the tail of a horse, hence its name the cauda equina (Figure 8.15).

The spinal cord is fed by radicular arteries and veins which pass in and out of the intervertebral foramina along the nerve roots except for the upper cervical cord. Radicular arteries and veins which pass through the intervertebral foramina of the lumbosacral spine, run along the cauda equina to reach the lumbar enlargement of the cord (Figure 8.16).

Three main arterial channels are formed on the surface of the spinal cord: (i) a single anterior median longitudinal arterial trunk of the spinal cord (anterior spinal artery), and (ii) paired posterolateral longitudinal arterial trunks of the spinal cord (paired posterior spinal arteries).

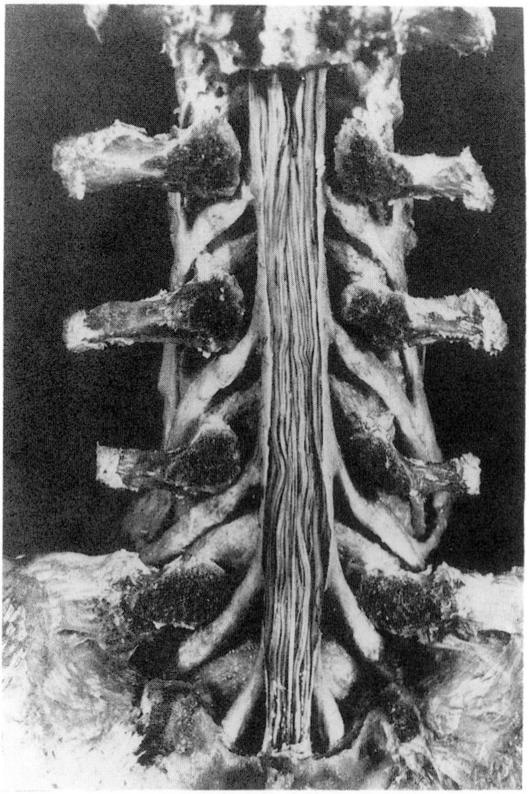

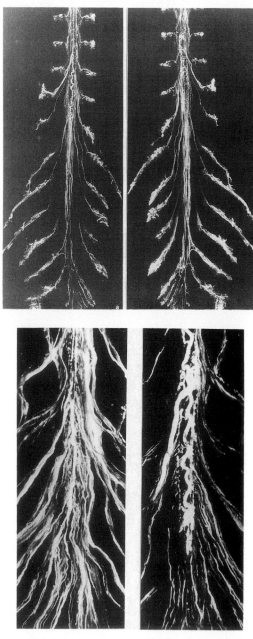

Figure 8.16 Arterial supply (top) and venous drainage (bottom) of the spinal cord. Anterior (left) and posterior (right) photographs of the spinal cord and the cauda equina. (Reproduced with permission from Crock, H.V. and Yoshizawa, H. (1977) *The Blood Supply of the Vertebral Column and Spinal Cord in Man*. New York, Springer-Verlag.)

Figure 8.15 The cauda equina nerve roots.

Controversy surrounds the questions of the site and number of contributing branches to these three main arterial channels throughout the length of the spinal cord.

Of the three sets of branches of each lumbar segmental artery which enter the spinal canal, the nervous system branches arise from each segmental artery, just medial to the site of origin of the anterior spinal canal branches, but still outside the spinal canal. Anterior and posterior radicular arteries course upward reaching the superior edge of the adjacent nerve root, running along the dural nerve root sleeve for a short distance before penetrating it. The artery accompanying the anterior nerve root is of larger caibre than that accompanying the posterior nerve root (Figure 8.17).

These radicular arteries, which vary considerably in size, join the anterior median longitudinal arterial trunk (anterior spinal artery) and the posterior longitudinal arterial trunks (posterior spinal arteries) of the spinal cord, respectively, at each segmental level of the vertebral column.

Despite this demonstration, many authors still believe that only thick radicular arteries supply blood

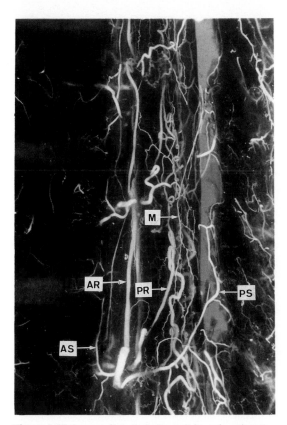

Figure 8.17 Intermediate (spinal canal) branches showing anterior (AS) and posterior (PS) spinal canal branches, anterior (AR) and posterior (PR) radicular arteries, and meningeal (M) branches.

to the spinal cord, and they have been called radiculomedullar arteries. The number and the location of these arteries differs among individuals. The average number of anterior radiculomedullar arteries is between five and six, and that of posterior radiculomedullar arteries is a little more. The percentage of right and left is 40–60%, respectively. Among radiculomedullar arteries, the strikingly thick artery, which feeds the spinal cord in the large area that covers the lower thoracic cord and the conus medullaris, is called the great anterior radiculomedullar artery (Adamkiewicz artery). In 80% of individuals this artery enters from the left, and in 85% the vessel enters along one of the nerve roots between T9 and T12. In 15% of people the artery enters along one of the nerve roots between T5 and T8 but they have other smaller radiculomedullar arteries entering the lower section of the spinal cord.

When more is known about the control of blood flow in small radicular arteries, further revision of the nomenclature of spinal arteries such as the artery of Adamkiewicz will be required. There may be many feeder arteries with diameters in neonates not less than 350 μm, and in older age groups not less than 450 μm, so that the significance of recognizing a single artery of Adamkiewicz may lose much of its currently imagined importance.

The arteries of the spinal cord

The spinal cord is penetrated around its circumference posteriorly by radially disposed arteries, branches of the posterolateral longitudinal arterial trunks (posterior spinal arteries) and of the pial plexus (Figure 8.18). Anteriorly, based on the anterior median longitudinal arterial trunk (anterior spinal artery), the cord is penetrated by a series of horizontally orientated central arteries. The number of these varies, being greatest in the cervical and lumbar enlargements. In the cervical area central arteries pass backward along a slightly oblique path, alternate branches usually passing to left and right just anterior to the central canal of the cord. Each branch then bifurcates to spread out laterally into the anterior column of gray matter in the pattern of branches of a closely cropped leafless tree (Figure 8.19).

In the region of the lumbar enlargement, the central arteries are most numerous. They pass backward in the horizontal plane in slightly wavy courses, being somewhat longer than their counterparts in the cervical region (Figure 8.20).

In the thoracic region, the central arteries are more widely spaced at their origins along the anterior median longitudinal arterial trunk (anterior spinal artery) of the cord. They course backward obliquely and break up into branches which form long ascending and descending loops within the anterior horns of

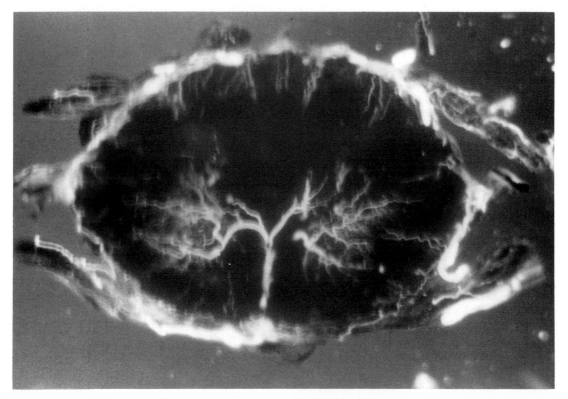

Figure 8.18 A transverse section of the cervical spinal cord showing intrinsic arteries.

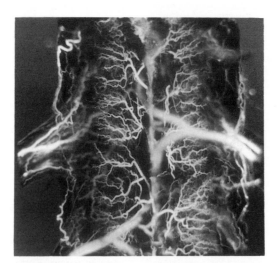

Figure 8.19 A coronal section of a segment of the cervical spinal cord showing distribution of central arteries. The section is cut just posterior to the bulbous anterior horns of gray matter. (Reproduced with permission from Crock, H.V. and Yoshizawa, H. (1977) *The Blood Supply of the Vertebral Column and Spinal Cord in Man*. New York, Springer-Verlag.)

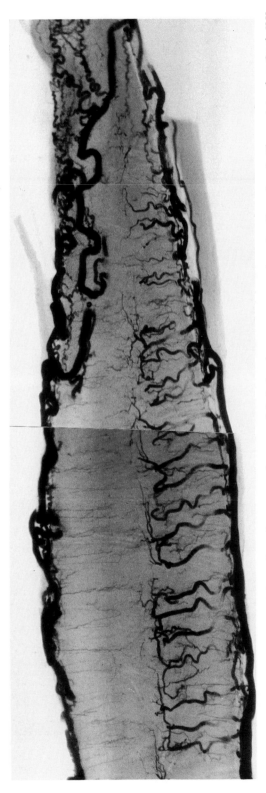

Figure 8.20 A median sagittal section of the lumbar enlargement and conus medullaris showing numerous central arteries. (Reproduced with permission from Crock, H.V. and Yoshizawa, H. (1977) *The Blood Supply of the Vertebral Column and Spinal Cord in Man.* New York, Springer-Verlag.)

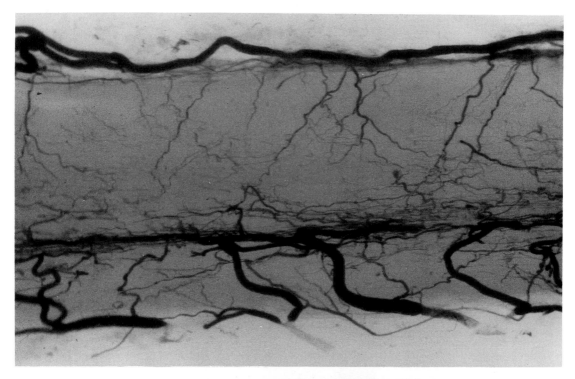

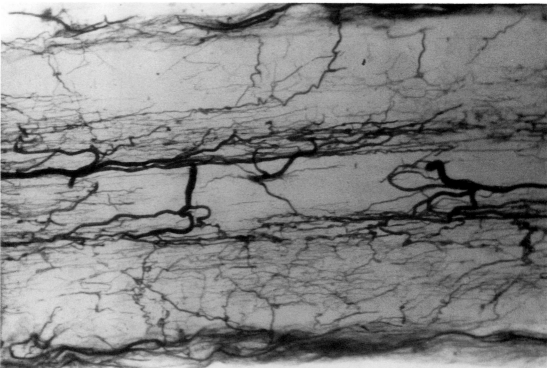

Figure 8.21 A median sagittal (top) and a coronal section (bottom) of the thoracic cord showing central arteries more widely spaced. (Reproduced with permission from Crock, H.V. and Yoshizawa, H. (1977) *The Blood Supply of the Vertebral Column and Spinal Cord in Man*. New York, Springer-Verlag.)

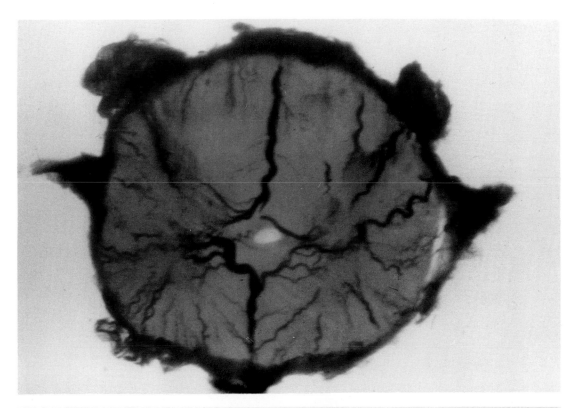

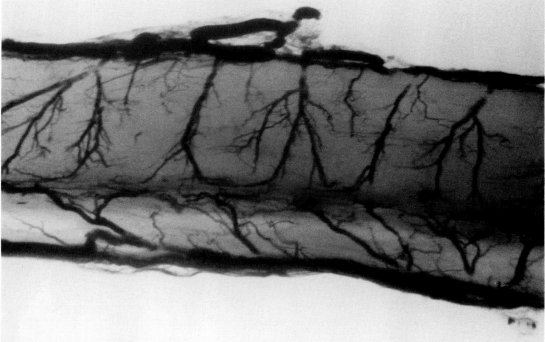

Figure 8.22 A transverse (top) and a median sagittal section (bottom) of the thoracic cord showing anterior and posterior median veins, the latter having no real arterial counterpart. (Reproduced with permission from Crock, H.V. and Yoshizawa, H. (1977) *The Blood Supply of the Vertebral Column and Spinal Cord in Man.* New York, Springer-Verlag.)

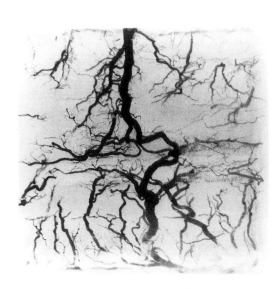

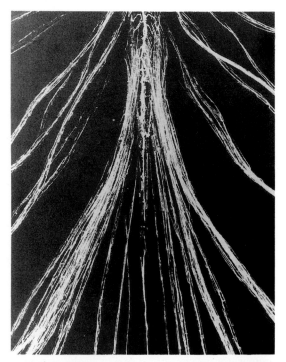

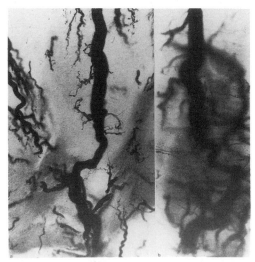

Figure 8.23 A continuous intrinsic venous channel formed in the midline by confluence of anterior and posterior median veins. A median sagittal section from a segment of the thoracic spinal cord (top). The transverse (bottom left) and the sagittal (bottom right) sections show the relationship of the median anteroposterior venous channel of the spinal cord to the central canal. (Reproduced with permission from Crock, H.V. and Yoshizawa, H. (1977) *The Blood Supply of the Vertebral Column and Spinal Cord in Man*. New York, Springer-Verlag.)

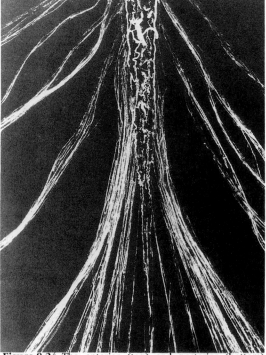

Figure 8.24 The anterior (top) and posterior (bottom) surfaces of the conus medullaris and the cauda equina showing arteries supplying them. (Reproduced with permission from Crock, H.V., Yamagishi, M. and Crock, M.C. (1986) *The Conus Medullaris and Cauda Equina in Man*. Wien, New York, Springer-Verlag.)

the cord, like grapevines after their leaves have fallen (Figure 8.21).

In intramedullary arteries, their anastamosis does not exist apart from capillaries, although duplication control may be seen.

Veins of the spinal cord

The spinal cord is drained by radiate veins which accompany the entrant arteries. There are a number of major differences between the two systems of vessels. Large anterior and posterior median veins are found within it which have no arterial counterparts.

The median veins, if separate, each bifurcate close to the central canal, collecting tributaries from both sides of the gray matter. In turn, the veins emerge onto the surface of the cord to join, respectively, the anterior median longitudinal venous trunk (anterior spinal vein), and the posterior median longitudinal venous trunk (posterior spinal vein). The other radiate veins join the venous pial plexus around the circumference of the cord (Figure 8.22).

There is often a continuous venous channel formed in the midline of the cord between these anterior and posterior median veins which deviate to one side around the central canal of the cord, or centrodorsolateral venous anastomosis linking the anterior median spinal vein with veins on the posterolateral surface of the cord (Figure 8.23). However, the clinical meaning of these intramedullary venous anastomoses is not yet well understood.

Blood supply of the nerve roots and ganglia

Corbin (1961) described anatomical details of radicular arteries and classified them into three groups: artères radiculo-grêles, artères radiculo-piemeriennes, and artères radiculo-medullaires. First, two arteries were named as distal and proximal radicular arteries by Parke *et al.* (1981) and were thought to be nutrient arteries of the nerve roots. The dorsal root ganglion has its own nutrient arteries branching directly from the spinal segmental artery.

Parke *et al.* (1981) describe each lumbosacral spinal nerve root as receiving its intrinsic blood supply from both distal and proximal radicular arteries, through which blood flows toward a mutual anastomosis in the proximal one-third of the root. They postulate that the region of relative hypovascularity formed below the conus by the combined areas of anastomoses in the cauda equina may provide an anatomical rationale for the suspected neuroischaemic manifestations concurrent with degenerative changes in the lumbar spine. However, based on our studies, *we hold a different view in that there is no area of hypovascu-*

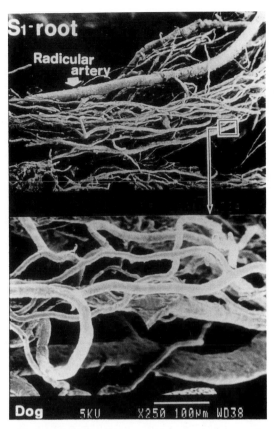

Figure 8.25 The vascular network in the nerve root of a dog (scanning electron microscope photographs).

larity in the region of the middle third of the cauda equina (Figure 8.24). We do not argue that the watershed stays in the blood stream of the radicular artery itself. Its fluid changes according to its posture, or the compression of the nerve root, so this watershed is not necessarily a weak point and the 'watershed' of the radicular artery does not have any particular clinical meaning. In compression radiculopathy, disorders of blood circulation in the area of the capillaries or venules, which control the nutrition of the nerve root, play a major role in radicular symptoms. Inside the nerve root, traversing capillaries which diverge from the radicular artery exist fully between funiculi, and the dense capillary network is formed along the total length of the nerve root (Figure 8.25). If we compare the intraradicular vascular plexus in the cauda equina with the intramedullary vascular plexus in the spinal cord at the level of the conus medullaris, the vascular plexus of the nerve root is dense compared with the vascular plexus of the white matter of the spinal cord, but sparse compared with the vascular plexus of the gray matter. Generally, the gray matter of the dorsal root ganglion, where many nerve cells exist, is denser in blood vessels than in the

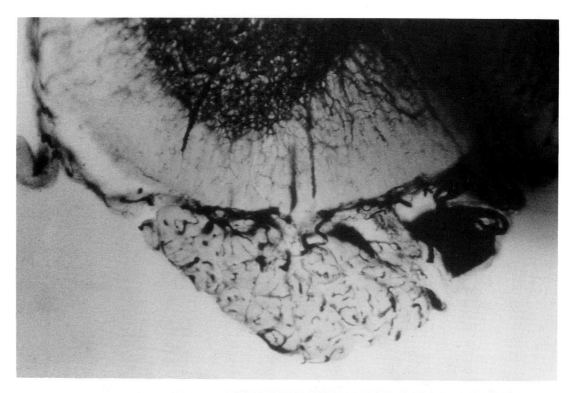

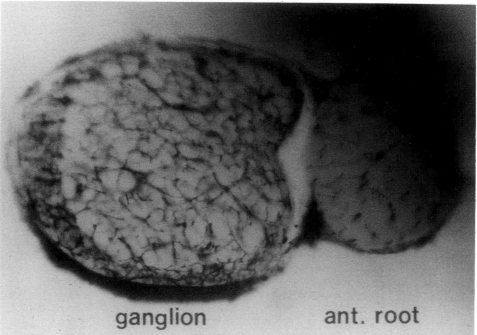

Figure 8.26 A transverse section of the conus medullaris and the anterior nerve root (top). The vascular plexus of the nerve root is denser compared with the vasculature of the white matter of the spinal cord but sparse compared with the gray matter. The bottom shows a transverse section of the anterior nerve root and the dorsal root ganglion. The latter, where many nerve cells exist, is denser in its blood vessels than the nerve root. (Reproduced with permission from Yoshizawa, H., Kobayashi, S. and Hachiya, Y. (1991) Blood supply of nerve roots and dorsal root ganglia. *Orthop. Clin. of North Am.* **22**, 195–211.)

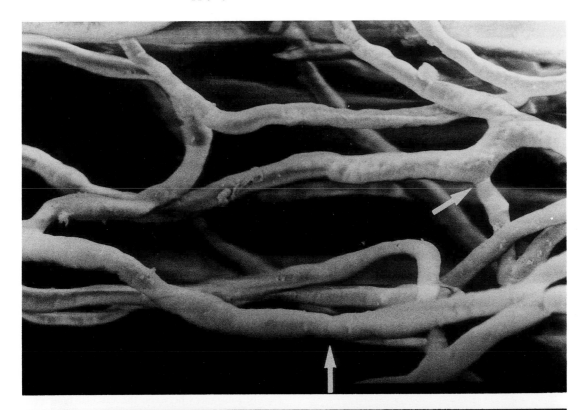

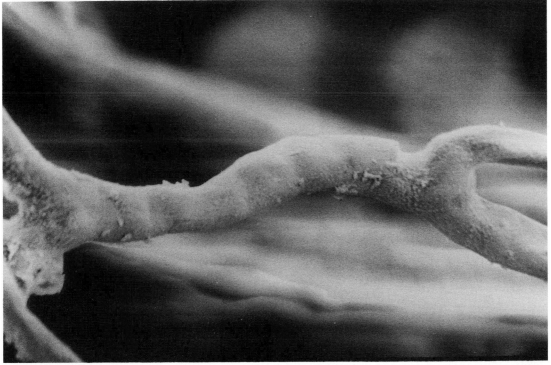

Figure 8.27 Scanning electron microscope photographs of the intraradicular capillary vessel. Ring-like compressions (top), and traces of compression due to vascular endothelial cells (bottom), are seen.

white matter, nerve roots, or peripheral nerves, where nerve fibres alone exist, and also the blood flow volume is apparently larger (Figure 8.26). In the intraradicular capillary vessel, as in the brain or the spinal cord, many ring-like compressions, which the vascular sphincters may cause, and many traces of compression which the vascular endothelial cells may cause, are observed. This fact suggests that the motor

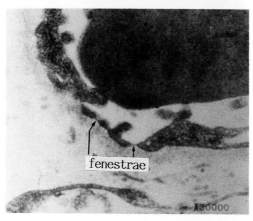

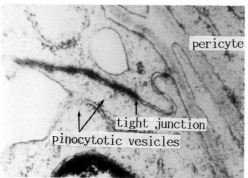

Figure 8.28 Difference of capillaries in the nerve root (top), the dorsal root ganglion (middle) and the sciatic nerve (bottom).

function of the vascular endothelial cell has something to do with the control of the bloodstream in the nerve root (Figure 8.27).

Within the nervous system a blood–brain (nerve) barrier exists which sustains the homeostasis of the environment in the nerve. Benett *et al.* (1959) classified the capillary into the continuous capillary, the fenestrated capillary, and the discontinuous capillary, by the shape of the vascular endothelium. Capillaries of the central and peripheral nervous system, except the dorsal root ganglion, are continuous capillaries. The area between the vascular endothelial cells is closed with tight junctions. Pinocytotic vesicles in the endothelial cell, which affect the transportation of substances, are few and the blood–brain (nerve) barrier which controls the shift of substances in the blood into the nervous tissue can be seen.

When we compare the nerve root and the peripheral nerve below the spinal nerve, the peripheral nerve pericytes surround the circumference of the vascular endothelial cell densely, whereas in the nerve root pericytes are few, and in many parts the vascular endothelial cell directly leads to the endoneurial space. In the nerve root, the tight junction closes the area between vascular endothelial cells but many pinocytotic vesicles are seen compared with the peripheral nerve, indicating that the transportation of substances between the vascular lumen and the endoneurial space in the nerve root is relatively active (Figure 8.28). In short, the blood–brain (nerve) barrier of the nerve root is weak compared with that of the peripheral nerve.

On the other hand, there are fenestrated capillaries which have about 70 nm diameter fenestra and continous capillaries which have gap junctions in the endothelium in the dorsal root ganglion. Thus, there is no blood–brain (nerve) barrier in the dorsal root ganglion.

References

Batson, O.V. (1940) The function of the vertebral veins and their role in the spread of metastases. *Arch. Surg.*, **112**, 138–149.

Benett H.S., Luft, J.H. and Humpton, J.C. (1959) Morphological classification of vertebrate blood capillaries. *Am J Physiol.*, **196**, 381–390.

Corbin, J.L. (1961) *Anatomie et Pathologie Arterielles de la Moelle*. Masson et Cie.

Crock, H.V. and Yoshizawa, H. (1976) The blood supply of the lumbar vertebral column. *Clin. Orthop.*, **115**, 6–21.

Crock, H.V. and Yoshizawa, H. (1977) *The Blood Supply of the Vertebral Column and Spinal Cord in Man*. Springer, Berlin, Heidelberg, New York.

Crock, H.V., Yoshizawa, H. and Kame, S.K. (1973) Observation on the venous drainage of the human vertebral body. *J. Bone Joint Surg.*, **55B**, 528–533.

Crock, H.V., Yamagishi, M. and Crock, M.C. (1986) *Conus Medullaris and Cauda Equina in Man.* Springer-Verlag, Berlin, Heidelberg, New York

Kobayashi, S., Yoshizawa, H., Hachiya, Y. *et al.* (1993) Vasogenic edema induced by compression injury to the spinal nerve root; distribution of intravenously injected protein tracers and gadolinium-enhanced magnetic resonance imaging. *Spine.*, **18**, 1410–1424.

Parke, W.W., Gemmell, K. and Rothman, R.H. (1981) Arterial vascularization of the cauda equina. *J. Bone Joint Surg.*, **63A**, 53–62.

Rydevik, B., Holm, S., Brown, M.D. *et al.* (1984) Nutrition of spinal nerve roots; The role of diffusion from the cerebrospinal fluid. *Trans. Orthop. Res. Soc.*, **9**, 276.

Yoshizawa, H., Kobayashi, S., Hachiya, Y. (1991) Blood supply of nerve roots and dorsal root ganglia. *Orthop. Clin. North Am.*, **22**, 195–211.

Yoshizawa, H., Kobayashi, S. and Kubota, K. (1989) Effects of compression on intraradicular blood flow in dogs. *Spine*, **14**, 1220–1225.

Yoshizawa, H., Kobayashi, S. and Morita, T. (1995) Chronic nerve root compression; pathophysiologic mechanism of nerve root dysfunction. *Spine*, **20**, 397–407.

9

Muscles and ligaments of the back

K.L. Moore

Most muscles in the back are concerned with maintenance of posture and movements of the vertebral column (spine). Superficial muscular layers are concerned with movement of the upper limbs and ribs.

Extrinsic back muscles

The superficial layer of extrinsic muscles in the back (trapezius, latissimus dorsi, levator scapulae, and rhomboids) connect the upper limb to the vertebral column (Moore, 1992). These muscles are related to movements of the upper limb and, as a consequence, are not discussed in this chapter. Ventral rami of spinal nerves supply these muscles in spite of their location in the back. This unusual innervation of these muscles results from their embryonic migration to the back to obtain attachment to the vertebral column (Moore and Persaud, 1993).

Deep to the limb muscles in the back there is a thin intermediate layer of extrinsic muscles. The serrati muscles move the ribs and are related to movements of the ribs and inspiration. The *serratus posterior superior* is a thin quadrilateral muscle that lies at the junction of the neck and trunk. It arises by a thin, broad aponeurosis from the inferior part of the ligamentum nuchae, the spinous processes (spines) of C7 and T1–T3 vertebrae, and the supraspinous ligament (Figure 9.1). This muscle runs inferolaterally to insert into the superior borders of the second to fourth (or fifth) ribs. The serratus posterior superior, innervated by ventral rami of the first four intercostal nerves, elevates the ribs. The *serratus posterior inferior* is broader than the superior muscle and is separated from it by about four ribs. This thin irregularly quadrilateral muscle lies at the junction of the thoracic and lumbar regions. The serratus posterior inferior arises by a thin aponeurosis from the

spinous processes of the last two thoracic and the first two or three lumbar vertebrae, and from the supraspinous ligament. This muscle runs superolaterally and attaches to the inferior borders of the inferior three or four ribs near their angles. The serratus posterior inferior, innervated by ventral rami of the ninth to twelfth intercostal nerves, draws the ribs inferolaterally.

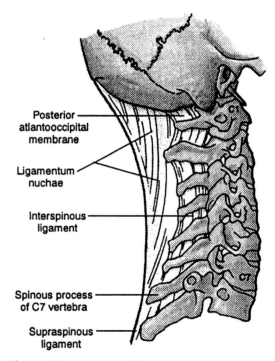

Posterior atlantooccipital membrane

Ligamentum nuchae

Interspinous ligament

Spinous process of C7 vertebra

Supraspinous ligament

Figure 9.1 Lateral view of the ligaments of the cervical region of the vertebral column. (From Moore, K.L. and Agur, A.M.R. (1996) *Essential Clinical Anatomy.* Williams & Wilkins, Baltimore.)

Intrinsic back muscles

Underlying the superficial limb and intermediate respiratory musculature are the intrinsic or *deep muscles of the back* and posterior aspect of the neck. The deep back muscles (*postvertebral muscles*) consist of a complex group of muscles extending from the pelvis to the skull that maintain posture and control movements of the vertebral column and head.

The deep muscles of the back are enclosed by fascia that attaches medially to the ligamentum nuchae, the tips of the spinous processes of the vertebrae, the supraspinous ligament, and the median crest of the sacrum. The fascia attaches laterally to the cervical and lumbar transverse processes and to the angles of the ribs. The thoracic and lumbar parts of the deep fascia constitute the *thoracolumbar fascia*, which forms a thin fibrous covering for the deep muscles in the thoracic region and separates them from the superficial muscles that connect the upper limb to the vertebral column. In the lumbar region the thoracolumbar (lumbar) fascia forms a strong thick covering for these muscles. The thoracolumbar fascia plays an essential role in the function of the lumbar region of the vertebral column. In the lumbar region the thoracolumbar fascia can be divided into posterior, middle, and anterior layers. The posterior layer is a thick, fibrous covering that is attached to the spinous processes of the lumbar and sacral vertebrae and to the supraspinous ligament.

The intrinsic back muscles are grouped according to their relationship to the surface.

Superficial layer of deep muscles

The *splenius muscles* (splenius capitis and splenius cervicis) are located on the lateral and posterior aspects of the neck and the posterior aspect of the upper thorax, somewhat like a bandage (G. *splenion*, bandage), which explains their name. The splenii lie directly under the trapezius muscles and are covered by the ligamentum nuchae and deep fascia. They arise from the ligamentum nuchae and the spinous processes from the seventh cervical to the sixth thoracic vertebrae. The muscle may be divided into two parts. The *splenius cervicis* extends superolaterally to the cervical vertebrae and the *splenius capitis* passes to the mastoid process of the temporal bone and the lateral third of the superior nuchal line of the occipital bone. The splenius muscles cover and hold the deep neck muscles in position (Figure 9.2A, Table 9.1). The splenius muscles also draw the head and neck posteriorly and rotate the head and neck so that the face moves toward the side of the muscle that is acting. When both muscles contract, they extend the head and neck. The splenius muscles are innervated by lateral branches of the dorsal rami of the second to fifth or sixth cervical nerves.

Intermediate layer of deep muscles

The *erector spinae* (sacrospinalis) is a massive and complex muscle that lies in a trough on each side of the spinous processes, and forms a prominent bulge on each side of the median plane. The erector spinae lies directly under the posterior layer of thoracolumbar fascia and stretches from the sacrum to the skull (Figure 9.2A, Table 9.1, see anatomical cross-section example: Figure 11.5. The *erector spinae*, the chief extensor of the vertebral column, begins inferiorly in a broad, thick aponeurosis. This tendinous origin is from the posterior aspect of the sacrum, the posterior part of the iliac crest, the lumbar spinous processes, and the supraspinous ligament. The muscular fibres can be divided into three vertical columns that are subdivided into parts according to their attachments:

1. Iliocostalis muscle, lateral column
   - Iliocostalis lumborum
   - Iliocostalis thoracis
   - Iliocostalis cervicis
2. Longissimus muscle, intermediate column
   - Longissimus thoracis
   - Longissimus cervicis
   - Longissimus capitis
3. Spinalis muscle, medial column
   - Spinalis thoracis
   - Spinalis cervicis
   - Spinalis capitis

See Table 9.1 for the attachments, nerve supply, and actions of these muscles.

Deep layer of deep back muscles

Deep to the erector spinae is an obliquely disposed group of muscles known as the *transversospinal group* (semispinalis, multifidus, and rotatores). This muscle group is so named because the fibres of most muscles extend superomedially from the transverse processes of vertebrae to the spinous processes of superior vertebrae. The semispinalis is superficial, the multifidus is deeper, and the rotatores are deepest (Figure 9.2B). The attachments, nerve supply, and actions of these muscles are described in Table 9.1.

The *semispinalis muscle*, as its name indicates, occupies half the length of the vertebral column (Figure 9.2B). It is divisible into three parts – semispinalis capitis, semispinalis cervicis, and semispinalis thoracis. The semispinalis capitis covers the

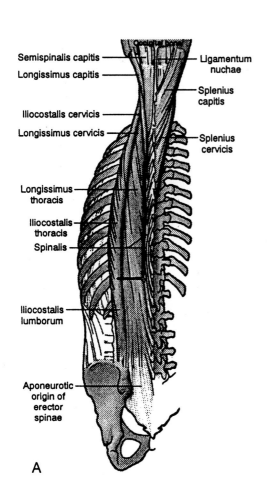

A

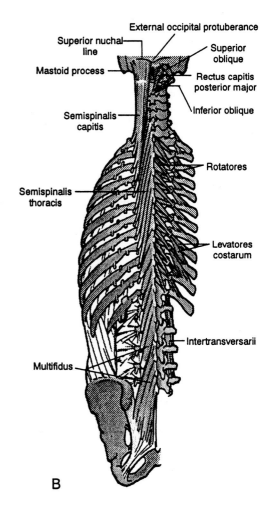

B

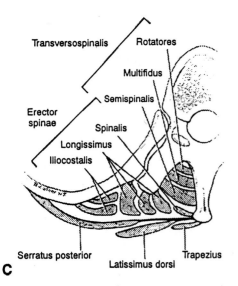

C

Figure 9.2 Intrinsic back muscles. (A). Erector spinae, splenius, and semispinalis. (B). Dissection of back showing transversospinalis. (C). Partial transverse section of the back. Note that the erector spinae muscle is formed by three columns, and that the transversospinalis muscle is composed of three layers. (From Moore, K.L. and Agur, A.M.R. (1996) *Essential Clinical Anatomy.* Williams & Wilkins, Baltimore.)

Table 9.1 *Intrinsic back muscles*

Muscles	Origin	Insertion	Nerve supply	Main actions
Superficial layer				
Splenius	Arises from ligamentum nuchae and spinous processes of C7–T3 or T4 vertebrae	*Splenius capitis:* Fibres run superolaterally to mastoid process of temporal bone and lateral third of superior nuchal line of occipital bone *Splenius cervicis:* Posterior tubercles of transverse processes of C1–C3 or C4 vertebrae		*Acting alone,* they laterally bend and rotate the head to the side of the active muscles *Acting together,* they extend the head and neck
Intermediate layer				
Erector spinae	Arises by a broad tendon from the posterior part of iliac crest, the posterior surface of the sacrum, the sacral and inferior lumbar spinous processes, and the supraspinous ligament	*Iliocostalis:* lumborum, thoracis, and cervicis Fibres run superiorly to the angles of lower ribs and cervical transverse processes *Longissimus:* thoracis, cervicis, and capitis Fibres run superiorly to ribs between tubercles and angles, to transverse processes in the thoracic and cervical regions, and to the mastoid process of the temporal bone *Spinalis:* thoracis, cervicis, and capitis Fibres run superiorly to spinous processes in the upper thoracic region and to the skull	Dorsal rami of spinal nn.[1]	*Acting bilaterally,* they extend the vertebral column and head. As the back is flexed they control the movement – by gradually lengthening their fibres *Acting unilaterally,* they laterally bend the vertebral column
Deep layer				
Transversospinal	Semispinalis arises from thoracic and cervical transverse processes	*Semispinalis:* thoracis, cervicis, and capitis Fibres run superomedially and attach to the occipital bone and spinous processes in the thoracic and cervical regions, spanning four to six segments		Extends the head and the thoracic and cervical regions of the vertebral column and rotates them contralaterally
	Multifidus arises from sacrum and ilium, transverse processes of T1 to T3, and articular processes of C4 to C7	Fibres pass superomedially to spinous processes, spanning two to four segments		Stabilizes vertebrae during local movements of the vertebral column
	Rotatores arise from transverse processes of vertebrae; best developed in thoracic region	Pass superomedially and attach to the junction of the lamina and transverse process of the vertebra of origin or into the spinous process above, their origin spanning one or two segments		Stabilize vertebrae and assist with local extension and rotary movements of the vertebral column
Minor deep layer				
Interspinales	Superior surfaces of spinous processes of cervical and lumbar vertebrae	Inferior surfaces of spinous processes of vertebrae superior to vertebrae of origin	Dorsal rami of spinal nn.	Aid in extension and rotation of vertebral column
Intertransversarii	Transverse processes of cervical and lumbar vertebrae	Transverse processes of adjacent vertebrae	Dorsal and ventral rami of spinal nn.	Aid in lateral bending of vertebral column Acting bilaterally they stabilize the column
Levatores costarum	Tips of transverse processes of C7 and T1 to T11 vertebrae	Pass inferolaterally and insert on the rib between its tubercle and angle	Dorsal rami of C8–T11 spinal nn.	Elevate the ribs, assisting inspiration Assist with lateral bending of the vertebral column

[1] Most back muscles are innervated by the dorsal rami of spinal nerves, but a few are innervated by ventral rami. The anterior intertransversarii of the cervical region are supplied by ventral rami. The levatores costarum were once said to be innervated by ventral rami, but current authors state that they are innervated by dorsal rami. (From Moore, K. L. (1992) *Clinically Oriented Anatomy,* 3rd edn, Williams & Wilkins, Baltimore)

semispinalis cervicis. The *multifidus muscle* extends throughout the length of the vertebral column, but is heaviest in the lumbar region. The multifidus is thick and prominent in the lumbopelvic region. It forms a large muscle mass between the lumbar transverse and spinous processes (see anatomical examples: Figures 3.11, 11.). The *rotatores muscles* are the shortest members of the transversospinal group.

There is a series of minor deep back muscles, the *interspinalis muscles* (interspinalis cervicis, interspinalis thoracis, and interspinalis lumborum) and the *intertransversarii muscles* (intertransversarii anterior cervicis, intertransversarii posterior cervicis, intertransversarii thoracis, and intertransversarii lumborum). These intersegmental muscles connect one intervertebral segment with another and are named after the parts of the vertebra to which they attach. Their functions can only be presumed from their anatomical position (Table 9.1).

The *levatores costarum* (12 on each side) represent the posterior intertransversarius in the thoracic region. As their name indicates they elevate the ribs, assisting in inspiration. They also assist with lateral bending of the vertebral column. The attachments, nerve supply and actions of these muscles are described in Table 9.1.

The deep back muscles in the thoracic region are supplied by the dorsal branches of the *posterior intercostal arteries*, which are branches of the thoracic aorta. The deep back muscles in the lumbar region are supplied by the dorsal branches of the *lumbar arteries*, which are branches of the abdominal aorta.

Muscles producing movements of intervertebral joints

The principal muscles producing movements of the cervical, thoracic, and lumbar intervertebral joints are summarized in Tables 9.2 and 9.3.

Suboccipital muscles

In the suboccipital region there is a triangular area called the *suboccipital triangle* between the occipital bone and the posterior aspects of C1 (atlas) and C2 (axis) vertebrae. The suboccipital triangle lies deep to the trapezius and semispinalis capitis muscles (Figure 9.3). The contents of the suboccipital triangle are the vertebral artery and suboccipital nerve. The four small muscles in the suboccipital region, two rectus capitis posterior and two obliquus capitis, are innervated by the dorsal ramus of C1, the *suboccipital nerve*. The suboccipital muscles are mainly postural muscles, but they also help to move the head. The actions of the suboccipital group of muscles is to extend the head on C1 vertebra and rotate the head on C1 and C2 vertebrae (Tables 9.4 and 9.5).

- *Rectus capitis posterior major* arises from the spinous process of C2 vertebra and inserts into the lateral part of the inferior nuchal line and the occipital bone.

Table 9.2 *Principal muscles producing movements of the cervical intervertebral joints*

Flexion	Extension	Lateral bending	Rotation
Bilateral action of:	Bilateral action of:	Unilateral action of:	Unilateral action of:
Longus coli	Splenius capitis	Iliocostalis cervicis	Rotatores
Scalene	Semispinalis capitis	Longissimus capitis and cervicis	Semispinalis capitis and cervicis
Sternocleidomastoid	and cervicis	Splenius capitis and cervicis	Multifidus
			Splenius cervicis

Table 9.3 *Principal muscles producing movements of the thoracic and lumbar intervertebral joints*

Flexion	Extension	Lateral bending	Rotation
Bilateral action of:	Bilateral action of:	Unilateral action of:	Unilateral action of:
Rectus abdominis	Erector spinae	Iliocostalis thoracis and lumborum	Rotatores
Psoas major	Multifidus	Longissimus thoracis	Multifidus
Gravity	Semispinalis thoracis	Multifidus	External oblique acting synchronously
		External and internal oblique	with the opposite internal oblique
		Quadratus lumborum	Semispinalis thoracis

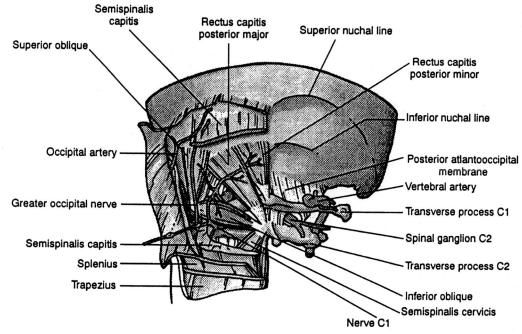

Figure 9.3 Muscles in suboccipital region. The trapezius, sternocleidomastoid, splenius, and semispinalis capitis muscles have been removed to expose the suboccipital muscles in the suboccipital triangle. (From Moore,K.L. and Agur, A.M.R. (1996) *Essential Clinical Anatomy.* Williams & Wilkins, Baltimore.)

Table 9.4 *Principal muscles producing movements of the atlantooccipital joints*

Flexion	Extension	Lateral bending
Longus capitis	Rectus capitis posterior major and minor	Sternocleidomastoid
Rectus capitis anterior	Obliquus capitis superior	Obliquus capitis superior and inferior
Anterior fibres of	Semispinalis capitis	Rectus capitis lateralis
sternocleidomastoid	Splenius capitis	Longissimus capitis
	Longissimus capitis	Splenius capitis
	Trapezius	

Table 9.5 *Principal muscles producing rotation at the atlantoaxial joints[1]*

Ipsilateral[2]	Contralateral
Obliquus capitis inferior	Sternocleidomastoid
Rectus capitis posterior, major and minor	Semispinalis capitis
Longissimus capitis	
Splenius capitis	

[1] Rotation is the specialized movement at these joints. Movement of one joint involves the other.
[2] The same side to which the head is rotated.

- *Rectus capitis posterior minor* arises from the posterior arch of C1 vertebra and inserts into the medial part of the inferior nuchal line.
- *Obliquus capitis inferior* arises from the spinous process of C2 vertebra and inserts into the transverse process of C1 vertebra.
- *Obliquus capitis superior* arises from the transverse process of C1 vertebra and inserts into the occipital bone between the superior and inferior nuchal lines.

The suboccipital muscles form the boundaries of the suboccipital triangle and its floor and roof:

- Superomedially - rectus capitis posterior major
- Superolaterally - obliquus capitis superior
- Inferolaterally - obliquus capitis inferior
- Floor - posterior atlantooccipital membrane and posterior arch of C1 vertebra
- Roof - semispinalis capitis

Ligaments of the back

The bodies of the vertebrae are held together by *intervertebral discs* and by anterior and posterior longitudinal ligaments (Figure 9.4).

The *intervertebral discs* consist of an *anulus fibrosus* composed of concentric lamellae of fibrocartilage, which surrounds a gelatinous and highly elastic *nucleus pulposus* (Figure 9.4A). The fibres of the anulus fibrosus insert into the smooth, rounded *epiphyseal rings* on the articular surfaces of the vertebral bodies. Greater stability is achieved because the fibres of each adjacent lamina of the anulus fibrosus pass in different directions, crossing each other like the limbs of the letter X (Clemente, 1985). There is no disc between C1 (atlas) and C2 (axis) vertebrae. The most inferior functional disc is between L5 and S1. The discs vary in thickness in different regions; they are thickest in the lumbar region and thinnest in the superior thoracic region. The discs are thicker anteriorly in the cervical and lumbar regions and more uniform in thickness in the thoracic region.

The *anterior longitudinal ligament* is a strong, broad fibrous band that covers and connects the anterior aspects of the vertebral bodies and intervertebral discs. It extends from the pelvic surface of the sacrum to the anterior tubercle of C1 (atlas) and the occipital bone anterior to the foramen magnum. Its extension to the occipital bone may be referred to as the *anterior atlantoaxial ligament*. The anterior longitudinal ligament broadens as it descends and is slightly thicker over the vertebral bodies than over the discs. This ligament maintains the stability of the joints between the vertebral bodies and helps prevent hyperextension of the vertebral column.

The *posterior longitudinal ligament* is a narrower, somewhat weaker band than the anterior longitudinal ligament. It is thicker in the thoracic region than in the cervical and lumbar regions. The posterior longitudinal ligament lies within the vertebral canal along the posterior aspect of the vertebral bodies (see anatomical example: Figure 3.5). It is continuous superiorly with the *tectorial membrane*. It is attached to the intervertebral discs and the posterior edges of the vertebral bodies from the C2 vertebra (axis) to the sacrum. This ligament helps prevent hyperflexion of the vertebral column and posterior protrusion of the discs.

The *ligamenta flava* join the laminae of adjacent vertebral arches from the C2 vertebra to the first segment of the sacrum (Figure 9.4A) (see anatomical and histological examples: Figures 3.5, 3.9, 3.11, 3.14 and 5.11). These broad elastic ligaments extend almost vertically from the lamina above to the lamina below. The ligamenta flava are thickest in the lumbar region. These ligaments help to preserve the normal curvature of the vertebral column and to straighten the column after it has been flexed. They also serve to preserve the upright posture.

Adjacent spinous processes are joined by weak *interspinous ligaments* (Figure 9.4B). The ligaments are thin, membranous bands that connect adjoining spinous processes. Their attachments extend from the roots to the apices of the spinous processes. They meet the ligamenta flava anteriorly and the supraspinous ligament posteriorly (see anatomical example: Figure 3.5). They are narrow and elongated in the thoracic region and broad, thick, and quadrilateral in the lumbar region.

The strong, cord-like *supraspinous ligament* merges superiorly with the ligamentum nuchae, the median ligament of the neck. The supraspinous ligament is thicker and broader in the lumbar region than in the thoracic region.

The *ligamentum nuchae* is a strong, fibroelastic membrane that is attached to the tips of the spinous processes of the cervical vertebrae (Figure 9.1). It corresponds to the supraspinous ligament of the vertebrae in the thoracic and lumbar regions. Because of the shortness of the C3–C5 spinous processes, the ligamentum nuchae substitutes for bone in providing muscular attachments for the splenius muscles (Table 9.1).

The *intertransverse ligaments*, connecting adjacent transverse processes (Figure 9.4B), consist of a few scattered fibres in the cervical region but form rounded cords in the thoracic region. In the lumbar region they are thin and membranous but more substantial.

The *costotransverse ligament* is a broad band of short fibres that connects the posterior aspect of the neck of a rib with the anterior surface of the adjacent transverse process.

The *lateral costotransverse ligament* passes obliquely from the apex of the transverse process to the non-articular part of the tubercle of the rib.

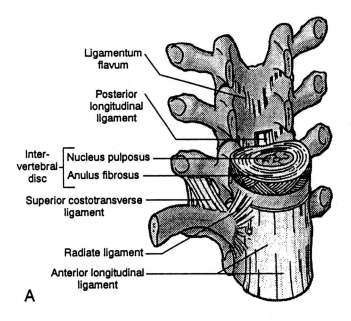

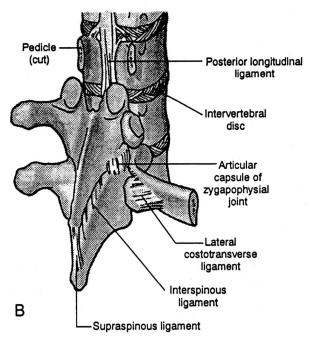

Figure 9.4 Ligaments of vertebral column. (A). Anterior view. Pedicles of upper vertebrae have been sawn through and their bodies have been removed. A rib and its costovertebral joint and associated ligaments are illustrated. (B). Dorsolateral view of two articulated thoracic vertebrae and their associated ligaments. The vertebral arch of the upper vertebra has been removed. (From Moore, K.L. and Agur, A.M.R. (1996) *Essential Clinical Anatomy.* Williams & Wilkins, Baltimore.)

The *superior costotransverse ligament* is a broad band of fibres that ascends laterally from the crest of the neck of a rib to the inferior border of the superior transverse process (Figure 9.4A). The radiate ligament consists of a band of fibres attaching the head of the rib to the costal facets of the thoracic vertebral bodies; a central band attaches the rib head directly onto the intervertebral disc (Figure 9.4A).

Surface anatomy of back muscles

In the median plane of the back there is a *posterior median furrow* that ends superiorly at the junction of the neck and scalp and inferiorly at the base of the sacrum. The furrow is deepest in the lower thoracic and upper lumbar regions.

Most of the cervical spinous processes are short and deep but the seventh cervical spinous process is long and easily palpable and visible, especially when the neck is flexed. Because of its prominent spinous process, C7 is referred to as the *vertebra prominens* (Figure 9.1).

All the thoracic spinous processes can be palpated. The tips of the lumbar spinous processes may be indicated by pits or depressions in the posterior median furrow. The *erector spinae* forms a prominent vertical bulge on each side of the furrow. The bulge is especially large in the lumbar region and the lateral margin of the muscle is indicated by a shallow groove about 10 cm lateral to the median plane. The highest point of the iliac crest indicates the level of L4 vertebra.

References

Clemente, C.D. (1985) *Gray's Anatomy*, 30th American edition. Lea & Febiger, Philadelphia.

Moore, K.L. (1992) *Clinically Oriented Anatomy*, 3rd edn. Williams & Wilkins, Baltimore.

Moore, K.L. and Agur, A.M.R. (1996) *Essential Clinical Anatomy*. Williams & Wilkins, Baltimore.

Moore, K.L. and Persaud, T.V.N. (1993) *The Developing Human. Clinically Oriented Embryology*, 5th edn. W.B. Saunders, Philadelphia.

10

Biomechanics of the lumbosacral spine

Mark J. Pearcy

Introduction

The lumbar spine provides a strong flexible link between the pelvis and thorax. It is a very complex structure that sustains large loads whilst providing considerable mobility to the trunk. Our upright posture frees the arms for manipulating tools and objects but this results in quite substantial forces being generated in the lumbar spine. A major part of these forces is produced by the spinal muscles themselves. They act on relatively short lever arms to counterbalance the moments produced by lifting objects and hence develop large compressive forces across the intervertebral joints. Many episodes of back pain are thought to have some component of mechanical overload or fatigue in their origin and so the study of spinal mechanics has great potential for illuminating the function of the spine and what loads might be acceptable before mechanical damage results.

The purpose of this chapter is not to give a detailed review of the spinal mechanics literature, which is covered comprehensively by White and Panjabi (1990), but to look at how the study of spinal mechanics has developed and to highlight the current understanding of how the back works mechanically. The literature quoted in this chapter is also not exhaustive but is designed to provide a starting point for research into the many areas of study of the mechanics and modelling of the spine. In addition, the aim is to indicate the directions that those involved in spinal research and modelling are heading in.

Knowledge of how a structure functions under certain conditions enables mathematical models to be developed which can then be used to predict how the structure will behave in different situations. Data from the literature on the mechanical properties of the individual elements of the spine can be combined with anatomical details of their morphology and connections to one another to provide a mathematical description of the spine. However, the accuracy of prediction from models produced in this way will only be as good as the information used to build them. If the information is incomplete, then the model can only be expected to be approximate and may only predict part of the back's behaviour, or give entirely erroneous information.

Development of spinal biomechanics

Interest in the mechanics of the spine can be traced back to ancient times from documents that describe how forces could be applied to the trunk to correct spinal deformities. The origins of modern concepts of spinal mechanics were in the 1950s with two different approaches investigating different aspects of the effects of loads on the spine.

Shortly before this the medical fraternity had described the pathological entity of the prolapsed intervertebral disc (Mixter and Barr, 1934). It was assumed that compressive overload on the intervertebral joint was responsible for causing the disc to prolapse but mechanical tests on intervertebral joints in the laboratory were unable to produce these lesions with axial compression (Perey, 1957). Fractures of the end-plates were produced but not herniation of the nucleus pulposus through the anulus fibrosus. The conclusion from this was that pure compression was not responsible for prolapse of the intervertebral discs, and other factors must be involved. It was not until the early 1980s that studies subjecting intervertebral joints to hyperflexion, combined with compression, produced these lesions in the laboratory (Adams and Hutton, 1982). It has also been shown that repetitive loading is most probably responsible for this type of lesion, causing what can be described as a fatigue failure of the anulus providing a channel through which the nucleus can migrate (Adams and Hutton, 1985). From these studies it is apparent that the intervertebral joints exhibit complex character-

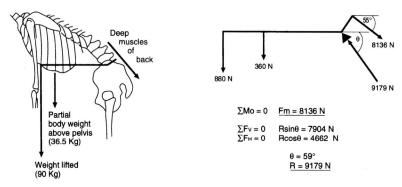

Figure 10.1 A diagram showing a simple lever arm system for the calculation of forces in the back during lifting.

istics and their mechanics have been, and still are being, studied extensively.

At the same time that Perey (1957) was discovering that the disc could not be caused to prolapse with the application of compressive force to the intervertebral joint, other groups were looking at the body as a whole. Principles of mechanics for static bodies were used to estimate the forces in the lumbar spine, considering the body as a simple lever system. Such analyses as that shown in Figure 10.1 were performed to calculate the muscle force and the consequent compressive force on the lumbosacral junction for a weight-lifter lifting 90 kg. This analysis indicates that, to counteract the moment of the weight being lifted together with body weight, which act on relatively long lever arms, the muscles acting on a much shorter arm would be required to produce a force of over 8000 N. This would produce a compressive force at the lumbosacral joint of over 9000 N. The muscle force required is probably higher than the muscles can produce and the compressive load is likely to crush the vertebrae (Brinckmann *et al.*, 1989). This being the case, it became obvious that such a simple model was not sufficient to describe the behaviour of the spine, and a search began for other physiological mechanisms that might reduce the forces.

Intra-abdominal pressure

The concept that the development of pressure in the abdominal cavity might be such a mechanism was described by Bartelink (1957) following observations that this pressure rose as the weight being lifted was increased. This theory was developed further by Morris *et al.* (1961). Intra-abdominal pressure is produced by contraction of the abdominal muscles. It is worth pointing out that, in their analyses, Morris *et al.* (1961) included the effect of the abdominal muscles acting to flex the spine during their contraction to produce an increase in intra-abdominal pressure. Hence the additional force shown in Figure 10.2 acting on the diaphragm assisting the back muscles to produce an extensor moment, is the net force produced by intra-abdominal pressure acting on the diaphragm and pelvic floor, minus the action of the oblique and longitudinal abdominal muscles acting to flex the spine. The resultant force required from the back muscles is reduced and, as a consequence, so is the compressive force. Intra-abdominal pressure appears to be a real mechanism but the forces do not always resolve this well and, indeed, even in this example, the required muscle force is still large.

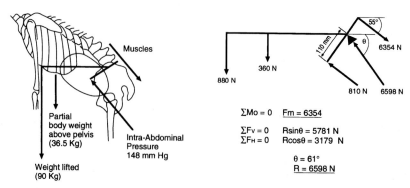

Figure 10.2 A diagram showing the moderation of the forces in the back with the inclusion of intra-abdominal pressure.

Posterior ligamentous system and thoracolumbar fascia

There was, and still is, some controversy about the true role of intra-abdominal pressure (Tesh *et al.*, 1987), so other mechanisms related to the complex anatomy of the trunk were proposed that might contribute to the strength of the back. The thoracolumbar (or dorsolumbar) fascia was suggested to have a role in developing an extensor moment on the spine (Figure 10.3) (Fairbank and O'Brien, 1980; Gracovetsky *et al.*, 1981). The fascia is tensed when the spine is flexed and can transmit forces from the pelvis to the thorax. Hence, if the spine is held flexed, the hip muscles can rotate the pelvis backwards with the posterior ligamentous system and fascia transferring force to the thorax to provide an extensor moment about the lower back. The back must remain flexed for this mechanism to work and this has been observed not to be the case in all circumstances. To cope with this, an active role was subscribed to the fascia by virtue of its attachments to the abdominal muscles (Fairbank and O'Brien, 1980). The action of the transverse abdominals, in particular, was proposed to cause tension in the fascia laterally, which would produce an extensor moment by virtue of the oblique orientation of the fibres in the fascia. The fibres in the superficial lamina of the fascia run caudomedially, while those in the deep lamina run craniomedially, from the lateral raphe to the midline. This triangulate structure will contract axially acting to extend the spine when pulled on laterally by the abdominal muscles. However, later studies have shown that this mechanism can only act on one or two levels of the spine and does not provide a major component to the extensor moment (Macintosh and Bogduk, 1987a; Tesh *et al.*, 1987; McGill and Norman, 1988).

What these studies highlight is that there was a growing awareness that, in order to understand the mechanics of the back, a much more detailed knowledge of the anatomy and its mechanical structure was required. This has led on to four areas of research: detailed descriptions of spinal anatomy, investigations of the mechanical characteristics of spinal structures, measurements of physiological function, and modelling studies that begin to integrate all of the information from the other three.

Anatomy

The startling feature about the anatomy of the spine is the order in its complexity. However, the standard anatomical texts neither describe the complexity required for mechanical modelling nor the organization of its structure. To be able to model the mechanical function of the spine it is essential to know the exact positions of the different elements in relation to each other, what the fibre orientation is in the ligaments and muscles, and where they are attached. Without this information it is not possible to model their mechanical function because it is impossible to determine what directions the forces that the ligaments and muscles produce will act in. Examples of where accurate data have become available only relatively recently will serve to highlight this problem, and indicate the detail required for accurate modelling.

The fibre direction in the interspinous ligament was, for many years, described erroneously because of a figure that was reversed in an original text (Fick, 1904; Heylings, 1978). This would have significant consequences and must be recognized when used in a mathematical model (McGill, 1988).

The remarkable complexity and organization of the back muscles has only been revealed in the last decade through the meticulous work of an Australian anatomist and his students (Macintosh *et al.*, 1986; Macintosh and Bogduk, 1987b, 1991; Bogduk *et al.*, 1992b; compiled in Bogduk and Twomey, 1991). In particular, their work has shown that each intervertebral level has complex muscular attachments (Figure 10.4). This implies that there may be control possible of individual intervertebral levels and casts doubt on models that combine muscle groups to give single large force components. In addition, a role other than motor function has been proposed for the small intersegmental muscles. These muscle are so small and so close to the centres of rotation of the intervertebral joints that they can have little mechanical effect. They are, however, in the ideal place to be sensors of joint position and motion (Bogduk, personal communication). If these small muscles were primarily sensors then it would provide an explanation for the spasm that is sometimes seen in the back muscles. If one of the sensors was injured, its signals would be erroneous and would disturb the control functions of the other muscles, causing them to contract in an inappropriate manner.

Modern imaging techniques of computer-aided tomographic radiography (CT radiography), and magnetic resonance imaging (MRI), are providing new insights into the anatomy of the trunk (see for example: McGill *et al.*, 1988; Singer *et al.*, 1989; Tracy

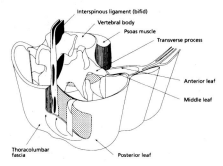

Figure 10.3 A diagrammatic representation of the thoracolumbar fascia. (Redrawn after Fairbank and O'Brien, 1980.)

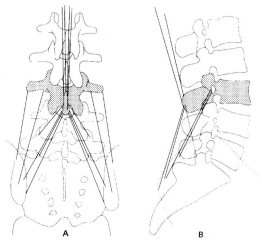

Figure 10.4 Diagrammatic sketches of the muscular attachments to the third lumbar vertebra. (A) Posterior view, (B) lateral view. (Redrawn after Bogduk *et al.*, 1992a.)

et al., 1989; Santaguida and McGill, 1995). However, care has to be taken in interpreting measurements taken from transverse sections of the trunk with these techniques to quantify muscle size and orientation. The obliquity of the muscles must be recognized and taken into account, and there are muscles of the trunk that act across the lumbar spine but are only present as tendons across the lumbar region.

Mechanical characteristics of spinal structures

The literature abounds with laboratory studies of the mechanical characteristics of individual spinal ligaments, intervertebral discs, vertebral bone and intervertebral joints. An introduction to this literature and a summary of information gleaned from it can be found in White and Panjabi's excellent book (*Clinical Biomechanics of the Spine*, 2nd edition, 1990).

Many early experiments were conducted on preserved or embalmed specimens and it has since been shown that this affects their mechanical properties (Viidik, 1973). Soft tissues are affected particularly, but bones are not unaffected and so this renders the results of these tests of little value. The mechanics of the soft tissues are susceptible to alteration due to other factors as well unless handled carefully. Once removed from the body, they are likely to dehydrate. The visco-elastic properties they exhibit are derived, in part, from the water retained in their structure and so loss of water will change their behaviour. It has been shown that if frozen to −20°C on removal from the body, and then kept moist with saline solutions when thawed and under test, the mechanics remain

constant (Viidik, 1973). Changes in temperature, and immersion in saline solutions also result in changes. It is thus recommended that, in order to simulate their behaviour in life, biological tissues should be tested in conditions of 100% relative humidity and at body temperature.

Unless the tissues are always tested in identical conditions, then the absolute values produced by one group of researchers will not be comparable directly to those from another group. In addition, to represent their true action, the tissues must be deformed *in vitro* as they are in life. If they are not, the results must be treated with caution. This is particularly the case when whole intervertebral joints are tested mechanically. Many experiments examining the mechanics of intervertebral joints constrain the vertebrae to rotate about a fixed axis. This is not how they behave in life as there is no fixed axis (Ogston *et al.*, 1986). This poses a problem as the variation in published data represents real biological variation plus differences due to the experimental conditions tests were conducted under. For the data to be used for modelling purposes careful scrutiny of the conditions tests were conducted under must be made to assemble information that is as compatible as possible. Having raised this concern, it is nevertheless true that, in recent years, *in vitro* experiments have produced information that is valuable and have cast dramatic light on the mechanics of the spinal tissues and the mechanisms of mechanical failure. In particular, the work of Adams and Hutton (1982, 1985) has shown that a combination of hyperflexion and axial compression may cause prolapse of the intervertebral disc, and that cyclic loading in flexion and side bending can produce fatigue failures of the intervertebral disc. It has also been shown that cyclic loading of the intervertebral joint in torsion can cause fatigue damage (Liu *et al.*, 1985).

These *in vitro* studies of the spine have shown that all components of the joints can be damaged through mechanical loading, either by a single overload event, or by multiple cycles of loading causing fatigue failure. All the components of the intervertebral joints are innervated and so are all potential sources of pain. The intervertebral disc, which was for long considered not to be innervated, has now been shown to have nerve endings in the outer third of the anulus (Yoshizawa *et al.*, 1980; Bogduk *et al.*, 1982). This implies that the disc can be a pain source without herniation or prolapse of the nucleus pulposus (Bogduk, 1991). As early as the beginning of the 1970s, mechanisms for producing internal disruption of the disc had been shown experimentally (Farfan *et al.*, 1970), but it has only been with the development of CT scanning that such lesions could be identified. It is still a further step to recognize that lesions such as circumferential delamination of layers of the anulus may be painful and amenable to some form of interventional therapy. There is now research underway to identify these internal disruptions of the disc and to investigate their clinical significance (Manthey *et al.*, 1994).

Physiological function

The mechanical function of the back during normal activities is the subject of much research. These studies generally examine movements of the spine and back and action of the back muscles during lifting tasks and other activities.

Movements

Measurement of the movements of the spine and intervertebral joints is problematical because of their inaccessibility. Simple clinical measures merely serve to give an index of back and trunk movement and are not very reliable (Portek *et al.*, 1983). Radiographic techniques to measure three-dimensional movements are as yet still only able to measure end of range positions, although developments in video-fluoroscopic radiography may enable active movements to be measured in the future. Techniques using devices attached to the skin can only record body segment movements, not vertebral movements, and are liable to artefact due to movement of the skin relative to the skeleton. Those studies in which pins have been inserted into the spinous processes are of limited value because it is not clear how such invasive procedures interfere with the ability of the subjects to act normally (Gunzberg *et al.*, 1991). Opto-electronic systems, developed primarily for gait analysis, also have been used for measuring back movements but rely on bulky rigs to obtain full three-dimensional analysis (Thurston and Harris, 1983) or only measure two-dimensional movement (see for example Holmes *et al.*, 1992; Barker and Atha, 1995). Nevertheless, there is useful information in the literature on the movements of the spine.

The normal range of voluntary movements of the intervertebral joints was determined using biplanar radiography (summarized in Table 10.1) (Pearcy, 1985). The spine is a three-dimensional structure which is symmetrical only in the sagittal plane hence, when side bending or twisting movements are performed, the intervertebral joints undergo movements in all three dimensions. For example, the general pattern is that, during side bending, normal subjects exhibit some flexion of the back plus twisting to the side opposite that to which they are bending. These patterns are described fully in the literature for radiographic measures (Pearcy, 1985) and using electromagnetic goniometers (Hindle *et al.*, 1990). In addition, the joints of the spine, like all joints in the body, exhibit circadian variation in their range of movement (Russell *et al.*, 1992; Dvorak *et al.*, 1995).

Table 10.1 *Representative values for the voluntary range of movements available at each intervertebral joint. The values are given in degrees and lateral bending and axial rotation are the total range from left to right, there being no difference in the range to either side*

Level	Flexion	Extension	Lateral Bending	Axial Rotation
L1–2	8	5	10	2
L2–3	10	3	11	2
L3–4	12	1	10	3
L4–5	13	2	6	3
L5–S1	9	5	3	2

Other studies have sought to show that the mobility of the spine depends on the posture adopted. For example, if the spine is flexed the intervertebral joints may have a greater range of motion available (Pearcy, 1993). This would suggest that the intervertebral disc is more vulnerable to injury from torsion when the spine is flexed. This information can be used to assess work place requirements and it can be expected that this type of study will become more common. However, more information on how the complex structure of the spine moves is required before mathematical models will be able to predict the full behaviour of the back. This will require further development of techniques to measure three-dimensional movements of the spine *in vivo*.

Electromyography (EMG)

Alongside movement studies, the action of the muscles has been investigated in order to estimate the forces that the lower back is subjected to during lifting tasks, and to develop models of the control strategies the body uses. The complex muscular anatomy of the spine renders interpretation of electromyographic signals from the back muscles problematical. Surface electrodes can only give a value for the activity of undifferentiated muscle groups. The use of needle or wire electrodes is necessarily restricted to small groups of subjects and cannot examine the action of all the muscles involved. Early work in this area is reviewed by Ortengren and Anderson (1977), who highlight that the information on the true action of the back muscles is incomplete. The use of EMG to provide data for models of how the back functions is becoming more sophisticated (see for example Thelen *et al.*, 1994; Cholewicki *et al.*, 1995). Mathematical techniques, including optimization strategies, are being developed to quantify EMG signals in relation to forces produced by the back. As these methods are improved, more confidence will develop in their predictions of forces imposed on the intervertebral joints.

Modelling

The information that is now available on the mechanical behaviour of the spine is extensive. Initial attempts to model the spine did not have such detailed information and were thus necessarily limited in their ability to predict the behaviour of the spine. A detailed bibliography of earlier models incorporating the mechanics of the different components of the spine was produced by King (1984). Nevertheless, the skills that have been developed have provided some insight into the function of the low back and have led to the models that are now being developed (Schultz, 1990).

Use of the Finite Element method of structural analysis has developed along with advances in the technique itself. The extent of the development of this method of modelling is demonstrated by a recent article describing an analysis of the whole lumbar spine in torsion (Shirazi-Adl, 1994). This work is the latest development of many years of work in three-dimensional modelling of the ligamentous spine. However, the author states that there is still a very large discrepancy among even the recent data reported on the mechanics of some of the ligaments, so assumptions had to be made as to their properties. Finite

element models do now offer the ability to model the spine, within the acknowledged limitations due to lack of precise data on some ligaments, and it can be expected that they will make valuable contributions to understanding mechanisms of injury to the passive components of the intervertebral joints.

Modelling the muscles is problematical because of their complex anatomy and the unknown nature of their control. Anatomical studies have been combined with motion analyses to predict the maximum forces that the back muscles can exert on the spine, and have highlighted some features of the available functions of the back muscles (Bogduk *et al.*, 1992a; Macintosh *et al.*, 1993a,b). Summaries of the estimated maximum moments and forces that the lumbar back muscles can produce on each of the lumbar intervertebral joints from these studies are given in Tables 10.2, 10.3, 10.4 and 10.5. The data show that the effect of flexion on these forces is generally small, except for the shear forces which may change direction (Table 10.4), and that the lumbar back muscles have little action in twisting the spine. In addition, the psoas muscle, with its lines of action so close to the centres of rotation of the intervertebral joints, can have little role in controlling motions of the spine (Bogduk *et al.*, 1992b). Rather its position is suited to acting on the hip, although in so doing, it

Table 10.2 *Estimations of the maximum moments that the lumbar erector spinae can produce about each level of the lumbar spine in the upright and fully flexed postures*

Level	Moments (Nm)		Difference %
	Upright	Flexed	
L1–2	14	13	–7
L2–3	34	28	–18
L3–4	57	47	–18
L4–5	75	66	–12
L5–S1	75	74	–1

Table 10.4 *Estimations of the maximum posterior shear forces that the lumbar erector spinae can produce on each level of the lumbar spine in the upright and fully flexed postures*

Level	Shear (Posterior +ve) (N)		Difference %
	Upright	Flexed	
L1–2	65	–44	–169
L2–3	192	–15	–108
L3–4	267	76	–72
L4–5	230	154	–33
L5–S1	–149	127	+185

Table 10.3 *Estimations of the maximum compression forces that the lumbar erector spinae can produce on each level of the lumbar spine in the upright and fully flexed postures*

Level	Compression (N)		Difference %
	Upright	Flexed	
L1–2	320	329	+3
L2–3	677	712	+5
L3–4	1117	1157	+4
L4–5	1511	1546	+2
L5–S1	1608	1646	+2

Table 10.5 *Estimations of the maximum axial torques that the lumbar erector spinae can produce about each level of the lumbar spine in the upright and fully flexed postures*

Level	Axial torque (Nm)	
	Upright	Flexed
L1–2	1.7	0.9
L2–3	2.7	1.2
L3–4	3.5	1.9
L4–5	4.2	3.1
L5–S1	1.8	1.5

does apply large compressive and translatory forces to the intervertebral joints.

The complexity of the back musculature has been incorporated in a recent model developed by Stokes and Gardener-Morse (1995). Their purpose was to examine strategies of muscle use for control of the spine and, in particular, to show that for equilibrium all of the muscles could not be working at their maximum at any one time. This was shown to be the case, as the muscles generally span several levels and muscle activations calculated for single intervertebral level analyses were not compatible with equilibrium at other levels. This highlights a dilemma in modelling studies in that the complexity of the structure results in models that have no single solution and hence the modeller has to choose optimization criteria to solve the equations. Further, when the true complexity of the spine is modelled, the computing power required to analyse the model becomes excessive and, at present, limits the applications that can be studied. However, as the models approximate to the complexity of the anatomy, they are able to begin to show which hypotheses of control are possible solutions.

Electromyographic studies combined with the anatomical knowledge are also providing new insights into the function of the back (see for example Cholewicki *et al.*, 1995). Studies of the action of the back muscles during activities are necessarily limited by the restricted access to the muscles that is possible with the electrodes. However, when combined with available information from other modelling studies, hypotheses of function can be developed and tested.

Compilations of data are now able to be used to form models to predict the loads on the lumbar spine. Recently Adams and Dolan (1991) have developed an elegant theory combining their group's previous studies on the mechanics of intervertebral joints with movement data to predict the bending moments experienced by the spine. They have then gone on to use this model, together with data from other studies, to predict the loads on the spine when lifting and give evidence that the lumbar spine should be kept only in a degree of moderate flexion when lifting heavy objects (Adams *et al.*, 1994).

Conclusion

This short review brings two main features to light. The first is that there is still no complete and comprehensive description of how the back functions mechanically. The second is that consideration of isolated components of the spine often masks their true function because their interaction with other elements of the spine and trunk are missing. However, recent studies are providing information that is being found of value in understanding the mechanisms of injury to the spine, and for the planning of therapeutic interventions.

The general functions of the different components of the spine may be summarized as follows.

The passive elements of the spine provide a flexible coupling between the pelvis and thorax whose complex structure is designed to allow mobility, principally in directions that the back muscles can control (principally flexion, extension plus side bending), but provide restraint to torsion.

The back muscles themselves provide postural support, and some extensor moment, during extension from the upright position. Their intricate attachments may provide the ability for the positions of the individual vertebrae to be controlled independently. The abdominal muscles provide a load-bearing system anterior to the spine and also contribute to the control of the spine through their attachments to the thoracolumbar fascia and, in particular, are responsible for torsional control of the spine.

To model the function of the back it has been shown that the full complexity of the spinal anatomy cannot be overlooked. It is necessary to consider how the individual elements of the spine and back interact in the trunk, as a whole, in order to understand how the back functions mechanically.

References

Adams, M.A. and Dolan, P. (1991) A technique for quantifying the bending moment acting on the lumbar spine in vivo. *J. Biomech.*, **24**, 117-126.

Adams, M.A. and Hutton, W.C. (1982) Prolapsed intervertebral disc - a hyperflexion injury. *Spine*, **7**, 184-191.

Adams, M.A. and Hutton, W.C. (1985) Gradual disc prolapse. *Spine*, **10**, 524-531.

Adams, M.A., McNally, D.S., Chinn, H. and Dolan, P. (1994) Posture and the compressive strength of the lumbar spine. *Clin. Biomech.*, **9**, 5-14.

Barker, K. and Atha, J. (1995) Reducing the biomechanical stress of lifting by training. *Appl. Ergon.*, **25**, 373-378.

Bartelink, D.L. (1957) The role of abdominal pressure in relieving the pressure on the lumbar intervertebral discs. *J. Bone Joint Surg.*, **39B**, 718-725.

Bogduk, N. (1991) The lumbar disc and low back pain. *Neurosurg. Clin. North Am.*, **2**, 791-806.

Bogduk, N. and Twomey, L.T. (1991) *Clinical Anatomy of the Lumbar Spine*, 2nd edn. Churchill Livingstone, Melbourne.

Bogduk, N., Tynan, W. and Wilson, A.S. (1982) The nerve supply to the human lumbar intervertebral discs. *J. Anat.*, **132**, 39-56.

Bogduk, N., Macintosh, J.E. and Pearcy, M.J. (1992a) A universal model of the lumbar back muscles in the upright position. *Spine*, **17**, 897-913.

Bogduk, N., Pearcy, M.J. and Hadfield, G. (1992b) Anatomy and biomechanics of psoas major. *Clin. Biomech.*, **7**, 109-119.

Brinckmann, P., Biggemann, M. and Hilweg, D. (1989) Prediction of the compressive strength of human lumbar vertebrae. *Clin. Biomech.*, **4**, S1-S27.

Cholewicki, J., McGill, S.M. and Norman, R.W. (1995) Comparison of muscle forces and joint load from an optimization and EMG assisted lumbar spine model: towards development of a hybrid approach. *J. Biomech.,* **28**, 321-331.

Dvorak, J., Vajda, E.G., Grob, D. and Panjabi, M.M. (1995) Normal motion of the lumbar spine as related to age and gender. *Euro. Spine J.,* **4**, 18-23.

Fairbank, J.C.T. and O'Brien, J.P. (1980) The abdominal cavity and thoracolumbar fascia as stabilisers in patients with low back pain. In *Engineering Aspects of the Spine*, CP-2. IMech E Publications, London, pp. 83-88.

Farfan, H.F., Cossette, J.W., Robertson, G.H., Wells, R.V. and Kraus, H. (1970) The effects of torsion on the lumbar intervertebral joints: the role of torsion in the production of disc degeneration. *J. Bone Joint Surg.,* **52A**, 468-497.

Fick, R. (1904) *Anatomie und Mechanik der Gelenk*. Verlag von Gustav Fischer, Jena.

Gracovetsky, S., Farfan, H.F. and Lamy, C. (1981) The mechanism of the lumbar spine. *Spine,* **6**, 249-262.

Gunzburg, R., Hutton, W. and Fraser, R. (1991) Axial rotation of the lumbar spine and the effect of flexion. An in vitro and in vivo biomechanical study. *Spine,* **16**, 22-28.

Heylings, D.J.A. (1978) Supraspinous and interspinous ligaments of the human lumbar spine. *J. Anat.,* **125**, 127-131.

Hindle, R.J., Pearcy, M.J., Cross, A.T. and Miller, D.H.T. (1990) Three-dimensional kinematics of the human back. *Clin. Biomech.,* **5**, 218-228.

Holmes, J.A., Damaser, M.S. and Lehman, S.L. (1992) Erector spinae activation and movement dynamics about the lumbar spine in lordotic and kyphotic squat-lifting. *Spine,* **17**, 327-334.

King, A.I. (1984) A review of biomechanical models. *J. Biomech. Eng.,* **106**, 97-104.

Liu, Y.K., Goel, V.K., Dejong, A., Njus, G., Hishiyama, K. and Buckwalter, J. (1985) Torsional fatigue of the lumbar intervertebral joints. *Spine,* **10**, 894-900.

Macintosh, J.E. and Bogduk, N. (1987a) The morphology of the lumbar erector spinae. *Spine,* **12**, 658-668.

Macintosh, J.E. and Bogduk, N. (1987b) The biomechanics of the thoracolumbar fascia. *Clin. Biomech.,* **2**, 78-83.

Macintosh, J.E. and Bogduk, N. (1991) The attachments of the lumbar erector spinae. *Spine,* **16**, 783-792.

Macintosh, J.E., Bogduk, N., Valencia, F. and Munro, R.R. (1986) The morphology of the human lumbar multifidus. *Clin. Biomech.,* **1**, 196-204.

Macintosh, J.E., Bogduk, N. and Pearcy, M.J. (1993a) The effects of flexion on the geometry and actions of the lumbar erector spinae. *Spine,* **18**, 884-893.

Macintosh, J.E., Pearcy, M.J. and Bogduk, N. (1993b) The axial torque of the lumbar back muscles: torsion strength of the back muscles. *Aust. N.Z. J. Surg.,* **63**, 205-212.

Manthey, B.A., Fazzalari, N.L. and Vernon-Roberts, B. (1994) A preliminary study of three-dimensional mapping of circumferential tears and annular fibre detachment in the disc. *J. Bone Joint Surg.,* **76B**, 117.

McGill, S.M. (1988) Estimation of force and extensor moment contributions of the disc and ligaments at L4-L5. *Spine,* **13**, 1395-1402.

McGill, S.M. and Norman, R.W. (1988) Potential of lumbo-dorsal fascia forces to generate back extensor moments during squat lifts. *J. Biomed. Eng.,* **10**, 312-318.

McGill, S.M., Patt, N. and Norman, R.W. (1988) Measurement of the trunk musculature of active males using CT scan radiography: implications for force and moment generat-

ing capacity about the L4/L5 joint. *J. Biomech.,* **21**, 329-341.

Mixter, W.J. and Barr, J.S. (1934) Rupture of the inter-vertebral disc with involvement of the spinal canal. *N. Engl. J. Med.,* **211**, 210-215.

Morris, J.M., Lucas, D.B. and Bresler, B. (1961) Role of the trunk in stability of the spine. *J. Bone Joint Surg.,* **43A**, 327-351.

Ogston, N.G., King, G.J., Gertzbein, S.D., Tile, M., Kapasouri, A. and Rubenstein, J.D. (1986) Centrode patterns in the lumbar spine. *Spine,* **11**, 591-595.

Ortengren, R. and Anderson, G.B.J. (1977) Electromyo-graphic studies of trunk muscles with special reference to the functional anatomy of the lumbar spine. *Spine,* **2**, 44-52.

Pearcy, M.J. (1985) Stereo radiography of lumbar spine motion. *Acta Orthop. Scand. (Suppl)*, **212**, 1-45.

Pearcy, M.J. (1993) Twisting mobility of the human back in flexed postures. *Spine,* **18**, 114-119.

Perey, O. (1957) Fracture of the vertebral end-plate in the lumbar spine. *Acta Orthop. Scand. (Suppl.)*, **25**, 1-101.

Portek, I., Pearcy, M.J., Reader, G.P. and Mowat, A.G. (1983) Correlation between radiographic and clinical measure-ment of lumbar spine movement. *Br. J. Rheumatol.,* **22**, 197-205.

Russell, P., Weld, A., Pearcy, M.J., Hogg, R. and Unsworth, A. (1992) Variation in lumbar spine mobility measured over a 24-hour period. *Br. J. Rheumatol.,* **31**, 329-332.

Santaguida, P.L. and McGill, S.M. (1995) The psoas major muscle: a three-dimensional geometric study. *J. Biomech.,* **28**, 339-345.

Schultz, A.B. (1990) Models for analyses of lumbar spine loads. *Appl. Mech. Rev.,* **43**, 119-125.

Shirazi Adl, A. (1994) Nonlinear stress analysis of the whole lumbar spine in torsion-mechanics of facet articulation. *J. Biomech.,* **27**, 289-299.

Singer, K.P., Breidahl, P.D. and Day, R.E. (1989) Posterior element variation at the thoracolumbar transition: a morphometric study using computed tomography. *Clin. Biomech.,* **4**, 80-86.

Stokes, I.A.F. and Gardner-Morse, M. (1995) Lumbar spine maximum efforts and muscle recruitment patterns pre-dicted by a model with multijoint muscles and joints with stiffness. *J. Biomech.,* **28**, 173-186.

Tesh, K.M., Shaw Dunn, J. and Evans, J.H. (1987) The abdominal muscles and vertebral stability. *Spine,* **12**, 501-508.

Thelen, D.G., Schultz, A.B. and Ashton-Miller, J.A. (1994) Quantitative interpretation of lumbar muscle myoelectric signals during rapid cyclic attempted trunk flexions and extensions. *J. Biomech.,* **27**, 157-167.

Thurston, A.J. and Harris, J.D. (1983) Normal kinematics of the lumbar spine and pelvis. *Spine,* **8**, 199-205.

Tracy, M.F., Gibson, M.J., Szypryt, E.P., Rutherford, A. and Corlett, E.N. (1989) The geometry of the lumbar spine determined by magnetic resonance imaging. *Spine,* **14**, 186-193.

Viidik, A. (1973) Functional properties of collagenous tissues. *Int. Rev. Connect Tissue Res.,* **6**, 127-215.

White, A.A. and Panjabi, M.M. (1990) *Clinical Biomechanics of the Spine*, 2nd edn. J.B. Lippincott, Philadelphia.

Yoshizawa, H., O'Brien, J.P., Thomas-Smith, W. and Trumper, M. (1980) The neuropathology of intervertebral discs removed for low back pain. *J. Pathol.,* **132**, 95-104.

11

Sacroiliac joint

L.G.F. Giles and C.M. Crawford

Gross anatomy

The bony structures of the pelvis are the two hip bones (innominates), the sacrum and the coccyx (Figure 11.1). The female bony pelvis has a larger pelvic inlet and a wider pubic arch than the male bony pelvis.

The medial aspect of the left hip bone is shown in Figure 11.2, which demonstrates the iliac, ischial and pubic parts of this bone, as well as its auricular surface.

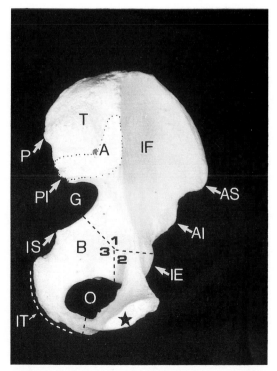

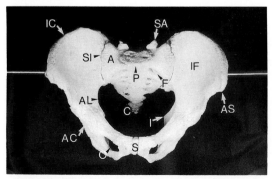

Figure 11.1 Anterior view of the bony pelvis showing the sacroiliac joints and some other labelled anatomical structures. A = ala of sacrum; AC = acetabulum; AL = arcuate line of ilium; AS = anterior superior iliac spine; C = coccyx; F = pelvic sacral foramen (anterior); I = ischial spine; IC = iliac crest; IF = iliac fossa; O = obturator foramen; P = promontory of sacrum; S = symphysis pubis (pubic symphysis) with interpubic 'disc'; SA = superior articular process of sacrum; SI = sacroiliac joint.

Figure 11.2 Medial aspect of the left hip bone. A= auricular surface; AI = anterior inferior iliac spine; AS = anterior superior iliac spine; B = body of ischium; G = greater sciatic notch; IE = iliopubic eminence; IF = iliac fossa; IS = ischial spine; IT = ischial tuberosity; P = posterior superior iliac spine; PI = posterior inferior iliac spine; T = tuberosity of ilium; star shows the articular surface of the symphysis pubis. The dotted lines approximately indicate the limits of the iliac (1), pubic (2), and ischial (3) parts of the bone.

The four bones of the pelvic girdle are held together by strong ligaments and articulate via four articulations: two *synovial* sacroiliac joints, and two secondary *cartilaginous* joints, the pubic symphysis and sacrococcygeal joints which are connected by fibrocartilaginous discs as well as by ligaments (Rickenbacher, 1985; Moore, 1992). Each articular surface of the pubic symphysis is covered by a thin layer of hyaline cartilage, which is connected to the cartilage of the other side by a thick fibrocartilaginous interpubic disc which is generally thicker in women than in men; the ligaments joining the pubic bones are the superior pubic and the arcuate pubic ligaments (Moore, 1992).

The three ligaments that stabilize the pelvis, sacrum, and the fifth lumbar vertebra are the iliolumbar, sacrotuberous and sacrospinous ligaments, respectively (Hanson and Sonesson, 1994) which have been well documented in anatomical texts. According to Bogduk and Twomey (1991), the iliolumbar ligament consists of five different parts but

Hanson and Sonesson (1994) found it to consist of only two, and Williams and Warwick (1980) found it to consist of three parts.

The radiograph in Figure 11.3 shows the two sacroiliac joints, the symphysis pubis, and the sacrococcygeal joint, as well as the associated hip and lumbosacral joints.

The strong sacroiliac articulations have irregular but reciprocal elevations and depressions between the auricular surfaces of the sacrum and ilium which may help to interlock the opposing surfaces of these joints. In addition, stability is provided by a strong articular capsule and the powerful interosseous and posterior sacroiliac ligaments (Figure 11.4), which tightly knit and strengthen the joint but allow minimal movement (Rickenbacher *et al.*, 1985).

The sacroiliac joint is an atypical synovial joint, possessing a joint cavity containing synovial fluid, cartilaginous surfaces, and a synovial lined capsule. It is atypical because the cartilage on the ilium is fibrocartilage whereas the cartilage on the sacral

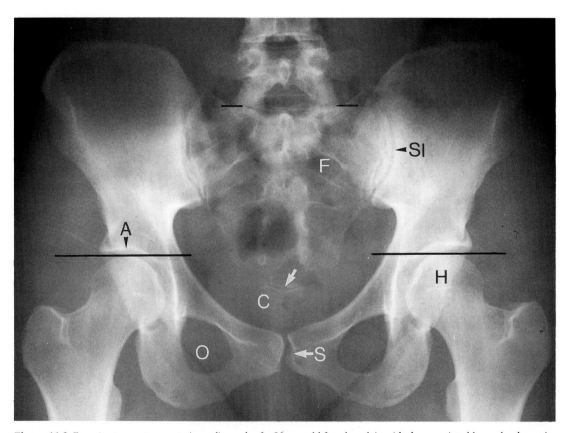

Figure 11.3 Erect posture anteroposterior radiograph of a 26-year-old female pelvis with the associated lower lumbar spine and hip joints. A = acetabulum (superior surface); C = coccyx; F = sacral foramen; H = head of femur; O = obturator foramen; S = symphysis pubis; SI = sacroiliac joint; white arrow = sacrococcygeal joint. The long and short black lines show the femur head heights and the superior sacral notch heights, respectively.

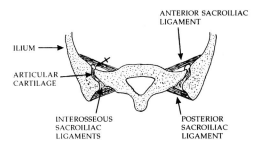

ANTERIOR SACROILIAC LIGAMENT

ILIUM

ARTICULAR CARTILAGE

INTEROSSEOUS SACROILIAC LIGAMENTS

POSTERIOR SACROILIAC LIGAMENT

Figure 11.4 This schematic representation of a horizontal section through the sacroiliac joints illustrates the powerful interosseous sacroiliac ligaments which assist in suspending the sacrum between the iliac bones. Also illustrated are the posterior and anterior sacroiliac ligaments. The anterior sacroiliac ligament lies just anterior to the capsule (tailed arrow). The sacroiliac joint consists of a ligamentous compartment posteriorly and an articular compartment anteriorly (Modified from Rickenbacher, J., Landolt, A.M. and Theiler, K. (1985) *Applied Anatomy of the Back.* Springer-Verlag, Berlin. Bernard, T.N. and Cassidy, J. D. (1991) The sacroiliac joint syndrome. Pathophysiology, diagnosis and management. In *The Adult Spine: Principles and Practice.* Raven Press, New York, pp 2107–2130. Moore, K.L. (1992) *Clinically Oriented Anatomy,* 3rd edn. Williams and Wilkins, Baltimore.

surface is hyaline articular cartilage. Typical synovial joints have hyaline articular cartilage on both surfaces of the joint.

The superior surface of a block of osteoligamentous tissues cut in the horizontal plane through the sacrum and parts of its adjacent ilia, at the level of the first left and right sacral intervertebral canals (foramina), and the lower margin of the first sacral intervertebral disc, is shown in Figure 11.5.

Part of a histological section, cut in the horizontal plane through the left side of the sacrum and the adjacent ilium at the level of the root of the superior articular process and the adjacent lamina of the first sacral segment (see reference line on Figures 3.3 and 11.3), is shown in Figure 11.6. This figure also shows part of the interosseous sacroiliac ligament in the sacroiliac joint cavity (Vleeming *et al.*, 1992) which is the main determinant of sacral movement (Vukicevic *et al.*, 1991). This histological section further illustrates how the massive and very strong interosseous sacroiliac ligaments unite the iliac and sacral tuberosities; they consist of short, strong bundles of fibres that blend with, and are supported by, the thick firm posterior sacroiliac ligaments (Moore, 1992). The

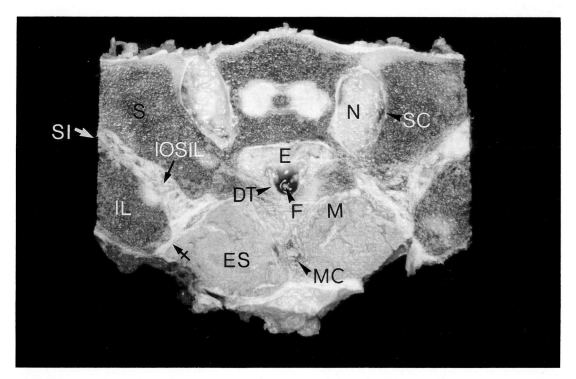

Figure 11.5 A block of osteoligamentous tissues cut in the horizontal plane through the sacrum (S) and adjacent ilia (IL) at the level of the first sacral intervertebral canals (foramina) (SC) containing neural structures (N) (51-year-old female). The sacral canal is seen centrally and contains epidural fat (E), vascular structures and the lower portion of the dural tube (DT) with its filum terminale internum (F). Parts of the left and right sacroiliac joints are shown at this level. ES = erector spinae muscle; IOSIL = interosseous sacroiliac ligament; M = multifidus muscle; MC = median sacral crest; tailed arrow = posterior sacroiliac ligament; SI = part of the sacroiliac joint. Same orientation as in Figure 11.4.

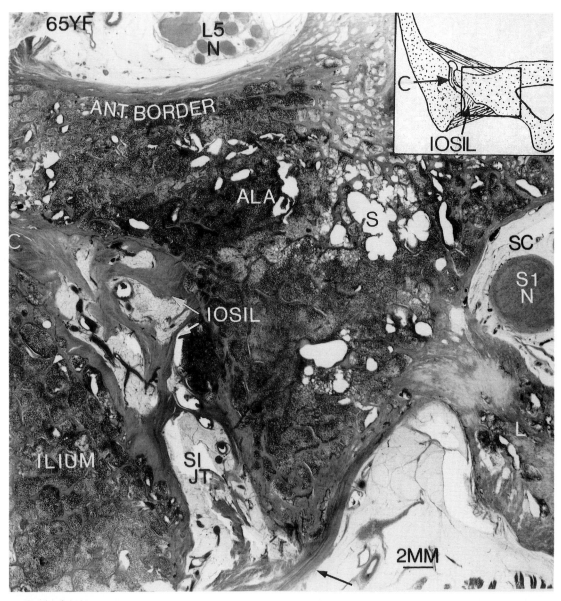

Figure 11.6 A 200 μm thick histological section cut in the horizontal plane showing the left side of the sacrum (S) and the adjacent ilium at the level of the root of the superior articular process and the adjacent lamina (L) of the first sacral segment. (65-year-old female) (See Figures 3.3 and 11.3 for reference line indicating the approximate level of this section). The anterior border of the sacral ala is shown, with adjacent neural structures forming part of the fifth lumbar nerve (L5N). The sacral canal (SC) contains neural structures forming part of the first sacral nerve (S1N), adipose tissue and vascular structures. Part of the posterior sacroiliac ligament (arrow) is seen bridging between the first sacral segment and the ilium at the posterior, i.e. non-synovial part of the sacroiliac joint (SI JT). IOSIL = interosseous sacroiliac ligament. Insert line drawing shows the approximate orientation of the histological section (rectangle). C = cartilage; IOSIL = interosseous sacroiliac joint ligament.

interosseous sacroiliac ligament, part of which is shown in Figure 11.6, fills the irregular space immediately above and behind the sacroiliac joint and is covered by the posterior sacroiliac ligament (Williams and Warwick, 1980).

The histological section (Figure 11.6) shows that there is also adipose tissue between the sacrum and the ilium, through which course quite large blood vessels. The synovial part of the sacroiliac joint is located more anterolaterally than is shown in this histological section, although its most posterior part is just visible on the left edge of the photomicrograph.

Part of the synovial region of a sacroiliac joint is shown in its superior to inferior length in Figure 11.7.

This figure shows the histological features of a section cut through the sacroiliac joint between the auricular surfaces of the sacrum and ilium, in which the sacral articular surface is covered by hyaline articular cartilage and the iliac articular surface is covered by fibrocartilage (Putschar, 1931; Schunke, 1938; Dijkstra *et al.*, 1989; Cassidy, 1992). The iliac auricular surface is covered by fibrocartilage (Dijkstra *et al.*, 1989), although Paquin *et al.* (1983) showed by collagen typing that the iliac cartilaginous surface had no collagen typical of fibrocartilage. Therefore, they concluded that this cartilage is more hyaline than fibrocartilage in nature but noted that the orientation of its collagen fibrils is abnormal in being organized parallel to the auricular surface throughout the

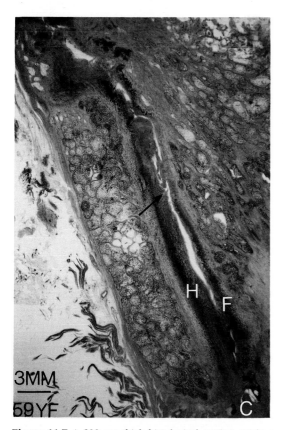

Figure 11.7 A 200 μm thick histological section cut in a slightly oblique plane through a sacroiliac joint from a 59-year-old female. C = fibrous articular capsule inferiorly; F = fibrocartilage on the iliac side of the joint; H = hyaline articular cartilage on the sacral articular surface, which shows osteoarthritic changes (arrow) in this specimen.

cartilage's depth. The depth of the cartilage on the sacral surface ranges from 0.2 to 2.4 mm, while on the sacral surface the range is 0.1–1.8 mm, indicating that the sacral cartilage is, on average, 1.7 times thicker than that of the iliac surface (Walker, 1986).

Vleeming *et al.* (1990a) showed the presence of cartilage covered ridges and depressions which are complementary on the opposing auricular surfaces of the sacroiliac joints. In Figure 11.7, it can be seen that the sacral hyaline articular cartilage is considerably thicker than the fibrocartilage on the iliac articular surface in this atypical synovial joint, confirming the findings of Rickenbacher *et al.* (1985). The fibrocartilage tends to degenerate early in life but the joint space most often remains patent throughout life (Cassidy, 1992) and there is still a demonstrable joint space well into the eighth and ninth decades (Greenman, 1992). The histological section in Figure 11.7 shows some evidence of *debris* within the upper one-third of the joint, which may correspond with the *debris* first described by Brooke (1924). The adult sacroiliac joint will accept a volume of 1–2 cc of injectate but the addition of more fluid distends the joint (Aprill, 1992).

The sacroiliac joint can undergo a small amount of anteroposterior rotatory movement (Weisl, 1955; Sturesson *et al.*, 1989) which appears to range from 2 degrees (Egund *et al.*, 1978) to 12 degrees (Lavignolle *et al.*, 1983); movement is now well accepted, and Vleeming *et al.* (1990b) state that small movements are indeed possible, and this is compatible with the findings of small, non-bridging anterior peripheral osteophytes which are found regularly (Dijkstra *et al.*, 1989). Rotation in a para-median plane (anterior, posterior and cranial caudal translation) has been identified, and rotation in the frontal plane has been shown (Stevens, 1992). Under abnormal loading conditions of sacroiliac joints with ridges and depressions, it is possible that a sacroiliac joint can be forced into a new position where the ridges and depressions are no longer complementary theoretically causing a blocked joint (Vleeming *et al.*, 1990b).

The sacroiliac joint is supplied by arterial branches derived from the superior gluteal, iliolumbar, and lateral sacral arteries (Moore, 1992).

The detailed dissections of Bradley (1974) illustrated not only the innervation of the posterior aspect of the sacrum but also the innervation of the zygapophysial joints. More recent authors (Bogduk, 1983; Giles, 1989) have confirmed the work of Bradley (1974) with regard to innervation of the lumbar zygapophysial joints after the medial branch passes under a ligament forming a tunnel approximately 6 mm long (Bradley, 1974), i.e., the mamillo-accessory ligament. A plexiform arrangement of nerves lying on the posterior surface of the sacrum, in contact with the interosseous sacroiliac ligament and the sacrotuberous ligament (Figure 11.8) was demonstrated by Bradley (1974). The fifth lumbar nerve (L5) descends vertically in a groove on the ala of the sacrum, immediately lateral to the articular facet, and can be traced downwards as the lateral division for a distance of approximately 6 cm before it joins the lateral division of the first sacral nerve (S1) (Bradley, 1974). The medial division of the L5 nerve curves under the lumbosacral zygapophysial joint, sending tiny branches to it; the lateral division of the L5 nerve, supplies the posterior sacroiliac ligament (Bradley, 1974).

The lateral branch of the S1 nerve is joined above with the L5 nerve, and below with the S2 nerve; the lateral division of the S2 nerve descends and courses downwards on the sacrum, just lateral to the third and fourth sacral foramina, where it joins with the lateral divisions of the S3 and S4 nerves (Bradley, 1974).

The medial divisions of the S1 to S4 nerves pass medially to the multifidus muscle (see Chapter 9), while the lateral divisions pass between the interosseous and overlying posterior sacroiliac ligaments which also receive several fine filaments from the lateral divisions of the L5 and S1-3 nerves (Bradley, 1974).

The anterior sacroiliac ligament is innervated by ventral branches from the sacral plexus (S1-4) (Rickenbacher *et al.*, 1985) and possibly small filaments of the obturator nerve (L2-4) (Sunderland, 1968).

In summary, all nerves adjacent to the sacroiliac joint supply small branches to the joint capsule, with the ventral branches coming largely from the sacral plexus; the inferior parts of the joint are supplied by a branch of the superior gluteal nerve (L4-S1 ventral rami). Posteriorly, the joint receives branches from the dorsal rami of S1 and S2 (Rickenbacher *et al.*, 1985).

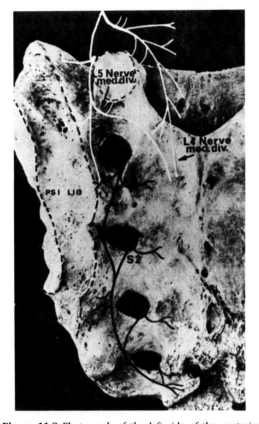

Figure 11.8 Photograph of the left side of the posterior surface of the sacrum showing the posterior sacral nerve plexus formed on the dorsum of the sacrum by the dorsal rami of the lower lumbar and sacral nerves. The proximity of the posterior sacral plexus to the posterior sacroiliac ligament (PSI LIG) and interosseous ligament is illustrated, as is the overlap of nerve branches from different cord segments. The pattern of the nerve supply of the lumbosacral joint is also shown. (Reproduced with permission from Bradley, K.C. (1974) The anatomy of backache. *Aust. N.Z. J. Surg.*, **44**, 227-232.)

Clinical

Sacroiliac joint dysfunction appears to be an overlooked condition which is not even considered a possibility by many clinicians involved in the diagnosis and treatment of patients with mechanical back pain (Aprill, 1992). This is in spite of the clinical observation that pain can be exacerbated by various physical manoeuvres which are thought to stress the joint (Mooney, 1992). The resulting syndrome is a common condition thought to result from a mechanical derangement of the joint (Kirkaldy-Willis, 1988). Sacroiliac joint dysfunction may be associated with a small degree of subluxation, based on the apparent success of manipulation directed at the sacroiliac joint (Allan and Waddell, 1989; Bernard and Cassidy, 1991). As early as 1905, Goldthwait and Osgood emphasized mobility of the sacroiliac joint and suggested that an acute or chronic slip, or subluxation, of the joint could cause pain and suggested that the variability of symptoms may be attributable to differing degrees of mobility.

As a major link in the connections between the trunk and the lower limbs, the sacroiliac joints are subject to heavy loads, both static and dynamic (Rickenbacher *et al.*, 1985). Numerous conditions can involve the sacroiliac joints (Table 11.1) and, in the last few years, the importance of sacroiliac syndrome in the causation of low back pain has gained increasing recognition, partly due to the clinical and radiological studies by Schmid (1980) which showed a larger range of movement in the sacroiliac joints than was previously supposed. Shaw (1992) states that sacroiliac joint dysfunction is a very common cause of low back pain.

Table 11.1 *Possible causes of sacroiliac joint pain*

Mechanical:
  Sacroiliac dysfunction
  Postural
    Pelvic obliquity; postural lumbar scoliosis; excessive
      lumbar lordosis; obesity
  Pregnancy with joint laxity

Degenerative:
  Sacroiliac osteoarthrosis
  Osteitis condensans ilii

Inflammatory (rheumatic):
  Sacroiliac arthritis
    Ankylosing spondylitis (Bechterew's disease); psoriatic
      arthritis; Reiter's syndrome; intestinal lipodystrophy
      (Whipple's disease); rheumatoid arthritis;
      ossification of the capsule in hyperostotic
      spondylosis (Forestier's disease); gouty arthritis

Infective:
  Tuberculosis; brucellosis, osteomyelitis, etc.

Osteopathies:
  Dystrophic
  Osteoporosis; osteomalacia; hyperparathyroidism;
    hypogonadism
  Hypertrophic
  Osteitis deformans (Paget's disease)

Neoplasms:
  Benign and malignant (primary and secondary)

Trauma

Dysplasias
  Hypoplasia of one sacroiliac joint

(Modified from Rickenbacher *et al.*, 1985.)

According to Schmid (1980), the main feature of the sacroiliac syndrome is the paroxysmal character of the pain which may fluctuate widely during rest and movement, and may not be confined to the vicinity of the sacroiliac joint, radiating into the groin, trochanteric area, or distal parts of the posterior thigh; occasionally, pain may be referred down the lateral or posterior areas of the calf to the ankle, foot and toes (Kirkaldy-Willis, 1988). A survey by Aprill (1992) revealed that 25–30% of non-specific back pain patients have symptomatic sacroiliac dysfunction in conjunction with other defined lesions (symptomatic anular fissures, symptomatic zygapophysial joint dysfunction). Pain on movement involving the sacroiliac, gluteal, inguinal and trochanteric regions, usually referring to the back, and pain in the lower abdomen and groin due to tension in the iliacus muscle, and sciatic-type pain, can be part of the sacroiliac syndrome (Rickenbacher *et al.*, 1985). In addition, there may be intermittent limping of the affected side, usually associated with fatigue pain (Rickenbacher *et al.*, 1985).

Clinical examination

Clinical examination of the sacroiliac joint must include inspection, assessment for leg length inequality and pelvic torsion, and palpation of the iliacus, adductor, gluteus major, and piriformis muscles (Rickenbacher *et al.*, 1985). Palpation should also include posterior superior iliac spines, sacrotuberous ligaments, as well as the origins and insertions of major muscles (glutei, piriformis, adductors) for both tenderness and increased tension (Aprill, 1992). Clinically, it is the region of the posterior surface of the sacrum immediately lateral to the line of the foramina, which is important, with respect to pain and tenderness, as this is where the interosseous and posterior sacroiliac ligaments receive nerve fibres which pass laterally between the ligaments (Bradley, 1974). Palpation for mobility of the sacroiliac joint has been advocated but the validity of this examination has yet to be established. Two out of three positive clinical provocation tests (Gaenslen's, Faber-Patrick and Yeoman's) are found in most cases of sacroiliac joint syndrome (Cassidy and Mierau, 1992). Rectal or vaginal examination complete the physical assessment (Rickenbacher *et al.*, 1985).

Pelvic obliquity and leg length inequality assessments are important (Aprill, 1992). The effect of significant (>9 mm) leg length inequality (Giles, 1989) on the sacroiliac joints is unknown but it is reasonable to assume that it may result in excessive unilateral stress on the sacroiliac joint capsule, its ligaments, and its articular cartilage (Dihlmann, 1980) (Figure 11.9).

In an electromyographic study, Taillard (1969) found anomalies of pelvic and spinal posture, as well as abnormalities in the dynamics of postural muscles when there was a leg length difference of 1 cm or more. Vink and Kamphuisen (1989) concluded that intrinsic lumbar back muscle electromyographic activity can increase at 15 mm leg length inequality and that 'small' (<35 mm) leg length inequalities may not be harmless. Jenner and Barry (1995) found that people with a leg length difference of at least 2 cm are more prone to back pain. Some clinicians still consider significant leg length inequality to be 2 cm or more (Guichet *et al.*, 1991) and arbitrarily dismiss leg length inequality between 1 and 2 cm (personal communication, J.P. Gofton, 1989) without any scientific basis, even though there is no final agreement on what leg length inequality is clinically significant (Krettek *et al.*, 1994). According to Hoffman and Hoffman (1994), levelling of the sacral base by shoe raise provides statistically significant relief from low back pain, often with spectacular reduction of symptoms (Williams, 1974). Tjernstrom and Rehnberg (1994) found that correction of leg length discrepancy of 3 cm and more improved patients' ability to work, walk and perform recreational activities. This issue requires clarification as surgical prophylactic intervention can correct leg

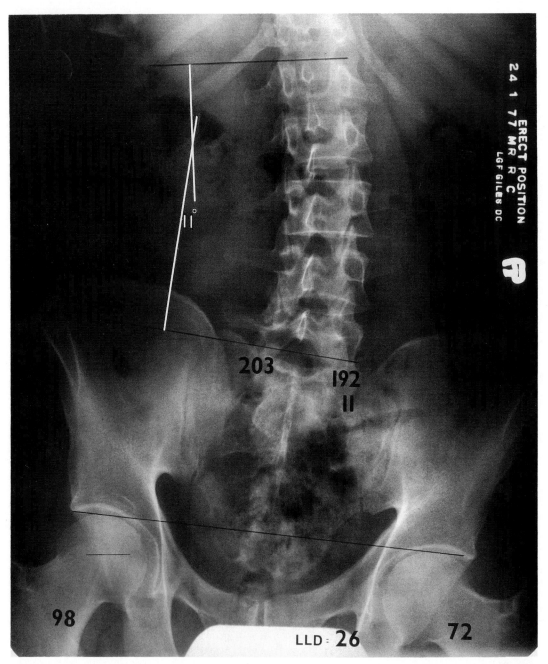

Figure 11.9 Radiograph of a 37-year-old male with a right leg length deficiency of 26 mm and a postural scoliosis of 11 degrees using the Cobb (1948) method of measurement. Note that the right pubic crest is slightly higher than the left which may indicate some degree of rotation between the sacrum and ilium on one or both sides. There is some wedging of the intervertebral discs, particularly at L4–5, with the discs being narrower on the left side. (Reproduced with permission from Giles, L.G.F. (1989) *Anatomical Basis of Low Back Pain*. Williams and Wilkins, Baltimore.)

length discrepancy before epiphyseal closure (Harcke and Mandell; 1993, Mattassi, 1993), whereas leg lengthening in adult life entails potential risks of serious complications (Tjernstrom *et al.*, 1993) in a high percentage (84.8%) of cases (Zippel and Lang, 1993; Dahl *et al.*, 1994).

The relationship of sacroiliac joint dysfunction, osteoarthrosis, and sacroiliac syndrome (Lewis, 1985; Bernard and Kirkaldy-Willis, 1987; Kirkaldy-Willis, 1988; Huskisson, 1990; Cassidy and Mierau, 1992; Dreyfuss *et al.*, 1994; Chaabane *et al.*, 1994) to leg length inequality is unknown.

In young individuals, bony structures are sometimes seen within the sacroiliac joint but are considered normal (Funke *et al.*, 1992). However, during old age, the sacroiliac joint often becomes, partially ossified, especially in men, and calcification in the anterior sacroiliac ligaments makes the joint cavities less visible on radiographs, even though they are still present (Moore, 1992). It should be noted that the sacroiliac joints are often asymmetrical (Dijkstra, 1992). Aprill (1992) has developed a diagnostic technique for consistent opacification of the joint space; contrast material is contained within the space of a 'normal' joint, implying the capsule is intact. However, periarticular spread of contrast material indicates disruption of the ventral capsule (Aprill, 1992).

References

Allan, D.B. and Waddell, G. (1989) An historical perspective on low back pain and disability. *Acta Orthop. Scand. (Suppl. 234)*, **60**, 1–23.

Aprill, C.N. (1992) The role of anatomically specific injections into the sacroiliac joint. In *First Interdisciplinary World Congress on Low Back Pain and its Relation to the Sacroiliac Joint* (A. Vleeming, V. Mooney, C. Snijders and T. Dorman, eds). ECO, Rotterdam, pp. 373–380.

Bernard. V. and Cassidy, J.D. (1981) Macroscopic and microscopic anatomy of the sacroiliac joint from embryonic life until the eighth decade. *Spine*, **6**, 620–628.

Bernard, T.N. and Kirkaldy-Willis, W.H. (1987) Recognising specific characteristics of non-specific low back pain. *Clin. Orthop. Rel. Res.*, **217**, 96.

Bradley, K.C. (1974) The anatomy of backache. *Aust. N.Z. J. Surg.*, **44**, 227–232.

Bogduk, N. (1983) The innervation of the lumbar spine. *Spine*, **8**, 286–293.

Bogduk, N. and Twomey, L.T. (1991) *Clinical Anatomy of the Lumbar Spine*, 2nd edition. Churchill Livingstone, Edinburgh.

Brooke, R. (1924) The sacroiliac joint. *J. Anat.*, **58**, 299–305.

Cassidy, J.D. (1992) The pathoanatomy and clinical significance of the sacroiliac joint. *J. Manipulative Physiol. Ther.*, **15**, 41–42.

Cassidy, J.D. and Mierau, D.R. (1992) Pathophysiology of the sacroiliac joint. In *Principles and Practice of Chiropractic* (S. Haldeman, ed.) 2nd edition. Appleton and Lange, Norwalk, pp. 211–224.

Chaabane, M., Abid, R., Hamza, K. *et al.* (1994) Etiologie inhabituelle de cruralgie. *J. Radiol.*, **75**, 283–285.

Cobb, J.R. (1948) Outline for the study of scoliosis. Instructional course lectures. *Am. Acad. Orthop. Surg.*, **5**, 261–275.

Dahl, M.T., Gulli, B. and Berg, T. (1994) Complications of limb lengthening. A learning curve. *Clin. Orthop.*, **301**, 10–18.

Dijkstra, P.F. (1992) Radiology of the normal sacroiliac joints; congenital variations and imaging techniques. In *First Interdisciplinary World Congress on Low Back Pain and its Relation to the Sacroiliac Joint* (A. Vleeming, V. Mooney, C. Snijders and T. Dorman, eds). ECO, Rotterdam, pp. 275–282.

Dijkstra, P.F., Vleeming, A. and Stoeckart, R. (1989) Complex motion tomography of the sacroiliac joint. *Fortschr. Röntgenstr.*, **150**, 635–642.

Dihlmann, W. (1980) *Diagnostic Radiology of the Sacroiliac Joints.* Year Book Medical Publishers, Chicago, pp. 92–93.

Dreyfuss, P., Dryer, S., Griffin, J. *et al.* (1994) Positive sacroiliac screening tests in asymptomatic adults. *Spine*, **15**, 1138–1143.

Egund, N., Ollson, T.H., Schmid, H. and Selvik, G. (1978) Movements in the sacroiliac joints demonstrated with roentgen stereophotogrammetry. *Acta Rad. Diagn.*, **19**, 833–846.

Funke, V.M., Gotz, W., Fischer, G. *et al.* (1992) Apophyses of the sacro-iliac joints on CT. *Fortschr. Geb. Rontgenstr. Neuen. Bildgeb. Verfahr.*, **157**, 43–46.

Giles, L.G.F. (1989) *Anatomical Basis of Low Back Pain.* Williams and Wilkins, Baltimore.

Goldthwait, J.E. and Osgood, R.B. (1905) A consideration of the pelvic articulations from an anatomical, pathological and clinical standpoint. *Boston Med. Surg. J.*, **152**, 593–601.

Greenman, P.E. (1992) Sacroiliac dysfunction in the failed low back pain syndrome.

Guichet, J.M., Spivak, J.M., Trouilloud, P. and Grammont, P.M. (1991) Lower limb-length discrepancy: an epidemiologic study. *Clin. Orthop. Rel. Res.*, **272**, 235–241.

Hanson, P. and Sonesson, B. (1994) The anatomy of the iliolumbar ligament. *Arch. Phys. Med. Rehabil.*, **75**, 1245–1246.

Harcke, H.T. and Mandell, G.A. (1993) Scintigraphic evaluation of the growth plate. *Semin. Nucl. Med.*, **23**, 266–273.

Hoffman, K.S. and Hoffman, L.L. (1994) Effects of adding sacral base leveling to osteopathic manipulative treatment of back pain: a pilot study. *J. Am. Osteopath. Assoc.*, **94**, 217–220, 223–226.

Huskisson, E.C. (1990) Back pain. In *Clinical Medicine. A Text-book for Medical Students and Doctors.* (P.J. Kumar and M.L. Clark, eds), 2nd edition. Baillière Tindall, London, p. 410.

Jenner, J.R. and Barry, M. (1995) Low back pain. *BMJ*, **310**, 929–932.

Kirkaldy-Willis, W.H. (1988) The site and nature of the lesion. In *Managing Low Back Pain* (W.H. Kirkaldy-Willis, ed.) 2nd edition. Churchill Livingstone, New York, pp. 133–154.

Lavignolle, B., Vital, J.M., Senegas, J. *et al.* (1983) An approach to the functional anatomy of the sacroiliac joints in vivo. *Anat. Clin.*, **5**, 169–176.

Lewis, T.L.T. (1985) Pelvis, pain in. In *French's Index of Differential Diagnosis* (D.F. Hart, ed.), 12th edition.

Wright, London, pp. 660–661.

Mattassi, R. (1993) Differential diagnosis in congenital vascular-bone syndromes. *Semin. Vasc. Surg.*, **6**, 233–244.

Mooney, V. (1992) Can we measure function in the sacroiliac joint? In *First Interdisciplinary World Congress on Low Back Pain and its Relation to the Sacroiliac Joint* (A. Vleeming, V. Mooney, C. Snijders and T. Dorman, eds). ECO, Rotterdam, pp. 407–421.

Moore, K.L. (1992) *Clinically Oriented Anatomy*, 3rd edn. Williams and Wilkins, Baltimore.

Paquin, J.D., van der Rest, M., Marie, P.J. *et al.* (1983) Biochemical and morphologic studies of cartilage from the adult human sacroiliac joint. *Arthritis Rheum.*, **26**, 887–895.

Putschar W. (1931) Entwicklung, Wachstum und Pathologie der Beckenverbin Lungen des Menschen mit besonderer Berucksichtigüng von Schwangerschaft, Geburt und ihren Folgen. Aus dem pathologischen Institute der Universität. Göttingen, Fischer Verlag, Stuttgart.

Rickenbacher, J., Landolt, A.M. and Theiler, K. (1985) *Applied Anatomy of the Back*. Springer-Verlag, Berlin.

Schmid, H. (1980) Das iliosakralgelenk in einer untersuchung mit rontgenstereophogrammetrie und einer klinischen studie. *Acta Rheumatol.*, **5**, 163.

Schunke, G.B. (1938) The anatomy and development of the sacroiliac joint in man. *Anat. Rec.*, **72**, 313–331.

Shaw, J.L. (1992) The role of the sacroiliac joint as a cause of low back pain and dysfunction. In *First Interdisciplinary World Congress on Low Back Pain and its Relation to the Sacroiliac Joint* (A. Vleeming, V. Mooney, C. Snijders and T. Dorman, eds). ECO, Rotterdam, pp. 67–80.

Stevens, A. (1992) Side-bending and axial rotation of the sacrum inside the pelvic girdle. In *First Interdisciplinary World Congress on Low Back Pain and its Relation to the Sacroiliac Joint* (A. Vleeming, V. Mooney, C. Snijders and T. Dorman, eds) ECO, Rotterdam, pp. 209–230.

Sturesson, B., Selvik, G. and Uden, A. (1989) Movements of the sacroiliac joints. A roentgen stereophotogrammetric analysis. *Spine*, **14**, 162–165.

Sunderland, S. (1968) *Nerves and Nerve Injuries*. E and S Livingstone, Edinburgh.

Taillard, W. (1969) Colonne lambaire et inegalite des membres inferieures. *Acta Orthop. Belg.*, **35**, 601–613.

Tjernstrom, B. and Rehnberg, L. (1994) Back pain and arthralgia before and after lengthening. 75 patients questioned after 6 (1–11) years. *Acta Orthop. Scand.*, **65**, 328–332.

Tjernstrom, B., Olerud, S. and Karlstrom, G. (1993) Direct leg lengthening. *J. Orthop. Trauma*, **7**, 543–551.

Vink, P. and Kamphuisen, H.A.C. (1989) Leg length inequity, pelvic tilt and lumbar back muscle activity during standing. *Clin. Biomech.*, **4**, 115–117.

Vleeming A., Stoechart, R. and Snijders, C.J. (1992) General introduction. In *First Interdisciplinary World Congress on Low Back Pain and its Relation to the Sacroiliac Joint* (A. Vleeming, V. Mooney, C. Snijders and T. Dorman, eds). ECO, Rotterdam, pp. 4–64.

Vleeming, A., Stoechart, R., Volkers, A.C.W. and Snijders, C.J. (1990a) Relation between form and function in the sacroiliac joint, Part 1: Clinical anatomical aspects. *Spine*, **15**, 130–132.

Vleeming, A., Volkers, A.C.W., Snijders, C.J. and Stoeckart, R. (1990b) Relation between form and function in the sacroiliac joint, Part 2: Biomechanical aspects. *Spine*, **15**, 133–136.

Vukicevic, S., Marusic, A., Stavljenic, A. *et al.* (1991) Holographic analyisis of the human pelvis. *Spine*, **16**, 209–214.

Walker, J.M. (1986) Age-related differences in the human sacroiliac joint: a histological study; implications for therapy. *J. Orthop. Sports Phys. Ther.*, **7**, 325–334.

Weisel, H. (1955) The movements of the sacro-iliac joints. *Acta Anat.*, **23**, 80–91.

Williams, P.C. (1974) *Low Back and Neck Pain*. Charles C Thomas, Springfield, p. 52.

Williams, P.L. and Warwick, T. (1980) *Gray's Anatomy*, 36th edn. Churchill Livingstone, London.

Zippel, H. and Lang, K. (1993) Operative extremitatenverlangerungen – erfahrugen und ergebnisse. *Zentralbl. Chir.* **118**, 646–657.

12

Pathoanatomy of the thoracolumbar transitional junction

K.P. Singer

Introduction

The human vertebral transitional junctions show the diversity of our anatomy (Schmorl and Junghanns, 1971). An appreciation of this diversity is important to the clinician of manual therapy as a majority of clinical presentations occur at the transitions. Despite an abundant early literature emphasizing the range of anatomies within the spine, most contemporary descriptions in anatomy and clinical sources imply that the vertebrae are symmetrical and highly consistent in number and regional morphology. In discussing the biomechanics of the thoracolumbar column, Kazarian (1972) noted the true idiosyncratic behaviour of the column when it was loaded. This reflects the subtle, and at times, marked asymmetries within and between vertebral segments.

This chapter will summarize investigations into the anatomy and mechanics of the thoracolumbar junction. It is hoped that this work will provide a framework for the clinician when assessing and treating this diverse and highly variable region of the spine.

The thoracolumbar junction is commonly represented in anatomical sources as showing an abrupt change in the configuration of the zygapophysial joints of the twelfth thoracic vertebrae (Figure 12.1). In most texts, this morphology was depicted by inferior articular processes which turned out to face laterally (Pick, 1890). This concept of a regular and predictable anatomy has been perpetuated in most sources. To appreciate the variations in this transitional region, the interested clinician needed to explore early, anatomical, anthropological and radiological literature.

A number of these reports described (i) cranial and caudal variations in the location of the thoracolumbar

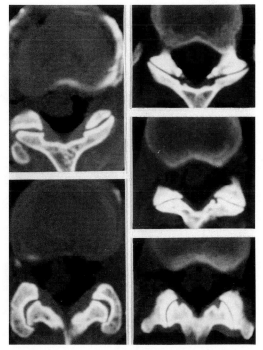

Figure 12.1 *Ex vivo* CT images depicting the two main patterns of change in zygapophysial joint configuration at the thoracolumbar junction. The transition (left), is the standard anatomical textbook description of an abrupt change from the coronal plane of the lower thoracic zygapophysial joints to the predominantly sagittal planes of the first lumbar segment. An angulation difference between adjacent paired joints of >120° was used as the criterion to separate these patterns. The gradual pattern (right) depicts an intermediate zygapophysial joint configuration interposed between the more coronally and sagittally orientated levels.

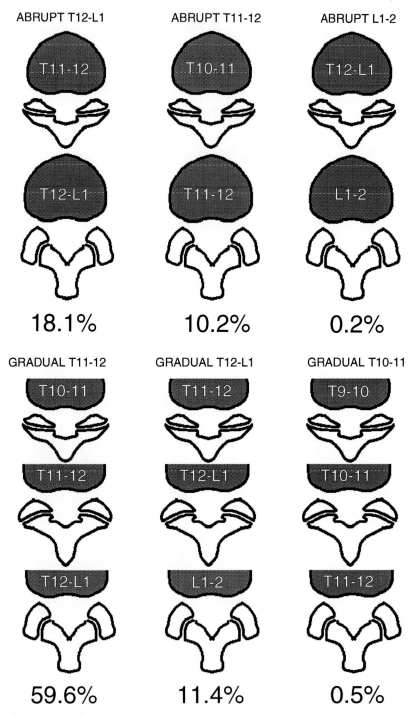

Figure 12.2 The textbook depiction of an abrupt transition in zygapophysial joint transitions at the thoracolumbar junction was evident in approximately 30% of cases. The presence of intermediately configured zygapophysial joints characterized the gradual transitions which were typically located between T10–11 and T12–L1. (Reproduced with permission from Singer, K.P., Breidahl, P.D. and Day, R.E. (1989) Posterior element variation at the thoracolumbar transition. A morphometric study using computed tomography. *Clin. Biomech.*, **4**: 80–86.)

junction (Humphry, 1858; Struthers, 1875; Hasebe, 1913; Schertlein, 1928; Kühne, 1932, Stewart, 1932; Lanier, 1939; Terry and Trotter, 1953; Allbrook, 1955), (ii) asymmetry of the TLJ zygapophysial joints (Barclay-Smith, 1911; Whitney, 1926; Shore, 1930), and (iii) a wrap-around configuration of the thoracolumbar junction zygapophysial joints in which the superior articular processes locked those from the vertebra above (Topinard, 1877; Le Double, 1912; Davis, 1955). Differences in thoracolumbar junction location and morphology were reported by Todd in 1922 to be so common that any attempt to categorize them was considered impractical.

As little specific investigation of this region had occurred since, this prompted a comprehensive examination of the lower thoracic and upper lumbar segments (i.e. T10–11, T11–12, T12–L1 and L1–2). This work was undertaken initially using CT archives from over 600 patient examinations, with histology performed on 75 cadaveric thoracolumbar junctions (Singer, 1989a). The major observation from this examination has been the dismissal of the notion that an abrupt transition is representative of the normal anatomy of the thoracolumbar junction (Singer *et al.*, 1989a) (Figure 12.1). Instead, a more gradual change from thoracic to lumbar morphology appears to be normal. Indeed, in 1875, Struthers described a transition pattern in which the thoracolumbar junction zygapophysial joints showed an intermediate configuration between the sagittal and coronal planes of adjacent thoracolumbar junction segments. The standard textbook description of an abrupt transition, as defined in these studies (Figure 12.2), would apply to about 30% of the population examined.

Having defined a gradual form of transition as the normal pattern, it was of interest to explore whether this morphology differed from the abrupt mode. It was surmised that the gradual pattern might serve to minimize stresses between the mobile segments of this transitional region and this would be evident in terms of articular histology, patterns of spinal injuries, and mechanics.

Developmental anatomy of the thoracolumbar junction

The sequence of ossification of the vertebral centra reveal a consistent pattern whereby the first sites are located in the lower two thoracic and first lumbar vertebral bodies; thereafter, a progressive cranial and caudal pattern of ossification commences in adjoining vertebrae (Noback and Roberston, 1951; Bagnall *et al.*, 1977; Birkner, 1978). Similarly, by about 2 years of postnatal life the vertebral ring apophyses from T10 to L1 appear to ossify first (Louis, 1983). These ossification patterns have prompted Bagnall *et al.*

(1977) to suggest that the use of trunk musculature and fetal movement *in utero* act to stimulate early skeletal development of the thoracolumbar junction elements in response to these mechanical stresses applied to the vertebral column. The thoracolumbar junction transition also shows an increase in the size of the vertebral bodies and intervertebral discs (Davis, 1980; Berry *et al.*, 1987), associated with a larger vertebral canal to accommodate the lumbar enlargement of the spinal cord and conus (Gonon *et al.*, 1975; Louis, 1983).

Thoracolumbar spinal curvature

The gradual thoracic kyphosis formed by the thoracic vertebrae and intervertebral discs (Kapandji, 1977) permits relatively little motion compared with the lordotic curves of the cervical and lumbar regions. The thoracic cage, with its anterior concavity, affords protection to the thoracic and upper abdominal viscera. Tension on the spinal cord is impeded due to the rib cage which restricts thoracic flexion (Humphry, 1858). Different physiological postures are evident in the thoracolumbar curvature and appear to vary widely in response to activity (Strasser, 1913), gender and to increasing age (Singer *et al.*, 1990e, 1994). Curvature characteristics are also influenced by spinal trauma, and gibbus deformity is a common sequel (Willén *et al.*, 1990). In the normal vertical posture, the location of the line of gravity with reference to the vertebral column often appears located through the transitional regions (Humphry, 1858; Nathan, 1962; Anderson, 1982). Despite changes in the magnitude of the curves from one region to another, they compensate each to maintain a 'balance' in relation to the line of gravity (Steindler, 1955). This reciprocal change in curvature from the thoracic kyphosis to lumbar lordosis produces an inflexion area which is found usually between T11 and L1 (Stagnara *et al.*, 1982; Singer *et al.*, 1990e).

The strategy of positioning an inflexion point at an area of mechanical and morphological transition might offer protection in the form of reduced localized bending stress, at least for sagittal plane motion. This contrasts with the curve apex which sustains the greatest deflection under static loading. Clinically, the mid-thoracic region is where there is an increased risk of anterior vertebral deformities (Kazarian, 1978; Lampmann *et al.*, 1984). In contrast, if the bending moment is applied suddenly, the thoracic column may tend to 'pivot' over the mechanically 'stiffened' thoracolumbar junctional region, often producing a compression fracture (Levine and Edwards, 1987).

When considering the significance of the thoracolumbar junction inflexion point, the dynamic role of the vertebral column as a whole must be examined. During static axial compression loads, the thoracolumbar junction shows little rotational deformity in the horizontal plane, compared to adjacent thoracic and lumbar regions (Kazarian, 1972). This mechanical characteristic appears to reflect the increased stability of this region during upright postures. The morphology of the thoracolumbar mortice joint, which will be described in this chapter, may aptly be described as an 'antitorsion' device, operating to resist torsional stresses at the thoracolumbar junction segments (Markolf, 1972; Singer *et al.*, 1989b). Any explanation which seeks to account for the localized incidence of vertebral body compression fractures at the thoracolumbar junction (Rehn, 1968) must consider not only the anatomical and aetiological factors contributing to the problem, but other factors such as the biomechanical capacities of the mobile segments and the change in curvature at the thoracolumbar junction.

Load-bearing by the thoracolumbar junction mobile segments

Weight transmission down the axial skeleton in the erect posture is predominantly through the vertebral bodies and intervertebral discs, which enlarge in size from C1 to L5 (Pooni *et al.*, 1986) to accommodate the increasing load. However, the zygapophysial joints also contribute to axial weight-bearing (El-Bohy *et al.*, 1989) relative to their orientation and position with the line of gravity. At the thoracolumbar junction, the upper lumbar vertebral bodies demonstrate a relatively marked increase in cross-sectional geometry compared with the thoracic vertebrae (Gonon *et al.*, 1975; Davis, 1980; Berry *et al.*, 1987). Cancellous bone density of the vertebral bodies shows greater average values for the lower thoracic compared with upper lumbar vertebral levels. However, the product of mid-vertebral body cross-sectional area and the associated vertebral cancellous density, is similar for each vertebra from T10 to L1 (Singer and Breidahl, 1990b; Singer *et al.*, 1995). This finding may suggest that, at the thoracolumbar junction, a relatively equal axial weight-bearing load may be accommodated by each vertebral segment, despite the increase in the physical morphology of the lumbar vertebrae. The tendency for the anterior aspect of each vertebral body to demonstrate a significantly higher trabecular density measure (Singer and Breidahl, 1990b) may relate to the habitual flexion loads sustained by the low thoracic and upper lumbar vertebrae.

In a qualitative anatomical study which attempted to estimate the proportion of load shared between the vertebral mobile segments, Pal and Routal (1987) suggested that those vertebrae crossing the line of gravity would sustain the highest axial loading. The vertebrae situated within a concavity would load the vertebral bodies and, reciprocally, the zygapophysial joints would be preferentially loaded in lordotic postures. While Nachemson (1960) has tended to discount the posterior elements as less significant contributors to direct transfer of axial loads, there is experimental evidence to the contrary. Yang and King (1984) have shown that lumbar zygapophysial joints can contribute up to 47% of axial load-bearing; this relationship is dependent on the location of the vertebrae from the line of gravity.

Similarly, the marked increase in pedicle cross-section area at the thoracolumbar junction (Zindrick *et al.*, 1986; Berry *et al.*, 1987) appears designed to allow the passage of forces between the anterior and posterior elements relative to changes in posture.

As each synovial joint is designed to sustain load transmission across the articular surfaces (Radin, 1976; Putz, 1985), the thoracolumbar junction zygapophysial joints were examined for their potential to sustain axial loads. A feature evident from frontal plane CT scans of the thoracolumbar junction zygapophysial joints was a medial taper and enclosure provided by the superior articular process (Singer, 1989b). This morphology, likened to a carpenter's 'mortice' joint (Davis, 1955), putatively locks the joint when loaded to resist axial plane stress. At the level of the mortice joint and above, the inferior articular processes would appear to stop against the lamina in axially loaded postures and in end-range spinal extension.

Zygapophysial joint asymmetry at the thoacolumbar junction

Differences in zygapophysial joint horizontal planes (tropism) is another common feature at the thoracolumbar junction in which tropism greater than 20° between left and right paired joint planes showed a two-fold higher frequency in males (Singer, 1989a). The rationales proposed to account for tropism are numerous. Debate exists between those who propose either a developmental or functional hypothesis, or both. Whitney (1926) suggested that manipulative tasks using the dominant upper limb produced a bias in trunk rotation which was manifest in thoracolumbar junction zygapophysial joint asymmetry. In contrast, Odgers (1933) suggested that the multifidus muscle controlled the sagittal development of lumbar zygapophysial joints and accounted for the diversity of articular plane configurations between joint pairs; a position supported by Pfeil (1971) and Lutz (1967). The view proposed by Putz (1976, 1985)

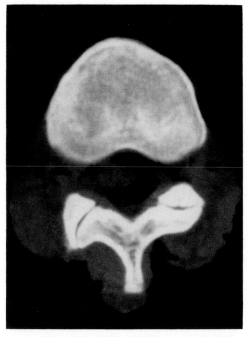

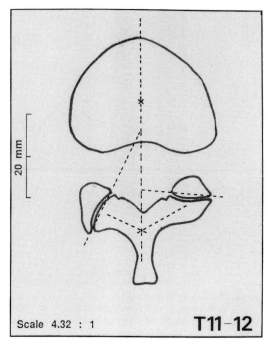

Figure 12.3 Right and left joint zygapophysial joint angles, at the level of the superior end-plate, were calculated by plotting a line of best fit through the joint margins in relation to the sagittal midline. In this CT example from T11–12, marked asymmetry in joint planes is evident.

describes lateral mechanical shear stresses on the articular surfaces which help to shape the zygapophysial joints. This latter view is supported with the model of scoliosis, as the articular surfaces appear to adapt their orientation in response to the deformity (Giles, 1982).

The embryological studies by Huson (1967), Reichmann (1971), Hadley (1976), Med (1980) and Cihak (1981), who examined zygapophysial joint configurations in the developing vertebral column, have usually recorded that all joints lie close to the coronal plane *in utero*. However, Reichmann (1971) did show variation in the *in utero* development of zygapophysial joints, with some individuals showing the eventual adult form and shape of the lumbar zygapophysial joints.

Zygapophysial joint tropism occurs most frequently at the T11–12 segment (Figure 12.3) (Malmivaara *et al.*, 1987; Singer *et al.*, 1989a) which has been described by Veleanu *et al.* (1972) as the headquarters for the thoracolumbar junction. The highly diverse orientations in the zygapophysial joints at this level may indicate an intermediate stage in the evolution of this transitional region. The gradual form of transition, which was found in the majority of cases, is probably the most likely form for this region (Singer *et al.*, 1989a).

Interlocking mortice-like thoracolumbar zygapophysial joints

Early descriptions of interlocking zygapophysial joints (Hildebrandt, 1816; Humphry, 1858), and the thoracolumbar junction 'mortaise' joint coined by Topinard (1877) and others (Le Double, 1912; Davis, 1955), have been extensively reported. Davis (1955, 1961) suggested that the 'mortice' effect could be gauged according to development of the mammillary processes and their projection behind the inferior articular processes. This morphological feature was examined radiographically, with the use of CT, and histologically, to provide a detailed review of the relationship between the mammillary processes to thoracolumbar junction zygapophysial joint orientation (Figure 12.4). The most common segmental level demonstrating mortice joints was T11–12, followed by T12–L1, consistent with reports by Davis (1955), Malmivaara *et al.* (1987) and Singer (1989b).

Unilateral mortice joints have been identified with zygapophysial joint asymmetry (Malmivaara *et al.*, 1987), usually formed by a mammillary process on the side of the coronally orientated joint (Singer *et al.*,

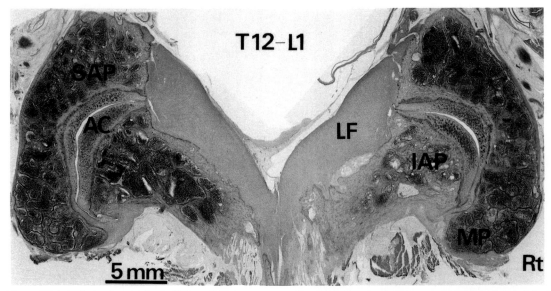

Figure 12.4 A photomicrograph of a 200 µm thick transverse section cut in the plane of the superior vertebral end-plate at T11–12 to illustrate a type I bilateral mortice joint formed by the embracing mammillary processes (MP) which are the posterior reflections off the superior articular process (IAP). The articular cartilage (AC) appears normal (LF) = ligamentum flavum. (Reproduced with permission from: Singer, K.P. and Giles, L.G.F. (1990) Manual therapy considerations at the thoracolumbar mortice joint. An anatomical and functional perspective. *J. Manipulative Physiol. Ther.,* **13**, 83–88.)

1990c). The mammillary process, located adjacent to the inferior articular process, may behave as a support for the zygapophysial joint. This concept was evident during functional CT scans of subjects who were positioned in unilateral side posture trunk rotation; separation of the joint appeared to be limited according to the proximity of the nearby mammillary process (Singer *et al.,* 1989b).

According to comparative anatomy reports by Vallois (1920) and Kaplan (1945), the mammillary processes are evident at the thoracolumbar junction in primates who adopt an orthograde position during ambulation. Both authors consider that these processes develop in response to the activity of multifidus which, from electromyographic studies performed by Donisch and Basmajian (1972), appears to behave as a stabilizer of adjacent vertebral segments during rotary motion. If the multifidus acted as an antagonist to rotation at the thoracolumbar junction, this would provide further support for the morphological role of the zygapophysial joints to resist torsion. The laminar fibres of multifidus, which attach to the mammillary processes immediately below, would tend to act closer to the axial plane, whereas the fibres passing superiorly to the spinous process of the cranial segments, might function as a 'brake' to flexion coupled with rotation. This may further ensure that the joints remain relatively approximated, as a tactic to limit segmental mobility.

Intra-articular synovial folds of zygapophysial joints

Histologically, intra-articular synovial folds were demonstrated consistently in the thoracolumbar junction zygapophysial joints (Singer *et al.,* 1990d). This observation complements previous reports on zygapophysial joints of the cervical regions (Töndury, 1940; Giles, 1986; Bland, 1992); thoracic (Ley, 1975); lumbar (Töndury, 1940; Dörr, 1958; Kirklaldy-Willis, 1984), and lumbosacral junction (Giles and Taylor, 1987). According to Töndury (1972), these intra-articular synovial folds act as deformable space-fillers which accommodate incongruities between the articular facets during normal joint motion. The relative change in configuration of the thoracolumbar junction zygapophysial joints may also account for differences in the morphology of these intra-articular synovial folds, as seen at the mid-joint level. Fibro-adipose folds were noted more in the frontal plane zygapophysial joints, which appeared suited to the marked translatory movements performed by these joints. In contrast, fibrous folds were more evident in the more sagittally orientated joints (Singer *et al.,* 1990d), occasionally showing histological evidence of fibrotic changes at their tips to suggest that they may have been compressed. This may occur due to sudden torsional forces, or compression, during joint approximation in flexion or extension postures.

Rudimentary ossification centres at the thoracolumbar junction

The development of the thoracolumbar junction zygapophysial joints has often been associated with the appearance of vertebral process variants (Hayek, 1932; Heise, 1933). Accessory ossification centres appearing adjacent to the spinous, transverse and mammillary-accessory processes are a relatively rare finding, found in approximately 1–2% of the populations studied by Pech and Haughton (1985) and Singer and Breidahl (1990a). Rib anomalies are more frequently noted, and appear to be more common in men than women (Schertlein, 1928). At times these variations may be confused with fractures at the TLJ (Keats, 1979; Singer and Breidahl, 1990a) or contribute to miscalculations of vertebral levels (Wigh, 1980); the latter having significance when only lumbar spinal radiographs are used to estimate the level(s) for surgery (Wigh, 1979).

Biomechanical considerations at the thoracolumbar junction

Limitation to regional spinal and segmental motion occurs through a combination of the shape of the vertebral bodies, the thickness of the intervertebral discs, and the configuration of the zygapophysial joints (Fick, 1911; Pearcy, 1986). In the thoracic region, the almost vertical alignment of the zygapophysial joints, together with the costovertebral joints and the splinting effect of the thoracic cage, precludes any marked flexion tendency. Similarly, thoracic rotation and extension is impeded by the constraint offered by the posteriorly projecting lamina and approximation of the spinous processes. The stabilizing role of the thoracic cage is lessened in the lower thoracic segments due to the greater mobility afforded by the floating ribs.

Investigations by White (1969), Kazarian (1972), Markolf (1972) and Oxland et al. (1992), have been performed on cadaveric thoracolumbar vertebral columns to determine the mobility of these segments. The influence of variation in transitional patterns (Singer et al., 1989a) has been largely ignored. The typical finding from these studies has been the restriction in segmental mobility due to the changing morphology of the thoracolumbar junction zygapophysial joints. Of these cadaveric studies, Kazarian (1972) drew attention to the idiosyncratic behaviour of the lower thoracic vertebral elements, particularly when loaded axially; he attributed this to the presence of the thoracolumbar junction mortice joint. Similarly, Markolf (1972) emphasized that torsional resistance was greatest at the thoracolumbar junction segments. Gregerson and Lucas (1967) examined mobility

patterns throughout the thoracolumbar spine affixing instrumented Steinmann pins into multiple spinous processes of male volunteers. Although the general trend showed greatest rotation within the middle thoracic segments, and least within the lumbar levels, no attempt was made to examine the thoracolumbar junction region specifically.

The change of zygapophysial joint configuration at the thoracolumbar junction has been considered by anatomists and clinicians as denoting an abrupt change in the mobility of these joints, particularly horizontal plane movements (Humphry, 1858; Levine and Edwards, 1987). In their summary of the literature, White and Panjabi (1978) base mobility estimates for the last thoracic segment on extrapolations from adjacent lower thoracic and upper lumbar levels. However, the almost preferential patterns of rotation of the thoracic segments, and sagittal range in the lumbar region, reflect regional orientations of the TLJ zygapophysial joints (Davis, 1959; Gregerson and Lucas, 1967; Evans, 1982). The upper lumbar joints, through approximation of the articular surfaces, also restrict mobility, particularly extreme extension (Davis, 1955; Singer, 1989), or flexion (Kummer, 1981); indeed, the posterior elements of the upper lumbar segments are positioned to afford stability in the plane of the intervertebral disc (Farfan, 1983) and appear to minimize excessive torsional forces (Stokes, 1988).

Computer tomography studies of subjects who were positioned in side posture rotation were used to consider the potential for segmental motion at the thoracolumbar junction (Singer et al., 1989b). These authors demonstrated ipsilateral compression, and contralateral separation, of the sagittally directed articular surfaces, whereas coronally directed joints tended to show translatory displacement of the articular facets (Singer et al., 1989b). Those subjects possessing a mortice type joint demonstrated little motion relative to adjacent segments (Figure 12.5).

Other anatomical, developmental and degenerative mechanisms would act to increase resistance to torsional displacement, for instance the ingrowth into the ligamentum flavum by laminar spicules (Davis, 1955; Allbrook, 1957) and, in some instances, ossification of the ligamentum flavum (Kudo et al., 1983; Maigne et al., 1992). The orientation of the laminar fibres of multifidus muscle may also serve to increase the axial 'stiffness' of the thoracolumbar junction (Donisch and Basmajian, 1972).

The notion that axial plane rotation is restricted in the upper lumbar region, due to predominantly sagittal orientation of the zygapophysial joints, is not new. Hildebrandt (1816), and numerous commentators over the ensuing decades, have described lumbar inter-segmental rotation as minimal (Humphry, 1858; Lewin et al., 1962; Kummer, 1981; Farfan, 1983; Putz, 1985). Rotation is induced through the displacement of adjacent vertebrae which produces lateral shear

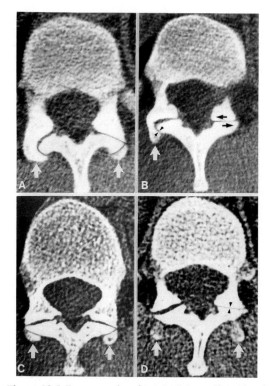

Figure 12.5 Four examples of mortice joints at T11–12 and their respective influences on transverse plane rotation. The variable presence of mammillary process (white arrows) adjacent to the inferior articular process appear to block movement or to facilitate slight separation of the articular surfaces (black arrows). (Reproduced with permission from: Singer, K.P., Day, R.E. and Breidahl, P.D. (1989) In vivo axial rotation at the thoracolumbar junction: an investigation using low dose CT in healthy male volunteers. *Clin. Biomech.*, **4**: 145–150.)

forces within the intervertebral disc (Gregerson and Lucas, 1967), flexibility of the neural arch (Farfan, 1983; Stokes, 1988) and, to a lesser extent, by compliance of the articular surfaces (Lewin *et al.*, 1962).

Vertebral extension at the thoracolumbar junction

At the thoracolumbar junction, an approximated joint position is achieved when the thoracolumbar column is extended, as a result of the medial taper of the zygapophysial joints (Singer, 1989b) and the 'mortice-like' configuration of the articular processes and their mammillary processes (Topinard, 1877). This approximation would act to 'lock' the thoracolumbar junction segments (Davis, 1955).

The tendency for the mortice joint to act as an 'axis', or pivot, can be demonstrated by loading

autopsy vertebral columns into extension and then examining the alteration in spinal curvature in relation to the unloaded upright position. In the loaded posture, a noticeable discontinuity of the thoracolumbar curve at the junctional region appears. The significance of this finding appears to suggest that a close-packed position is achieved at the thoracolumbar junction when the inferior articular processes come into contact with the laminae of the vertebra below (Grieve, 1981).

Mechanics of spinal injuries at the thoracolumbar junction

The thoracolumbar junction has been the focus for many clinical and surgical reports, due to the high frequency of serious spinal trauma located within the lower thoracic and upper lumbar mobile segments (Rehn, 1968; Rostad *et al.*, 1969; Schmorl and Junghanns, 1971; Denis, 1983; Larson, 1986). In this context, the transition has been classically considered mechanically disposed to trauma; being less capable of attenuating axial and torsional stresses at a point of marked anatomical and mechanical change (Humphry, 1858; Macalister, 1889). The localization of injury to the TLJ has been attributed to the difference in mobility between the thoracic and lumbar regions, given the tendency, during rapid flexion, for the 'stiff' thoracic segments to act as a long 'lever' which pivots over the lumbar spine fulcrum (Jefferson, 1927; Levine *et al.*, 1988). The majority of traumatic injuries at the TLJ involve the vertebral bodies, usually producing a compression or burst fracture (Rehn, 1968; Denis, 1983; Lindahl *et al.*, 1983; Willén *et al.*, 1990).

Most descriptions of thoracolumbar junction injuries do not appear to have considered the influence that transitional variations of the zygapophysial joints might have in the mechanism of injury and the type of trauma sustained. Although limited by a small series, an abrupt transition pattern at the thoracolumbar junction was shown to confine trauma to these segments, particularly when rotation was a known contributor to the injury mechanism (Singer *et al.*, 1989c).

Pathoanatomical relationships at the thoracolumbar junction

Whether the thoracolumbar junction motion segments were susceptible to stress resulting in early degenerative changes has been considered by a number of researchers. Of these, Veleanu *et al.* (1972) noted similar patterns of osteoarthritis in the lower thoracic and uper lumbar zygapophysial joints, and he proposed that these elements must sustain similar stresses as the lumbar spine. Lewin (1964) had previously speculated that the thoracolumbar mortice joint morphology might predispose to the early development of osteoarthritis. In a preliminary study into the effects of zygapophysial joint osteoarthritic changes in macerated specimens, Malmivaara *et al.* (1987) noted that the more sagittally orientated joints showed greater signs of degeneration compared with more coronally disposed joints. However, a subsequent histological examination of hyaline articular cartilage by Singer *et al.* (1990c) failed to reveal any correlation between articular cartilage degeneration and tropism. Evidence suggested that zygapophysial joint tropism and the presence of a well developed mammillary process ensured the integrity of the articular surfaces (Singer *et al.*, 1990c); mortice joints appeared, therefore, to act in a protective fashion.

Davis (1955) suggested that the mortice joint morphology might act as fulcrum, localizing flexion forces and producing thoracolumbar junction vertebral compression fractures, a theory which may also relate to the high frequency of vertebral end-plate lesions (Schmorl's nodes) in this region (Resnick and Niwayama, 1978; Hilton, 1980). In the absence of marked torsional forces, usually producing fracture/dislocation trauma, the thoracolumbar junction vertebral bodies are susceptible to intravertebral disc herniation through the end-plates. According to Malmivaara *et al.* (1987), these end-plate lesions appear most commonly in the lower thoracic vertebrae. The lower thoracic and upper lumbar zygapophysial and costovertebral joints have been associated with a high frequency of osteoarthritis (Shore, 1935; Nathan *et al.*, 1964; Tan, 1993). Recent studies by Malmivaara and co-workers have concentrated on the pathologies involving the vertebral bodies and intervertebral discs of the thoracolumbar junction (Malmivaara, 1987; Malmivaara *et al.*, 1987). Their reports on investigations of 24 cadaveric thoracolumbar spines and have described the pathoanatomic relationships between Schmorl's nodes, costovertebral joint osteoarthritis, vertebral body osteophytosis, and intervertebral disc degeneration. They propose that patterns of thoracolumbar junction degeneration are closely linked to the transitional characteristics of the anterior and posterior elements depending on their respective capabilities for resisting torsional and compressive forces applied to this region; they describe a shift from anterior degenerative patterns in the low thoracic vertebrae, to posterior degeneration in the upper lumbar segments.

Clinical anatomy of the thoracolumbar junction

Multiple vertebral anomalies may be present at several transitional junctions (Kühne, 1932; Schmorl and Junghanns, 1971; MacGibbon and Farfan, 1979; Wigh, 1980; Singer, 1989a). These can be represented by, for example, transitional asymmetries in zygapophysial joint configuration, and rib and accessory ossification anomalies. Wigh (1979) noted that surgical patients with thoracolumbar, and or lumbosacral, transitional variations were more likely to have inappropriate surgery. In part, the problem associated with identifying the symptomatic level related to incorrect classification of accessory ossification centres and vestigial ribs (Singer and Breidahl, 1990a).

Some pain syndromes appear to be specific to the thoracolumbar junction. For example, investigations reported by McCall *et al.* (1979) and Maigne (1980, 1981) have suggested that irritation to the lateral branches of the dorsal rami from the thoracolumbar junction segments may be mistaken for low back pain syndromes, as these nerves are cutaneous over the buttocks and the region of the greater trochanter.

Manual therapy recommendations about the mechanical capability and treatment of the thoracolumbar junction mobile segments contrast with biomechanical data which indicates that this region acts to resist torsional forces (Singer *et al.*, 1989b). Therefore, the appropriateness of the manipulative treatment of this transitional region may need to be reappraised (Singer and Giles, 1990).

Using mechanical evidence, Markolf (1972) has suggested that the first segment above the transitional level with coronally-orientated zygapophysial joints would be more susceptible to torsional stress. This speculation could not be confirmed within the context of a preliminary study of thoracolumbar junction spinal injuries (Singer *et al.*, 1989c). However, clinical evidence shows that thoracic disc herniations appear more frequently in the lower thoracic segments compared with the middle and upper thoracic region (Ryan *et al.*, 1988). In slight contrast, using an unselected sample of cadaveric cases, the trend showed both middle and lower segments to be equally affected by prolapse (Crawford, 1994). The incidence of thoracic discal herniation is approximately 4% (Bury and Powell, 1989); however, the relationship between level of lesion and the nature of the thoracolumbar junction transition has not been explored comprehensively. Mechanical factors are, according to Russell (1989), often implicated in the production of thoracic disk symptoms.

Intra-articular synovial folds have been demonstrated in the superior and inferior joint recesses of the thoracolumbar junction zygapophysial joints and, less commonly, at the middle third of the joint (Singer *et al.*, 1990d). The presence of free nerve endings in the substance of similar synovial folds within lower lumbar zygapophysial joints have been recorded by Giles and Taylor (1987). Using immunohistology techniques to study these nerves, Giles and Harvey (1987) showed the presence of small substance P immunofluorescent nerves in the synovial folds of human lumbosacral zygapophysial joints. Therefore, it may be assumed that compression or traction of intra-articular synovial fold structures could produce pain. The variable morphology of the thoracolumbar junction and zygapophysial joints is reflected in the type and location of intra-articular synovial folds (Singer *et al.*, 1990d). Therefore, forceful manual therapy techniques which compress or apply torsion to these joints may provoke symptoms. Similarly, the pain centralization phenomenon described by Donelson *et al.* (1990), following repeated or sustained thoracolumbar extension, may well evoke symptoms from the zygapophysial joints due to the compression of intra-articular structures.

From the foregoing discussion, it would appear that conservative treatment of painful disorders arising from the thoracolumbar junction may be appropriate over some of the recommended mechanical therapies (Grieve, 1981; Singer and Giles, 1990). The clinical impression advanced by Lewit (1986) that the thoracolumbar junction is designed for rotation appears to contradict the anatomical and biomechanical studies reported on this region (Singer, 1989b; Singer *et al.*, 1989b).

A review of the anatomy of the thoracolumbar junction reveals that, in a majority of individuals studied, the thoracolumbar junction exhibits features which attempt to gradually change the anatomy from thoracic to lumbar type in an area of considerable morphological and functional variation. This is achieved primarily through a gradual transition in the configuration of the zygapophysial joints. This finding challenges the notion that the thoracolumbar junction is necessarily a 'weak point' of the vertebral column. It was evident that the conventional description of an abrupt transition produced a more demarcated pattern of segmental rotation and that this transition type was associated with a higher proportion of severe spinal injuries.

The thoracolumbar junction represents the most variable of the vertebral transitional junctions in terms of zygapophysial joint orientation, asymmetry, and in the segmental level of transition. The mortice arrangement at the T11-12 and T12-L1 zygapophysial joints appears to restrict rotation and extension. Assessment procedures, and any manual therapy interventions, should consider these issues for the effective management of patients with mechanical disorders of the thoracolumbar transition.

Acknowledgements

The collegial assistance from Drs Peter Breidahl, R.E. Day and access to facilities provided by Professor Charles Oxnard (Anatomy and Human Biology Dept UWA), Clinical Professors T.M.H. Chakera and B. Kakulas (Royal Perth Hospital) is gratefully acknowledged.

References

Allbrook, D. (1955) The East African vertebral column. *Am. J. Phys. Anthrop.*, **13**, 489–511.

Allbrook, D. (1957) Movements of the lumbar spinal column. *J. Bone Joint Surg.*, **39B**, 339–345.

Anderson, J. (1982) The thoracolumbar spine. *Clin. Rheum. Dis.*, **8**, 631–653.

Bagnall, K., Harris, P. and Jones, P. (1977) A radiographic study of the human fetal spine. [2] The sequence of development of ossification centres in the vertebral column. *J. Anat.*, **124**, 791–798.

Barclay-Smith, E. (1911) Multiple anomaly in a vertebral column. *J. Anat.*, **45**, 144–171.

Berry, J., Moran, J., Berg, W. and Steffee, A. (1987) A morphometric study of human lumbar and selected thoracic vertebrae. *Spine*, **12**, 362–367.

Birkner, R. (1978) *Normal Radiologic Patterns and Variances of the Human Skeleton*. Urban and Schwarzenberg, Baltimore.

Bland, J. (1992) *Disorders of the Cervical Spine.*, 2nd edn, W.B. Saunders, Philadelphia.

Bury, R. and Powell, T. (1989) Prolapsed thoracic intervertebral disc. The importance of CT assisted myelography. *Clin. Radiol.*, **40**, 416–421.

Cihak, R. (1981) Die morphologie und entwicklung der wirbelbogengelenke. *Die Wirbel. Forsch. Praxis*, **87**, 13–28.

Crawford, R. (1994) Normal and degenerative anatomy of the thoracic intervertebral discs and vertebral bodies: age and gender relationships. Honours Thesis. Curtin University of Technology, Perth.

Davis, P. (1955) The thoraco-lumbar mortice joint. *J. Anat.*, **89**, 370–377.

Davis, P. (1959) The medial inclination of the human thoracic intervertebral articular facets. *J. Anat.*, **93**, 68–74.

Davis, P. (1961) The thoraco-lumbar mortice joint in West Africans. *J. Anat.*, **95**, 589–593.

Davis, P. (1980) Engineering aspects of the spine. In *Mechanical Aspects Of The Spine*. Mechanical Engineering Publications, London, pp. 33–36.

Denis, F (1983) The three column spine and its significance in the classification of acute thoracolumbar spinal injuries. *Spine*, **8**, 817–831.

Donelson, J., Silva, G. and Murphy, K. (1990) Centralization phenomenon. Its usefulness in evaluating and treating referred pain. *Spine*, **153**, 211–213.

Donish, E. and Basmajian, J. (1972) Electromyography of deep muscles in man. *Am. J. Anat.*, **133**, 25–36.

Dörr, W. (1958) Über die anatomie der wirbelgelenke. *Arch. Orthop. Unfallc.*, **50**, 222–243.

El-Bohy, A., Yang, K.-H. and King, A. (1989) Experimental verification of facet load transmission by direct measurement of facet lamina contact. *J Biomech.*, **22**, 931–941.

Evans, D. (1982) Biomechanics of spinal injuries. In *Biomechanics of Musculoskeletal Injury* (E. Gonza and I. Harrington, eds), Williams and Wilkins, Baltimore, pp. 163–224.

Farfan, H. (1983) Biomechanics of the lumbar spine. In *Managing Low Back Pain*. (W. Kirkaldy-Willis, ed.), Churchill Livingstone, New York, pp. 9–21.

Fick, R. (1911) Spezielle gelenke und muskelmechanik. In *Handbuch der Anatomie und Mechanik der Gelenke*. Gustav Verlag Fischer, Jena.

Gehweiler, J., Osborne, R. and Becker, R. (1980) *The*

Radiology of Vertebral Trauma. Saunders, Philadelphia.

Giles, L.G.F. (1982) *Leg Length Inequality with Postural Scoliosis, Its Effect on Lumbar Apophyseal Joints*. MSc Thesis, The University of Western Australia.

Giles, L.G.F. (1986) Lumbo-sacral and cervical zygapophysial joint inclusions. *Man. Med.*, 2, 89–92.

Giles, L.G.F. and Harvey, A. (1987) Immunohistochemical demonstration of nociceptors in the capsule and synovial folds of human zygapophysial joints. *Br. J. Rheumatol.*, 26, 362–364.

Giles, L.G.F. and Taylor, J.R. (1987) Human zygapophysial joint capsule and synovial fold innervation. *Br. J. Rheumatol.*, 26, 93–98.

Gonon, G., Rousson, B., Fischer, L., Morin, A. *et al.* (1975) Donnes metriques concernant l'arc posterieur au niveau du rachis dorso-lombarire de D8 a L5. *Assoc. Anat. Compt. Rendus*, 58, 867–875.

Gregersen, G.G. and Lucas, D. (1967) An in vivo study of the axial rotation of the human thoraco-lumbar spine. *J. Bone Joint Surg.*, 49A, 247–262.

Grieve, G. (1981) *Common Vertebral Joint Problems*. Churchill Livingstone, Edinburgh, p. 14.

Hadley, L. (1976) *Anatomico-Roengentgenographic Studies of the Spine*. CC Thomas, Illinois.

Hasebe, K. (1913) Die wirbelsäule der japaner. *Z. Morph. Jahr.*, 43, 449–476.

Hayek, H. (1932) Über lendenrippen. Fortschritte auf dem gebiete der rontgenstrahlen und der Nuklearmedizin. *Erganzungsband*, 45, 582–592.

Heise, H. (1933) Über anomalien der lendenwirbelsäule. *Deut. Z. Chir.*, 227, 349–367.

Hildebrandt, G. (1816) *Handbuch der Anatomie*. Cited in Humphry, 1858.

Hilton, R. (1980) Systematic studies of spinal mobility and Schmorl's nodes. In *The Lumbar Spine and Back Pain* (M, Jayson, ed.). Pitman, Bath, pp. 115–134.

Humphry, G. (1858) *A Treatise on the Human Skeleton*. MacMillan, London, pp. 169–171.

Huson, A (1967) Les articulations intervertébrales chez les foetus humain. *Comptes Rendus des Association D'Anatomists*, 138, 676–683.

Jefferson, G. (1927) Discussion on spinal injuries. *Proc. R. Soc. Med.*, 20, 625–637.

Kapandji, I. (1977) The trunk and vertebral column, vol. 3. *The Physiology of the joints*. 2nd edn. Churchill Livingstone, Edinburgh, pp. 16–17.

Kaplan, E. (1945) The surgical and anatomic significance of the mammillary tubercle of the last thoracic vertebra. *Surgery*, 17, 78–92.

Kazarian, L. (1972) Dynamic response characteristics of the human vertebral column. *Acta Orthop. Scand.*, Suppl 146.

Kazarian, L. (1978) Identification and classification of vertebral fractures following emergency capsule egress from military aircraft. *Aviat. Space. Environ. Med.*, 49, 150–157.

Keats, T. (1979) *An Atlas of Normal Roentgen Variants That Simulate Disease*. 2nd edn. Year Book Medical Publishers, Chicago.

Kirkaldy-Willis, W. (1984) The relationship of structural pathology to the nerve root. *Spine*, 9, 49–52.

Kudo, S., Ono, M. and Russell, W. (1983) Ossification of thoracic ligamenta flava. *Am. J. Roentgenol.*, 141, 117–121.

Kühne, K. (1932) Die vererbung der variationen der menschlichen. *Wirbelsäule Z. Morph. Anthropol.*, 30,

1–221.

Kummer, B. (1981) Biomechanik der wirbelgelenke. *Wirbel. Forsch. Praxis*, 87, 29–34.

Lampmann, L., Duursmar, S. and Ruys, J. (1984) *CT Densiometry on Osteoporosis*. Martinus Nijhoff, Boston.

Lanier, R. (1939) The presacral vertebrae of American white and Negro males. *Am. J. Phys. Anthrop.*, 3, 341–420.

Larson, S. (1986) The thoracolumbar junction. In *The Unstable Spine* (S.B. Dunsker, H. Schmidek, J. Frymoyer and A. Kahn, eds). Grune and Stratton, Orlando, pp. 127–152.

Le Double, A.-F. (1912) *Traite des Variations de la Colonne Vertébrale de l'Homme*. Vignot-Freres, Paris.

Levine, A. and Edwards, C. (1987) Lumbar spine trauma. In *The Lumbar Spine* (E. Camins and P. O'Leary, eds). Raven Press, New York, pp. 183–212.

Levine, A., Bosse, M. and Edwards, C. (1988) Bilateral facet dislocations in the thoracolumbar spine. *Spine*, 13, 630–640.

Lewin, T. (1964) Osteoarthritis in lumbar synovial joints. *Acta Orthop. Scand.*, Suppl 73.

Lewin, T., Moffett, B. and Viidik, A. (1962) The morphology of the lumbar synovial intervertebral joints. *Acta Morph. Neerl. Scand.*, 4, 299–319.

Lewit, K. (1986) Muscular pattern in thoraco-lumbar lesions. *Man. Med.*, 2, 105–107.

Ley, F. (1975) Contribution a l'étude des cavités articulaires interapophysaires vertébrales thoraciques. *Arch. D'Anat. D'Hist. D'Embryol.*, 57, 61–114.

Lindahl, S., Willén, J., Nordwall, A. and Irstam, L. (1983) The 'crush-cleavage' fracture. A 'new' thoracolumbar unstable fracture. *Spine*, 8, 181–186.

Louis, R. (1983) *Surgery of the Spine*. Springer-Verlag, Berlin, p. 10.

Lutz, G. (1967) Die entwicklung der kleinen wirbelgelenke. *Z. Orthop. Grenz.*, 104, 19–28.

Macalister, A. (1889) *A Textbook on Human Anatomy*. Griffin, London, p. 129.

MacGibbon, B. and Farfan, H. (1979) A radiologic survey of various configurations of the lumbar spine. *Spine*, 4, 258–266.

Maigne, J.Y., Ayral, X. and Guèrin-Surville, H. (1992) Frequency and size of ossifications in the caudal attachments of the ligamentum flavum of the thoracic spine. Role of rotatory strains in their development. *Surg. Radiol. Anat.*, 14, 119–124.

Maigne, R. (1980) Low back pain of thoracolumbar origin. *Arch. Phys. Med. Rehabil.*, 61, 389–395.

Maigne, R. (1981) The thoracolumbar junction syndrome. Low back pain, pseudo-visceral pain, pseudo-hip pain and pseudo-pubalgia. *Sem. Hop. Paris*, 57, 545–554.

Malmivaara, A. (1987) Disc degeneration in the thoracolumbar junctional region. Evaluation by radiography and discography in autopsy. *Acta Radiol.*, 28, 755–760.

Malmivaara, A., Videman, T., Kuosma, E. and Troup, J. (1987) Facet joint orientation facet and costovertebral joint osteoarthrosis, disc degeneration, vertebral body osteophytosis and Schmorl's nodes in the thoracolumbar junctional region of cadaveric spines. *Spine*, 12, 458–463.

Markolf, K. (1972) Deformation of the thoracolumbar intervertebral joints in response to external loads. *J. Bone Joint Surg.*, 54A, 511–533.

McCall, I., Park, W. and O'Brien, J. (1979) Induced pain referral from posterior lumbar elements in normal subjects. *Spine,* **4**, 441–446.

Med, M. (1980) Prenatal development of intervertebral articulation in man and its association with ventrodorsal curvature of the spine. *Folia Morphol.,* **28**, 264–267.

Nachemson, A. (1960) Lumbar intradiscal pressure. *Acta Orthop. Scand.,* Suppl 43.

Nathan, H. (1962) Osteophytes of the vertebral column. An anatomical study of their development according to age, race and sex, with considerations as to their etiology and significance. *J. Bone Joint Surg.,* **44A**, 243–268.

Nathan, H., Weinberg, H., Robin, G. and Aviad, I. (1964) The costovertebral joints. Anatomico-clinical observations in arthritis. *Arth. Rheum.,* **7**, 228–240.

Noback, C. and Roberston, G. (1951) Sequences of appearance of ossification centres in the human skeleton during the first five prenatal months. *Am J. Anat.,* **89**, 1–28.

Odgers, P. (1933) The lumbar and lumbo-sacral diarthrodial joints. *J. Anat.,* **67**, 301–317.

Oxland, T.R., Lin, R.-M. and Panjabi, M.M. (1992) Three-dimensional mechanical properties of the thoracolumbar junction. *J. Orthop. Res.,* **10**, 573–580.

Pal, G., Routal, R. (1987) Transmission of weight through the lower thoracic and lumbar regions of the vertebral column in man. *J. Anat.,* **152**, 93–105.

Pearcy, M. (1986) Measurement of back and spinal mobility. *Clin. Biomech.,* **1**, 44–51.

Pech, R. and Haughton, V. (1985) CT appearance of unfused ossicles in the lumbar spine. *Am. J. Neuroradiol.,* **6**, 629–631.

Pfeil, E. (1971) Stellungsvarianten der gelenkfortsätze am lendenkreuzbein-übergang. *Z. Chir.,* **93**, 10–17.

Pick, T. (1890) *Gray's Anatomy, Descriptive and Surgical.* Longmans, London.

Pooni, J., Hukins, D., Harris, P. *et al.* (1986) Comparison of the structure of human intervertebral discs in the cervical, thoracic and lumbar regions of the spine. *Surg. Radiol. Anat.,* **8**, 175–182.

Putz, R. (1976) Beitrag zur morphologie und rotationsmechanik der kleinen gelenke der lendenwirbelsäule. *Z. Orthop.,* **114**, 902–912.

Putz, R. (1985) The functional morphology of the superior articular processes of the lumbar vertebrae. *J. Anat.,* **143**, 181–187.

Radin, E. (1976) Aetiology of osteoarthrosis. *Clin. Rheum. Dis.,* **2**, 509–522.

Rehn, J. (1968) Die knöcheren verletzungen der wirbelsäule bedeutung des erstbefundes für die spätere begutachtung. *Wirbel. Forsch. Praxis,* **40**, 131–138.

Reichmann, S. (1971) The postnatal development of form and orientation of the lumbar intervertebral joint surfaces. *Z. Anat. Entwick.,* **133**, 102–123.

Resnick, D. and Niwayama, G. (1978) Intravertebral disk herniations, cartilaginous Schmorl's nodes. *Radiology,* **126**, 57–65.

Rostad, H., Solheim, K., Siewers, P. and Lie, M. (1969) Fracture of the spine. *Acta Orthop. Scand.,* **40**, 664–665.

Russell, T. (1989) Thoracic intervertebral disc protrusion, experience of 76 cases and review of the literature. *Br. J. Neurosurg.,* **3**, 153–160.

Ryan, R., Lally, J., Kozic, Z. (1988) Asymptomatic calcified herniated thoracic disks, CT recognition. *Am. J. Neuroradiol.,* **9**, 363–366.

Schertlein, A. (1928) Über die haufigsten anomalien an der Brustlendenwirbelsäulengrenze. *ROFO,* **38**, 478–488.

Schmorl, G. and Junghanns, H. (1971) *The Human Spine In Health And Disease,* 2nd American edition. Grune and Stratton, New York, pp. 55–60.

Shore, L. (1930) Abnormalities of the vertebral column in a series of skeletons of Bantu natives of South Africa. *J. Anat.,* **64**, 206–238.

Shore, L. (1935) On osteo-arthritis in the dorsal intervertebral joints. A study in morbid anatomy. *Br. J. Surg.,* **22**, 833–849.

Singer, K. (1989a) Variations at the Human Thoracolumbar Transitional Junction with Reference to the Posterior Elements. Ph.D. Thesis, The University of Western Australia.

Singer, K. (1989b) The thoracolumbar mortice joint. Radiological and histological observations. *Clin. Biomech.,* **4**, 137–143.

Singer, K. and Breidahl, P. (1990a) Accessory ossification centres at the thoracolumbar junction. *Surg. Radiol. Anat.,* **12**, 53–58.

Singer, K. and Breidahl, P. (1990b) Vertebral body trabecular density at the thoracolumbar junction using quantitative computed tomography. A post-mortem study. *Acta Radiol.,* **31**, 37–40.

Singer, K. and Giles, L. (1990) Manual therapy considerations at the thoracolumbar junction. An anatomical and functional perspective. *J. Manipulative Physiol. Ther.,* **13**, 83–88.

Singer, K., Breidahl, P. and Day, R. (1988) Variations in zygapophysial orientation and level of transition at the thoracolumbar junction. A preliminary CT survey. *Surg. Radiol. Anat.,* **10**, 291–295.

Singer, K., Breidahl, P. and Day, R. (1989a) Posterior element variation at the thoracolumbar transition. A morphometric study using computed tomography. *Clin. Biomech.,* **4**, 80–86.

Singer, K., Day, R. and Breidahl, P. (1989b) In vivo axial rotation at the thoracolumbar junction, an investigation using low dose CT in healthy male volunteers. *Clin. Biomech.,* **4**, 145–150.

Singer, K., Willén, J., Breidahl, P. and Day, R. (1989c) A radiologic study of the influence of zygapophysial joint orientation on spinal injuries at the thoracolumbar junction. *Surg. Radiol. Anat.,* **11**, 233–239.

Singer, K., Edmondston, S., Day, R. and Breidahl, W. (1994). Computer-assisted curvature assessment and Cobb angle determination of the thoracic kyphosis: an in-vivo and in-vitro comparison. *Spine,* **19**, 1381–1384.

Singer, K., Giles, L. and Day, R. (1990c) Influence of zyagapophyseal joint orientation on hyaline cartilage at the thoracolumbar junction. *J. Manipulative Physiol. Ther.,* **13**, 207–214.

Singer, K., Giles, L. and Day, R. (1990d) Intra-articular synovial folds of the thoracolumbar junction zygapophysial joints. *Anat. Rec.,* **226**, 147–152.

Singer, K., Jones, T. and Breidahl, P. (1990e) A comparison of radiographic and computer-assisted measurements of thoracic and thoracolumbar sagittal curvature. *Skel. Radiol.,* **19**, 21–26.

Sobotta, J. and Uhlenhuth, J. (1957) *Atlas of Descriptive Anatomy,* 7th English edition. Hafner, New York, p. 24.

Stagnara, P., Mauroy, J., de Dran, G. *et al.* (1982) Reciprocal angulation of vertebral bodies in a sagittal plane. Approach to references for the evaluation of kyphosis and lordosis. *Spine,* **7**, 335–342.

Steindler, A. (1955) *Kinesiology of the Human Body, Under*

Normal and Pathological Conditions. CC Thomas, Illinois.

Stewart, T. (1932) The vertebral column of the Eskimo. *Am. J. Phys. Anthrop.,* **16**, 51-62.

Stokes, I. (1988) Mechanical function of facet joints in the lumbar spine. *Clin. Biomech.,* **3**, 101-105.

Strasser, H. (1913) *Die Rumpfhaultungen. Lehrbuch der Muskel und Gelenkmechanik.* Springer, Berlin, pp. 244-320.

Struthers, J. (1875) On variations of the vertebrae and ribs in man. *J. Anat. Physiol.,* **9**, 17-96.

Tan, B.-K. (1993) Histomorphometry of the lower thoracic costovertebral joints: normal and pathological anatomy. Honours Thesis, Curtin University of Technology, Perth.

Terry, R. and Trotter, M. (1953) Osteology. In *Morris' Human Anatomy.* (J.P. Schaeffer, ed.). McGraw-Hill, New York, p. 102.

Testut, L. and Latarjet, A. (1948) *Traité d'Anatomie Humaine,* vol. 1, 9th edn. Dion, Paris, p. 69.

Todd ,T. (1922) Numerical significance in the thoracolumbar vertebrae of the mammalia. *Anat. Rec.,* **24**, 261-286.

Töndury, G. (1940) Beitrag zur kentniss der Kleinen wirbelgelenke. *Z. Anat. Ent.,* **110**, 568-575.

Töndury, G. (1972) Anatomie functionelle des petites articulations de rachis. *Anal. Med. Phys.,* **15**, 173-191.

Topinard, P. (1877) Des anomalies de nombre de la colonne vertebrale chez l'homme. *Rev. D'Anthropol.,* **6**, 577-649.

Vallois, H. (1920) La signification des apophyses mammillaires et accessories des vertébres lombaires. *Compt. Rend. Soc. Biol.,* **83**, 113-115.

Veleanu, C., Grün, U., Diaconescu, M. and Cocota, E. (1972) Structural peculiarities of the thoracic spine. Their functional significance. *Acta Anat.,* **82**, 97-107.

White, A.A. (1969) Analysis of the mechanics of the thoracic spine in man. *Acta Orthop. Scand.,* Suppl **127**.

White, A. and Panjabi, M.M, (1978) Basic kinematics of the spine. *Spine,* **3**, 12-29.

Whitney, C. (1926) Asymmetry of vertebral articular processes and facets. *Am. J. Phys. Anthrop.,* **9**, 451-455.

Wigh, R. (1979) Phylogeny and the herniated disc. *South. Med. J.,* **72**, 1138-1143.

Wigh, R. (1980) The thoracolumbar and lumbosacral transitional junctions. *Spine,* **5**, 215-222.

Willén, J., Anderson, J., Tomooka, K. and Singer, K. (1990) The natural history of burst fractures in the thoracolumbar spine T12 and L1. *J. Spinal Dis.,* **3**, 39-46.

Williams, P. and Warwick, R. (1980) Osteology. In *Gray's Anatomy.* 3rd edn. Churchill Livingstone, London, pp. 277, 284.

Yang, K. and King, A. (1984) Mechanism of facet load transmission as a hypothesis for low back pain. *Spine,* **9**, 557-565.

Zindrick, M., Wiltse, L., Doornik, A., Widell, E. *et al.* (1986) Analysis of the morphometric characteristics of the thoracic and lumbar pedicles. *Spine,* **12**, 160-166.

13

Miscellaneous pathological and developmental (anomalous) conditions

L.G.F. Giles

This chapter will review the following conditions viz: tethered cord, Baastrup's disease, ununited ossification centres of articulating processes, transitional lumbosacral vertebrae, ligamentum flavum hypertrophy, pars interarticularis defects, spondylolisthesis, and facet tropism. The incidence of these conditions and their association with mechanical back pain will be reported.

Tethered cord syndrome

The tethered cord is defined as a low state of the conus medullaris below the second lumbar vertebra after the neonatal period. This tethering results in stretching as growth occurs (Kavukcu et al., 1993). The normal filum terminale, which is usually less than 2 mm thick, is a 20 cm long delicate fibrous connective tissue structure which descends from the apex of the conus medullaris, and its proximal 5–6 mm contains the central canal. The cranial 15 cm of the filum terminale, the filum terminale internum, is surrounded by tubular extensions of the dural and arachnoid membranes and reaches as far as the lower border of the second sacral vertebra (S2). Beyond this, its final 5 cm, the filum terminale externum, is closely united with the investing sheath of dura mater, and it descends to become attached to the dorsal aspect of the first coccygeal segment (Williams and Warwick, 1980; Sarwar et al., 1984).

Because skeletal growth is greater than neural growth, the conus medullaris of the spinal cord normally migrates from the tip of the coccyx in the fetus at 3 months to the upper border of the third lumbar vertebra at birth, the level of the second lumbar vertebra by 5 years, and the lower border of the first lumbar vertebra by adulthood (Reinmann

and Anson, 1944; Keim and Kirkaldy-Willis, 1987; Bullough and Boachie-Adjei, 1988). When the conus medullaris does not migrate cephalad, the tethered cord may occur, some possible causes of which are a short thickened filum terminale, fibrotic ligaments, or intradural lipomas (Weissert et al., 1989; Kavukcu et al., 1993; Chong et al., 1994; Reigel et al., 1994; Wakata et al., 1994).

The tethered cord syndrome is produced by traction of the lumbosacral spinal cord (Horton et al., 1989) and can be associated with spinal dysraphism (Flanigan et al., 1989) in which a short, thickened filum terminale prevents the ascent of the conus medullaris, and intraspinal lipoma causes compression upon the caudal part of the spinal cord (Compobasso et al., 1988). However, according to Sarwar et al. (1984), the origins of the primary tethered cord syndrome have not been satisfactorily explained and the syndrome is an entirely different entity from overt myelomeningocele and associated Arnold–Chiari type II malformation. They postulate that primary tethered cord syndrome is a manifestation of local dysmorphogenesis of all three germ layers at the lumbosacral area, possibly triggered by a haemorrhagic, inflammatory, or other local lesion occurring in embryogenesis.

The primary tethered cord syndrome, and spinal dysraphism, i.e. spina bifida (in which there is failure of the posterior walls of the vertebral canal to meet), which frequently present with clinical symptoms during infancy, childhood and adolescence, are rarely encountered in adults (Adams, 1968; Zumkeller et al., 1989). However, generally accepted features of the syndrome can include presentation at any age with a clinical spectrum including backache, sensorimotor deficit, bladder and bowel dysfunction, leg atrophy, foot deformity, and scoliosis (Sarwar et al., 1984; Weissert et al., 1989). Radicular pain, apparently restricted to a single dermatome and mimicking lumbar disc disease, is seldom seen (Piatt and Hoffman, 1987b). In some cases, no skin changes can be detected over the affected area (Bode *et al.*, 1985), and it should be noted that there is some controversy regarding the importance of spinal anomalies being associated with tethered cord syndrome. According to Beeger and Roos (1989), the tethered cord syndrome occurs regularly in patients with spina bifida occulta and spina bifida aperta but, according to James and Lassman (1981) and Piatt and Hoffman (1987b), spina bifida at L5 or S1 is so common in the general population, with a prevalence of 5–36%, that it carries no specificity of tethered spinal cord and it can be considered an anatomic variant of normal that rarely causes serious pain problems in adult life (Keim and Kirkaldy-Willis, 1987). However, according to Avrahami *et al.* (1994), spina bifida occulta of S1 is not an innocent finding as patients with this condition have a higher incidence of posterior intervertebral disc herniation which increases with age.

Spina bifida is a congenital malformation which occurs during the first weeks after conception (Gabay *et al.*, 1989) due to posterior cleavage of the vertebral arch; when only the bony elements are involved the condition is referred to as spina bifida occulta but where the meninges and/or the spinal cord are affected (0.2% of the population), the condition is known as spina bifida cystica (myelodysplasia) (Bullough and Boachie-Adjei, 1988).

In normal humans, lumbar nerve roots exhibit a downward oblique course. However, in primary tethered cord syndrome, caudal nerve root angulation may be horizontal or upward-slanting (Sarwar *et al.*, 1984). The spinal cord is a viscoelastic tissue with limited elasticity, and traction at the cauda equina causes elongation predominantly in the lumbosacral cord (Sarwar *et al.*, 1983; Tani *et al.*, 1987). This is supported by the investigations of Reimann and Anson (1944), Barry *et al.* (1957), Emery and Naik (1968), and Naik and Emery (1968), who have shown that, in clinical and experimental cases of cord tethering, the maximal elongation occurs in the lumbosacral cord. The confinement of stretch to the lumbosacral cord may suggest a bracing action of the dentate ligaments in the lumbar region (Emery and Naik, 1968; Tani *et al.*, 1987) as seen in the cervical region (Emery and Naik, 1968). In an experimental study of the pathophysiology of spinal cord traction in dogs, Fujita and Yamamoto (1989) found that traction caused vulnerability of the spinal cord to compression and concluded that tethered cord syndrome is caused by impairment of the spinal cord and lumbosacral roots due to traction.

In this syndrome, the degree of clinical neurologic deficit and the surgical outcome (Hoffman *et al.*, 1976; Linder *et al.*, 1982; Pang and Wilberger, 1982) are probably related to (i) tolerance to stretch of the neural tissue in each individual, (ii) locomotion (neck flexion stretches lumbar nerve roots and can exacerbate pain in primary tethered cord patients), and (iii) the length of time the cord has been subjected to the abnormal stretching. The greater the percentage of elongation of the spinal cord the greater the impairment of the oxidative metabolism in the lumbosacral cord and the severity of neurological deficit (Tani *et al.*, 1987).

Giles (1991) examined the prevalence of tethered cord in 50 cadavers, aged 35–92 years (mean = 64 years); 36 males and 14 females, in which lumbosacral spines were carefully removed during routine autopsy examinations. One example of tethered cord was found and is presented here.

Of the 50 spines radiographed, five (10%) (three males; two females) were found to have spina bifida occulta at the L5 level (two specimens) or S1–2 level (three specimens). However, only one set of radiographs showed spina bifida occulta involving the S1 and S2 levels in conjunction with an enlarged spinous process of the fifth lumbar vertebra (Figure 13.1).

Lateral view radiographs and the corresponding bisected spines of the lumbosacral level of this specimen clearly show the enlarged spinous process of L5 (Figure 13.2). The gross anatomical specimen shows that the conus medullaris terminates at the S1 level and that some of the nerve roots run cephalad from the tethered spinal cord.

Part of the histology of the right side of the lumbosacral level showing the tethered cord is shown in Figure 13.3.

This case of tethered cord, in which the spinal cord terminates at the S1 level in a 78-year-old male cadaver with no evidence of surgical intervention or record to indicate any neurological dysfunction, indicates that a tethered cord should be considered as a possibility in patients whose plain film radiographs show spina bifida occulta. When neurological signs and symptoms indicate such a possibility, plain CT or MRI should be performed (Gado *et al.*, 1984; Beeger and Roos, 1989) in order to establish the exact dimensions of the subarachnoid space around the cord in case a pattern suggestive of a tethered cord is shown. Even though the inability of CT without contrast to show anatomical structures inside the lumbar dural sac is well known (Caverni *et al.*, 1987), McLendon *et al.* (1988) suggest that fatty tissue in the area of the filum may be an indicator for tethering of the spinal cord, although Raco *et al.* (1987) consider CT diagnostic investigation for tethered cord syndrome should be performed with contrast medium. However, MRI makes it easier to detect anomalies associated with spina bifida (Beeger and Roos, 1989) and MRI findings are very important for a clear understanding of the tethered cord process and preoperative evaluation of potential sites of tethering (Tamaki *et al.*, 1988), while MRI has the advantage of no radiation and no contrast administration is necessary; also the production of sagittal images, or images in any other plane, can be obtained without loss of anatomical detail (Piatt and Hoffman, 1987b) making MRI the procedure of choice (Chong *et al.*, 1994; Wakata *et al.*, 1994).

According to Roy *et al.* (1986), imaging procedures and urodynamic studies are useful for establishing a diagnosis, while electrophysiological recording of

posterior tibial nerve somatosensory evoked potential offers a sensitive diagnostic tool for the detection of the development of neurological deficits in patients with tethered cord syndrome.

It should be remembered that the onset of tethered cord syndrome in a 28-year-old male (Fain *et*

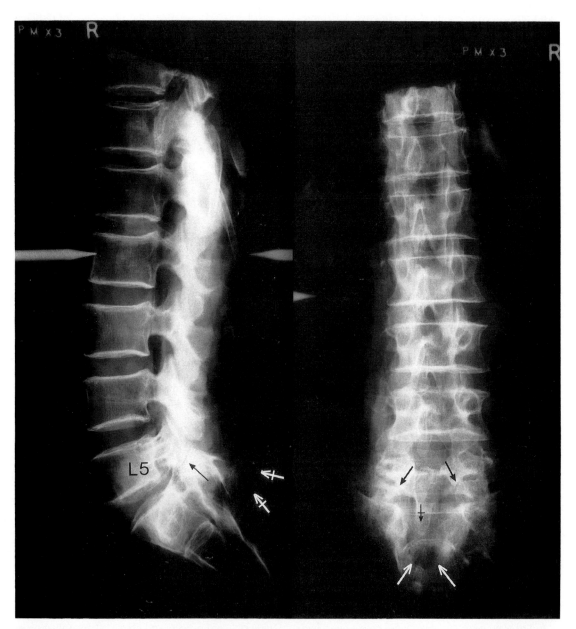

Figure 13.1 Lateral and posteroanterior radiographs of a 78-year-old male cadaver showing the enlarged spinous process (tailed arrow) of the fifth lumbar vertebra (L5). The posteroanterior view also shows the sacral spina bifida occulta (white arrow heads >). Both views show fractures of the L5 pars interarticulares (arrow) which are seen more clearly in Figure 13.2. (Reproduced with permission from Giles, L.G.F. (1991) Review of tethered cord syndrome with a radiological and anatomical study: case study. *Surg. Radiol. Anat.*, **13**, 339–343. Copyright Springer-Verlag.)

al., 1985) a 40-year-old male (Wakata *et al.*, 1994) and 11 other adults (Chong *et al.*, 1994) confirms the finding of Kaplan and Quencer (1980) that this syndrome is not restricted to children and adolescents and that, in adults, neural structures already taut due to a tethered cord may only cause symptoms with the development of spondylosis and hypertrophied zygapophysial joint facets which further compromise the neural structures (Sostrin *et al.*, 1977), that is, as a result of injury with associated degenerative changes leading to mechanical back pain. Furthermore, James and Lassman (1962) reported that a 67-year-old patient, who had no neurological abnormality or deformity, was found at autopsy to have a cord tethered at L5. Thus, these documented findings, coupled with the fact that the 78-year-old male cadaver in this study did not undergo surgery for tethered spinal cord, suggest that this condition should be considered in the differential diagnosis of adult patients who have radiological evidence of spina bifida.

When tethered spinal cord causes a disturbance of neuronal physiology, this can usually be remedied by appropriate surgical techniques (Piatt and Hoffman, 1987a). The incidence of tethered cord in adults is unknown at this time.

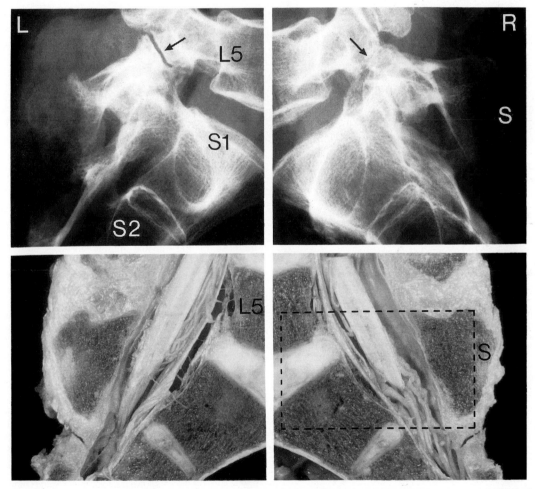

Figure 13.2 Radiographs showing the left (L) and right (R) halves of the lower lumbosacral spine (L5, S1 and S2 spinal levels) following its bisection in the median plane. The large spinous process (S) of L5 is clearly shown, as are the left and right pars interarticularis defects (arrows). The corresponding anatomical structures are shown for each radiograph. Note that the conus medullaris terminates at the S1 level and that some of the spinal nerve roots run in a cephalad direction. The rectangle shows the region from which the histological section in Figure 13.3 was obtained. (Reproduced with permission from Giles, L.G.F. (1991) Review of tethered cord syndrome with a radiological and anatomical study: case study. *Surg. Radiol. Anat.*, **13**, 339–343. Copyright Springer-Verlag.)

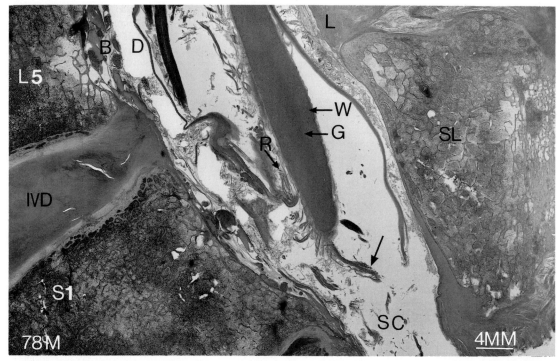

Figure 13.3 A 200 μm thick histological section through part of the right lumbosacral intervertebral joint and the adjacent tethered cord. IVD = intervertebral disc; SL = sacral lamina; D = dural tube; L = ligamentum flavum; B = Batson's venous plexus; L5 = fifth lumbar vertebral body; S1 = first sacral body; SC = spinal canal; W = white matter; G = gray matter; R = nerve root trunks of cauda equina running cephalad. Arrow shows part of the filum terminale.

Knife clasp deformity

The radiographs in Figure 13.1 also demonstrate a radiographic example of the knife clasp deformity in which spina bifida occulta is associated with an increased vertical dimension of the fifth lumbar spinous process (Rich, 1965a,b; Starr, 1971; Guebert *et al.*, 1987). During extension of the lumbar spine in such patients, the enlarged spinous process may invade the sacral neural canal resulting in the knife clasp syndrome, with symptoms varying with the degree of invasion (Rich, 1965b).

In Giles' (1991) cadaveric study, 1 out of 50 (2%) lumbosacral spines showed the knife clasp deformity.

Interspinous osteoarthritis (Baastrup's disease)

Baastrup (1933) described a clinical syndrome in which the lumbar spinous processes impinge upon each other in lumbar extension – the so-called 'kissing spines', which leads to interspinous periostitis and osteoarthritis (see Figure 18.4).

This clinical syndrome can occur due to (i) an increase in the normal lumbar lordosis, and (ii) enlargement of the superior to inferior dimensions of a spinous process, both of which may produce approximation and contact of the 'tips' of the spinous processes, which can result in trauma and injury to the interspinous tissues with bursa formation (Anderson, 1983), as well as the formation of osteoarthrosis showing sclerosis and osteophytosis (Schmorl and Junghanns, 1971; Epstein, 1976). Free nerve endings, conforming with the generally accepted morphology

Figure 13.4 Radiograph of the anatomical specimen shown in Figure 13.5. The elongated fifth lumbar spinous process articulates with the adjacent sacral tubercle (arrow). Sclerotic changes are noted at the tip of the fifth spinous process and the adjacent sacral tubercle. Thinning of the lumbosacral intervertebral disc space is noted with a minor osteophytic spur on the sacral promontory, minor subluxation of the L5–S1 facet surfaces with associated changes consistent with sclerosis and eburnation of the superior and inferior articular processes and part of the pedicle. The left lumbosacral intervertebral canal 'foramen' shows more encroachment by the osteoarthritic superior articular process of the sacrum than does the right. (Compare with Figure 6.7, sacral articular facets.)

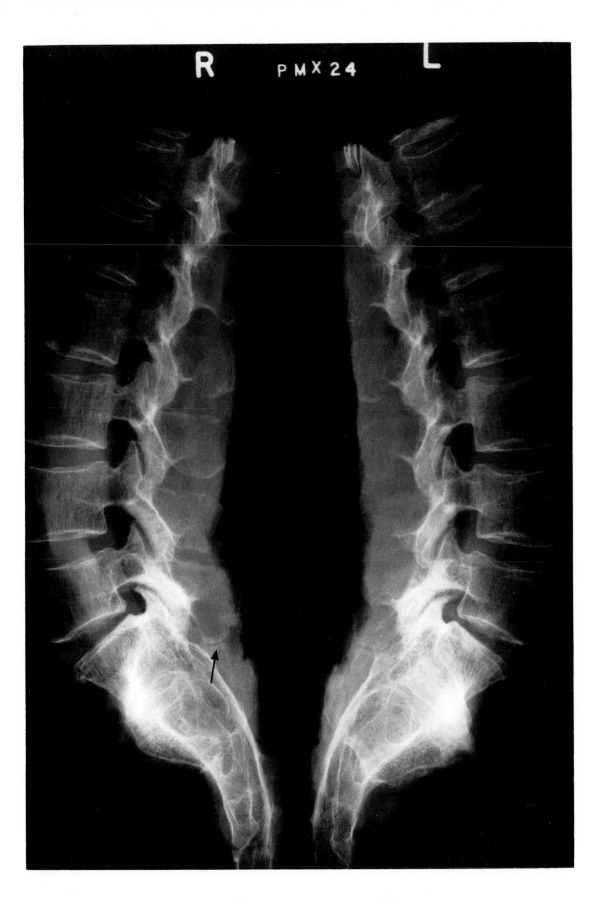

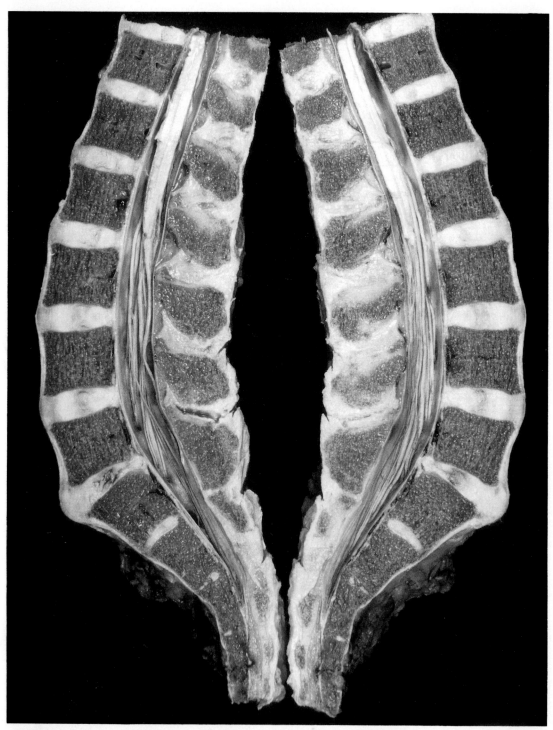

Figure 13.5 Anatomical specimen of the sagittally sectioned spine shown radiographically in Figure 13.4. Note the approximation of the elongated fifth lumbar spinous process and the adjacent sacral spinous tubercle, in spite of the normal lumbar lordosis in this 70-year-old female. The L5 intervertebral disc shows degenerative changes which include (i) anterior 'bulging' of the disc, and (ii) posterior herniation of the disrupted nucleus pulposus which has elevated the posterior longitudinal ligament above and below this disc level.

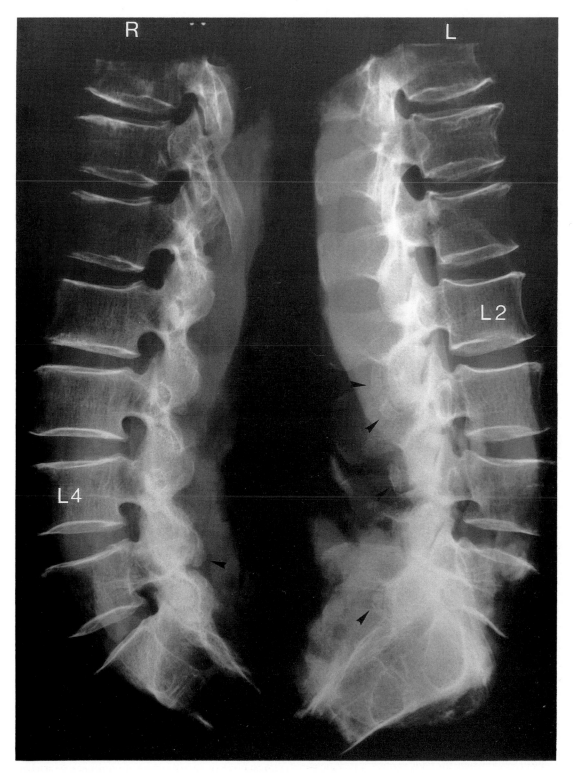

Figure 13.6 Radiograph of a 62-year-old male showing ununited secondary ossification centres adjacent to (a) the right inferior articular process of L4 vertebra, and (b) the left inferior articular processes of L2, L3, and L5, respectively.

of pain receptors, have been demonstrated in the interspinous ligament by Yahia *et al.* (1988) thus providing one mechanism for nociception when the interspinous ligament is pinched, causing pressure damage and chronic mechanical low back pain (Epstein, 1976; Woo, 1987; Beks, 1989; Beckers and Bekaert, 1991).

A radiographic example of a fifth lumbar spinous process which has an elongated superior to inferior dimension, and which articulates with the spinous tubercle of the sacral median crest, is shown in Figure 13.4. The 'kissing' of these osseous structures has lead to sclerotic changes with some eburnation in this 70-year-old female.

Figure 13.5 shows the sagittally sectioned spine, from the thoracolumbar junction to, and including, the sacrum in this 70-year-old female. The lumbar lordosis is within normal limits but the excessive superior to inferior elongation of the fifth lumbar spinous process has resulted in its inferior margin articulating with the adjacent spinous tubercle of the sacral median crest, as shown in the radiograph of this specimen (Figure 13.4). Compare with Figures 3.5 and 3.6 which show fifth lumbar spinous processes with normal superior to inferior dimensions.

Normal spinous processes are covered by periosteum but, according to Bywaters and Evans (1982), bursae develop between the kissing spinous processes as a result of a repeated shearing movement, frequently in older people (Francois *et al.*, 1985). However, according to Hadley (1964), kissing spinous processes destroy the interspinous ligament and bumper-fibrocartilage can develop where the spinous processes are subjected to intermittent pressure, and only an adventitious bursa may develop.

According to Hadley (1964), Schmorl and Junghanns (1971), and Epstein (1976), this impingement of adjacent spinous processes can cause chronic and sometimes severe pain, which may be aggravated by rotational movement or bending forward or backward. Patients should be advised to avoid activities which cause hyperlordosis of the lumbar spine and to avoid poor posture. The incidence of this condition is thought to be approximately 20% in the elderly adult population (Dr P. Breidahl, 1995, personal communication).

Ununited ossification centres of articulating processes

Three ossification centres are found in each vertebra, one for the body and two for the arch; the arch centres appearing earlier than the vertebral body centres, except in the lower thoracic and upper lumbar regions where the body centres appear first as described in detail by Rickenbacher *et al.* (1982). Additional accessory ossification centres (apophyses)

appear in children aged 11–14 years on the articular processes and the tips of the spinous and transverse processes as well as on the mamillary and accessory processes (Schmorl and Junghanns, 1971; Rickenbacher *et al.*, 1982). These small accessory ossification centres develop at the cartilaginous tips of the individual arch processes, covering them like a cap, at first separated from the tips of the processes by cartilage which then gradually disappears; normally the accessory ossification centres unite completely with the osseous processes at about the completion of spinal growth at approximately 25 years of age (Schmorl and Junghanns, 1971). The apophyses at the tips of the superior and inferior articular processes can remain separated from the articular processes by a fine cleft and the majority are located at the inferior articular processes (Schmorl and Junghanns, 1971). These anomalous variants (Keats, 1973) are shown in Figure 13.6, a radiograph of a sagittally bisected spine

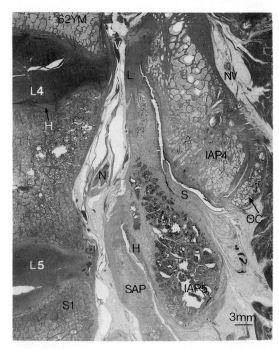

Figure 13.7 A 200 μm thick histological section cut in the parasagittal plane through the right L4 and L5 intervertebral levels showing an ununited secondary ossification centre (OC) adjacent to the inferior articular process in a 62-year-old male. Note the cleft between these two structures which is lined by cartilage at this level. H = hyaline articular cartilage of end-plate (arrow) and osteoarthritic hyaline articular cartilage on facet surfaces; IAP4 = inferior articular process of fourth lumbar vertebra; IAP5 = inferior articular process of L5; L = ligamentum flavum; L4 = fourth lumbar intervertebral disc; L5 = fifth lumbar intervertebral disc; N = neural structure; NV = neurovascular structures; S = synovial fold; S1 = first sacral segment; SAP = superior articular process of sacrum.

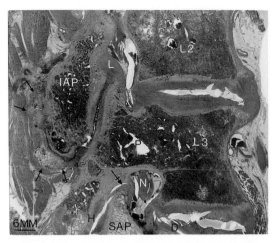

Figure 13.8 A 200 µm thick histological section cut in the parasagittal plane through the left L2 and L3 levels showing an adjacent ununited secondary ossification centre (arrows) which has become partly fused with the adjacent inferior articular process posteriorly, but not inferiorly where a small cleft is noted between these two structures; the cleft is lined by cartilage. D = intervertebral disc; H = hyaline articular cartilage; IAP = inferior articular process of second lumbar vertebra (L2); L = ligamentum flavum; L3 = third lumbar vertebra; N = neural structure; P = pedicle; SAP = superior articular process of fourth lumbar vertebra. Tailed arrow indicates a fibrotic synovial fold projecting from the superior recess of the joint towards the joint 'space'.

(eleventh thoracic to second sacral levels) of a 62-year-old male. Ununited secondary ossification centres are seen in close proximity to (a) the right inferior articular process of the fourth lumbar vertebra, and (b) the left inferior articular processes of the second, third and fifth lumbar vertebrae, respectively.

Histological sections showing the ununited secondary ossification centres at the right L4, and left L2 levels are shown in Figures 13.7 and 13.8, respectively.

The incidence of ununited secondary ossification centres of the articular processes is thought to occur 'frequently' (Hadley, 1964) but their possible role in mechanical back pain must remain speculative, as it is not known if they cause pain (Schmorl and Junghanns, 1971).

Transitional lumbosacral vertebrae

Transitional vertebrae occur at regions of the spine where the morphological characteristics of the vertebrae normally change markedly from one region to the next, i.e., lumbosacral, thoracolumbar and cervicothoracic regions (Guebert *et al.*, 1987). When the L5 vertebra is partly or completely incorporated into the sacrum, the condition is known as hemisacralization or sacralization, respectively; when the S1 vertebra is more or less separated from the sacrum and is partly or completely fused with the L5 vertebra the condition is known as lumbarization of the S1 vertebra (Moore, 1992). A change in the number of mobile vertebrae in the lumbar spine is a significant vertebral anomaly that can cause low back pain (Keim and Kirkaldy-Willis, 1987) and as shown in Figure 13.9, osteoarthritic changes can occur between the enlarged transverse process of the presacral segment and the sacral ala (Resnick, 1985; Guebert *et al.*, 1987).

The histology of part of this bilateral lumbarization is shown in Figure 13.10, and it can be seen that cartilage has developed between these pseudoarticulations.

The incidence of transitional lumbosacral vertebrae is 4-8% of the general population (Elster, 1989). Lumbosacral transitional vertebrae can be associated with mechanical back pain, possibly because of

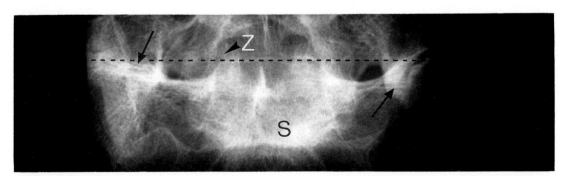

Figure 13.9 Trimmed block of osteoligamentus tissues, photographed in the posteroanterior position, showing (i) bilaterally enlarged transverse processes of the last presacral vertebra articulating with the lateral mass of the sacrum, i.e. lumbarization of the presacral segment (arrows), and (ii) small anomalous diarthrodial zygapophysial joints (Z). Note the osteoarthritic changes which are seen as sclerosis of the anomalous articulations. S = sacral segment.

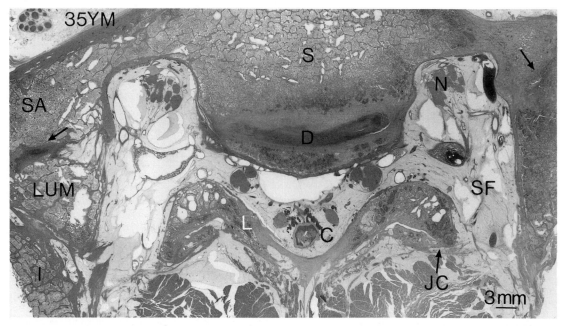

Figure 13.10 A 200 μm thick histological section cut in the horizontal plane through the level of the bilateral lumbarization of a 35-year-old male (see broken line in Figure 13.9). The arrows show the hyaline articular cartilage lining these anomalous joints between the enlarged transverse process of the presacral lumbar (LUM) segment and the sacral ala (SA). On the right side, fibrillation of the cartilage indicates osteoarthritic changes. C = cauda equina in the dural tube; D = intervertebral disc (rudimentary) at the presacral joint; I = ilium; JC = fibrous joint capsule of the right small zygapophysial joint of this anomalous presacral segment – both zygapophysial joints have osteoarthritic hyaline articular cartilage; L = lamina of first sacral segment; N = neural structures; S = first sacral segment; SF = sacral foramen. (Ehrlich's haematoxylin and light green counterstain.)

osteoarthritic degenerative changes within the anomalous joints. Disc bulge or herniation is extremely rare at the interspace below the transitional vertebra but, when it occurs, is nearly nine times more common at the interspace immediately above the transitional vertebra than at any other level, and spinal stenosis and nerve root canal stenosis occur more commonly at or near the interspace above the transitional vertebra (Elster, 1989).

Ligamentum flavum

In young persons the ligamenta flava bulge little or not at all into the spinal canal, but with advancing age the ligamenta flava sometimes undergo liquefaction necrosis and oedema in association with disc degeneration and spondylosis, and this can be a contributory factor in the sciatica of some patients who have normal-sized spinal canals (McRae, 1977) as the hypertrophy can cause spinal stenosis.

Lumbar spinal stenosis is defined as an abnormal narrowing of the lumbar spinal canal, or regions thereof, and has a large variety of causes and is due to congenital stenosis or acquired stenosis (Penning,

1992). The initial work describing the importance of spinal stenosis as a cause of neural dysfunction was by Verbiest (1954). The most common cause of spinal stenosis is zygapophysial joint facet osteoarthritis with hypertrophy and thickening of the ligamentum flavum, while other causes are synovial cysts (Jackson *et al.*, 1989), spondylotic spurs (Teng and Papatheodorou, 1963), vertebral misalignment and trauma, bony expansile lesions (Herzog *et al.*, 1991, Ross *et al.*, 1987; Weisz, 1983) and intervertebral disc herniation.

The ligamentum flavum can undergo hyperplastic change with replacement of the normal yellow elastic tissue with white fibrous tissue containing calcareous deposits (Spurling *et al.*, 1937). Furthermore, it can become thickened, buckled inward, depressed by enlarged or overriding laminae, or incorporated into articular osteophytes at the site of its attachment to the zygapophysial joint capsule (Weinstein *et al.*, 1977). Ligamentum flavum thickening may result in a width ranging from 4 to 8 mm (Love and Walsh, 1940; Pennal and Schatzker, 1971) which can cause spinal canal stenosis.

According to Dockerty and Love (1940), in the case of thickened ligamentum flavum, there is no true hypertrophy but rather thickening and fibrosis, and

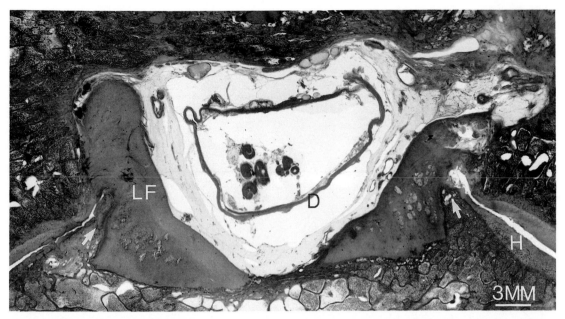

Figure 13.11 A 200 μm thick histological section cut slightly obliquely in the horizontal plane showing hypertrophy of the ligamentum flavum (LF) on the left side of this lumbosacral joint from a 76-year-old male. The hypertrophy in this specimen caused considerable stenosis of the spinal canal, as shown, as well as stenosis of the lateral recess. Large osteophytes (arrows) on the left and right inferior articular processes of the L5 vertebra are seen adjacent to the facets. D = dural tube; H = hyaline articular cartilage on the zygapophysial joint facet surfaces. (Ehrlich's haematoxylin and light green counterstain.)

according to Farfan (1978) ligamentum flavum thickening is a natural sequel of the shortening of an elastic structure. Nachemson and Evans (1968) state that an increase in width of the ligamentum flavum is always secondary to severe disc degeneration. Thickening of the ligamentum flavum due to disc thinning, with approximation of the pedicles and subluxation of the zygapophysial joint facets, can lead to compromise of the nerve root in the intervertebral foramen as demonstrated by Hadley (1951) and Giles (1994) (see Figure 6.4).

An example of hypertrophy of the ligmentum flavum at the lumbosacral level of the spine of a 76-year-old male is shown in Figure 13.11.

Patients with lumbar spinal canal stenosis may present with a variety of clinical symptoms, including back pain, radiculopathy, and neurogenic claudication (Herzog *et al.*, 1991). The initial size of the spinal and intervertebral canals is an important factor in determining whether degenerative changes will cause neural impingement or compression (Herzog, 1990).

As noted by Singer *et al.* (1990), in a study of intra-articular synovial folds of thoracolumbar junction zygapophysial joints, the ligamentum flavum passing around the anteromedial margin of lumbar zygapophysial joints can also occasionally be penetrated by an extension of epidural fat extending through the ligamentum flavum. An example of this is shown in Figure 13.12 but whether it has clinical significance in mechanical back pain is unknown.

Pars interarticularis defect

A pars interarticularis defect, or isthmus defect, is frequently due to a stress fracture causing a cleft in the vertebral arch. It occurs in 5–7% of Caucasians (Wolfers and Hoeffken, 1974) and is also known as isthmic spondylolysis (Herzog, 1990). Spondylolysis can be a unilateral or bilateral defect in the vertebral isthmus and has no associated vertebral body slippage (Keim and Kirkaldy-Willis, 1987) and is often asymptomatic.

The pars interarticularis cross-sectional area normally shows a gradual increase from L1 (approximately 62 mm^2) to L4 (approximately 81 mm^2) and L5 (approximately 82 mm^2) (Panjabi *et al.*, 1992). However, the pars interarticlaris width, and therefore cross-sectional area, may vary considerably in size from one vertebra to the next and between paired interarticulares at a given spinal level (Figure 13.13), presumably affecting the strength of individual pars

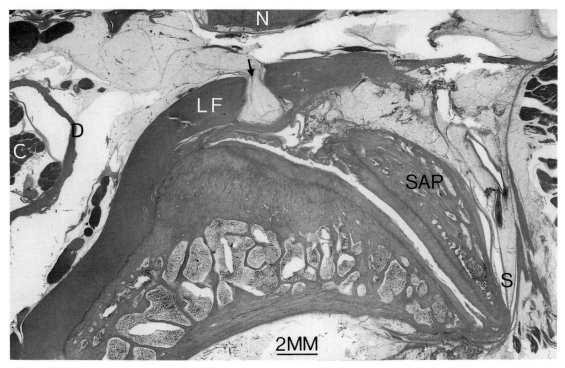

Figure 13.12 Histological section cut in the horizontal plane through the lumbosacral zygapophysial joint of an 83-year-old male. The ligamentum flavum (LF) is separated at this level by a 'herniation' of epidural fat (arrow) through the ligament. The ligamentum flavum has also become separated from the superior articular process (SAP) of the lumbosacral zygapophysial joint. C = cauda equina within the dural tube (D); N = spinal ganglion; S = synovial fold (fibrotic) projecting into the joint from the fibrous capsule. (Ehrlich's haematoxylin and light green counterstain.)

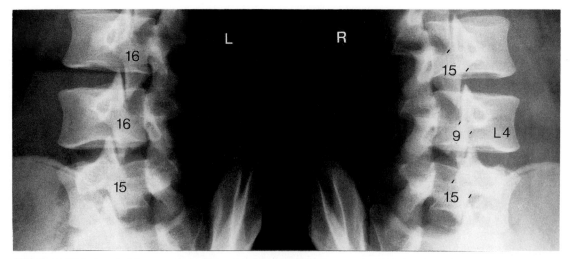

Figure 13.13 Left and right posterior oblique view radiographs of a 17-year-old male which show that there can be considerable variation in size between the paired pars interarticulares at a given level. At L4, there is a pars interarticularis width of 9 mm on the right side, whereas the width is 16 mm on the left side. The short lines on the right view show how and where the measurements were made.

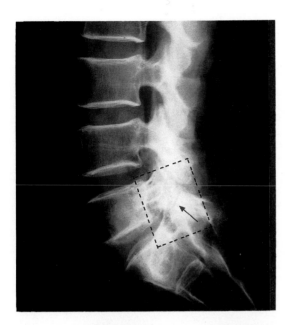

Figure 13.14 Bilateral fractures of the pars interarticularis of the fifth lumbar vertebra are seen superimposed on this lateral view radiograph of a 78-year-old male. There is spondylolysis with virtually no forward displacement of the L5 vertebral body on the sacrum. A histological section from the area within the rectangle is shown in Figure 13.15.

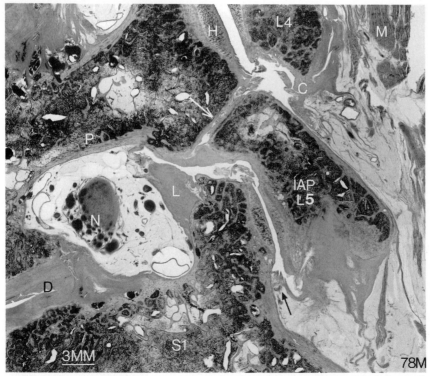

Figure 13.15 A 200 µm thick histological section cut in the parasagittal plane from the rectangle shown on the radiograph in Figure 13.14. This includes the right pars interarticularis (isthmus) defect (white arrow) which has developed fibrocartilagenous type tissue on both bony surfaces. There is no true hyaline articular cartilage but there is some fibrous tissue crossing the pars defect. There is a distinct cortex on each side of the isthmic defect. C = fibrous joint capsule (disrupted); D = intervertebral disc; H = hyaline articular cartilage; IAPL5 = inferior articular process of 5th lumbar vertebra; L = ligamentum flavum (disrupted due to the pars defect); L4 = inferior articular process of 4th lumbar vertebra; M = muscle; N = neural structures within the intervertebral canal; P = pedicle of L5; S1 = first sacral segment. Black arrow shows synovial fold. (Ehrlich's haematoxylin and light green counterstain.)

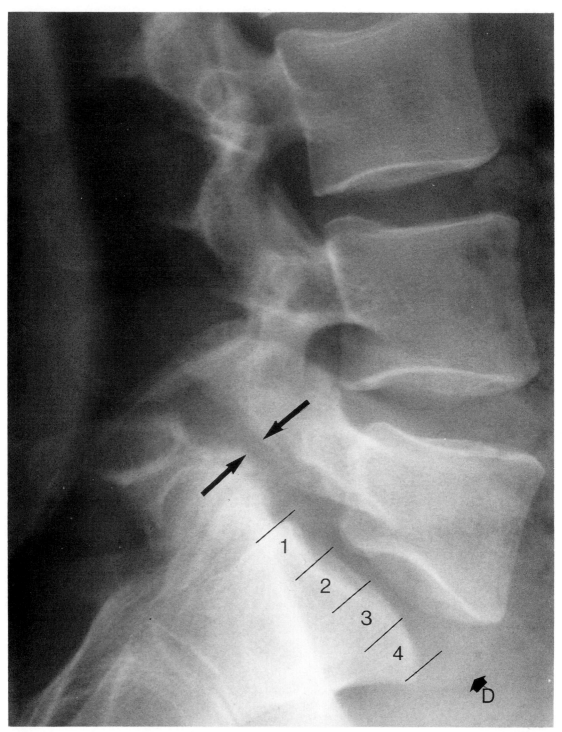

Figure 13.16 The arrows show the bilateral isthmus defect and that there is a grade 1 spondylolisthesis of L5 on S1. The degree of spondylolisthesis is found by dividing the sacral base into four equal parts, as shown, then noting where the posterior part of the vertebral body is located in relation to these parts as suggested by Meyerding (1932). Some anterior bulging of the L5–S1 intervertebral disc (D) is seen as a soft tissue shadow in this 25-year-old male. See Figure 13.18 for possible neural involvement.

interarticulares. A pars interarticularis defect (or isthmus of the vertebral arch) is best seen on 45 degree oblique view radiographs (Figure 13.13).

Historically, controversy existed in the literature for many years regarding the development of spondylolysis (Schmorl and Junghanns, 1971). Two schools of thought debated the issue of whether a pars interarticularis defect is the result of developmental changes (Taillard, 1954) or of an acquired fracture cleft (Rowe and Roche, 1953; Brauer, 1955; Hadley, 1964). However, it is now accepted that when the spine is subjected to excessive mechanical stresses, it may suffer a unilateral or bilateral fatigue fracture of the pars interarticularis at one or more spinal levels (Wiltse *et al.*, 1975). From a radiographic study of the lumbosacral spines of 143 non-ambulatory patients, Rosenberg *et al.* (1981) concluded that spondylolysis and isthmus spondylolisthesis represent a fatigue fracture resulting from activities associated with ambulation, as no case of spondylolysis or spondylolisthesis was detected when compared to the 5.8% incidence in the general population.

Bilateral pars interarticularis fractures are illustrated in Figure 13.14. The histology of the right pars defect/fracture in Figure 13.14 is shown in Figure 13.15.

Spondylolisthesis is a condition in which the vertebral body and transverse processes of a vertebra with bilateral pars interarticularis fractures slip anteriorly, leaving the posterior elements, i.e., spinous process and laminae, in their normal position. A radiological example of spondylolisthesis of L5 on S1 is shown in Figure 13.16.

Spondylolisthesis usually causes occasional back pain but, in active teenagers, the condition can be serious, especially if symptoms are progressive and there is radiographic evidence of increased slippage (Keim and Kirkaldy-Willis, 1987). Once skeletal maturity is reached, further forward displacement is very rare (Keim and Kirkaldy-Willis, 1987). However, in a magnetic resonance imaging study of entrapment of lumbar nerve roots in spondylolytic spondylolisthesis, Jinkins and Rauch (1994) found a strong association between apparent nerve root impingement and clinical evidence of radiculopathy.

A radiographic example of a grade 1–2 spondylolisthesis of L5 on S1 in a 73-year-old female is shown in Figures 13.17 and 13.18, which show the radiographic appearance of the isthmus defects bilaterally in the lateral and posteroanterior projections. Histological studies of the spinal nerves in this particular case of spondylolisthesis show that nerve impingement, due to bony entrapment, can occur. Histological sections cut in the coronal plane through the isthmus defects in Figures 13.17 and 13.18 are shown in Figures 13.19 and 13.20. These figures show how the inferior articular process of the fourth lumbar vertebra can impinge upon the posterior 'rim' of the first sacral segment, causing impingement of the fifth lumbar

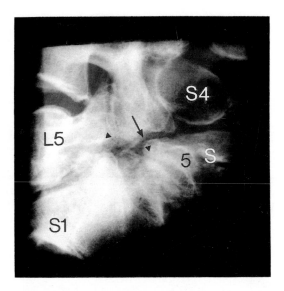

Figure 13.17 Lateral radiographic view showing a grade 1–2 spondylolisthesis of L5 on S1 in a 73-year-old female. The arrow heads show the relative displacement of the two sides of the pars interarticularis fracture. L5 = fifth vertebral body, the inferior articular process (5) of which remains adjacent to the superior articular process of the first sacral segment (S1); S = spinous process of L5 vertebra; S4 = spinous process of L4 vertebra. The black arrow shows the proximity between the L4 inferior articular process and the isthmus defect adjacent to the lamina of the fifth lumbar vertebra.

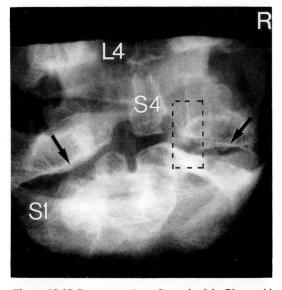

Figure 13.18 Posteroanterior radiograph of the 73-year-old female with grade 1–2 spondylolisthesis of L5 on S1 showing the bilateral pars interarticularis fractures (arrows). L4 = fourth vertebral body; R = right side; S1 = first sacral segment; S4 = spinous process of L4 vertebra.

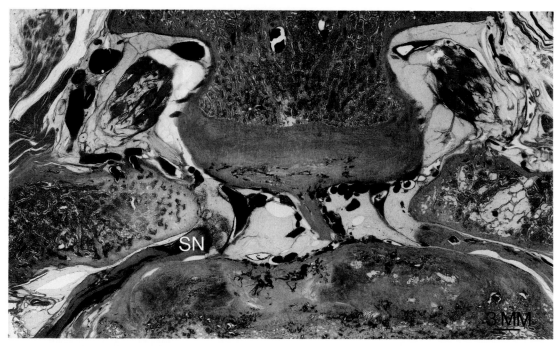

Figure 13.19 A 200 μm thick histological section, cut in the coronal plane, from the block of tissue in Figures 13.17 and 13.18. Bilaterally, the fifth spinal nerves (SN) are impinged (arrows) due to osseous pressure between bony structures as a result of the pars interarticularis defects and the grade 1–2 spondylolisthesis. The nerves are highly vascular, so their associated blood vessels are also compromised. This section is from the approximate area shown between the two parallel lines in Figure 13.18. (Ehrlich's haematoxylin and light green counterstain.)

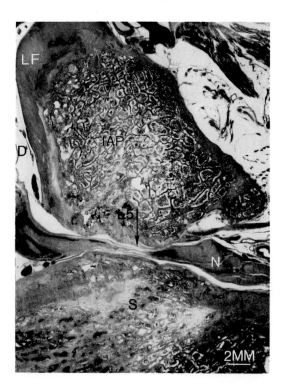

Figure 13.20 A 200 μm thick histological section, cut in the coronal plane (from the rectangle shown in Figure 13.18) through the right pars interarticularis region of the 73-year-old female specimen shown in Figures 13.17 and 13.18. This shows how the fifth lumbar (L5↓) spinal nerve (N) at this level can be severely compressed between the inferior articular process (IAP) of the fourth lumbar vertebra and the posterior rim of the first sacral segment (S). D = dura mater of the root sleeve; LF = ligamentum flavum.

nerve and its dural sheath, as well as its radicular arteries.

The incidence of spondylolysis and spondylolisthesis varies in different populations, suggesting that inherited anatomic variations may predispose to the injury (Keim and Kirkaldy-Willis, 1987).

Management of spondylolisthesis can be conservative in uncomplicated cases, with attention being paid to conservative exercises, good posture, and loss of weight in obese patients. In addition, because spondylolisthesis is frequently complicated by a posterior joint syndrome one level above the lesion, or by a sacroiliac joint syndrome, manipulation of these other joints may result in improvement in the patient's symptoms (Cassidy and Kirkaldy-Willis, 1988). However, if pain persists or muscle spasm causes loss of normal lumbar lordosis, with associated hamstring spasm, spinal fusion may be necessary (Keim and Kirkaldy-Willis, 1987), although few topics generate more debate among spinal surgeons than the best manner to surgically treat spondylolisthesis (Zindrick, 1991). Contemporary thinking is that degenerative spondylolisthesis, which is due to (i) osteoarthritis of the zygapophysial joints, or (ii) congenital malformation of the articular processes in rare cases, can frequently be accompanied by spinal instability (Dupuis *et al.*, 1985) but lytic spondylolisthesis usually is not (Pearcy and Shepherd, 1985).

According to Poussa and Tallroth (1993), who presented the case histories of three patients with a painful lumbar disc herniation in spondylolytic spondylolisthesis, painful lumbar disc herniation is rare in this condition. However, pressure upon spinal nerves and their associated blood vessels may well result in venous stasis causing ischaemia of the neural structures and accumulation of metabolic waste products with pain, as postulated in Chapter 5, and summarized in Figure 5.26.

Facet tropism

In some spines, paired facets at one spinal level do not have a symmetrical orientation, i.e. one facet may be in the sagittal plane while the other is in the coronal plane. When there is a difference of 5 degrees or more between the horizontal planes of the left and right zygapophysial joints, this is known as tropism (Cihak, 1970), as described in Chapter 5 (see Figure 13.21).

Tropism is found in 21–37% of the population (Brailsford, 1928; Farfan, 1973). The importance of tropism as a cause of low back pain has been discussed in the literature for many years (Fullenlove and Williams, 1957; Farfan and Sullivan, 1967; Hagg and Wallner, 1990; Cassidy *et al.*, 1992; Vanharanta *et al.*, 1993). It is currently a subject of intense interest because marked tropism has the potential to markedly alter the biomechanics of lumbar spinal movements and precipitate early degenerative changes either in the zygapophysial joint or adjacent intervertebral discs, abnormalities that may contribute to back pain (Tulsi and Hermanis, 1993).

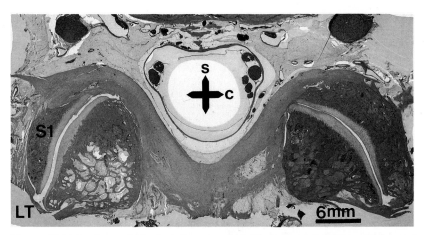

Figure 13.21 Lumbosacral histological section cut in the horizontal plain at a thickness of 100 μm. There is evidence of early fibrillation in the left hyaline articular cartilage, particularly of the superior articular process of the sacrum (S1) in this 35-year-old female specimen, with 11 degrees of tropism. The right cartilages appear relatively normal, apart from minor tinctorial changes in the cartilage at the anteromedial portion of the joint. S = sagittal plane; C = coronal plane; LT = left side of specimen. (Ehrlich's haematoxylin stain with light green counterstain.) (Reproduced with permission from Giles, L.G.F. (1987) Lumbosacral zygapophysial joint tropism and its effect on hyaline cartilage. *Clin. Biomechan.*, **1**, 2–6. Copyright John Wright, Bristol.)

It is thought that zygapophysial joint facet tropism, which is quite common, is clinically significant because it adds rotational stresses to the zygapophysial joints (Keim and Kirkaldy-Willis, 1987). In a small histological study, Giles (1987) suggested that there appeared to be greater interfacet forces in the more sagittally orientated facets, in keeping with the work of Cyron and Hutton (1980). At the zygapophysial joint centre, the more sagittal facing facets were found to have less cross-sectional cartilage area and thickness than did the coronal facing facets (Giles, 1987). More sagittal facing facets showed a greater tendency to osteoarthrosis with its characteristic changes of fibrillation, loss of cartilage, and greater subchondral sclerosis.

The clinical finding of low back pain associated with tropism may be due to several factors. For example, tropism may result in instability of the motion segment (Cyron and Hutton, 1980) causing (i) strain on the innervated joint capsule (Giles and Taylor, 1987), (ii) pinching of the highly vascular and innervated intra-articular synovial folds (Giles and Taylor, 1987; Giles and Harvey, 1987), and (iii) osteoarthritis of the zygapophysial joint facets. In osteoarthritic zygapophysial joints, erosion channels extend from the hyaline articular cartilage through the calcified cartilage into the subchondral bone; these channels contain substance P positive nerve fibres which implicates these joints in low back pain (Beaman *et al.*, 1993). This is particularly significant as substance P is the most well-documented neurotransmitter for nociception (Ahmed *et al.*, 1993).

Although some authors have suggested a possible relationship between lumbar tropism and unilateral intervertebral disc herniation (Farfan and Sullivan, 1967; Farfan *et al.*, 1972), others have not been able to support this relationship (Hagg and Wallner, 1990; Cassidy *et al.*, 1992; Vanharanta *et al.*, 1993).

References

Adams, J.C. (1968) *Outline of Orthopaedics*, 6th edn. Livingstone, Edinburgh, p. 174.

Ahmed, M., Bjurholm, A., Kreicbergs, A. *et al.* (1993) Sensory and autonomic innervation of the facet joint in the rat lumbar spine. *Spine*, **18**, 2121-2126.

Anderson, J.E. (1983) *Grant's Atlas of Anatomy*, 8th edn. Williams and Wilkins, Baltimore.

Avrahami, E., Frishman, E., Fridman, Z. *et al.* (1994) Spina bifida occulta is not an innocent finding. *Spine*, **19**, 12-15.

Baastrup, C.H. (1933) On the spinous processes of the lumbar vertebrae and the soft tissues between them, and on pathological changes in that region. *Acta Radiol. (Stockb.)*, **14**, 52.

Barry, A., Patten, B.M. and Steward, B.H. (1957) Possible factors in the development of the Arnold-Chiari malformation. *J. Neurosurg.*, **14**, 285-301.

Beaman, D.N., Graziano, G.P., Glover, R.A. *et al.* (1993) Substance P innervation of lumbar spine facet joints. *Spine*, **18**, 1044-1049.

Beckers, L. and Bekaert, J. (1991) The role of lordosis. *Acta Orthop. Belg.*, **57**, 198-202.

Beeger, J.H. and Roos, R.A. (1989) Spinal dysraphia and tethered cord syndrome. Current developments. *Tijdschr. Kindergeneeskd.*, **57**, 93-96.

Beks, J.W. (1989) Kissing spines: fact or fancy? *Acta Neurochir. (Wien)*, **100**, 134-135.

Bode,, H., Sauer, M., Strassburg, H.M. *et al.* (1985) The tethered cord syndrome. *Klin. Padiatr.*, **197**, 409-414.

Brailsford, J.F. (1928-29) Deformities of the lumbosacral region of the spine. *Br. J. Surg.*, **16**, 562-568.

Brauer, W. (1955) Beitrag zur kasuistik der kontorsionstenschäden. *Z. Orthop.*, **86**, 140.

Bullough, P.G. and Boachie-Adjei, O. (1988) *Atlas of Spinal Diseases*. J.B. Lippincott, Philadelphia, pp. 53, 84-97.

Bywaters, E.G.L. and Evans, S. (1982) The lumbar interspinous bursae and Baastrup's syndrome. *Rheumatol. Int.*, **2**, 87-96.

Cailliet, R. (1968) *Low Back Pain Syndrome*. F.A. Davis, Philadelphia, p. 124.

Cassidy, J.D. and Kirkaldy-Willis, W.H. (1988) Manipulation. In *Managing Low Back Pain* (W.H. Kirkaldy-Willis, ed.). 2nd edn. Churchill Livingstone, New York, p. 293.

Cassidy, J.D., Loback, D., Yong-Hing, K. and Tchang, S. (1992) Lumbar facet joint asymmetry. Intervertebral disc herniation. *Spine,* **17**, 570-574.

Caverni, L., Giombelli, E., Brambilla, P. *et al.* (1987) Tethered cord syndrome in an adult: clinical and neuroradiological features. *Ital. J. Neurol. Sci.*, **8**, 157-160.

Chong, C., Molet, J., Oliver, B. *et al.* (1994) The tethered cord syndrome: a review of causes. *Neurologia*, **9**, 12-18.

Cihak, R. (1970) Variations of lumbosacral joints and their morphogenesis. *Acta Univ. Carol. [Med. Monogr.] [Praha]*, **16**, 145-165.

Compobasso, P., Galiani, E., Verzerio, A. *et al.* (1988) A rare cause of occult neuropathic bladder in children: the tethered cord syndrome. *Pediatr. Med. Chir.*, **10**, 641-645.

Cyron, B.M. and Hutton, W.C. (1980) Articular tropism and stability of the lumbar spine. *Spine*, **5**, 168-172.

Dockerty, M.B. and Love, J.G. (1940) Thickening and fibrosis (so-called hypertrophy) of the ligamentum flavum: a pathological study of fifty cases. *Proc. Staff Meet. Mayo Clin.*, **15**, 161-166.

Dupuis, P.R., Yong-Hing, K., Cassidy, J.D. *et al.* (1985) Radiologic diagnosis of degenerative lumbar spinal instability. *Spine*, **10**, 262.

Elster, A.D. (1989) Bertolotti's syndrome revisited: transitional vertebrae of the lumbar spine. *Spine*, **14**, 1373-1377.

Emery, J.L. and Naik, D.R. (1968) Spinal cord segment lengths in children with meningomyelocele and the Cleland-Arnold-Chiari malformation. *Br. J. Radiol.*, **41**, 287-290.

Epstein, B. (1976) *The Spine: A Radiological Text and Atlas*, 4th edn. Lea and Febiger, Philadelphia, p. 417.

Fain, B., Vellet, D. and Hertzanu, Y. (1985) Adult tethered cord syndrome. A case report. *S. Afr. Med. J.*, **67**, 985-986.

Farfan, H.F. (1973) *Mechanical Disorders of the Low Back*. Lea and Febiger, Philadelphia.

Farfan, H.F. (1978) The biomechanical advantage of lordosis and hip extension for upright man as compared with other anthropoids. *Spine*, **3**, 336-345.

Farfan, H.F. and Sullivan, J.D. (1967) The relation of facet orientation to intervertebral disc failure. *Can. J. Surg.*, **10**, 179-185.

Farfan, H.F., Huberdeau, R.M. and Dubow, H. (1972) Lumbar intervertebral disc degeneration. The influence of geometrical features on the pattern of disc degeneration - a postmortem study. *J. Bone Joint Surg.*, **54A**, 492-510.

Flanigan, R.C., Russell, D.P. and Walsh, J.W. (1989) Urologic aspects of tethered cord. *Urology*, **33**, 80-82.

Francois, R.J., Bywaters, E.G.L. and Aufdermaur, M. (1985) Illustrated glossary for spinal anatomy. *Rheumatol. Int.*, **5**, 241-245.

Fujita, Y. and Yamamoto, H. (1989) An experimental study on spinal cord traction effect. *Spine*, **14**, 698-705.

Fullenlove, T.M. and Williams, A.J. (1957) Comparative roentgen findings in symptomatic and asymptomatic backs. *Radiology*, **68**, 572-574.

Gabay, C., van Linthoudt, D. and Orr, H. (1989) Lumbosacral spina bifida associated with an intraspinal lipoma. *Schweiz Med. Wochenschr.*, **119**, 1604-1608.

Gado, M., Hodges, F. and Patel, J. (1984) CT of the spine with metrizamide. In *CT of the Spine* (J.F. Post, ed.). Williams and Wilkins, Baltimore.

Giles, L.G.F. (1987) Lumbo-sacral zygapophysial joint tropism and its effect on hyaline cartilage. *Clin. Biomech.*, **2**, 2-6.

Giles, L.G.F. (1991) Review of tethered cord syndrome with a radiological and anatomical study. *Surg. Radiol. Anat.*, **13**, 339-343.

Giles, L.G.F. (1994) A histological investigation of human lower lumbar intervertebral canal (foramen) dimensions. *J. Manipulative Physiol. Ther.* **15**, 551-555.

Giles, L.G.F. and Harvey, A.R. (1987) Immunohistochemical demonstration of nociceptors in the capsule and synovial folds of human zygapophysial joints. *Br. J. Rheumatol.*, **26**, 362-364.

Giles, L.G.F. and Taylor, J.R. (1987) Human zygapophysial joint capsule and synovial fold innervation. *Br. J. Rheumatol.*, **26**, 93-98.

Guebert, G.M., Yochum, T.R. and Rowe, L.J. (1987) Congenital anomalies and normal skeletal variants. In *Essentials of Skeletal Radiology* (T.R. Yochum, and L.J. Rowe, eds), vol. 1. Williams and Wilkins, Baltimore, pp. 122-125.

Hadley, L.A. (1951) Intervertebral joint subluxation, bony impingement and foramen encroachment with nerve root changes. *Am. J. Roentgenol.*, **65**, 377.

Hadley, L.A. (1964) *Anatomico-Roentgenographic Studies of the Spine*. Charles C. Thomas, Springfield, IL., pp. 32, 179, 130.

Hagg, O. and Wallner, A. (1990) Facet joint asymmetry and protrusion of the intervertebral disc. *Spine*, **15**, 356-359.

Herzog, R.J. (1990) State of the art imaging studies of spinal disorders. In *Physical Medicine and Rehabilitation: State of the Art Reviews*, vol. 4, No. 2. Hanley and Belfus, Philadelphia, pp. 221-269.

Herzog, R.J., Kaiser, J.A., Saal, J.A. *et al.* (1991) The importance of posterior epidural fat pad in lumbar central canal stenosis. *Spine*, **16**, S227-S233.

Hoffman, H.J., Hendrick, E.B. and Humphreys, R.P. (1976) The tethered spinal cord: its protean manifestations diagnosis and surgical correction. *Childs Brain*, **2**, 145-155.

Horton, D., Barnes, P., Pendleton, B.D. *et al.* (1989) Spina bifida occulta: early clinical and radiologic diagnosis. *J. Okla. State Med. Assoc.*, **82**, 15-19.

Jackson, Jr D.E., Atlas, S.W., Mani, J.R. *et al.* (1989) Intraspinal synovial cysts: MR imaging. *Radiology*, **170**, 527-530.

James, C.C. and Lassman, L.P. (1962) Spinal dysraphism. The diagnosis and treatment of progressive lesions in spina bifida occulta. *J. Bone Joint Surg.*, **44B**, 828-840.

James, C.C. and Lassman, L.P. (1981) *Spina Bifida Occulta. Orthopaedic Radiological and Neurosurgical Aspects.* Academic Press, London.

Jinkins, J.R. and Rauch, A. (1994) Magnetic resonance imaging of entrapment of lumbar nerve roots in spondylolytic spondylolisthesis. *J. Bone Joint Surg.*, **76A**, 1643-1648.

Kaplan, J.O. and Quencer, R.M. (1980) The occult tethered conus syndrome in the adult. *Radiology*, **237**, 387-391.

Kavukcu, S., Ozaksoy, D., Turkmen, M. *et al.* (1993) The urological manifestations of the tethered spinal cord. *Turk. J. Pediatr.*, **35**, 313-317.

Keats, T.E. (1973) *An Atlas of Normal Roentgen Variations that may Simulate Disease*. Year Book Medical Publishers, Chicago, p. 98.

Keim, H.A. and Kirkaldy-Willis, W.H. (1987) Low back pain. In *Clinical Symposia*. 32(6) Ciba-Geigy Corp., New Jersey.

Linder, M., Rosenstein, J. and Sklar, F.H. (1982) Functional improvement after spinal surgery for the dysraphic malformation. *Neurosurgery*, **11**, 622-624.

Love, J.G. and Walsh, M.N. (1940) Intraspinal protrusion of intervertebral discs. *Arch. Surg.*, **40**, 454.

McLendon, R.E., Oakes, W.J., Heinz, E.R. *et al.* (1988) Adipose tissue in the filum terminale: a computed tomographic finding that may indicate tethering of the spinal cord. *Neurosurgery*, **22**, 873-876.

McRae, D.L. (1977) Radiology of the lumbar spinal canal. In *Lumbar Spondylosis, Diagnosis, Management and Surgical Treatment* (P.R. Weinstein, G. Ehni and C.B. Wilson, eds). Year Book Medical Publishers, Chicago, pp. 92-114.

Meyerding, H.W. (1932) Spondylolisthesis. *Surg. Gynecol. Obstet.*, **54**, 371-377.

Moore, K.L. (1992) *Clinically Oriented Anatomy*, 3rd edn. Williams and Wilkins, Baltimore.

Nachemson, A.L. and Evans, J.H. (1968) Some mechanical properties of the third human lumbar interlaminar ligament (ligamentum flavum). *J. Biomech.*, **1**, 211.

Naik, D.R. and Emery, J.L. (1968) The position of the spinal cord segments related to the vertebral bodies in children with meningomyelocele and hydrocephalus. *Dev. Med. Child. Neurol. (Suppl.)*, **16**, 62-68.

Pang, D. and Wilberger, J.E. (1982) Tethered cord syndrome in adults. *J. Neurosurg.*, **57**, 32-47.

Panjabi, M.M., Goel, V., Oxland, T. *et al.* (1992) Human lumbar vertebrae: quantitative three-dimensional anatomy. *Spine*, **17**, 299-306.

Pearcy, M. and Shepherd, J. (1985) Is there instability in spondylolisthesis? *Spine*, **10**, 175-177.

Pennal, G.F. and Schatzker, J. (1971) Stenosis of the lumbar spinal canal. *Clin. Neurosurg.*, **6**, 86.

Penning, L. (1992) Functional pathology of lumbar spinal stenosis. *Clin. Biomech.*, **7**, 3-17.

Piatt, J.H. Jr and Hoffman, H.J. (1987a) The tethered spinal cord with focus on the tight filum terminale. (I)

Introduction, nosology and pathology, developmental aspects, biomechanical aspects. *Neuro-Orthopedics*, **3**, 67-75.

Piatt, J.H. Jr and Hoffman, H.J. (1987b) The tethered spinal cord with focus on the tight filum terminale. (II) Clinical presentations, diagnostic investigations, radiological features, urological investigations, electrophysiological evaluation, results. *Neuro-Orthopedics*, **4**, 1-11.

Poussa, M. and Tallroth, J. (1993) Disc herniation in lumbar spondylolisthesis: report of 3 symptomatic cases. *Acta Orthop. Scand.*, **64**, 13-16.

Raco, A., Ciappetta, P. and Mariottine, A. (1987) Lumbosacral lipoma causing tethering of the conus: case report. *Ital. J. Neurol. Sci.*, **8**, 59-62.

Reigel, D.H., Tchernoukha, K. and Bazmi, B. (1994) Change in spinal curvature following release of tethered spinal cord associated with spina bifida. *Pediatr. Neurosurg.*, **20**, 30-42.

Reimann, A.F. and Anson, B.J. (1944) Vertebral level of termination of the spinal cord with report of a case of sacral cord. *Anat. Rec.*, **88**, 127-138.

Resnick, D. (1985) Degenerative diseases of the vertebral column. *Radiology*, **156**, 3-14.

Rich, E.A. (1965a) *Atlas of Clinical Roentgenology.* RAE Publishing Co., Indianapolis, p. 192.

Rich, E.A. (1965b) *Manual of Radiography and Diagnostic Roentgenology.* RAE Publishing Co., Indianapolis, p. 165.

Rickenbacher, J., Landolt, A.M. and Theiler, K. (1982) *Applied Anatomy of the Back.* Springer-Verlag, Berlin, pp. 15-16.

Rosenberg, N.J., Bargar, W.L. and Friedman, B. (1981) The incidence of spondylolysis and spondylolisthesis in non-ambulatory patients. *Spine*, **6**, 35-38.

Ross, J.S., Masaryk, T.J., Modic, M.T. *et al.* (1987) Vertebral hemangiomas: MR imaging. *Radiology*, **164**, 165-169.

Rowe, G.G. and Roche, M.B. (1953) The etiology of separate neural arch. *J. Bone Joint Surg.*, **35A**, 102-110.

Roy, M.W., Gilmore, R. and Walsh, J.W. (1986) Evaluation of children and young adults with tethered spinal cord syndrome. Utility of spinal and scalp recorded somatosensory evoked potentials. *Surg. Neurol.*, **26**, 241-248.

Sarwar, M., Crelin, E.S., Kier, E.L. *et al.* (1983) Experimental cord stretchability and the tethered cord syndrome. *AJNR*, **4**, 641-643.

Sarwar, M., Virapongse, C. and Bhimani, S. (1984) Primary tethered cord syndrome: a new hypothesis of its origin. *AJNR*, **5**, 235-242.

Schmorl, G. and Junghanns, H. (1971) *The Human Spine in Health and Disease*, 2nd edn. Grune and Stratton, New York.

Singer, K.P., Giles, L.G.F. and Day, R.E. (1990) Intra-articular synovial folds of thoracolumbar junction zygapophysial joints. *Anat. Rec.*, **226**, 147-152.

Sostrin, R.D., Thompson, J.R., Rouhe, S.A. *et al.* (1977) Occult spinal dysraphism in the geriatric patient. *Radiology*, **125**, 165-169.

Spurling, R.G., Mayfield, F.H. and Rogers, J.B. (1937) Hypertrophy of the ligamenta flava as a cause of low back pain. *JAMA*, **109**, 928.

Starr, W.A. (1971) Spina bifida occulta and engagement of the fifth lumbar spinous process. *Clin. Orthop.*, **81**, 71.

Taillard, W. (1954) Le spondylolisthesis chez l'enfant et l'adolescent. *Acta Orthop. Scand.*, **24**, 115.

Tamaki, N., Shirataki, K., Kojima, N. *et al.* (1988) Tethered cord syndrome of delayed onset following repair of myelomeningocele. *J. Neurosurg.*, **69**, 393-398.

Tani, S., Yamada, S. and Knighton, R.S. (1987) Extensibility of the lumbar and sacral cord. Pathophysiology of the tethered spinal cord in cats. *J. Neurosurg.*, **66**, 116-123.

Teng, P. and Papatheodorou, C. (1963) Lumbar spondylosis with compression of cauda equina. *Arch. Neurol.*, **8**, 221-229.

Tulsi, R.S. and Hermanis, G.M. (1993) A study of the angle of inclination and facet curvature of superior lumbar zygapophysial facets. *Spine*, **18**, 1311-1317.

Vanharanta, H., Floyd, T., Ohnmeiss, D.D. *et al.* (1993) The relationship of facet tropism to degeneratirve disc disease. *Spine*, **18**, 1000-1005.

Verbiest, H. (1954) A radicular syndrome from developmental narrowing of the lumbar vertebral canal. *J. Bone Joint Surg.*, **36B**, 230-237.

Wakata, N., Araki, Y., Murabayashi, K. *et al.* (1994) Tethered cord syndrome accompanied by unilateral muscle atrophy in the calf muscle. *Int. Med.*, **33**, 60-63.

Weinstein, P.R., Ehni, G. and Wilson, C.B. (1977) Clinical features of lumbar spondylosis and stenosis. In *Lumbar Spondylosis: Diagnosis, Management and Surgical Treatment* (P.R. Weinstein, G. Ehni and C.B. Wilson, eds). Year Book Medical Publishers, Chicago, pp. 115-133.

Weissert, M., Gysler, R. and Sorenson, N. (1989) The clinical problem of the tethered cord syndrome: a report of 3 personal cases. *Z. Kinderchir.*, **44**, 275-279.

Weisz, G.M. (1983) Lumbar spinal canal stenosis in Paget's disease. *Spine*, **8**, 192-198.

Williams, P.L. and Warwick, T. (1980) *Grays Anatomy*, 36th edn. Churchill Livingstone, London, p. 865.

Wiltse, L.L., Widell, E.H. and Jackson, D.W. (1975) Fatigue fracture: the basic lesion in isthmic spondylolisthesis. *J. Bone Joint Surg.*, **57A**, 17-22.

Wolfers, H. and Hoeffken, W. (1974) Fehlbildungen der wirbelbogen. In *Handbuch der medizinischen Radiologie, Bd 6, Teil 1: Rontgendiagnostik der Wirbelsaule, 1* (L. Diethelm, F. Heuck, O. Olsson *et al.*, eds). Springer, Berlin, pp. 265-389.

Woo, C.C. (1987) Hyperostosis of lumbar spinous process; a radiological feature in a young acromegalic. *J. Manipulative Physiol. Ther.*, **10**, 111-115.

Yahia, L.H., Newman, N. and Rivard C.-H. (1988) Neurohistology of lumbar spine ligaments. *Acta Orthop. Scand.*, **59**, 508-512.

Zindrick, M.R. (1991) The role of transpedicular fixation systems for stabilization of the lumbar spine. *Orthop. Clin. North Am.*, **22**, 333-344.

Zumkeller, M., Seifert, V. and Stolke, D. (1989) Spinal dysraphia and disordered ascension of the spinal cord in adults. *Z. Orthop.*, **127**, 336-342.

Spinal Clinical Neuroanatomy and Neurophysiology

14

Innervation of spinal structures

L.G.F. Giles

Formation of the spinal nerve

Each spinal nerve is formed by the union of the anterior and posterior roots which are attached in series to the sides of the spinal cord (Williams and Warwick, 1980). A histological section cut in the horizontal plane at the lumbosacral level (Figure 14.1) shows part of the spinal canal and how the anterior and posterior nerve root trunks leave the cauda equina within the subarachnoid space, and pass towards the intervertebral canal where they will unite to form the fifth lumbar spinal nerve.

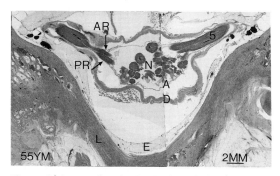

Figure 14.1 Note that the dural tube, which contains the cauda equina nerve root trunks (N), is surrounded by epidural fat (E) within the spinal canal. A = arachnoid membrane; D = dural membrane. The anterior nerve root (AR) and posterior nerve root (PR) trunks at the fifth (5) spinal level pass from the dural tube, within a dural sleeve, to the intervertebral canal. L = lamina. 55-year-old male. (Ehrlich's haematoxylin and light green counterstain.)

The nerve roots within the extensions of the dural tube, i.e. root sleeves, are accompanied by blood vessels (Figure 14.2).

Once the spinal nerves pass through the intervertebral canal they immediately divide to form anterior and posterior primary rami (Vick, 1976; Moore, 1992; Tortora and Grabowski, 1993). The posterior root carries sensory fibres whose cell bodies lie in the spinal ganglion (Moore, 1992). The anterior root is predominantly motor but, according to Bogduk and Twomey (1991), there is some controversy regarding the contribution made by different fibre-types and Dripps *et al.* (1977) have shown that some afferent fibres enter the cord via this pathway. According to Coggeshall *et al.* (1977), who examined rat anterior roots, the anterior nerve roots contain both myelinated and unmyelinated nerve fibres but, according to Schaumburg and Spencer (1975), the anterior roots are composed only of myelinated fibres. The nerve roots, spinal nerves and their branches compose the various parts of long cellular extensions from nerve cell bodies, located in the anterior horn of the spinal cord or in the posterior nerve root ganglion (Rydevik *et al.*, 1984).

Extracapsular distribution of the posterior primary ramus

In this text, the anatomy of the anterior primary ramus, which forms the lumbosacral plexus, is not reviewed; however, the distribution of the medial branch of the posterior primary ramus, which is of

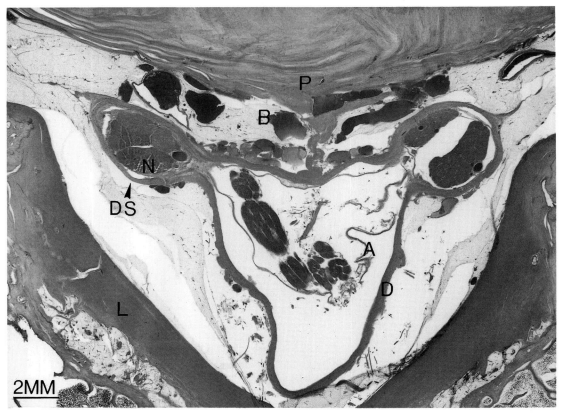

Figure 14.2 This figure shows how the fifth lumbar nerve root trunks (N) within the dural sleeve (DS) become separated from the nerve root trunks of the cauda equina within the dural tube. A = arachnoid membrane; D = dural membrane; L = ligamentum flavum; B = Batson's venous plexus; P = posterior longitudinal ligament. 69-year-old female. (Ehrlich's haematoxylin and light green counterstain.)

paramount clinical relevance because of its distribution to the zygapophysial joints (Bogduk and Twomey, 1991) and, therefore, has frequently been implicated in low back pain, is reviewed in detail.

The posterior primary rami have a diameter of 2 mm or less and are quite small compared with the anterior primary ramus (Sunderland, 1975; Bradley, 1980). Figures 14.3 and 14.4 show the course and branches of the posterior primary rami in simplified diagrams which are not drawn to scale.

As the posterior primary rami pass from the intervertebral canal into the posterior compartment of the back, each is accompanied by an artery and its associated vein forming a neurovascular bundle. The posterior primary ramus runs downward and backwards across the lateral surface of the adjacent superior articular process of the zygapophysial joint, then passes backward above the origin of the transverse process where it divides into medial and lateral branches; the finer medial branch which is less than 1 mm in diameter (Sunderland, 1975; Bradley, 1980) establishes important relationships with zygapophysial joints (Sunderland, 1975; Bradley, 1980).

From its inferolateral aspect, before it passes beneath the mamillo-accessory ligament, the posterior primary ramus gives off a lateral branch (Figures 14.2 and 14.3) which supplies the iliocostalis lumborum muscle.

The medial branch descends beneath the mamillo-accessory ligament, which bridges the mamillary and accessory processes (Bogduk, 1981), and which consists of a tight bundle of collagen fibres of various thickness (Bogduk and Twomey, 1991). It is only the medial branch which supplies zygapophysial joints although, according to Lazorthes and co-workers (1956, 1964), approximately six articular rami arise directly from the posterior primary ramus and run towards the superior and inferior articular processes. As the medial branch reaches the inferior aspect of the joint it may be embedded in the capsule for a distance of 2–3 mm, at which point it lies directly superficial to the communication between the fat-filled inferior recess and the synovial cavity of the joint (Lewin *et al.*, 1961). Within the capsule, nerves break up into large numbers of diffusely ramifying branches containing sensory fibres (Sunderland, 1978; Wyke, 1981).

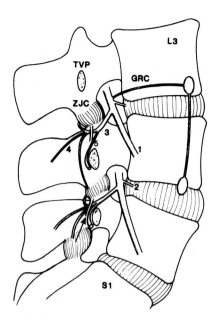

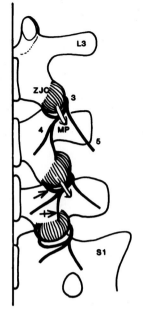

Figure 14.3 Part of the lower spinal innervation (lateral view). 1 = anterior primary ramus of the spinal nerve; 2 = anterior primary ramus branch to the intervertebral disc; 3 = posterior primary ramus of the spinal nerve; 4 = medial branch of the posterior primary ramus with an adjacent zygapophysial joint capsule (articular) branch, and a descending branch to the zygapophysial joint capsule (articular branch) one joint lower; 5 = lateral branch of the posterior primary ramus; A = autonomic ganglion; GRC = gray ramus communicans; TVP = transverse process; ZJC = zygapophysial joint capsule; arrow = part of the mamillo-accessory ligament. (Reproduced with permission from Giles, L.G.F. (1989) *Anatomical Basis of Low Back Pain*. Williams and Wilkins, Baltimore.)

Figure 14.4 Part of the lower spinal innervation (posterior view). 3 = posterior primary ramus of the spinal nerve; 4 = medial branch of the posterior primary ramus with an adjacent zygapophysial joint capsule (articular) branch (arrow), and a descending branch to the zygapophysial joint capsule (articular branch) one joint lower (bisected arrow); 5 = lateral branch of the posterior primary ramus; MP = part of the mamillo-accessory ligament passing caudally towards the accessory process at the posteroinferior aspect of the root of the transverse process; ZJC = zygapophysial joint capsule. (Reproduced with permission from Giles, L.G.F. (1989) *Anatomical Basis of Low Back Pain*. Williams and Wilkins, Baltimore.)

Most authors regard each zygapophysial joint capsule as being innervated by medial branches of only two spinal nerves (Fick, 1904; Zuckschwerdt *et al.*, 1955; Pedersen *et al.*, 1956; Lewin *et al.*, 1961; Lazorthes, 1972; Bradley, 1974, 1980; Sunderland, 1975; Bogduk, 1976; Edgar and Ghadially, 1976; Reilly *et al.*, 1978; Bogduk and Long, 1979; Sunderland, 1979; Bogduk *et al.*, 1982; Auteroche, 1983; Lynch and Taylor, 1986; Giles, 1989; Moore, 1992). The claims of Wyke (1980b, 1981), Paris *et al.* (1980) and Paris (1983) that each zygapophysial joint is innervated from no less than three nerve roots do not appear to have been substantiated by other studies.

The *superior portion of the joint capsule* is innervated by 'distal' branches arising from the nerve one level higher and the *inferior portion of the joint capsule* is innervated by 'proximal' branches arising from the nerve as it emerges from the intervertebral canal adjacent to the zygapophysial joint in question. This gives an overlap of innervation. Bogduk *et al.*

(1982), found the anatomy of the L1–4 posterior rami to be different from that of L5, in that the L1–4 posterior rami tend to form three branches (medial, lateral and intermediate), whereas the L5 posterior ramus forms only a medial and an intermediate branch.

A histological study using blocks of L3 and L4 spinal tissues, serially sectioned in the coronal plane as shown in Figure 14.5, confirmed the extracapsular course of the posterior primary ramus (Figure 14.6) as previously described by gross dissection.

The medial branch of the posterior primary ramus passes beneath the mamillo-accessory ligament, in a notch containing an adequate protective reserve cushion of adipose tissue. It does not appear likely that this nerve could become trapped, under normal circumstances, as it passes beneath the mamillo-accessory ligament (Giles, 1991). However, Maigne *et al.* (1991) have shown that ossification of the mamillo-accessory ligament can occur in adult spines

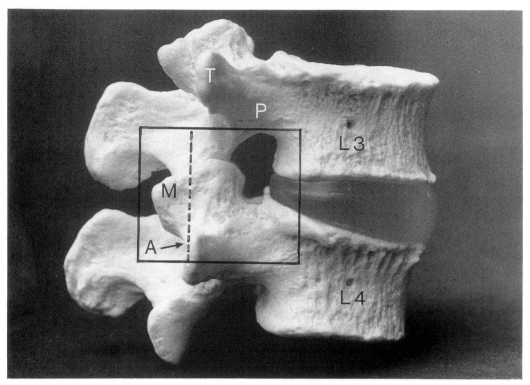

Figure 14.5 The rectangle shows how each osteoligamentous 'block' of tissue was trimmed for histological processing and sectioning. The approximate plane of coronal sectioning for Figure 14.6 is shown by the 'dashed' line A. M = mamillary process; P = pedicle; T = transverse process. (Reproduced with permission from Giles, L.G.F. (1991) The relationship between the medial branch of the lumbar posterior primary ramus and the mamillo-accessory ligament. *J. Manipulative Physiol. Ther.*, **14**, 189–192.)

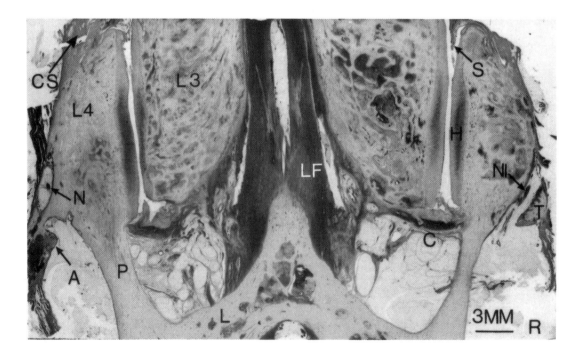

with osteoarthritis, resulting in bony foramina 1–5 mm wide, particularly at L5, which they suggest may be associated with low back pain.

The medial branch then divides into three separate branches. The first branch goes to the adjacent zygapophysial joint capsule in the region of the inferior recess (Figure 14.3).

Intracapsular distribution of the posterior primary ramus terminations

Using surgical specimens (Figure 14.7) to follow the intracapsular distribution of the nerve, it appears to divide into several small twigs as it penetrates the capsule (Figures 14.8 and 14.9).

The small twigs of the medial branch of the posterior primary ramus which penetrate the capsule (Figures 14.8 and 14.9) then pass to the synovial fold (Figures 14.10 and 14.11).

Part of a silver impregnated synovial fold lining membrane, with a very small nerve fibre, which runs in a paravascular situation for part of its course in the surface of the synovial lining membrane, closely associated with blood vessels, is demonstrated in Figure 14.11.

These findings are of interest because, although Gardner (1950), Hadley (1964), Wyke (1972, 1981, 1982) and Nade *et al.* (1980) were unable to find any nerves in human zygapophysial joint synovial folds of 'mature individuals', small diameter nerve fibres were found in human lower lumbar zygapophysial joint synovial folds of healthy human zygapophysial joint capsules, their synovium, and their intra-articular synovial fold tissue, removed during laminectomy (Figures 14.8 and 14.10) (Giles *et al.*, 1986; Giles and Taylor, 1987a,b; Giles, 1989; Gronblad *et al.*, 1991a,b). The immunohistochemical studies by Giles and Harvey (1987) and Gronblad *et al.* (1991a,b) showed that some of the small diameter nerves in these tissues most likely have a nociceptive function. Therefore, Wyke's conclusion that there is no mechanism whereby articular pain can arise directly from the synovial tissues (Wyke, 1981) is challenged. Kuslich *et al.* (1991) concluded that zygapophysial joint synovium was never sensitive to stimulation by means of mechanical force using blunt surgical instruments or by the application of low voltage electrical current. However, this may be because the synovium tested was 'so closely applied to the capsule' (Kuslich, 1994, personal communication) which implies that the large highly vascular and innervated intra-articular synovial *folds*

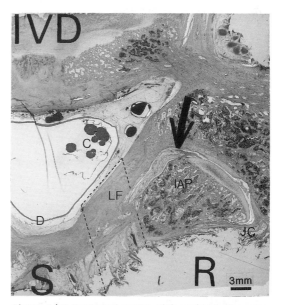

Figure 14.6 A histological section cut in the coronal plane as shown by the line on Figure 14.5, from a 36-year-old woman. The histological section is slightly oblique as the mammillo-accessory ligament is clearly seen enclosing the medial branch of the posterior primary ramus (N) on the left of the specimen, whereas on the right side the medial branch of the posterior primary ramus (N1) is seen coursing behind part of the transverse process (T). A = part of the accessory process; C = fibrous capsule inferiorly meshing with the ligamentum flavum (LF). The ligamenta flava join at the junction of the laminae, but the left and right ligaments are separate between spinous processes. CS = fibrous capsule superiorly; H = hyaline articular cartilage on the superior articular process of the L4 vertebra forming part of the zygapophysial joint; L = lamina of the L4 vertebra; P = pars interarticularis of the L4 vertebra; S = synovial fold. (Ehrlich's haematoxylin and light green counterstain.) (Reproduced with permission from Giles, L.G.F. (1991)The relationship between the medial branch of the lumbar posterior primary ramus and the mamillo-accessory ligament. *J. Manipulative Physiol. Ther.*, **14**, 189–192.)

Figure 14.7 Horizontal section of the right L5–S1 zygapophysial joint from a 54-year-old male. The rectangle represents the approximate extent of surgical material removed during laminectomy, i.e. part of the inferior joint recess comprising the posteromedial (accessory) fibrous capsule and adjacent ligamentum flavum with the adjoining synovial fold. C = cauda equina; D = dura mater; IAP = inferior articular process of L5; IVD = intervertebral disc; JC = posterolateral fibrous joint capsule; LF = ligamentum flavum; S = remains of the spinous process. The black arrow indicates a highly vascular connective tissue structure projecting between the right lumbosacral zygapophysial joint facets, i.e. an intra-articular synovial fold. (Ehrlich's haematoxylin stain wih light green counterstain.) (Reproduced with permission from Giles, L.G.F., Taylor, J.R. and Cockson, A. (1986) Human zygapophysial joint synovial folds. *Acta Anat.*, **126**, 110–114.)

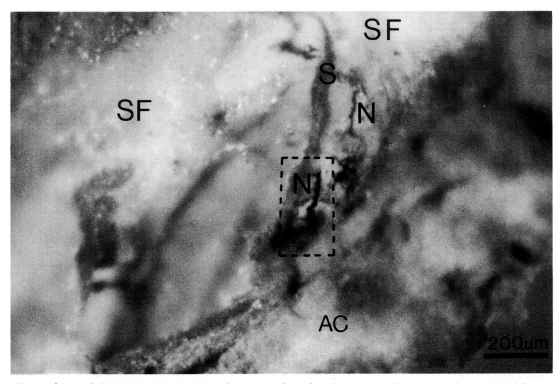

Figure 14.8 A whole mount silver impregnated specimen from the L5-S1 zygapophysial joint of a 27-year-old female, showing the inferior joint recess postero-medial (accessory) capsule (AC) (see rectangle in Figure 14.7) with nerve fasciculi (N) projecting from it into the synovial folds (SF), adjacent to a small fibrous 'septum' (S). The average diameter of the nerve fasciculi is 11.4 μm. The nerve fasciculus in the rectangle, which was resected then serially sectioned (at a thickness of 30 μm) is shown in Figure 14.9 (modified Schofield's silver impregnation). (Reproduced with permission from Giles, L.G.F. and Taylor, J.R. (1987a) Innervation of lumbar zygapophysial joint synovial folds. *Acta Orthop. Scand.*, **58**, 43–46. Copyright Munksgaard International Publishers, Denmark.)

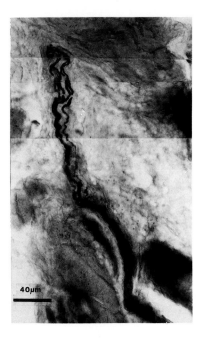

Figure 14.9 This shows a montage of a nerve fasciculus containing six axons; its average diameter is 11.4 μm. The average diameter of each axon is approximately 1.5 μm. (Reproduced with permission from Giles, L.G.F. and Taylor, J.R. (1987a) Innervation of lumbar zygapophysial joint synovial folds. *Acta Orthop. Scand.*, **58**, 43–46. Copyright Munksgaard International Publishers, Denmark.)

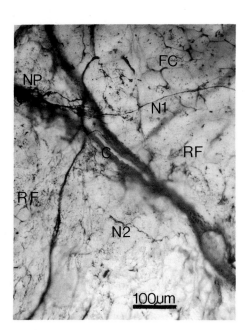

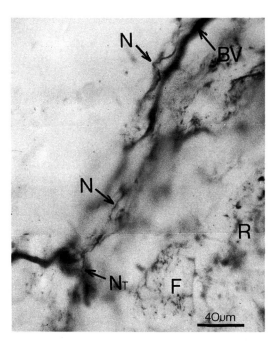

Figure 14.10 This is a highly magnified view of a synovial fold. Note (i) the extensive paravascular nerve plexus (NP) on the capillary (C), (ii) the synovial fold fat cells (FC), (iii) the single nerve fibre (N1), with an average diameter of 1.7 μm, traversing the synovial fold, and which is not related to any blood vessels, (iv) the silver stained structure (N2) which consists of one or two nerve fibres, and (v) the reticular fibres (RF) adjacent to the fat cells. (Reproduced with permission from Giles, L.G.F. and Taylor, J.R. (1987a) Innervation of lumbar zygapophysial joint synovial folds. *Acta Orthop. Scand.,* **58**, 43–46. Copyright Munksgaard International Publishers, Denmark.)

Figure 14.11 This montage of the L4–5 zygapophysial joint synovial fold, from a 49-year-old male, shows the extremely small nerve fibre (N) which appears to terminate as a 'free ending' (NT) in the synovial lining membrane. The average diameter of the nerve fibre between N and N is 1.1 μm. BV = blood vessel; F = fat cell; R = reticular fibres (modified Schofield's silver impregnation). (Reproduced with permission from Giles, L.G.F. (1988) Human zygapophysial joint inferior recess synovial folds: a light microscope examination. *Anat. Rec.,* **220**, 117–124. Copyright A.R. Liss, New York.)

which are not closely applied to the capsule (Figure 14.7) were not stimulated.

One branch of the posterior primary ramus goes to the adjacent multifidus muscles (Figure 14.3), then branches of the medial branch of the posterior primary ramus go to the zygapophysial joint capsules one segment caudad, and one segment cephalad, where they divide into several terminal twigs and penetrate the capsule.

Summary of distribution of nerves within the fibrous capsule and ligamentum flavum

Joint capsule

According to Resnick (1985), human zygapophysial joint fibrous capsules have a rich innervation. Immersion of human capsular material in methylene blue

showed these nerves to consist of myelinated and unmyelinated fibres, with a 'full triad' of nerve endings, i.e. (a) fine free fibres, (b) complex unencapsulated endings, and (c) small encapsulated endings (Hirsch *et al.*, 1963). Nerve endings classified as 'pain sensitive', on the basis of their histological appearance, have also been described in: (a) the fibrous capsule (Ikari, 1954; Pedersen *et al.*, 1956), (b) the ligamentum flavum, and (c) the adjacent interspinous ligaments (Hovelacque, 1925; Jung and Brunschwig, 1932; Bridge, 1959; Hirsch *et al.*, 1963).

Pedersen *et al.* (1956) combined their histological studies with physiological studies on decerebrate cats. They used mechanical (crushing) stimuli, as well as injections of hypertonic saline, to assess what effect these stimuli had on respiration and blood pressure. The cat's response varied from mild hyperpnoea to a 'gasping' inspiratory shift, with or without minor blood pressure changes. From these experiments, Pedersen *et al.* (1956) concluded that the posterior primary rami, in addition to their cutaneous and muscular distribution, give sensory fibres to spinal ligaments and fasciae, vertebral periosteum and all intervertebral joints. Pedersen *et al.*'s (1956) view is generally applicable to all joints so far examined and is in accord with Hilton's Law (1891). This law states that the nerves supplying a joint also supply the muscles moving the joint and the skin covering the insertion of these muscles.

Histological studies performed by Gardner (1950), Dee (1978), Gardner (1978), and Wyke (1979) reported myelinated and unmyelinated nerve fibres in normal human zygapophysial joint capsules.

According to Lewinnek (1983), only two kinds of nerve endings are found in the fibrous joint capsule: (a) complex unencapsulated endings and (b) smaller encapsulated endings. Other workers have found free nerve endings in the zygapophysial joint capsule by histologic investigation (Hadley, 1964; Reilly *et al.*, 1978) and these endings are generally regarded as related to pain sensation (Haldeman, 1980; Kandel and Schwartz, 1981; Daube *et al.*, 1986).

According to Wyke and Polacek (1975) and Wyke (1980a, 1981), all the synovial joints of the body in mature individuals, including the zygapophysial joints, are provided with four varieties of receptor nerve endings. Wyke (1981) has classified these as follows:

Type I: mechanoreceptors which consist of clusters of thinly encapsulated globularcorpuscles embedded in the outer layers of the fibrous capsule.

Type II: mechanoreceptors which are thickly encapsulated conical corpuscles embedded in the deeper layers of the fibrous capsule.

Type III: mechanoreceptors which are much larger, thinly encapsulated corpuscles applied to the surfaces of joint ligaments, but which are absent from the spinal ligaments.

Type IV: a receptor system in the fibrous capsules of joints which is represented by a plexus of unmyelinated nerve fibres, which weave in three dimensions throughout the entire thickness of the joint capsule, but are entirely absent from synovial tissue and intra-articular menisci; the irritation of this system is said to be responsible for evoking joint pain.

Wyke's statements, relating these four types of articular nerve receptor endings to particular function, are repeated in several of his papers (1972, 1975, 1979, 1980a, 1981). He states that a correlation between fibre size and function does occur (Wyke, 1969). He appears to base his statements on the results of 'neurohistological studies considered in combination with (i) oscillographic analyses of the impulse traffic in the articular nerves, (ii) electrical

stimulation procedures, and (iii) other neurophysiological investigations' (Wyke, 1967). However, it is unclear if his conclusions are based entirely on work with cats or also apply to humans.

Ligamentum flavum

Accounts of innervation in the ligamentum flavum are variable, contradictory and inconclusive. Doubt remains regarding both the source of its innervation and which parts of it are innervated. According to Bogduk (1983), the medial branches of the posterior rami are the most likely source of innervation of the ligamenta flava because of their proximity to the posterior surfaces of the ligament. Fine free nerve fibres and endings were described by Pedersen *et al.* (1956), and Hirsch *et al.* (1963) on the outermost posterior surface of the ligamenta flava, but it is claimed that nerves have never been demonstrated in its deeper regions (Dockerty and Love, 1940; Hirsch *et al.*, 1963; Jackson *et al.*, 1966; Ramsey, 1966; Reilly *et al.*, 1978). On the other hand, Bridge (1959) made the surprising observation that in a few cases, the ligamentum flavum, which is a highly elastic structure, contained many nerves in its deep region, as well as on its surface, in thoracolumbar specimens. According to Pedersen *et al.* (1956), the nerve filaments on the posterior surface are derived from the posterior rami, while the sinuvertebral nerves may supply the anterior surface but no neural structures were found in the deeper part of the ligamentum flavum included in their surgical specimens. Korkala *et al.* (1985) and Konttinen *et al.* (1990) found no immunoreactivity for substance P in small pieces of the ligamentum flavum and therefore concluded that no nociceptive type nerves were present in the ligamenta flava.

The pattern of innervation of articular vessels is basically similar to that of other blood vessels, with both myelinated and unmyelinated fibres participating (Gardner, 1950). The myelinated fibres are afferent, and the unmyelinated fibres are both afferent and postganglionic sympathetic efferent (Woollard, 1926).

Sinuvertebral nerve distribution

The sinuvertebral nerve is briefly reviewed here because (a) it is possible that some branches may pass to the vertebral arches and to the zygapophysial joints (Bradley, 1980), and (b) the proximity of the sinuvertebral nerve to the zygapophysial joints may permit its paravascular twigs to reach these joints 'indirectly'. At or immediately distal to its origin, the ventral ramus of each spinal nerve is joined by a gray ramus communicans from the corresponding ganglion of the sympathetic trunk (Figure 14.12).

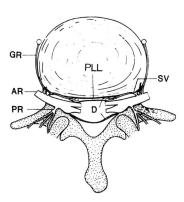

Figure 14.12 Transverse view of the distribution of a typical lumbar spinal nerve. AR = anterior primary ramus; D = dura mater; GR = gray ramus communicans; PLL = posterior longitudinal ligament; PR = posterior primary ramus; SV = sinuvertebral nerve. (Modified from Bogduk, N. (1984) The rationale for patterns of neck and back pain. *Patient Mangement*, **8**, 13–21.) Compare with more detailed figure in Chapter 17. (Reproduced with permission from Giles, L.G.F. (1989) *Anatomical Basis of Low Back Pain*. Williams and Wilkins, Baltimore.)

The sinuvertebral nerves are recurrent branches of the anterior primary rami that re-enter the intervertebral canal (Bogduk, 1983) and are present at all vertebral levels (Kimmel, 1961a,b). They contain autonomic and somatic sensory fibres (Allbrook, 1974). The sinuvertebral nerve was first described by von Luschka (1850), and each nerve is described as arising by two roots: one from the anterior ramus, and another from the gray ramus communicans (Bogduk, 1980) (Figure 14.12) at all spinal levels (Williams and Warwick, 1980).

At this stage the sinuvertebral nerve is 0.5–1 mm thick (Wiberg, 1949; Reilly *et al.*, 1978); it re-enters through the intervertebral foramen (von Luschka 1850; Hovelacque, 1925; Pedersen *et al.*, 1956; Bridge, 1959; Edgar and Ghadially, 1976; Bogduk, 1980), before dividing into a series of short and long terminal branches which may ascend and descend in variable ways (Hovelacque, 1925; Spurling and Bradford, 1939; Pedersen *et al.*, 1956; Bridge, 1959; Edgar and Nundy, 1966; Bogduk *et al.*, 1981). The short branches supply the walls of extradural veins (Hovelacque, 1925), and the posterior longitudinal ligament up to two vertebral levels lower than the nerve's origin (Spurling and Bradford, 1939). The longer terminal branches pass into the epidural space; some are described as penetrating bone on the posterior aspects of the vertebral bodies and the adjacent outer layer of the anulus fibrosus, and the anterior aspects of the laminae (Hovelacque, 1925); others are said to reach the flaval ligaments (Roofe, 1940; Wyke, 1970), with free nerve endings which probably mediate pain sensation (Reilly *et al.*, 1978). In some cases a sinuvertebral nerve is said to join

across the midline with the contralateral sinu-vertebral nerve (Pedersen *et al.*, 1956; Kimmel, 1961a; Lewinnek, 1983), but other investigators were unable to find such anastamoses (Hovelacque, 1925; Spurling and Bradford, 1939; Wiberg, 1949).

The ventral rami of the thoracic and the *first and second lumbar nerves* each contribute a *white ramus communicans* joining the corresponding sympathetic ganglion. The S2–4 sacral nerves also give off visceral branches; these, however, are not connected with the ganglia of the sympathetic trunk, but belong to the parasympathetic part of the autonomic system and run directly into the pelvic plexuses (Williams and Warwick, 1980).

Pain sensitive structures in the lumbosacral spine

Some spinal structures, e.g. the nucleus pulposus, cartilage plates and articular cartilages, have not been shown to have nerves despite repeated attempts to demonstrate them (Hirsch *et al.*, 1963; Rhodin, 1974; Stockwell, 1979). However, most anatomical structures in the spine have a sensory innervation, including the zygapophysial joint capsules, the outer anulus fibrosus, the major ligaments, the vertebral body, and all the posterior osseous structures (White and Panjabi, 1978). Sensory nerves are described in the periosteal covering of the vertebrae (Ikari, 1954; Pedersen *et al.*, 1956; Jackson *et al.*, 1966; Gronblad *et al.*, 1984), and in parts of the dura mater and epidural adipose tissue (Hovelacque, 1925; Pedersen *et al.*, 1956; Bridge, 1959; Edgar and Nundy, 1966; Wyke, 1970; Wyke, 1980b). Small diameter nerves, that are both paravascular and remote from blood vessels, that have free nerve endings, have been described in the synovial folds of the lumbar zygapophysial joints (Giles and Taylor, 1987a; Giles, 1988, 1989; Gronblad *et al.*, 1991a). Nervi nervorum are located on the dorsal root ganglion, as well as the peripheral nerves (Weinstein, 1991), and nerve fibres are seen in the walls of arteries and arterioles supplying spinal and paraspinal tissues (Hirsch *et al.*, 1963), adventitial sheaths of the epidural and paravertebral veins (Pedersen *et al.*, 1956; Bridge, 1959), cancellous bone of the vertebral bodies and their arches (Hovelacque1925; Roofe, 1940), and the paraspinal muscles (Iggo, 1961; Lim *et al.*, 1961).

It has frequently been claimed that in the adult, no nerve endings can be found in the intervertebral disc except for some free nerve endings located at the point where the superficial posterior fibres of the anulus fibrosus blend with the fibres of the posterior longitudinal ligament (Jung and Brunschwig, 1932; Tsukada, 1939; Roofe, 1940; Lazorthes *et al.*, 1947; Wiberg, 1949; Kuhlendahl, 1950; Kuhlendahl and Richter, 1952; Hirsch and Schajowicz, 1952; Ikari,

1954; Pedersen *et al.*, 1956; Malinsky, 1959; Ferlic, 1963; Hirsch *et al.*, 1963; Jackson *et al.*, 1966; Shinohara, 1970; Kumar and Davis, 1973; Bogduk *et al.*, 1981). It seems likely from clinical experience involving the injection of hypertonic saline (11%) under fluoroscopic control into the L4–5 and L5–S1 intervertebral discs in patients with low back pain (Hirsch *et al.*, 1963) that the disc is a source of pain. This view is supported by the observation that a patient's pain may be reproduced by discography (Holt, 1968) and that such pain is eliminated by injections of local anaesthetic into the disc (Bogduk, 1984). This may provide evidence of the presence of nociceptors in the intervertebral disc if the hypertonic saline does not leak out of the disc and irritate other pain sensitive structures, such as the posterior longitudinal ligament, which is rich in nociceptors (Dixon, 1980) and has been shown to contain substance P-positive profiles by Korkala *et al.* (1985). Holt (1968) performed discography, using sodium diatrizoate, on asymptomatic volunteers and noted that severe back pain resulted in 15% of the examinations as a result of extravasation of the sodium diatrizoate into the epidural space from the nucleus in 37% of patients.

Similar evidence of the presence of nociceptors in zygapophysial joints is provided by the observation that the injection of saline into zygapophysial joints produces both local and referred pain (Hirsch *et al.*, 1963), while local anaesthetic injections eliminate this pain (Kirkaldy-Willis, 1983; Aprill, 1986). According to Sherman (1963), a rich nerve supply can be demonstrated in human bones of any age, but the nerve fibres, which are usually associated with arterial vessels, are mostly unmyelinated, are probably derived from the autonomic nervous system, and are concerned with the regulation of blood flow. Duncan and Shim (1977) found that the intraosseous vessels in rabbits are richly supplied by adrenergic nerve fibres. In bone, there is a nerve supply to the endosteal surfaces of the medullary trabeculae and to the bone marrow, but none has been demonstrated in bone matrix (Miller and Kasahara, 1963; Reimann and Christensen, 1977). Sherman (1963) maintains that bone is relatively insensitive to painful 'stimuli' and is not usually a source of pain. On the other hand, localized expanding tumours in vertebrae, e.g. osteoid osteomas, are associated with both pain and local muscle spasm (Robbins, 1974; Parsons, 1980; Keim and Kirkaldy-Willis, 1987).

The clinical significance of these findings will be discussed in Chapter 15.

References

Allbrook, D. (1974) The intervertebral disc. In *Low Back Pain: Proceedings of a Conference on Low Back Pain* (L.T. Twomey, ed.). Western Australia, Institute of Technology, pp. 14–19.

Aprill, C. (1986) Lumbar facet joint arthrography and injection in the evaluation of painful disorders of the low back. (abstract.) *Presented at the International Society for the Study of the Lumbar Spine*, Dallas.

Auteroche, P. (1983) Innervation of the zygapophysial joints of the lumbar spine. *Anat. Clin.*, **5**, 17–28.

Bogduk, N. (1976) The anatomy of the lumbar intervertebral disc syndrome. *Med. J. Aust.*, **1**, 878–881.

Bogduk, N. (1980) The anatomy and physiology of lumbar back disability. *Bulletin of the Postgraduate Committee in Medicine*, University of Sydney, pp. 2–17.

Bogduk, N. (1981) The lumbar mamillo-accessory ligament: its anatomical and neurosurgical significance. *Spine*, **6**, 162–167.

Bogduk, N. (1983) The innervation of the lumbar spine. *Spine*, **8**, 286–293.

Bogduk, N. (1984) The rationale for patterns of neck and back pain. *Patient Management*, **8**, 13–21.

Bogduk, N. and Long, D.M. (1979) The anatomy of the so-called 'articular nerve'. *J. Neurosurg.*, **51**, 172–177.

Bogduk, N. and Twomey, L.T. (1991) *Clinical Anatomy of the Lumbar Spine*. Churchill Livingstone, Melbourne.

Bogduk, N., Tynan, W. and Wilson, A. S. (1981) The nerve supply to the human lumbar intervertebral disc. *J. Anat.*, **132**, 39–56.

Bogduk, N., Wilson, A.S. and Tynan, W. (1982) The lumbar dorsal rami. *J. Anat.*, **134**, 383–397.

Bradley, K.C. (1974) The anatomy of backache. *Aust. N.Z. J. Surg.*, **44**, 227–232.

Bradley, K.C. (1980) The posterior primary rami of segmental nerves. In *Aspects of Manipulative Therapy, Proceedings of a Multidisciplinary International Conference on Manipulative Therapy* (D. Dewhurst, E. F. Glasgow, P. Tahan *et al.* eds). Ramsay Ware Stockland, Melbourne, pp. 56–59.

Bridge, C.J. (1959) Innervation of spinal meninges and epidural structures. *Anat. Rec.*, **133**, 553–561.

Coggeshall, R.E., Emery, D.G., Ito, H. *et al.* (1977) Unmyelinated and small myelinated axons in rat ventral roots. *J. Comp. Neurol.*, **172**, 601–608.

Daube, J.R., Reagan, T.J., Sandok, B.A. *et al.* (1986) *Medical Neurosciences. An Approach to Anatomy Pathology and Physiology by Systems and Levels*, edn 2. Little, Brown Boston, p. 119.

Dee, R. (1978) The innervation of joints. In *The Joints and Synovial Fluid* (L. Sokoloff, ed.), Vol. 1. Academic Press, New York, pp. 177–204.

Dixon, A.St. (1980) Diagnosis of low back pain – sorting the complainers. In *The Lumbar Spine and Back Pain* (M. Jayson, ed.), 2nd edn. Pitman Medical, Kent, pp. 135–156.

Dockerty, M.B. and Love, J.G. (1940) Thickening and fibrosis (so-called hypertrophy) of the ligamentum flavum: a pathological study of fifty cases. *Proc. Staff Meet. Mayo Clin.*, **15**, 161–166.

Dripps, R.D., Eckenhoff, J.E. and Vandam, L.D. (1977) *Introduction to Anaesthesia: The Principles of Safe Practice*. W.B. Saunders, Philadelphia, pp. 358–360.

Duncan, C.P. and Shim, S.S. (1977) The autonomic nerve supply of bone. *J. Bone Joint Surg.*, **59B**, 323–330.

Edgar, M.A. and Ghadially, J.A. (1976) Innervation of the lumbar spine. *Clin. Orthop.*, **115**, 35–41.

Edgar, M.A. and Nundy, S. (1966) Innervation of the spinal dura mater. *J. Neurol. Neurosurg. Psychiatry* **29**, 530–534.

Ferlic, D.C. (1963) The nerve supply of the cervical intervertebral disc in man. *Johns Hopkins Hospital Bulletin*, **113**, 347-351.

Fick, R. (1904) *Handbuch der Anatomie und Mechanik der Gelenke*, Vol. 2. Verlag G. Fischer, Jena, pp. 77-89.

Gardner, D.L. (1978) Structure and function of connective tissue and joints. In *Copeman's Textbook of the Rheumatic Diseases* (J.T. Scott, ed.), 5th edn. Churchill Livingstone, London, pp. 78-124.

Gardner, E. (1950) Physiology of movable joints. *Physiol. Rev.*, **30**, 127-176.

Giles, L.G.F. (1988) Human lumbar zygapophysial joint inferior recess synovial folds: a light microscope examination. *Anat. Rec.*, **220**, 117-124.

Giles, L.G.F. (1989) *Anatomical Basis of Low Back Pain*. Williams and Wilkins, Baltimore, pp. 45, 60.

Giles, L.G.F. (1991) The relationship between the medial branch of the lumbar posterior primary ramus and the mamillo-accessory ligament. *J. Manipulative Physiol. Ther.,s* **14**, 189-192.

Giles, L.G.F. and Harvey, A.R. (1987) Immunohistochemical demonstration of nociceptors in the capsule and synovial folds of human zygapophysial joints. *Br. J. Rheumatol.*, **26**, 362-364.

Giles, L.G.F. and Taylor, J.R. (1987a) Human zygapophysial joint capsule and synovial fold innervation. *Br. J. Rheumatol.*, **26**, 993-998.

Giles, L.G.F. and Taylor, J.R. (1987b) Innervation of human lumbar zygapophysial joint synovial folds. *Acta Orthop. Scand.*, **58**, 43-46.

Giles, L.G.F., Taylor, J.R. and Cockson, A. (1986) Human zygapophysial joint synovial folds. *Acta Anat.*, **126**, 110-114.

Gronblad, M., Liesi, P., Korkala, O. *et al.* (1984) Innervation of human bone periosteum by peptidergic nerves. *Anat. Rec.*, **209**, 297-299.

Gronblad, M., Weinstein, J.N. and Santavirta, S. (1991a) Immunohistochemical observations on spinal tissue innervation. *Acta Orthop. Scand.*, **62**, 614-622.

Gronblad, M., Korkala, O., Konttinen, Y.T. *et al.* (1991b) Silver Impregnation and immunohistochemical study of nerves in lumbar facet joint plical tissue. *Spine*, **16**, 34-38.

Hadley, L.A. (1964) *Anatomico-Roentgenographic Studies of the Spine*. Charles C. Thomas, Springfield, IL, pp. 186,189,190.

Haldeman, S. (1980) The neurophysiology of spinal pain syndromes. In *Modern Developments in the Principles and Practice of Chiropractic* (S. Haldeman, ed.). Appleton-Century-Crofts, New York, pp. 119-141.

Hilton, J. (1891) *Rest and Pain. A Course of Lectures*, 2nd edn (reprinted from the last London edition.) P.W. Gardfield, Cincinnati, OH.

Hirsch, C., Ingelmark, B.E. and Miller, M. (1963) The anatomical basis for low back pain. *Acta Orthop. Scand.*, **33**, 1-17.

Hirsch, H. and Schajowicz, F. (1952) Studies on structural changes in the lumbar anulus fibrosus. *Acta Orthop. Scand.*, **22**, 184-231.

Holt, A.P. (1968) A question of lumbar discography. *J. Bone Joint Surg.*, **50A**, 720-725.

Hovelacque, A. (1925) Le nerf sinuvertebral. *Ann. d'Anat. Path.*, **5**, 435-443.

Iggo, A. (1961) Non-myelinated afferent fibres from mammalian skeletal muscle. *J. Physiol. (Lond.)*,**155**, 52P.

Ikari, C. (1954) A study of the mechanism of low back pain. The neurohistological examination of the disease. *J. Bone Joint Surg.*, **36A**, 1272-1281.

Jackson, H.C., Winklemann, R.K. and Bickel, W.H. (1966) Nerve endings in the human lumbar spinal column and related structures. *J. Bone Joint Surg.*, **48A**, 1272-1281.

Jung, A. and Brunschwig, A. (1932) Recherches histologique des articulations des corps vertébraux. *Presse Med.*, **40**, 316-317.

Kandel, E.R. and Schwartz, J.H. (1981) *Principles of Neural Science*. Elsevier/North-Holland, New York, p. 168.

Keim, H.A. and Kirkaldy-Willis, W.H. (1987) Low back pain. *Ciba Clinical Symposia* **39**, Ciba-Geigy.

Kimmel, D.L. (1961a) Innervation of spinal dura mater and dura mater of the posterior cranial fossa. *Neurology*, **11**, 800-809.

Kimmel, D.L. (1961b) The nerves of the cranial dura mater and their significance in dural headache and referred pain. *Chicago Medical School Quarterly*, **22**, 16-26.

Kirkaldy-Willis, W.H. (1983) A comprehensive outline of treatment. In *Managing Low Back Pain* (W.H. Kirkaldy-Willis, ed.). Churchill Livingstone, New York, pp. 147-160.

Konttinen, Y.T., Gronblad, M., Antti-Poika, I. *et al.* (1990) Neuroimmunohistochemical analysis of peridiscal nociceptive neural elements. *Spine*, **15**, 383-386.

Korkala, O., Gronblad, M., Liesi, P. *et al.* (1985) Immunohisto chemical demonstration of nociceptors in the ligamentous structures of the lumbar spine. *Spine*, **10**, 156-157.

Kuhlendahl, H. (1950) Uber die beziehungen zwischen anatomischer und funktioneller Laision der lumbalen zwischenwirbelscheiben. *Artzl Wschr.*, **5**, 281.

Kuhlendahl, H. and Richter, H. (1952) Morphologie und funktionelle pathologie der lendenbandlscheiben. *Langenbecks Arch. Klin. Chir.*, **272**, 519.

Kumar, S. and Davis, P.R. (1973) Lumbar vertebral innervation and intra-abdominal pressure. *J Anat.*, **114**, 47-53.

Kuslich, S.D., Ulstrom, C.L. and Michael, E.J. (1991) The tissue origin of low back pain and sciatica: a report of pain response to tissue stimulation during operations on the lumbar spine using local anesthesia. *Orthop. Clin. North Am.*, **22**, 181-187.

Lazorthes, G. (1972) Les branches postérieures des nerfs rachidiens et le plan articulaire vertébral posterieur. *Ann. Med. Phys.*, **15**, 192-202.

Lazorthes, G. and Gaubert, J. (1956) *Innervation des Articulations Interapophysaires Vertébrales*. C R Assoc Anat, Lisbon.

Lazorthes, G. and Juskiewenski, S. (1964) Etude comparative des branches postérieures des nerfs dorsaux et lombaires et de leurs rapports avec les articulations interapophysaires vertébrales. *Bull. Assoc. Anat. ILIXe Réunion Madrid*, 10 Septembere, pp. 1025-1033.

Lazorthes, G., Poulhes, J. and Espagno, J. (1947) Etude sur les nerfs sinu-vertébraux lombaires. Le Nerf de Roofe éxiste-t-il? *Compte Rendu de l'Association des Anatomistes*, **34**, 317-320.

Lewin, T., Moffett, B. and Viidik, A. (1961) The morphology of the lumbar synovial intervertebral arches. *Acta Morphol Neerlando-Scandinavica*, **4**, 299-319.

Lewinnek, G.E. (1983) Management of low back pain and sciatica. *Int. Anaesthesiol. Clin.*, **21**, 61-78.

Lim, R.K.S., Guzman, F. and Rodgers, D.W. (1961) Note on the muscle receptors concerned with pain. In *Symposium on Muscle Receptors* (D. Barker, ed.). Hong Kong University Press, Hong Kong.

Lynch, M.C. and Taylor, J.F. (1986) Facet joint injection for low back pain. *J. Bone Joint Surg.*, **68B**, 138-141.

Maigne, J-Y., Maigne, R. and Guerin-Surville, H. (1991) The lumbar mamillo-accessory foramen: a study of 203 lumbosacral spines. *Surg. Radiol. Anat.*, **13**, 29-32.

Malinsky, J. (1959) The ontogenetic development of nerve terminations in the intervertebral discs of man. *Acta Anat.*, **38**, 96-113.

Miller, M.R. and Kasahara, M. (1963) Observations on the innervation of human long bones. *Anat. Rec.*, **145**, 13.

Moore, K.L. (1992) *Clinically Oriented Anatomy*, 3rd edn. Williams and Wilkins, Baltimore.

Nade, S., Bell, E. and Wyke, B.D. (1980) The innervation of the lumbar spinal joints and its significance. *Proc. Rep. JBJS*, **62B**, 255.

Paris, S.V. (1983) Anatomy as related to function and pain. *Orthop. Clin. North Am.*, **14**, 475-489.

Paris, S.V., Nyberg, R., Mooney, V. *et al.* (1980) What's new for low back pain and just plain pain? *Medical World News*, **21**, 2128-2143.

Parsons, V. (1980) *A Colour Atlas of Bone Disease*. Wolfe Medical Publications, Holland, p. 61.

Pedersen, H.E., Blunck, C.F.J. and Gardner, E. (1956) The anatomy of lumbosacral posterior rami and meningeal branches of spinal nerves (sinu-vertebral nerves) with an experimental study of their function. *J. Bone Joint Surg.*, **38A**, 377-391.

Ramsey, R.H. (1966) The anatomy of the ligamenta flava. *Clin. Orthop.*, **44**, 129-140.

Reilly, J., Yong-Hing, K., MacKay, R.W. *et al.* (1978) Pathological anatomy of the lumbar spine. In *Disorders of the Lumbar Spine* (A.J. Helfet and D.M. Gruebel, eds). J.B. Lippincott, Philadelphia, pp. 26-50.

Reimann, I. and Christensen, S.B. (1977) A histological demonstration of nerves in subchondral bone. *Acta Orthop. Scand.*, **48**, 345-352.

Resnick, D. (1985) Degenerative diseases of the vertebral column. *Radiology*, **156**, 3-14.

Rhodin, J.A.G. (1974) *Histology: A Text and Atlas*. Oxford University Press, London.

Robbins, S.L. (1974) *Pathologic Basis of Disease*. W.B. Saunders, Philadelphia, p. 1451.

Roofe, P.G. (1940) Innervation of anulus fibrosus and posterior longitudinal ligament. *Arch. Neurol. Psychiatry*, **44**, 100-103.

Rydevik, B., Brown, M.D. and Lundborg, G. (1984) Pathoanatomy and pathophysiology of nerve root compression. *Spine*, **9**, 7-15.

Schaumburg, H.H. and Spencer, P.S. (1975) Pathology of spinal root compression. In *The Research Status of Spinal Manipulative Therapy (Monograph No. 15)* (M. Goldstein, ed.). National Institute of Neurological and Communicative Disorders and Stroke, Bethesda, MD, pp. 141-148.

Sherman, M.S. (1963) Nerves of bone. *J. Bone Joint Surg.*, **45A**, 522-528.

Shinohara, H. (1970) A study on lumbar disc lesions. *J. Jpn Orthoped. Assoc.*, **44**, 553.

Spurling, R.G. and Bradford, F.K. (1939) Neurologic aspects of herniated nucleus pulposus. *JAMA*, **113**, 2019-2022.

Stockwell, R.A. (1979) *Biology of Cartilage Cells*. Cambridge University Press, Cambridge, p. 1.

Sunderland, S. (1975) Anatomical perivertebral influences on the intervertebral foramen. In *The Research Status of Spinal Manipulative Therapy (Monograph No. 15)* (M.

Goldstein, ed.). National Institute of Neurological and Communicative Disorders and Stroke, Bethesda, MD, pp. 129-140.

Sunderland, S. (1978) Traumatized nerves, roots, and ganglia: musculoskeletal factors and neuro-pathological consequences. In *The Neurobiologic Mechanisms in Manipulative Therapy* (M. Korr, ed.). Plenum Press, New York, pp. 137-166.

Sunderland, S. (1979) Advances in diagnosis and treatment of root and peripheral nerve injury. *Adv. Neurol.*, **22**, 271-305.

Tortora, G.J. and Grabowski, N.P. (1993) *Principles of Anatomy and Physiology*, 5th edn. Harper and Row, New York, pp. 292-294.

Tsukada, K. (1939) Histologische studien uber die zwischenwirbelscheibe des menschen altersvanderungen. *Mitt. Akad. Kioto*, **25**, 1-29.

Vick, N.A. (1976) The peripheral nervous system. In *Grinker's Neurology*, 7th edn. Charles C. Thomas, Springfield, IL, pp. 101-111.

Von Luschka, H. (1850) *Die nerven des menschlichen wirbelkanales*. Laupp and Siebeck, Tubingen.

Weinstein, J.N. (1991) Anatomy and neurophysiologic mechanisms of spinal pain. In *The Adult Spine: Principles and Practice* (J.N. Frymoyer, ed.). Raven Press, New York, pp. 593-610.

White, A.A., III and Pinjabi, M.M. (1978) *Clinical Biomechanics of the Spine*. J.B. Lippincott, Philadelphia, p. 279.

Wiberg, C. (1949) Back pain in relation to the nerve supply of the intervertebral disc. *Acta Orthop. Scand.*, **18–19**, 214.

Williams, P.L. and Warwick, T. (1980) *Gray's Anatomy*, 36th edn. Churchill Livingstone, London, pp. 1086, 1131.

Woollard, H.H. (1926) The innervation of the heart. *J. Anat.*, **60**, 345-373.

Wyke, B.D. (1967) The neurology of joints. *Ann. R. Coll. Surg. Engl.*, **41**, 25.

Wyke, B.D. (1969) *Principles of General Neurology*. Elsevier, Amsterdam, pp. 48-49.

Wyke, B.D. (1970) The neurological basis of thoracic spinal pain. *Rheumatol. Phys. Med.*, **10**, 356-367.

Wyke, B.D. (1972) Articular neurology: a review. *Physiotherapy*, **58**, 94-99.

Wyke, B.D. (1975) Neurology of the cervical spinal joints. *Physiotherapy*, **65**, 72-76.

Wyke, B.D. (1979) Neurological mechanisms in the experience of pain. *Acupunct. Electrother. Res. Int. J.*, **4**, 27-35.

Wyke, B.D. (1980a) Articular neurology and manipulative therapy. *Aspects of Manipulative Therapy*, Lincoln Institute of Health, Melbourne, pp. 67-74.

Wyke, B.D. (1980b) The neurology of low back pain. In *The Lumbar Spine and Back Pain* (M.I.V. Jayson, ed.), 2nd edn. Pitman Medical, Kent, pp. 265-339.

Wyke, B.D. (1981) The neurology of joints: a review of general principles. *Clin. Rheum. Dis.*, **7**, 223-239.

Wyke, B.D. (1982) Receptor systems in lumbosacral tissues in relation to the production of low back pain. In *Symposium on Idiopathic Low Back Pain* (A.A. White, S.L. Gordon, eds). CV Mosby, St Louis, pp. 97-107.

Wyke, B.D. and Polacek, P. (1975) Articular neurology: the present position. *J. Bone Joint Surg.*, **57B**, 401.

Zukschwerdt, L., Emminger, E., Biedermann, F. *et al.* (1955) *Wirbelgelenk und Bandscheibe*. Hippokrates-Verlag, Stuttgart.

15

Nerves, neuropeptides and inflammation in spinal tissues: mechanisms of back pain

Mats Grönblad and Johanna Virri

Introduction

There is currently a need for further basic knowledge regarding the innervation of spinal tissues and neurotransmitter and neuromodulator substances present in both uninjured and injured spinal tissues (Weinstein *et al.*, 1988a; Grönblad *et al.*, 1991; Weinstein, 1992; Kääpä *et al.*, 1994). Basic science research should be directed at answering questions such as: How do the nerves and nerve chemicals present in spinal tissues react to tissue injury and inflammation? Is there a difference in the type of inflammatory reaction in various types of spinal tissue injury? Does injury in the intervertebral disc, in particular, lead to an immunologic response and which are the cells and chemicals mediating such a response? What is, ultimately, the role of all the above in mechanisms of back pain, spinal tissue healing and degradation (Grönblad *et al.*, 1991; Weinstein, 1992; Tolonen *et al.*, 1995)?

As was pointed out by Wyke (1982), pain in the low back may originate in one or several of a number of different tissues. Due to the intricate innervation of these tissues and of the low back as a whole (Bogduk, 1983; Bogduk *et al.*, 1989; Gillette *et al.*, 1994), localizing such low back pain in a clinical setting to a particular tissue will generally prove difficult. In most back pain patients the specific pathophysiology or the pathoanatomic correlate of the pain will remain unknown (Nachemson, 1992; Frymoyer, 1992) (Figure 15.1).

However, in several recent elegant injection studies (Aprill, 1991; Barnsley *et al.*, 1993; Bogduk and Aprill, 1993; Schwarzer *et al.*, 1994a,b) investigators have

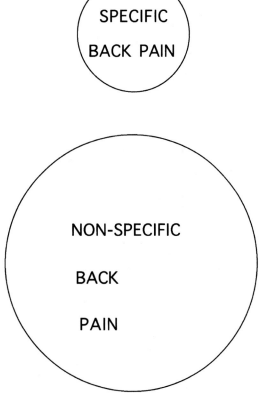

Figure 15.1 Most low back pain is non-specific. The pain generator is difficult to localize and the mechanism of pain difficult to characterize.

been successful in their attempts to discriminate between pain originating in the intervertebral disc and in the facet joint. Similar studies have also implicated the sacroiliac joint as a source of back pain symptoms (Fortin *et al.*, 1994; Schwarzer *et al.*, 1995). Moreover, convincing experimental evidence has been presented that alterations of the intradiscal chemical microenvironment (Weinstein *et al.*, 1988a) and, perhaps mechanical influence, e.g. exposure to vibration (Weinstein, 1986; Weinstein *et al.*, 1988b; McLain and Weinstein, 1991, 1993), will have an effect on local nerves/nerve endings present and, possibly through neural circuitry, result in alterations in dorsal root ganglion neuropeptide levels. There may also, of course, be various more direct effects on the ganglion (Howe *et al.*, 1977; Rydevik *et al.*, 1984), which has been shown to be uniquely mechanosensitive even in an uninjured state (Howe *et al.*, 1976, 1977, 1979). Important sensory cells of the dorsal root ganglia are specifically sensitive to capsaicin, indicating involvement in pain modulation, and are also known to be excited or sensitized by various inflammatory substances, e.g. bradykinin (Figure 15.2) and prostaglandin E2 (Baccaglini and Hogan, 1983; Åkerman and Grönblad, 1992; Grönblad and Åkerman, 1992).

These capsaicin sensitive sensory neurons of the dorsal root ganglion are also sensitive to an acid environment (Bevan and Yeats, 1991; Petersen and LaMotte, 1993), which may be important in, e.g. inflammation-induced back pain syndromes and sciatica. Such tissue and chemical interactions may be linked to both mechanisms of back pain and to basic tissue properties, including responses to injury of spinal tissues (Grönblad, 1991). Disruption of the end-plate may be an additional mechanism of back pain (Hsu *et al.*, 1988) and may be linked to back pain caused by disc degeneration.

New knowledge of spinal tissue innervation based upon information from recent immunocytochemical studies

There is presently a consensus of opinion, including that based upon immunocytochemical studies, that only the outermost part of the anulus is innervated in a normal, uninjured and non-degenerated disc, whereas no nerves can be observed in the nucleus pulposus (Roofe, 1940; Hirsch *et al.*, 1963; Yoshizawa *et al.*, 1980; Bogduk *et al.*, 1981, 1988; Bogduk, 1985; Grönblad *et al.*, 1991; Ashton *et al.*, 1992) (Figure 15.3). In the recent immunohistochemical study on human disc tissue by Ashton and coworkers (1992), nerve fibres were most predominant in the outermost 4 mm of the anulus. Substance P fibres were noted deeper in the anulus (Ashton *et al.*, 1992). In younger subjects (juvenile discs) both blood vessels and nerves may penetrate deep into the disc and also substance P nerves can be observed (Figure 15.4). They are, however, mostly associated with the blood vessels and are probably mostly involved in vasoregulation. It has been suggested (Coppes *et al.*, 1990), although not yet confirmed, that nerves could

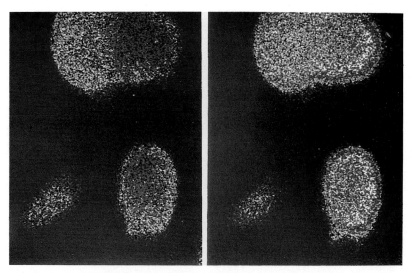

Figure 15.2 Rat dorsal root ganglion (DRG) sensory neurons (left) respond to stimulation by bradykinin and other inflammatory agents *in vitro*. Following such stimulation an increase in intracellular free Ca^{2+} (right) can be demonstrated (Grönblad and Åkerman, 1992).

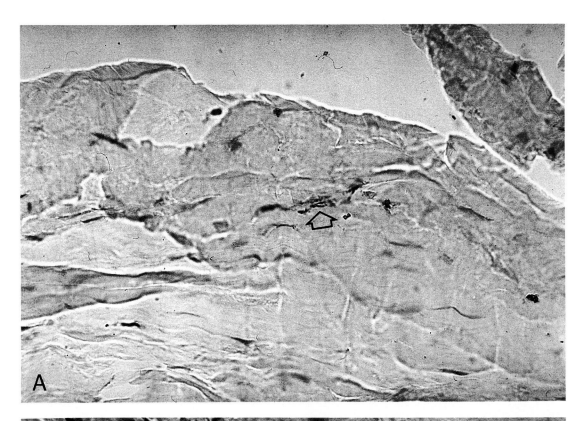

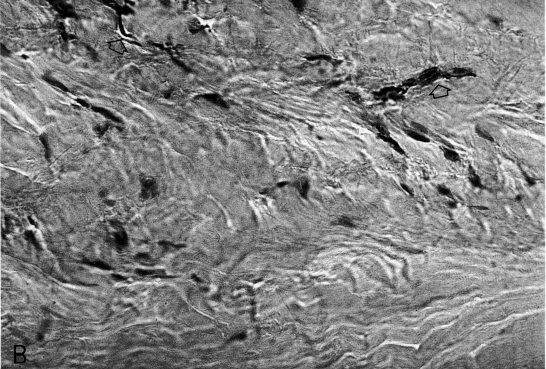

Figure 15.3 Nerves (arrows) shown with an antibody to protein gene product (PGP) 9.5, a general neural marker, in the (A) anterior, and (B) posterior, part of an intact, non-degenerated human lumbar intervertebral disc. Avidin-biotin-peroxidase complex (ABC) immunostaining, haematoxylin counterstaining. Original magnification ×370.

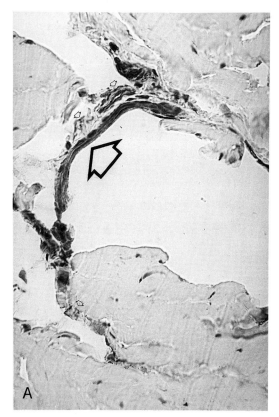

Figure 15.4 In juvenile intervertebral discs, blood vessels (large arrow) and accompanying nerves (small arrows) (A, B; PGP antibody) are present in deeper parts of the anulus. Substance P immunoreactive nerves (arrows) (C) also accompany blood vessels. ABC immunostaining, haematoxylin counterstaining. Original magnification ×370.

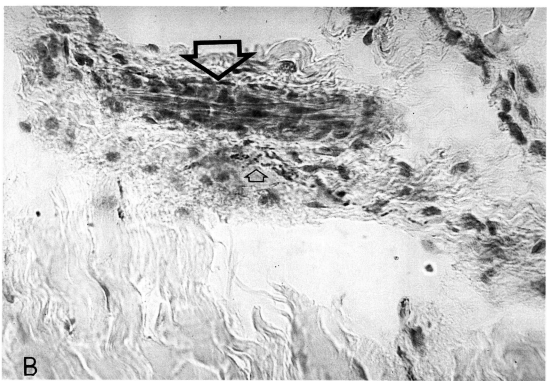

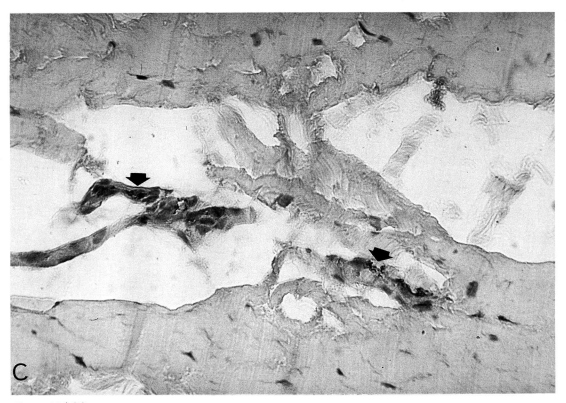

Figure 15.4 (C)

be present in deeper parts of discs that have undergone severe degeneration. In our studies on a limited number of degenerated discs we have not, so far, observed any nerves deeper in the disc, even if they may be abundant on and near blood vessels that have presumably grown through the periphery of the disc. It is our impression, however, that nerves can more easily be demonstrated in degenerated discs than in macroscopically normal discs. Further detailed immunocytochemical studies on degenerated painful and painless discs will be of great importance in this respect. It should also be further determined how different types of discal nerves (Weinstein *et al.*, 1988a; Ashton *et al.*, 1992) (Figures 15.5 and 15.6) respond to disc tissue injury (Kääpä *et al.*, 1994).

In disc herniations, small newly formed blood vessels are often very abundant. They may even form large capillary networks on the surface of, or penetrating deep into, the herniated disc tissue (Figure 15.7). Our results suggest that such blood vessels may be present in 80% or more of disc herniations (Virri *et al.*, 1994), and that they are often numerous. In herniated discs it has also been possible to demonstrate small dot-like nerve terminals, not only nerve fibres, and both sensory and sympathetic nerve

endings (Figure 15.8). Such nerve terminals are presumably involved in mechanisms of discogenic pain and in the vasoregulation of the newly formed small blood vessels (Ashton *et al.*, 1994). They strongly implicate the disc, at least the injured disc, as a source of low back pain symptoms.

There are also now several published immunocytochemical and neurophysiological studies on the demonstration of various types of nerves and neuropeptides in facet joint tissues (Giles, 1989; Yamashita *et al.*, 1990; Grönblad *et al.*, 1991), particularly the joint capsule and synovial folds (Giles, 1987; Giles and Harvey, 1987; Ashton *et al.*, 1992; McLain, 1994), which through mechanisms of stretching, pinching or, perhaps, chemical irritation may contribute to low back pain. There is also recent immunocytochemical evidence of substance P nerves, suggested to be involved in low back pain, in erosion channels of subchondral bone in degenerated facet joints, but not in non-degenerated facet joint specimens (Beaman *et al.*, 1993). Synovial folds within the joint may by irritation of local sensory nerves (Grönblad *et al.*, 1991; Giles, 1987; Giles and Harvey, 1987) by, for example inflammation, perhaps as a result of impingement (Giles, 1986; Konttinen *et al.*, 1990), contribute to back pain. This is supported by several

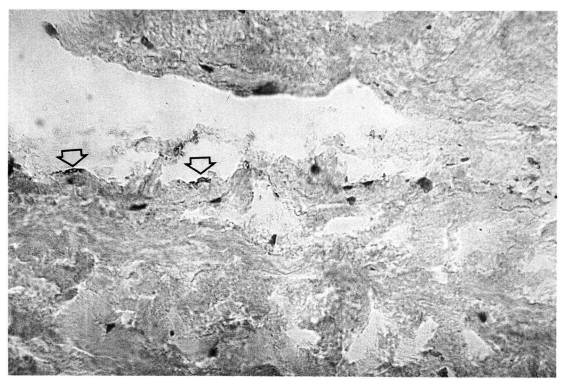

Figure 15.5 Posterior part of a degenerated human L5/S1 disc. Tiny substance P nerves (arrows). ABC immunostaining, haematoxylin counterstaining. Original magnification ×370.

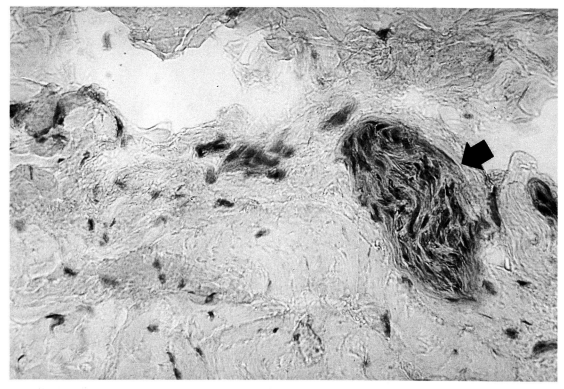

Figure 15.6 A larger mechanoreceptor nerve (arrow) stains with the PGP antibody in the anterior part of an intact human lumbar disc. ABC immunostaining, haematoxylin counterstaining. Original magnification ×370.

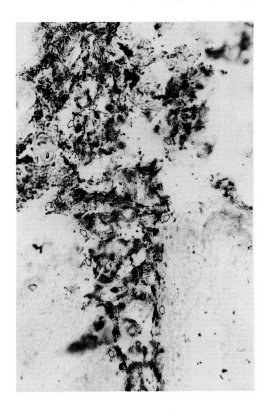

Figure 15.7 A large capillary network penetrating into a herniated disc. Abundant endothelial cells (arrows) can be demonstrated due to their specific intense staining with a monoclonal antibody to Ulex Europaeus. Immune staining with alkaline phosphatase anti-alkaline phosphatase (APAAP), haematoxylin counterstaining. Original magnification ×370.

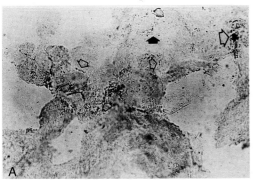
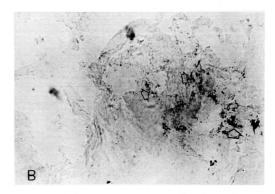

Figure 15.8 Herniated disc tissue. (A) Tiny substance P nerve terminals and thin varicose nerves can be observed (open arrows). Note also a separate cluster comprised of a few very tiny sensory nerve endings (black arrow). (B) Similar tiny dot-like sympathetic nerve terminals (arrows) can be observed after immunostaining with a C-flanking peptide of neuropeptide Y (CPON) antibody. ABC immunostaining, enhancement of peroxidase reaction product with glucose oxidase-nickel sulphate-3,3′ diaminobenzidine (DAB), haematoxylin counterstaining. Original magnification ×370. (Courtesy of Dr Tove Palmgren, Spine Research Unit research team, Helsinki, Finland.)

recent clinical pain provocation studies on patients with intractable low back pain syndromes (Aprill *et al.*, 1990; Aprill and Bogduk, 1992; Bogduk and Aprill, 1993; Schwarzer *et al.*, 1994), even if results from several recent randomized clinical studies have suggested that much of the observed therapeutic effect with such injections is non-specific or due to factors other than the injection *per se* (Jackson *et al.*, 1988;

Lilius *et al.*, 1989; Carette *et al.*, 1991; Jackson, 1992). The extent of observable abnormal illness behaviour (Waddell *et al.*, 1980; Hirsch *et al.*, 1991; Chan *et al.*, 1993; Pilowsky, 1993) is evidently one such important predictor for treatment response (Lilius *et al.*, 1989) and has to be taken into consideration when assessing patients with prolonged back pain (Hirsch *et al.*, 1991).

Nerves and nerve endings can also be demonstrated in tissue samples that have been removed from around symptomatic nerve roots (Murphy, 1977) (Figure 15.9), but to date, the determination of free sensory nerve endings, unrelated to blood vessels, has not been the subject of detailed studies in this important spinal area. Possibly such nerve endings, located in the epidural space, could react to local mechanical and chemical (inflammatory) stimulation, and contribute to back pain in addition to the adjacent nerve root. Furthermore, local inflammation in a herniated disc could perhaps irritate neural elements both in the disc itself and in the epidural space, in addition to effects on the nerve root. In this respect, the dorsal root ganglion

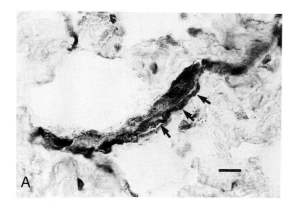

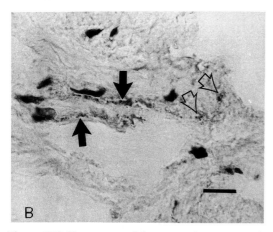

Figure 15.9 Tissue removed from around a symptomatic nerve root. (A) A PGP immunoreactive nerve (arrows) follows a tortuous course around a blood vessel. (B) Non-vascular varicose nerves and tiny dot-like nerve terminals (black arrows) can be observed after immunostaining with a synaptophysin antibody. Note also small clusters of dot-like free nerve terminals (open arrows). Note morphological similarity to nerve terminals observed in herniated disc tissue (Figure 15.8). ABC immunostaining, haematoxylin counterstaining. Bar = 10 micrometers.

(Weinstein *et al.*, 1988a) could also be an important focus causing low back pain, perhaps depending on its anatomical location in the nerve root canal (Hasue *et al.*, 1989).

Inflammation in spinal tissues – possible relation to low back pain and sciatica

Inflammation may be an important mechanism in both sciatica and discogenic back pain. It has been suggested by several investigators (Pankovich and Korngold, 1967; Marshall and Trethewie, 1973; Naylor *et al.*, 1975; Gertzbein, 1977; Marshall *et al.*, 1977) that disc tissue, perhaps following injury or degenerative alterations, may cause an immunologic, perhaps even an autoimmune, tissue reaction (Bobechko and Hirsch, 1965; Gertzbein *et al.*, 1975). However, such mechanisms are presently poorly understood. It has been reported that intradiscally injected steroids are not necessarily more effective than a local anesthetic, even though discs are painful at discography (Simmons *et al.*, 1992). Interestingly, porcine disc nucleus pulposus tissue was recently shown to cause an inflammatory reaction (Olmarker *et al.*, 1994a,b) and also in the dog, disc tissue implanted epidurally caused an observable local inflammation (McCarron *et al.*, 1987). Similarly, in herniated disc tissue there is biochemical evidence of inflammation (Saal *et al.*, 1990; Franson *et al.*, 1992) and also inflammatory cell infiltration (Table 15.1), presumably from the newly-formed numerous small blood vessels (Grönblad *et al.*, 1994; Virri *et al.*, 1994; Tolonen *et al.*, 1995). This tissue reaction was observed to be dominated by macrophages, which are numerously present in about 50% of disc herniations (Grönblad *et al.*, 1994) (Figure 15.10). In about 20% of disc herniations there are abundant lymphocytes (Figure 15.11), also activated T lymphocytes expressing interleukin-2 receptor, suggesting an active immune response in at least some of the herniated discs. This inflammatory response is often

Table 15.1 *Monoclonal antibodies used for studying inflammatory cells in herniated disc tissue (Grönblad et al., 1994; Virri et al., 1994, 1995)*

CD-code	Cell type
CD68	Macrophage
Ber-MaC3	Activated monocyte/macrophage
CD2	T-lymphocyte
CD25	Activated T-lymphocyte
CD22	B-lymphocyte
CD15	Granulocyte/neutrophil
IL-1β	Cytokine

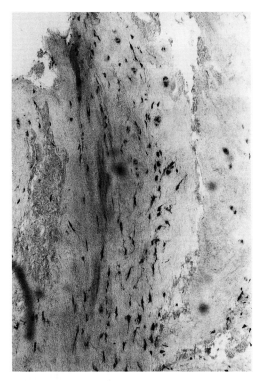

Figure 15.10 Macrophage cells are often abundant in disc herniations. APAAP immunostaining with a monoclonal CD68 antibody, haematoxylin counterstaining. Original magnification ×93.

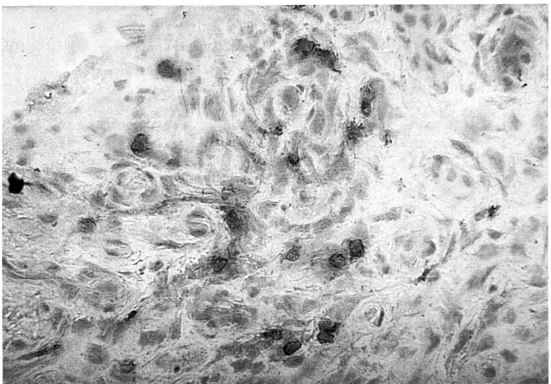

Figure 15.11 T cells in a disc herniation. APAAP immunostaining with CD2 antibody, haematoxylin counterstaining. Original magnification ×370.

accompanied by the presence of interleukin-1 beta immunoreactive cells, which contribute to the local inflammatory reaction (Grönblad *et al.*, 1994). It is not presently known, however, which type of inflammation occurs, if at all, in degenerated discs that have not yet progressed to the stage of herniation. We presently know, however, that inflammatory lymphocytes, both T and B cells, suggesting both a cell-mediated and a humoral immune reaction, are more prevalent in sequestrated discs than in extrusions, and evidently totally absent in protrusions (Virri *et al.*, 1995). We do not, however, fully comprehend the implications of such findings at the cellular and tissue level with respect to the clinically often observed decrease in disc herniation size and the resolution of symptoms with time (Saal *et al.*, 1990; Maigne *et al.*, 1992). It is our impression that pathophysiologically, at the cellular and molecular level, there may be variation between disc herniations. Our results also suggest a correlation between a tight straight leg raising test (SLR) and inflammatory cell occurrence in disc herniations (Virri *et al.*, 1995). Interestingly, we have repeatedly observed such a significant correlation between the SLR and the presence of activated T lymphocytes in particular (Virri *et al.*, 1995).

Taken together, all these new observations suggest inflammation, and perhaps an immune reaction, as possible components in the tissue response that follows disc tissue injury. In further support of an immune reaction we have, in our ongoing studies, obtained immunocytochemical evidence of immunoglobulin (Ig) deposition in herniated disc tissue (Tolonen *et al.*, 1995). IgM deposits particularly seem to be often present in herniated discs (Figure 15.12), supporting prior reports based upon biochemical measurement (Spiliopoulou *et al.*, 1994). Finally, the interaction between nerves, neuropeptides and inflammation in the production of low back pain and sciatica will require further study.

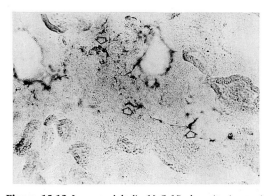

Figure 15.12 Immunoglobulin M (IgM) deposits (arrows) in a sequestrated disc. ABC immunostaining, haematoxylin counterstaining. Original magnification ×370. (Courtesy of Dr Aklilu Habtemariam, Spine Research Unit research team, Helsinki, Finland.)

Acknowledgements

Financial support from the following foundations is gratefully acknowledged: The Paulo Foundation, The Yrjö Jahnsson Foundation, The Memorial Foundation of Dorothea Olivia, Jarl Walter and Karl Walter Perklen, Helsinki, Finland. We also wish to acknowledge research funding from Helsinki University Central Hospital. For kind support and advice during our studies of neuropeptide nerves in human spinal tissues we wish to thank Professor Julia M. Polak, Department of Histochemistry, Royal Postgraduate Medical School, Hammersmith Hospital, London, UK.

References

Åkerman, K.E.O. and Grönblad, M. (1992) Intracellular free Ca^{2+} and Na+ in response to capsaicin in cultured dorsal root ganglion cells. *Neurosci. Lett.*, **147**, 13–15.

Aprill, C.N. (1991) Diagnostic disc injection. In *The Adult Spine: Principles and Practice* (J.W. Frymoyer, ed.). Raven Press, New York, pp. 403–442.

Aprill, C. and Bogduk, N. (1992) The prevalence of cervical zygapophysial joint pain: a first approximation. *Spine*, **17**, 744–747.

Aprill, C., Dwyer, A. and Bogduk, N. (1990) Cervical zygapophysial joint pain patterns. II: a clinical evaluation. *Spine*, **15**, 458–461.

Ashton, I.K., Ashton, B.A., Gibson, S.J. *et al.* (1992) Morphological basis for back pain: the demonstration of nerve fibers and neuropeptides in the lumbar facet joint capsule but not in ligamentum flavum. *J. Orthop. Res.*, **10**, 72–78.

Ashton, I.K., Roberts, S., Jaffray, D.C. *et al.* (1992) Immunochemical demonstration of innervation and neurotransmitters in the human intervertebral disc. Presented at the annual meeting of the *International Society for the Study of the Lumbar Spine*, May 20–24, Chicago, Illinois.

Ashton, I.K., Walsh, D.A., Polak, J.M. and Eisenstein, S.M. (1994) Substance P binding sites in the human intervertebral disc. Presented at the annual meeting of the *International Society for the Study of the Lumbar Spine*, June 21–25, Seattle, WA.

Baccaglini, P.I. and Hogan, P.G. (1983) Some rat sensory neurons in culture express characteristics of differentiated pain sensory cells. *Proc. Natl. Acad. Sci. USA*, **80**, 594–598.

Barnsley, L., Lord, S. and Bogduk, N. (1993) Comparative local anaesthetic blocks in the diagnosis of cervical zygapophysial joint pain. *Pain*, **55**, 99–106.

Beaman, D.N., Graziano, G.P., Glover, R.A. *et al.* (1993) Substance P innervation of lumbar spine facet joints. *Spine*, **18**, 1044–1049.

Bevan, S. and Yeats, J. (1991) Protons activate a cation conductance in a subpopulation of rat dorsal root ganglion neurones. *J. Physiol.*, **433**, 145–161.

Bobechko, W.P. and Hirsch, C. (1965) Auto-immune response to nucleus pulposus in the rabbit. *J. Bone Joint Surg.*, **47B**, 574–580.

Bogduk, N. (1983) The innervation of the lumbar spine. *Spine*, **8**, 286-293.

Bogduk, N. (1985) The innervation of the vertebral column. *Aust. J. Physiother.*, **31**, 89-94.

Bogduk, N. and Aprill, C. (1993) On the nature of neck pain, discography and cervical zygapophysial joint blocks. *Pain*, **54**, 213-217.

Bogduk, N., Tynan, W. and Wilson, A.S. (1981) The nerve supply to the human lumbar intervertebral discs. *J. Anat.*, **132**, 39-56.

Bogduk, N., Windsor, M. and Inglis, A. (1988) The innervation of the cervical intervertebral discs. *Spine*, **13**, 2-8.

Carette, S., Marcoux, S., Truchon, R. *et al.* (1991) A controlled trial of corticosteroid injections into facet joints for chronic low back pain. *N. Engl. J. Med.*, **325**, 1002-1007.

Chan, C.W., Goldman, S., Ilstrup, D.M. *et al.* (1993) The pain drawing and Waddell's nonorganic physical signs in chronic low-back pain. *Spine*, **18**, 1717-1722.

Coppes, M.H., Marani, E., Thomeer, R.T.W.M. *et al.* (1990) Innervation of anulus fibrosis in low back pain. *Lancet* (Letter), **336**, 189-190.

Fortin, J.D., Aprill, C.N., Ponthieux, B. *et al.* (1994) Sacroiliac joint: pain referral maps upon applying a new injection/arthrography technique. Part II: clinical evaluation. *Spine*, **19**, 1483-1489.

Franson, R.C., Saal, J.S. and Saal, J.A. (1992) Human disc phospholipase A2 is inflammatory. *Spine*, **17**, S129-S132.

Frymoyer, J.W. (1992) Predicting disability from low back pain. *Clin. Orthop.*, **279**, 101-109.

Gertzbein, S.D. (1977) Degenerative disk disease of the lumbar spine: immunological implications. *Clin. Orthop.*, **129**, 68-71.

Gertzbein, S.D., Tile, M., Gross, A. and Falk, R. (1975) Autoimmunity in degenerative disc disease of the lumbar spine. *Orthop. Clin. North Am.*, **6**, 67-73.

Giles, L.G.F. (1986) Pressure related changes in human lumbosacral zygapophysial joint articular cartilage. *J. Rheumatol.*, **13**, 1093-1095.

Giles, L.G.F. (1987) Innervation of zygapophysial joint synovial folds in low-back pain. *Lancet* (Letter), **2**, 692.

Giles, L.G.F. (1989) *Anatomical Basis of Low Back Pain*. Williams and Wilkins, Baltimore.

Giles, L.G.F. and Harvey, A.R. (1987) Immunohistochemical demonstration of nociceptors in the capsule and synovial folds of human zygapophysial joints. *Br. J. Rheumatol.*, **26**, 362-364.

Gillette, R.G., Kramis, R.C. and Roberts, W.J. (1994) Sympathetic activation of cat spinal neurons responsive to noxious stimulation of deep tissues in the low back. *Pain*, **56**, 31-42.

Grönblad, M. and Åkerman, K.E. (1992) Changes in intracellular free Ca2+ and Na+ upon stimulation of dorsal root ganglion (DRG) cells. Presented at the annual meeting of the *International Society for the Study of the Lumbar Spine*, May 20-24, Chicago, Illinois.

Grönblad, M., Korkala, O., Konttinen, Y.T. *et al.* (1991) Silver impregnation and immunohistochemical study of nerves in lumbar facet joint plical tissue. *Spine*, **16**, 34-38.

Grönblad, M., Weinstein, J.N. and Santavirta, S. (1991) Immunohistochemical observations on spinal tissue innervation. A review of hypothetical mechanisms of back pain. *Acta Orthop. Scand.*, **62**, 614-622.

Grönblad, M., Virri, J., Tolonen, J. *et al.* (1994) A controlled immunohistochemical study of inflammatory cells in disc herniation tissue. *Spine*, **19**, 2744-2751.

Hasue, M., Kunogi, J., Konno, S. and Kikuchi, S. (1989) Classification by position of dorsal root ganglia in the lumbosacral region. *Spine*, **14**, 1261-1264.

Hirsch, C., Ingelmark, B.-E. and Miller, M. (1963) The anatomical basis for low back pain. *Acta Orthop. Scand.*, **33**, 1-17.

Hirsch, G., Beach, G., Cooke, C. *et al.* (1991) Relationship between performance on lumbar dynamometry and Waddell score in a population with low-back pain. *Spine*, **16**, 1039-1043.

Howe, J.F. (1979) A neurophysiological basis for the radicular pain of nerve root compression. In *Advances in Pain Research And Therapy* (J. Bonica, ed.). Raven Press, New York, pp. 647-657.

Howe, J.F., Calvin, W.H. and Loeser, J.D. (1976) Impulses reflected from dorsal root ganglia and from focal nerve injuries. *Brain Res.*, **116**, 139-144.

Howe, J.F., Loeser, J.D. and Calvin, W.H. (1977) Mechanosensitivity of dorsal root ganglia and chronically injured axons: a physiological basis for the radicular pain of nerve root compression. *Pain*, **3**, 25-41.

Hsu, K.Y., Zucherman, J.F., Derby, R. *et al.* (1988) Painful lumbar end-plate disruptions: a significant discographic finding. *Spine*, **13**, 76-78.

Jackson, R.P. (1992) The facet syndrome myth or reality? *Clin. Orthop.*, **279**, 110-121.

Jackson, R.P., Jacobs, R.R. and Montesano, P.X. (1988) Facet joint injection in low back pain: a prospective statistical study. *Spine*, **13**, 966-971.

Kääpä, E., Grönblad, M., Holm, S. *et al.* (1994) Neural elements in the normal and experimentally injured porcine intervertebral disk. *Eur. Spine J.*, **3**, 137-142.

Konttinen, Y.T., Grönblad, M., Korkala, O. *et al.* (1990) Immunohistochemical demonstration of subclasses of inflammatory cells and active, collagen producing fibroblasts in the synovial plicae of lumbar facet joints. *Spine*, **15**, 387-390.

Lilius, G., Laasonen, E.M., Myllynen, P. *et al.* (1989) Lumbar facet joint syndrome: a randomised clinical trial. *J. Bone Joint Surg.*, **71B**, 681-684.

Maigne, J.-Y., Rime, B. and Deligne, B. (1992) Computer tomography follow-up study of forty-eight cases of nonoperatively treated lumbar intervertebral disc herniation. *Spine*, **17**, 1071-1074.

Marshall, L.L. and Trethewie, E.R. (1973) Chemical irritation of nerve-root in disc prolapse. *Lancet* (Letter), **2**, 320.

Marshall, L.L., Trethewie, E.R. and Curtain, C.C. (1977) Chemical radiculitis: a clinical, physiological and immunological study. *Clin. Orthop.*, **129**, 61-67.

McCarron, R.F., Wimpee, M.W., Hudkins, P.G. and Laros, G.S. (1987) The inflammatory effect of nucleus pulposus: a possible element in the pathogenesis of low-back pain. *Spine*, **12**, 760-764.

McLain, R.F. (1994) Mechanoreceptor endings in human cervical facet joints. *Spine*, **19**, 495-501.

McLain, R.F. and Weinstein, J.N. (1991) Ultrastructural changes in the dorsal root ganglion associated with whole body vibration. *J. Spinal Dis.*, **4**, 142-148.

McLain, R.F. and Weinstein, J.N. (1993) Morphometric model of normal rabbit dorsal root ganglia. *Spine*, **18**, 1746-1752.

Murphy, R.W. (1977) Nerve roots and spinal nerves in degenerative disk disease. *Clin. Orthop.*, **129**, 46-60.

Nachemson, A. (1992) Newest knowledge of low back pain. A critical look. *Clin. Orthop.*, **279**, 8-20.

Naylor, A., Happey, F., Turner, R.L. *et al.* (1975) Enzymic and immunological activity in the intervertebral disc. *Orthop. Clin. North Am.*, **6**, 51-58.

Olmarker, K., Blomquist, J., Strömberg, J. *et al.* (1994a) Inflammatogenic properties of nucleus pulposus. Presented at the annual meeting of the *International Society for the Study of the Lumbar Spine*, June 21-25, Seattle, WA.

Olmarker, K., Byröd, G., Cornefjord, M. *et al.* (1994b) Effects of methylprednisolone on nucleus pulposus-induced nerve root injury. *Spine*, **19**, 1803-1808.

Pankovich, A.M. and Korngold, L. (1967) A comparison of the antigenic properties of nucleus pulposus and cartilage protein polysaccharide complexes. *J. Immunol.*, **99**, 431-437.

Petersen, M. and LaMotte, R.H. (1993) Effect of protons on the inward current evoked by capsaicin in isolated dorsal root ganglion cells. *Pain*, **54**, 37-42.

Pilowsky, I. (1993) Aspects of abnormal illness behaviour. *Psychother. Psychosom.*, **60**, 62-74.

Roofe, P.G. (1940) Innervation of anulus fibrosus and posterior longitudinal ligament. *Arch. Neurol. Psychiat.*, **44**, 100-103.

Rydevik, B., Brown, M.D. and Lundborg, G. (1984) Patho-anatomy and pathophysiology of nerve root compression. *Spine*, **9**, 7-15.

Saal, J.A., Saal, J.S. and Herzog, R.J. (1990) The natural history of lumbar intervertebral disc extrusion treated non-operatively. *Spine*, **15**, 683-686.

Saal, J.S., Franson, R.C., Dobrow, R. *et al.* (1990) High levels of inflammatory phospholipase A2 activity in lumbar disc herniations. *Spine*, **15**, 674-678.

Schwarzer, A.C., Aprill, C.N. and Bogduk, N. (1995) The sacroiliac joint in chronic low back pain. *Spine*, **20**, 31-38.

Schwarzer, A.C., Aprill, C.N., Derby, R. *et al.* (1994a) Clinical features of patients with pain stemming from the lumbar zygapophysial joints. Is the lumbar facet syndrome a clinical entity? *Spine*, **19**, 1132-1137.

Schwarzer, A.C., Aprill, C.N., Derby, R. *et al.* (1994b) The relative contributions of the disc and zygapophysial joint in chronic low back pain. *Spine*, **19**, 801-806.

Simmons, J.W., McMillin, J.N., Emery, S.F. and Kimmich, S.J. (1992) Intradiscal steroids. A prospective double-blind clinical trial. *Spine*, **17**, S172-S175.

Spiliopoulou, I., Korovessis, P., Konstantinou, D. and Dimitracopoulos, G. (1994) IgG and IgM concentration in the prolapsed human intervertebral disc and sciatica etiology. *Spine*, **19**, 1320-1323.

Tolonen, J., Grönblad, M., Virri, J. *et al.* (1995a) Basic fibroblast growth factor immunoreactivity in blood vessels and cells of disc herniations. *Spine*, **20**, 271-276.

Tolonen, J., Grönblad, M., Virri, J. *et al.* (1995b) Localization of immunoglobulins in disc herniation tissue. Presented at the annual meeting of the *International Society for the Study of the Lumbar Spine*, June 18-22, Helsinki, Finland.

Virri, J., Sikk, S., Grönblad, M. *et al.* (1994) Concomitant immunocytochemical study of macrophage cells and blood vessels in disc herniation tissue. *Eur. Spine J.*, **3**, 336-341.

Virri, J., Grönblad, M., Tolonen, J. *et al.* (1995) Immunocytochemical analysis of lymphocytes in disc herniations. Presented at the annual meeting of the *International Society for the Study of the Lumbar Spine*, June 18-22, Helsinki, Finland.

Waddell, G., McCulloch, J.A., Kummel, E. and Venner, R.M. (1980) Nonorganic physical signs in low-back pain. *Spine*, **5**, 117-125.

Weinstein, J.N. (1986) Mechanisms of spinal pain: the dorsal root ganglion and its role as a mediator of low-back pain. *Spine*, **11**, 999-1001.

Weinstein, J.N. (1992) The role of neurogenic and non-neurogenic mediators as they relate to pain and the development of osteoarthritis. A clinical review. *Spine*, **17**, S356-S361.

Weinstein, J., Claverie, W. and Gibson, S. (1988a) The pain of discography. *Spine* **13**, 1344-1348.

Weinstein, J., Pope, M., Schmidt, R. *et al.* (1988b) Neuropharmacologic effects of vibration on the dorsal root ganglion. An animal model. *Spine*, **13**, 521-525.

Wyke, B. (1982) Receptor systems in lumbosacral tissues in relation to the production of low back pain. In *American Academy of Orthopaedic Surgeons Symposium on Idiopathic Low Back Pain* (A.A. White III and S.L. Gordon, eds). Mosby, St Louis, pp. 97-107.

Yamashita, T., Cavanaugh, J.M., El-Bohy, A. A. *et al.* (1990) Mechanosensitive afferent units in the lumbar facet joint. *J. Bone Joint Surg.*, **72A**, 865-870.

Yoshizawa, H., O'Brien, J.P., Thomas-Smith, W. *et al.* (1980) The neuropathology of intervertebral discs removed for low back pain. *J. Pathol.*, **132**, 95-104.

16

Anatomy and physiology of spinal nerve roots and the results of compression and irritation

Kjell Olmarker, Shinichi Kikuchi and Bjorn Rydevik

The nerve roots form an anatomically unique region with characteristics of both the central and the peripheral nervous system. Topographically, the nerve roots may be considered to be part of the central nervous system due to their location in the centre of the spine and due to their close connection to the spinal cord. However, functionally the nerve roots are more similar to peripheral nerves. The distribution of symptoms will also be more closely related to injuries in the peripheral nervous system than to injuries in the central nervous system. However, the nerve roots are not so well protected by connective tissues as are the peripheral nerves. Therefore, pathological conditions involving the spinal canal will put the unprotected nerve roots at high risk of injury, even at what might be considered as moderate injuries outside the spine. The nerve roots may thus be involved in the pathophysiology of conditions like disc herniation, spine trauma, intraspinal tumours and degenerative changes of the spine. During recent years there has been a remarkable increase of research regarding the nerve roots. This chapter will include an introduction to the anatomy and the physiology of the nerve roots as well as reviewing the current knowledge on nerve root pathophysiologic changes as induced by mechanical deformation and irritation.

Macro- and microscopic anatomy of the spinal nerve roots

The nerve roots are the parts of the nervous system located outside the spinal cord and surrounded by cerebrospinal fluid and meninges (Figure 16.1). 'Nerve root' and 'spinal nerve root' are two different names for the same structure. The nerve roots terminate at the level of the dorsal root ganglion (Figure 16.2). Distal to this point, the ventral and the dorsal nerve root will blend and exchange axons. The microscopic organization will also change to that of a peripheral nerve at this point. The nerve root will subsequently be transformed to the spinal nerve, and will thus become part of the peripheral nervous system.

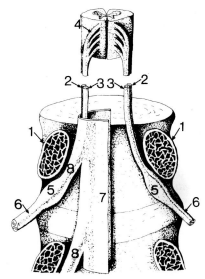

Figure 16.1 Drawing of the intraspinal course of a human lumbar spinal nerve root segment. The vertebral arches have been removed, by cutting the pedicles (1), and the opened spinal canal can be viewed from behind. The ventral (2) and dorsal (3) nerve roots leave the spinal cord as small rootlets (4) that caudally converge into a common nerve root trunk. Just prior to leaving the spinal canal, there is a swelling of the dorsal nerve root called the dorsal root ganglion (5). Caudal to the dorsal root ganglion, the ventral and the dorsal nerve roots mix and form the spinal nerve (6). The spinal dura encloses the nerve roots both as a central cylindrical sac (7), and as separate extensions called root sleeves (8). (Reproduced with permission from Olmarker, K., Thesis, 1990.)

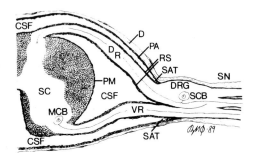

Figure 16.2 Cross-section of a segment of the spinal cord (SC), a ventral (VR) and a dorsal (DR) spinal nerve root. The cell bodies (MCB) of the motor axons, which run in the ventral nerve root, are located in the anterior horn of the gray matter of the spinal cord. The cell bodies (SCB) of the sensory axons, which run in the dorsal nerve root, are located in the dorsal root ganglion (DRG). The ventral and dorsal nerve roots blend just caudal to the dorsal root ganglion, and form the spinal nerve (SN). The spinal cord is covered with the pia mater (PM). This sheath continues out on the spinal nerve roots as the root sheath (RS). The root sheath reflects to the pia-arachnoid (PA) at the subarachnoid triangle (SAT). Together with the dura (D), the pia-arachnoid forms the spinal dura. The spinal cord and nerve roots are floating freely in the cerebrospinal fluid (CSF) in the subarachnoid space. (Reproduced with permission from Olmarker, K., Thesis, 1990.)

In the early embryonic phases, the spinal cord has the same length as has the spinal column. Each segmental cord level in the spine is thus located to the corresponding vertebral level. However, when the spine grows, the spinal cord cannot compensate for this elongation, and will in the adult be considerably shorter than the fully grown spinal column. The result of this *ascensis spinalis* is that the segmental levels of the spinal cord are located much more cranial than is the corresponding vertebral level. The termination of the spinal cord is called the *conus medullaris,* and is, due to this relative elevation of the spinal cord, located at thoracic vertebrae 11 and 12. The nerve roots of the lumbar and sacral levels therefore have to pass a considerable distance caudally in the spinal canal before reaching their exit level. Below the level of the conus medullaris there is thus only a bundle of nerve roots in the spinal canal and no spinal cord. This bundle of nerve roots has been named 'cauda equina' due to its resemblance to the tail of a horse.

Information between the spinal cord and the periphery travels in both directions. Motor or efferent impulses travel in nerve roots that leave the spinal cord from its anterior aspect, and sensory or afferent information reach the spinal cord via nerve roots that join the spinal cord on its posterior aspect (Figures 16.1 and 16.2). The ventral nerve roots are therefore also referred to as 'motor nerve roots' and the posterior roots as 'sensory nerve roots'. This separa-

tion of in and out-going information to motor and sensory nerve roots is generally known as 'the law of Magendie'. The cell bodies of the axons in the motor roots are located in the anterior horn of the gray matter of the spinal cord. The corresponding cell bodies for the axons in the sensory roots are located in an enlargement of the sensory roots, called the dorsal root ganglion (DRG), which is located in or near the intervertebral foramen (Hasue *et al.*, 1989). Each dorsal root ganglion is enclosed by a capsule formed by both a multi-layered connective tissue sheath similar to the perineurium of the peripheral nerve, and a loose connective tissue layer called epineurium (Andres, 1967; McCabe and Low, 1969).

The axons of the nerve root are located in the endoneural space (Figure 16.3). The endoneurium is similar between the nerve roots and the peripheral nerves (Gamble, 1964). However, the amount of collagen in nerve roots is five times less than in peripheral nerves, but six times more than in the spinal cord (Stodieck *et al.*, 1986). There are also

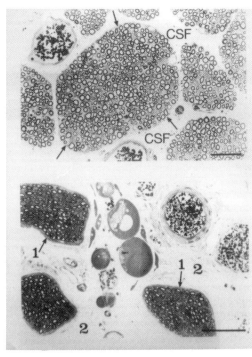

Figure 16.3 (Top) The axons of the spinal nerve roots are located in the endoneurium, which is enclosed only by the thin root sheath (arrows) and cerebrospinal fluid (CSF) (cauda equina from pig, stain: Richardson, bar = 100 μm). (Bottom) The endoneurium of the peripheral nerves is similar to that of the nerve roots. In the peripheral nerve, however, the axons are enclosed by the perineurium (1) and the epineurium (2). Blood vessels are located between the different nerve fascicles in the epineurium (N tibialis from rabbit, stain: Richardson, bar = 100 μm). (Reproduced with permission from Olmarker, K., Thesis, 1990.)

blood vessels, fibroblasts and collagen fibres in the endoneurium (Gamble and Eames, 1966). The presence of lymphatic vessels within the endoneurium has not been defined (Sunderland, 1978).

Outside the endoneurium of the nerve root, and thus separating the endoneurium from the cerebrospinal fluid, is the root sheath. The root sheath is a structure with certain similarities to the pia mater of the spinal cord. Usually there are two to five cellular layers, which differ histologically between the outer and the inner layers (Haller and Low, 1971; Steer, 1971). The cells of the outer layers resemble the pia cells of the spinal cord in the proximal part and arachnoid cells in the distal part of the nerve roots. These layers form a loose connective tissue sheath. The inner cell layers are more similar to the perineurium of peripheral nerves, with histologic characteristics of a structure with barrier properties (McCabe and Low, 1969). There is also an interrupted basement membrane which encloses the different cells. However, the root sheath is probably not an efficient diffusion barrier. In recent experiments, it has been shown that there is almost a free passage even of relatively large molecules across the root sheath (Rydevik *et al.*, 1990; Yoshizawa *et al.*, 1991).

The spinal dura mater encloses the nerve root with its endoneurium and root sheath, as well as the cerebrospinal fluid. The spinal dura is formed by an extension of the inner layer of the cranial dura mater that continues down the spinal canal. The outer layer of the cranial dura mater will mix with the periosteum of the part of the lamina of the cervical vertebrae facing the vertebral canal. The inner dura layer is tightly joined with the arachnoid and thus forms the spinal dura. There is a diffusion barrier located between the collagen lamellae of the dura and the cells of the arachnoid, called the neurothelium (Andres, 1967). The neurothelium shows a certain resemblance to the perineurium of the peripheral nerves.

Vascular anatomy of the spinal nerve roots

When the segmental arteries approach the intervertebral foramen they divide into three different branches; a) an anterior branch which supplies the posterior abdominal wall and lumbar plexus, b) a posterior branch which supplies the paraspinal muscles and facet joints, and c) an intermediate branch which supplies the content of the spinal canal (Crock and Yoshizawa, 1976). A branch of the intermediate branch joins the nerve root at the level of the dorsal root ganglion. There are usually three branches from this vessel; one to the ventral root, one to the dorsal root and one to the vasa corona of the spinal cord. The branch to the vasa corona of the spinal cord,

called the medullary feeder artery, is variable. There are only seven or eight remaining of the original 128 from the embryologic period of life. These vessels thus each supply more than one segment of the spinal cord (Lazorthes *et al.*, 1971). The main medullary feeder artery in the thoracic region of the spine, which is predominant for the vascular supply of the spinal cord, was discovered by Adamkiewicz in 1881 and still bears his name (Adamkiewicz, 1881). The medullary feeder arteries run parallel to the nerve roots but do not directly participate in the blood supply to the nerve root since there are no connections between these vessels and the vascular network of the nerve roots (Parke and Watanabe, 1985). They have therefore been referred to as the 'extrinsic vascular system' of the cauda equina (Parke *et al.*, 1981).

The vascular system of the nerve roots is formed by branches from the intermediate branch of the segmental artery distally, and by branches from the vasa corona of the spinal cord proximally. As opposed to the medullary feeder arteries, this vascular network has been named the 'intrinsic vascular system' of the cauda equina (Parke and Watanabe, 1985; Petterson and Olsson, 1989). The distal branch to the dorsal root first forms the ganglionic plexus within the dorsal root ganglion. The vessels run within the outer layers of the root sheath, called 'epi-pial tissue' (Waggener and Beggs, 1967). The vessels from the periphery and from the spinal cord anastomose in the proximal one-third of the nerve roots (Parke *et al.*, 1981). The anastomosing region has been suggested to have a less developed vascular network and could under such circumstances be a particularly vulnerable site of the nerve roots (Parke *et al.*, 1981). However, this is an issue of some controversy in the literature (Crock *et al.*, 1986).

The main intrinsic vessels of the nerve root, located in the root sheath, send steep branches into the nerve root, which form new vessels that run parallel to the axons and in turn provide branches to the capillary networks (Figure 16.4). Unlike peripheral nerves, the venules do not course together with the arteries in the nerve roots but instead usually have a 'spiralling course' in the deeper parts of the nerve tissue (Parke and Watanabe, 1985).

Between the lumen of the capillaries and the axons in the endoneurial space there is a barrier. This is located to the endothelial cells of the capillaries and is thus similar to the blood–nerve barrier seen in peripheral nerves (Waksman, 1961). However, the barrier in the nerve root has been found to be relatively weak (Olsson, 1968, 1971). There is experimental evidence that normal leakage of serum albumin from nerve root capillaries to the endoneurium does exist, but such leakage is less than in the dorsal root ganglion and in the epineurium of peripheral nerves (Olsson, 1968, 1971; Olmarker *et al.*, 1989a). However, the capillaries in the dorsal root

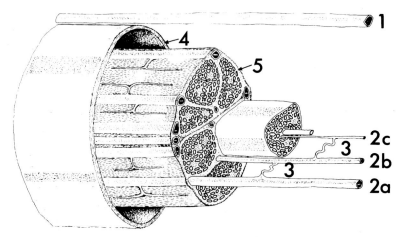

Figure 16.4 The arterioles within the cauda equina may be referred to either the extrinsic (I) or the intrinsic (2) vascular system. From the superficial intrinsic arterioles (2a) there are branches that continue almost at right angles down between the fascicles. These vessels often run in a spiralling course, thus forming vascular 'coils' (3). When reaching a specific fascicle they branch in a T-like manner, with one branch running cranially and one caudally, forming interfascicular arterioles (2b). From these inter-fascicular arterioles there are small branches that enter the fascicles where they supply the endoneurial capillary networks (2c). The arterioles of the extrinsic vascular system run outside the spinal dura (4) and have no connections with the intrinsic system by local vascular branches. The superficial intrinsic arterioles (2a) are located within the root sheath (5). (Reproduced with permission from, Olmarker, K., Thesis, Gothenburg, 1990.)

ganglion are fenestrated (Olsson, 1971; Jacobs *et al.*, 1976; Arvidsson, 1979), and the barrier present in the capillaries in the epineurium of peripheral nerves is less efficient than in the endoneurium (Lundborg, 1975; Rydevik and Lundborg, 1977). Thus, the blood–nerve barrier of nerve roots does not seem to be as well developed as in peripheral nerves, which implies that oedema may be formed more easily in nerve roots.

Compression pathophysiology of the nerve roots of the lumbar spine

Enclosed by the vertebral bones, the spinal nerve roots are relatively well protected from external trauma. However, since the nerve roots do not possess the same amounts and organization of protective connective tissue sheaths as do the periph-eral nerves, the spinal nerve roots are probably particularly sensitive to mechanical deformation due to intraspinal disorders such as disc herniations/protrusions, spinal stenosis, degenerative disorders and tumours (Murphy, 1977; Rydevik *et al.*, 1984). There has been a moderate interest in the past to

study nerve root compression in experimental mod-els. Gelfan and Tarlov in 1956 and Sharpless in 1975 performed some initial experiments on the effects of compression on nerve impulse conduction. Although, no calibration was performed of the compression devices used, the results of both papers indicated that nerve roots were more susceptible to compression than peripheral nerves (Gelfan and Tarlov, 1956; Sharpless, 1975). During recent years, however, the interest in nerve root pathophysiology has increased considerably and a number of studies have been performed and will be reviewed below.

Experimental nerve root compression

Some years ago, a model was presented for compres-sion of the cauda equina in pigs, that for the first time allowed for experimental, graded compression of cauda equina nerve roots at known pressure levels (Olmarker *et al.*, 1991a,b). In this model, the cauda equina was compressed by an inflatable balloon that was fixed to the spine (Figure 16.5). The cauda equina could also be observed through the trans-lucent balloon. This model made it possible to study the flow in the intrinsic nerve root blood vessels at various pressure levels (Olmarker *et al.*, 1989b, 1991c). The experiment was designed in a way that

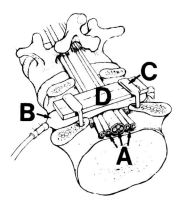

Figure 16.5 Schematic drawing of experimental model. The cauda equina (A) is compressed by an inflatable balloon (B) that is fixed to the spine by two L-shaped pins (C) and a Plexiglas plate (D). (Reproduced with permission from *Spine*, Olmarker *et al.*, 1989a.)

the pressure in the compression balloon was increased by 5 mmHg every 20 seconds. The blood flow and vessel diameters of the intrinsic vessels could simultaneously be observed through the balloon, using a vital microscope. The average occlusion pressure for the arterioles was found to be slightly below and directly related to the systolic blood pressure. The blood flow in the capillary networks was intimately dependant on the blood flow of the adjacent venules. This corroborates the assumption that venular stasis may induce capillary stasis and thus changes in the microcirculation of the nerve tissue, and which has been suggested as one of the mechanisms in the carpal tunnel syndrome (Sunderland, 1976). The mean occlusion pressures for the venules demonstrated large variations. However, a pressure of 5–10 mmHg was found to be sufficient for inducing venular occlusion. Due to retrograde stasis, it is not unlikely that the capillary blood flow will be affected as well in such situations.

In the same experimental set-up, the effects of gradual decompression, after initial acute compression maintained for only a short while, were studied (Olmarker *et al.*, 1991c). It was seen that the average pressure for starting the blood flow was slightly lower for arterioles, capillaries and venules. However, with this protocol it was found that there was not a full restoration of the blood flow until the compression was lowered from 5 mmHg to 0 mmHg. This observation further stresses the previous impression that vascular impairment is present even at low pressure levels.

A compression-induced impairment of the vasculature may thus be one mechanism for nerve root dysfunction since the nutrition of the nerve root will be affected. However, the nerve roots will also derive a considerable nutritional supply via diffusion from

the cerebrospinal fluid (Rydevik *et al.*, 1990). To assess the compression-induced effects on the total contribution to the nerve roots an experiment was designed where 3H-labelled methyl-glucose was allowed to be transported to the nerve tissue in the compressed segment both via blood vessels and via cerebrospinal fluid diffusion after systemic injection (Olmarker *et al.*, 1990a). The results showed that no compensatory mechanism from cerebrospinal fluid diffusion could be expected at the low pressure levels. On the contrary, 10 mmHg compression was sufficient to induce a 20–30% reduction of the transport of methyl-glucose to the nerve roots, as compared to control.

It is known from experimental studies on peripheral nerves that compression also may induce an increase in the vascular permeability, leading to an intraneural oedema formation (Rydevik and Lundborg, 1977). Such oedema may increase the endoneurial fluid pressure (Low and Dyck, 1977; Lundborg *et al.*, 1983; Myers and Powell, 1984; Rydevik *et al.*, 1989a), which in turn may impair the endoneurial capillary blood flow and in such way jeopardize the nutrition of the nerve roots (Low *et al.*, 1982, 1985; Myers *et al.*, 1982; Myers and Powell, 1984). Since the oedema usually persists for some time after the removal of a compressive agent, oedema may negatively affect the nerve root for a longer period than the compression itself. The presence of an intraneural oedema is also related to subsequent formation of intraneural fibrosis (Rydevik *et al.*, 1976), and may in such a way contribute to the slow recovery seen in some patients with nerve compression disorders. To assess if intraneural oedema may form also in nerve roots as the result of compression, the distribution of Evan's blue-labelled albumin (EBA) in the nerve tissue was analysed after compression at various pressures and at various durations (Figure 16.6, Olmarker *et al.*, 1989a). The study showed that oedema was formed even at low pressure levels. The predominant location was at the edges of the compression zone.

The function of the nerve roots has been studied by direct electrical stimulation and recordings either on the nerve itself or in the corresponding muscular segments (Olmarker *et al.*, 1990b; Pedowitz *et al.*, 1991; Rydevik *et al.*, 1991; Garfin *et al.*, 1993). During a 2-hour compression period, a critical pressure level for inducing a reduction of MAP-amplitude seems to be located between 50–75 mmHg (Figure 16.7). Higher pressure levels (100–200 mmHg) may induce a total conduction block with varying degrees of recovery after compression release. To study the effects of compression on sensory nerve fibres, the electrodes in the sacrum were instead used to record a compound nerve action potential after stimulating the sensory nerves in the tail, i.e. distal to the compression zone. The results showed that the sensory fibres are slightly more susceptible to compression than the motor fibres (Pedowitz *et al.*, 1991; Rydevik *et al.*,

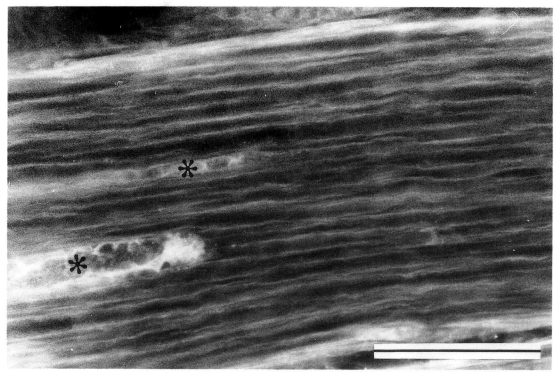

Figure 16.6 Photograph of a longitudinal section of a single nerve root with intraneural oedema. The EBA (white) is located between the axons (black) in all parts of the endoneurium visible in the picture. Two endoneurial vessels to the left of the picture (asterisks) contain EBA (white) and blood cells (black) (bar = 100 μm). (Reproduced with permission from *Spine*, Olmarker *et al.*, 1989a.)

1991). Also, the nerve roots are more susceptible to compression injury if the blood pressure is lowered pharmacologically (Garfin, 1990). This further implies the importance of the blood supply to maintain the functional properties of the nerve roots.

Onset rate of compression

When discussing the effects of compression on nerve tissue there is one thing that must be kept in mind that has not been considered until lately; the onset rate of the compression. The onset rate, i.e. the time from compression start until full compression, may vary clinically from fractions of seconds in traumatic conditions to months or years in association with degenerative processes. Even in the clinically rapid onset rates there may be a wide variation of onset rates. With the presented model it was possible to vary the onset time of the applied compression. Two onset rates have been investigated. Either the pressure is preset and compression is started by flipping the switch of the compressed-air system used to inflate the balloon, or the compression pressure level is slowly increased during 20 seconds. The first onset rate was

measured to be 0.05–0.1 seconds, which thus provides a rapid inflation of the balloon and a rapid compression onset.

Such a rapid onset rate was found to induce more pronounced effects on oedema formation (Olmarker *et al.*, 1989a), methyl-glucose transport (Olmarker *et al.*, 1990a), and impulse propagation (Olmarker *et al.*, 1990b) than the slow onset rate. Regarding methyl-glucose transport, the results are presented in Figure 16.7 and show that the levels within the compression zone is more pronounced at the rapid than at the slow onset rate at corresponding pressure levels. There was also a striking difference between the two onset rates when considering the segments outside the compression zones. In the slow onset series the levels approached base-line values closer to the compression zone than in the rapid onset series. This may indicate the presence of a more pronounced edge-zone oedema in the rapid onset series, with a subsequent reduction of the nutritional transport also in the nerve tissue adjacent to the compression zone.

For the rapid onset compression, which of course is more closely related to spinal trauma or disc herniation than to spinal stenosis, it has been seen that a pressure of 600 mmHg maintained only for one

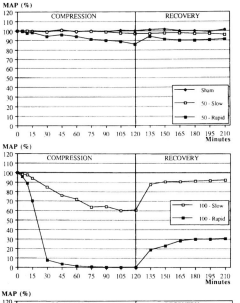

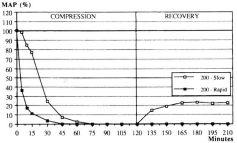

Figure 16.7 Average amplitude of fastest conducting nerve fibres expressed in percent of baseline value. The diagrams show the results of 2 hours of compression and 1.5 hours of recovery for sham compression and for rapid and slow onset of compression at 50 mmHg, 100 mmHg and 200 mmHg. (Reproduced with permission from *Spine*, Olmarker *et al.*, 1990b.)

second is sufficient to induce a gradual impairment of nerve conduction during the 2 hours studied after the compression was ended (Olmarker *et al.*, 1991d). Overall, the mechanisms for these pronounced differences between the different onset rates are not clear, but may be related to differences in displacement rates of the compressed nerve tissue towards the uncompressed parts, due to the viscoelastic properties of the nerve tissue (Rydevik *et al.*, 1989b). Such phenomena may lead to, not only structural damage to the nerve fibres, but also structural changes in the blood vessels with subsequent oedema formation. The gradual formation of intraneural oedema may also be closely related to the described observations of a gradually increasing difference in nerve conduction impairment between the two onset rates (Olmarker *et al.*, 1990b, 1991d).

Multiple levels of nerve root compression

Patients with double levels of spinal stenosis seem to have more pronounced symptoms than patients with a stenosis only at one level (Porter and Ward, 1992). The presented model was modified to address this interesting clinical question. Using two balloons at two adjacent disc levels, which produced a 10 mm uncompressed nerve segment between the balloons, resulted in a much more pronounced impairment of nerve impulse conduction than had been previously found at corresponding pressure levels (Olmarker *et al.*, 1992). For instance, a pressure of 10 mmHg in two balloons induced a 60% reduction of nerve impulse amplitude during 2 hours of compression, whereas 50 mmHg in one balloon showed no reduction.

The mechanism for the difference between single and double compression may not simply be based on the fact that the nerve impulses have to pass more than one compression zone at double level compression. There may also be a mechanism based on the local vascular anatomy of the nerve roots. Unlike peripheral nerves, there are no regional nutritive arteries from surrounding structures to the intraneural vascular system in spinal nerve roots (Lundborg, 1975; Parke *et al.*, 1985; Petterson and Olsson, 1989; Olmarker *et al.*, 1991a). Compression at two levels might therefore induce a nutritionally impaired region between the two compression sites. In this way, the segment affected by the compression would be widened from one balloon diameter (10 mm) to two balloon diameters including the interjacent nerve segment (30 mm). This hypothesis was partly confirmed in an experiment on continuous analyses of the total blood flow in the uncompressed nerve segment located between two compression balloons. The results showed that a 64% reduction of total blood flow was induced when both balloons were inflated to 10 mmHg (Takahashi *et al.*, 1993). At a pressure close to the systemic blood pressure there was complete ischaemia in the nerve segment. Preliminary data from a study on the nutritional transport to the nerve tissue at double level compression has demonstrated that there is a reduction of this transport to the uncompressed nerve segment located between the two compression balloons, that was similar to the reduction within the two compression sites (Cornefjord *et al.*, 1992). There is thus experimental evidence that the nutrition to the nerve segment located between two compression sites in nerve roots is severely impaired although this nerve segment itself is uncompressed.

Regarding nerve conduction (Olmarker *et al.*, 1992), it was also evident that the effects were much enhanced if the distance between the compression balloons was increased from one vertebral segment to two vertebral segments. However, this was not the case in the nutritional transport study where the methyl-glucose levels in the compression zones and in the uncompressed intermediate segment were similar between double compression over one and two vertebral segments (Cornefjord *et al.*, 1992). This indicates that the nutrition to the uncompressed nerve segment located between two compression sites is affected almost to the same extent as at the compression sites, regardless of the distance between the compression sites, but that functional impairment may be directly related to the distance between the two compression sites. The impairment of the nutrition to the nerve segment between the two compression balloons thus seems to be a more important mechanism, than the fact that the nerve impulses have to overcome two compression sites in double level compression.

Chronic experimental nerve root compression

The discussion of compression-induced effects on nerve roots has so far been dealing with acute compression, i.e. compression which lasts for some hours and with no survival of the animal. To mimic better the clinical situation, compression must be applied over longer periods of time. There are probably many changes in the nerve tissue, such as adaptation of axons and vasculature, that will occur in patients but cannot be studied in experimental models using only 1-6 hours of compression. Another important factor in this context is the onset rate that was discussed previously. In clinical syndromes with nerve root compression, the onset time may probably in many cases be quite slow. For instance, a gradual remodelling of the vertebrae to induce a spinal stenosis probably requires an onset time of many years. It will of course be difficult to mimic such a situation in an experimental model. It will also be impossible to have control over the pressure acting on the nerve roots in chronic models due to the remodelling and adaptation of the nerve tissue to the applied pressure. However, knowledge of the exact pressures is probably of less importance in chronic than in acute compression situations. Instead, chronic models should induce a controlled compression with a slow onset time that is easily reproducible. Such models may be well suited for studies on pathophysiologic events as well as intervention by surgery or drugs. Some attempts have been made to induce such compression.

Delamarter and collaborators presented a model on the dog cauda equina in which they applied a constricting plastic band (Delamarter *et al.*, 1990). The band was tightened around the thecal sac to induce a 25, 50, or 75% reduction of the cross-sectional area. The band was left in its place for

various times. Analyses were performed and showed both structural and functional changes that were proportional to the degree of constriction.

To induce a slower onset and more controlled compression, Cornefjord and collaborators used a constrictor to compress the nerve roots in the pig (Cornefjord *et al.*, 1995b). The constrictor was initially intended for inducing vascular occlusion in experimental ischaemic conditions in dogs. The constrictor consists of an outer metal shell that on the inside is covered with a material called ameroid that expands when in contact with fluids. Because of the metal shell the ameroid expands inwards with a maximum of expansion after 2 weeks, resulting in a compression of a nerve root placed in the central opening of the constrictor. Compression of the first sacral nerve root in the pig has resulted in a significant reduction of nerve conduction velocity and axonal injuries using a constrictor with a defined original diameter (Cornefjord *et al.*, 1995b). It has also been found that there is an increase in substance P in the nerve root and the dorsal root ganglion following such compression (Cornefjord *et al.*, 1995a). Substance P is a neurotransmitter that is related to pain transmission. The study may thus provide experimental evidence that compression of nerve roots produces pain. The constrictor model has also been used to study blood flow changes in the nerve root vasculature (Sato *et al.*, 1994). It could then be observed that the blood flow is not reduced just outside the compression zone, but significantly reduced in parts of the nerve roots located inside the constrictor.

One important aspect in clinical nerve root compression conditions is that the compression level is probably not stable but varies as the result of changes in posture and movements (Takahashi *et al.*, 1995, Konno *et al.*, 1995a). Konno and collaborators recently introduced a model where the pressure could be changed after some time of initial chronic compression (Konno *et al.*, 1995b). An inflatable balloon was introduced under the lamina of the seventh lumbar vertebrae in the dog. The normal anatomy and the effects of acute compression using compressed air was first evaluated in previous studies (Sato *et al.*, 1995). By inflating the balloon at a known pressure slowly over 1 hour with a viscous substance that would harden in the balloon, a compression of the cauda equina could be induced with a known initial pressure level. The compression was verified by myelography. Since the 'balloon' under the lamina comprised a twin set of balloons, the second balloon component could be connected to compressed-air and could be used to add compression to the already chronically compressed cauda equina.

In conclusion, acute nerve root compression experiments have been performed that have established critical pressure levels for interference with various physiologic parameters in the spinal nerve roots. However, studies on chronic compression may provide knowledge that will be more applicable to the clinical situation.

Nucleus pulposus-induced nerve root injury

Although it is well known clinically and also experimentally that mechanical deformation such as compression or elongation may induce changes in nerve root impulse conduction and structure, it has often been recognized that mechanical deformation alone can not be responsible for the symptomatology in many cases (Murphy, 1977; Rydevik *et al.*, 1984; Olmarker *et al.*, 1993). It has thus been suggested that components of the intervertebral discs, mainly the nucleus pulposus, may induce some 'non-mechanical' effects on the nerve roots. A new interesting field of research has been on-going for some years and the current knowledge will be reviewed.

Rydevik and collaborators applied autologous nucleus pulposus, obtained from a lumbar disc in the same animal, onto the tibial nerve of rabbits (Rydevik *et al.*, 1983). However, no changes in nerve function or structure could be observed. McCarron and collaborators applied autologous nucleus pulposus from discs of the dogs tail in the epidural space of the animal (McCarron *et al.*, 1987). They could observe that there was an epidural inflammatory reaction that did not occur when saline was injected as control. However, the nerve tissue was never assessed in this study.

Recently, Olmarker and collaborators presented a study that demonstrated that autologous nucleus pulposus may induce a reduction in nerve conduction velocity and light microscopic structural changes in a model of the pig cauda equina (Olmarker *et al.*, 1993). However, these axonal changes had a focal distribution and were too limited to be responsible for the significant neurophysiologic dysfunction observed. A follow-up study on the light microscopically normal areas revealed that there were significant injuries of the Schwann cells with vacuolization and disintegration of the Schmidt–Lanterman incisures (Olmarker *et al.*, 1996). These Schmidt-Lanterman incisures are essential for the normal exchange of ions between the axon and the surrounding tissues. An injury to this structure would therefore result in changes in the normal impulse conduction properties of the axons. However, these changes were also too limited to fully explain the neurophysiological dysfunction observed.

From these experiments, the mechanisms for the nucleus pulposus-induced nerve root injury could not be fully understood. However, there were indications in these studies that inflammatory reactions were present, at least epidurally. This initiated a study where a potent anti-inflammatory agent, methylprednisolone, was administered at different times intravenously after nucleus pulposus-application (Olmarker *et al.*, 1994). The results showed clearly that the nucleus pulposus-induced reduction in nerve conduction velocity was eliminated if methyl-prednisolone was administered within 24 hours of application. If methylprednisolone was administered within 48 hours the effect was not eliminated, but significantly lower than if no drug was used. This observation indicates that the negative effect does not occur immediately but will develop during the first 24 hours after application. However, if methyl-prednisolone is administered within 24 hours, there are still areas in the nerve roots, demonstrating normal impulse conduction properties that have light microscopic axonal changes in the same magnitude as in the previous study (Olmarker *et al.*, 1993). This further corroborates the impression that the structural nerve injury inducing nerve dysfunction may not be found at the light microscopic level but must be sought for at the subcellular level.

Although methylprednisolone may intervene with the pathophysiologic events of the nucleus pulposus-induced nerve root injury, it was not clear if this was due to the anti-inflammatory properties of the methylprednisolone or some other property. To establish if the presence of autologous nucleus pulposus could initiate a leukotactic response from the surrounding tissues a study was initiated that assessed the potential inflammatogenic properties of the nucleus pulposus (Olmarker *et al.*, 1995). Autologous nucleus pulposus and autologous retroperitoneal fat were placed in separate small perforated titanium chambers and placed subcutaneously, together with a sham chamber, in the pig. Seven days later, the number of leukocytes were assessed for the chambers. The number of leukocytes was the same in both the fat and the sham chambers. However, the nucleus pulposus-containing chambers had a number of leukocytes that exceeded the two others by 250%. Also, when injected locally in contact with the microvasculature of the hamster cheek-pouch, nucleus pulposus induced an increase in permeability for macromolecules that was not present if the animals were simultaneously treated with indomethacin (Blomquist *et al.*, 1995; Olmarker *et al.*, 1995).

These two latter studies thus indicate that inflammatory mediators may be produced when nucleus pulposus is in contact with other tissues. However, it is at present not evident if these mediators are produced and released by cells in the nucleus pulposus itself or by cells in the surrounding structures. It has been suggested that since the nucleus pulposus is avascular and thus 'hidden' from the systemic circulation, a presentation of the nucleus pulposus could result in an auto-immune reaction directed to antigens present in the nucleus pulposus, and that bioactive substances from this reaction may injure the nerve tissue (Naylor, 1962, 1971, 1975; Bobechko *et al.*, 1965; LaRocca, 1971; Gertzbein, 1977; Gertzbein *et al.*, 1975, 1977; Bisla *et al.*, 1976). However, no clear data exist as to whether this is a clinical reality or not. It seems more likely that substances should be produced by the cells of the nucleus pulposus. Recent studies have also confirmed that these cells may produce metalloproteases such as collagenase or gelatinase, as well as interleukin-6 and prostaglandin E2 (Kang *et al.*, 1995). Using the same pig model as described, Olmarker and coworkers have assessed the possible role of the nucleus pulposus cells for the nucleus pulposus-induced nerve injury (Olmarker *et al.*, l995c). In a blinded fashion, autologous nucleus pulposus was subjected to 24 hours of freezing at -20°C, digestion by hylauronidase or just to a heating-box at 37°C for 24 hours. The treated nucleus pulposus was reapplied after 24 hours and analyses were performed 7 days later. It was then evident that in animals where the nucleus pulposus had been frozen, and the cells thus killed, there were no changes in nerve conduction velocity, whereas in the other two series, the results were similar to the previous study (Olmarker *et al.*, 1993). It therefore seems reasonable to believe that the cells have been responsible in some way for inducing the nerve injury.

There will probably be rapid progress in this area in the coming years that eventually could lead to better methods for both diagnosis and treatment of nerve root-related spinal pain syndromes.

References

Adamkiewicz, A. (1881) Die Blutgefasse des menschlichen Ruckenmarkes. I. Die Gefasse der Ruckenmarkssubstanz. Sitzungsb. d. k. Akad. d. Wissensch. in Wien. math.naturw. CI., **84**, 469-502.

Andres, K.H. (1967) Uber die feinstruktur der arachnoidea und dura mater von mammalia. *Z. Zellforsch.*, **79**, 272-295.

Arvidson, B. (1979) Distribution of intravenously injected protein tracers in peripheral ganglia of adult mice. *Exp. Neurol.*, **63**, 388-410.

Bisla, R.S., Marchisello, P.J., Lockshin, M.D. *et al.* (1976) Autoimmunological basis of disk degeneration. *Clin. Orthop.*, **123**, 149-154.

Blomquist, J., Stromberg, J., Zachrisson, P. *et al.* (1995) Indomethacin blocks nucleus pulposus-induced macromolecular leakage. Manuscript.

Bobechko, W.P. and Hirsch, C. (1965) Auto-immune response to nucleus pulposus in the rabbit. *J. Bone Joint Surg.*, **47B**, 574-580.

Cornefjord, M., Takahashi, K., Matsui, H. *et al.* (1992) Impairment of nutritional transport at double level cauda equina compression. An experimental study. *Neuroorthopaedics*, **13**, 107-112.

Cornefjord, M., Olmarker, K., Farley, D. *et al.* (1995a) Neuropeptide changes in compressed spinal nerve roots. *Spine*, **20**, 670-673.

Cornefjord, M., Sato, K., Olmarker, K. *et al.* (1995b) A model for chronic nerve root compression studies. Presentation of a porcine gradual onset compression model with analyses of nerve root conduction velocity. *Spine* (in press).

Crock, H.V. and Yoshizawa, H. (1976) The blood supply of the lumbar vertebral column. *Clin. Orthop.*, **115**, 6-21.

Crock, H.V., Yamagishi, M. and Crock, M.C. (1986) *The Conus Medullaris and Cauda Equina in Man.* Springer-Verlag, New York.

Delamarter, R.B., Bohlman, H.H., Dodge, L.D. and Biro, C. (1990) Experimental lumbar spinal stenosis. Analysis of the cortical evoked potentials, microvasculature and histopathology. *J. Bone Joint Surg.*, **72A**, 110-120.

Gamble, H.J. (1964) Comparative electron-microscopic observations on the connective tissues of a peripheral nerve and a spinal nerve root. *J. Anat. (Lond.)*, **98**, 17-25.

Gamble, H.J. and Eames, R.A. Electron microscopy of human spinal-nerve roots. *Arch. Neurol.*, **14**, 50-53.

Garfin, S.R., Cohen, M.S., Massie, J.B. *et al.* (1990) Nerve-roots of the cauda equina. The effects of hypotension and acute, graded compression on function. *J. Bone Joint Surg.*, **72A**, 1185-1192.

Gelfan, S. and Tarlov, I.M. (1956) Physiology of spinal cord, nerve root and peripheral nerve compression. *Am. J. Physiol.*, **185**, 217-229.

Gertzbein, S.D. (1977) Degenerative disk disease of the lumbar spine. Immunological implications. *Clin. Orthop.*, **129**, 69-71.

Gertzbein, S.D., Tile, M., Gross, A. and Falk, R. (1975) Autoimmunity in degenerative disc disease of the lumbar spine. *Orthop. Clin. North Am.*, **6**, 67-73.

Gertzbein, S.D., Tait, J.H. and Devlin, S.R. (1977) The stimulation of lymphocytes by nucleus pulposus in patients with degenerative disk disease of the lumbar spine. *Clin. Orthop.*, **123**, 149-154.

Haller, F.R. and Low, F.N. (1971) The fine structure of the peripheral nerve root sheath in the subarachnoid space in the rat and other laboratory animals. *Am. J. Anat.*, **131**, 1-20.

Hasue, M., Kunogi, J., Konno, S. and Kikuchi. S. (1989) Classification by position of dorsal root ganglia in the lumbosacral region. *Spine*, **14**, 1261-1264.

Jacobs, J.M., MacFarlane, R.M. and Cavanagh, J.B. (1976) Vascular leakage in the dorsal root ganglia of the rat, studied with horseradish peroxidase. *J. Neurol. Sci.*, **29**, 95-107.

Kang, J.D., Georgescu, H.I., Larkin, L. *et al.* (1995) Herniated lumbar and cervical intervertebral discs spontaneously produce matrix metalloproteinases, nitric oxide, interleukin-6 and prostaglandin E2. *Trans. Orthopaedic Research Society*, Orlando, Florida, February.

Konno, S., Olmarker, K., Byrod, G. *et al.* (1995a) Intermittent cauda equina compression. An experimental study on the porcine cauda equina with analyses of nerve impulse conduction properties. *Spine*, **20**, 1223-1226

Konno, S., Sato, K., Yabuki, S. *et al.* (1995b) A model for acute, chronic and delayed, graded compression. Presentation of gross-, microscopic-, and vascular anatomy and accuracy in pressure transmission of the compression model. *Spine*, **20**, 2386-2391.

LaRocca, H. (1971) New horizons in research on disc disease. *Orthop. Clin. North Am.*, **2**, 521.

Lazorthes, G., Gouaze, A., Zadeh, J.O. *et al.* (1971) Arterial vascularization of the spinal cord. Recent studies of the anastomtic substitution pathways. *J. Neurosurg.,* **35**, 253-262.

Low, P.A. and Dyck, P.J. (1977) Increased endoneurial fluid pressure in experimental lead neuropathy. *Nature,* **269**, 427-428.

Low, P.A., Dyck, P.J. and Schmelzer, J.D. (1982) Chronic elevation of endoneurial fluid pressure is associated with low-grade fiber pathology. *Muscle Nerve,* **5**, 162-165.

Low, P.A., Nukada, H., Schmelzer, J.D. *et al.* (1985) Endoneurial oxygen tension and radial topography in nerve oedema. *Brain Res.,* **341**, 147-154.

Lundborg, G. (1975) Structure and function of the intraneural microvessels as related to trauma, oedema formation, and nerve function. *J. Bone Joint Surg.,* **57A**, 938-948.

Lundborg, G., Myers, R. and Powell, H. (1983) Nerve compression injury and increased endoneurial fluid pressure: a 'miniature compartment syndrome'. *J. Neurol. Neurosurg. Psychiatry,* **46**, 1119-1124.

McCabe, J.S. and Low, F.N. (1969) The subarachnoid angle: an area of transition in peripheral nerve. *Anat. Rec.,* **164**, 15-34.

McCarron, R.F., Wimpee, M.W., Hudkins, P. and Laros, G.S. (1987) The inflammatory effect of nucleus pulposus. A possible element in the pathogenesis of low-back pain. *Spine* **12**, 8, 760-764.

Murphy, R.W. (1977) Nerve roots and spinal nerves in degenerative disk disease. *Clin. Orthop.,* **129**, 46-60.

Myers, R.R. and Powell, C.C. (1984) Galactose neuropathy: impact of chronic endoneurial oedema on nerve blood flow. *Ann. Neurol.,* **16**, 587-594.

Myers, R.R., Mizisin, A.P., Powell, H.C. and Lampert, P.W. Reduced nerve blood flow in hexachlorophene neuropathy. Relationship to elevated endoneurial fluid pressure. *J. Neuropathol. Exp. Neurol.,* **41**, 391-39.

Naylor, A. (1962) The biophysical and biochemical aspects of intervertebral disc herniation and degeneration. *Ann. R. Coll. Surg. Engl.,* **31**, 91-114.

Naylor, A. Biochemical changes in human intervertebral disk degeneration and prolapse. *Orthop. Clin. North Am.,* **2**, 343.

Naylor, A., Happey, F. and Turner, R.L. (1975) Enzymatic and immunological activity in the intervertebral disc. *Orthop. Clin. North Am.,* **6**, 51-58.

Olmarker, K. (1991) Spinal nerve root compression. Acute compression of the cauda equina studied in pigs. *Acta Orthop. Scand.,* **62**, Suppl 242.

Olmarker, K. and Rydevik, B. (1992) Single versus Double Level Compression. An experimental study on the porcine cauda equina with analyses of nerve impulse conduction properties. *Clin. Orthop.,* **279**, 35-39.

Olmarker, K., Rydevik, B. and Holm, S. (1989a) Oedema formation in spinal nerve roots induced by experimental, graded compression. An experimtnal study on the pig cauda equina with special reference to differences in effects between rapid and slow onset of compression. *Spine,* **14**, 579-563.

Olmarker, K., Rydevik, B., Holm, S. and Bagge, U. (1989b) Effects of experimental graded compression on blood flow in spinal nerve roots. A vital microscopic study on the porcine cauda equina. *J. Orthop. Res.,* **7**, 817-823.

Olmarker, K., Rydevik, B., Hansson, T. and Holm, S. (1990a) Compression-induced changes of the nutritional supply to the porcine cauda equina. *J. Spinal Dis.,* **3**, 25-29.

Olmarker, K., Holm, S. and Rydevik, B. (1990b) Importance of compression onset rate for the degree of impairment of impulse propagation in experimental compression injury of the porcine cauda equina. *Spine,* **15**, 416-419.

Olmarker, K., Holm, S., Rosenqvist, A-L. and Rydevik, B. (1991a) Experimental nerve root compression. Presentation of a model for acute, graded compression of the porcine cauda equina, with analyses of neural and vascular anatomy. *Spine,* **16**, 61-69.

Olmarker, K., Holm, S., Rydevik, B. and Bagge, U. (1991b) Restoration of blood flow during gradual decompression of a compressed segment of the porcine cauda equina. A vital microscopic study. *Neuro Orthopaedics,* **10**, 83-87.

Olmarker, K., Lind, B., Holm, S. and Rydevik, B. (1991c) Continued compression increase impairment of impulse propagation in experimental compression of the porcine cauda equina. *Neuro Orthopaedics,* **11**, 75-81.

Olmarker, K., Rydevik, B. and Nordborg, C. (1993) Autologous nucleus pulposus induces neurophysiologic and histologic changes in porcine cauda equina nerve roots. *Spine,* **18**, 1425-1432.

Olmarker, K., Byrod, G., Cornefjord, M. *et al.* (1994) Effects of methylprednisolone on nucleus pulposus-induced nerve root injury. *Spine,* **19**, 1803-1808.

Olmarker, K., Blomquist, J. and Stromberg, J. *et al.* (1995) Inflammatogenic properties of nucleus pulposus. *Spine,* **20**, 665-669.

Olmarker, K., Rydevik, B. and Nordborg, C. (1996) Ultrastructural changes in spinal nerve roots induced by autologous nucleus pulposus. *Spine,* **21**, 411-414.

Olsson, Y. (1968) Topographical differences in the vascular permeability of the peripheral nervous system. *Acta Neuropathol.,* **10**, 26-33.

Olsson, Y. (1971) Studies on vascular permeability in peripheral nerves. IV Distribution of intravenously injected protein tracers in the peripheral nervous system of various species. *Acta Neuropathol. (Berl.),* **17**, 114-126.

Parke, W.W. and Watanabe, R. (1985) The intrinsic vasculature of the lumbosacral spinal nerve roots. *Spine,* **10**, 508-515.

Parke, W.W., Gamell, K. and Rothman, R.H. (1981) Arterial vascularization of the cauda equina. *J. Bone Joint Surg.,* **63A**, 53-62.

Pedowitz, R.A., Garfin, S.R., Hargens, *et al.* (1992) Effects of magnitude and duration of compression on spinal nerve root conduction. *Spine,* **17**, 194-199.

Petterson, C.A.V. and Olsson, Y. (1989) Blood supply of spinal nerve roots. An experimental study in the rat. *Acta Neuropathol.,* **78**, 455-461.

Porter, R.W. and Ward, D. (1992) Cauda equina dysfunction: the significance of multiple level pathology. *Spine,* **17**, 9-15.

Rydevik, B. and Lundborg, G. (1977) Permeability of intraneural microvessels and perineurium following acute, graded nerve compression. *Scand. J. Plast. Reconstr. Surg.,* **11**, 179-187.

Rydevik, B., Lundborg, G. and Nordborg, C. (1976) Intraneural tissue reactions induced by internal neurolysis. *Scand. J. Plast. Reconstr. Surg.,* **10**, 3-8.

Rydevik, B., Brown, M.D., Ehira, T. *et al.* (1983) Effects of graded compression and nucleus pulposus on nerve tissue: an experimental study in rabbits. *Acta Orthop. Scand.*, **54**, 670-671.

Rydevik, B., Brown, M.D. and Lundborg, G. Pathoanatomy and pathophysiology of nerve root compression. *Spine*, **9**, 7-15.

Rydevik, B., Myers, R.R. and Powell, H.C. (1989a) Pressure increase in the dorsal root ganglion following mechanical compression. Closed compartment syndrome in nerve roots. *Spine*, **14**, 574-576.

Rydevik, B., Lundborg, G. and Skalak, R. (1989b) Biomechanics of peripheral nerves. In *Basic Biomechanics of the Musculoskeletal System* (M. Nordin and V.H. Frankel, eds). Lea and Febiger, Philadelphia, pp. 75-87.

Rydevik, B., Holm, S., Brown, M.D. and Lundborg, G. (1990) Diffusion from the cerebrospinal fluid as a nutritional pathway for spinal nerve roots. *Acta Physiol. Scand.*, **138**, 247-248.

Rydevik, B.L., Pedowitz, R.A., Hargens, A.R. *et al.* (1991) Effects of acute graded compression on spinal nerve root function and structure: an experimental study on the pig cauda equina. *Spine*, **16**, 487-493.

Sato, K., Olmarker, K., Cornefjord, M. *et al.* (1994) Changes of intraradicular blood flow in chronic nerve root compression. An experimental study on pigs. *Neuro Orthopaedics*, **16**, 1-7.

Sato, K., Yabuki, S., Konno, S. *et al.* (1995) A model for acute, chronic and delayed, graded compression. Neurophysiologic changes induced by acute, graded compression. *Spine,* **20**, 2386-2391.

Sharpless, S.K. (1975) Susceptibility of spinal nerve roots to compression block. In *The Research Status of Spinal Manipulative Therapy.* NIH workshop, February 2-4, 1975. NINCDS Monograph no.15 (M. Goldstein, ed.), pp. 155-161.

Steer, J.M. (1971) Some observations on the fine structure of rat dorsal spinal nerve roots. *J. Anat.*, **109**, 467-485.

Stodieck, L.S., Beel, J.A. and Luttges, M.W. (1986) Structural properties of spinal nerve roots: protein composition. *Exp. Neurol.*, **91**, 41-51.

Sunderland, S. (1976) The nerve lesion in the carpal tunnel syndrome. *J. Neurol. Neurosurg. Psychiatry,* **39**, 615-626.

Sunderland, S. (1978) *Nerves and Nerve Injuries.* 2nd edition. Churchill Livingstone, Edinburgh.

Takahashi, K., Olmarker, K., Holm, S. *et al.* (1993) Double level cauda equina compression. An experimental study with continuous monitoring of intraneural blood flow in the porcine cauda equina. *J. Orthop. Res.*, **11**, 104-109.

Takahashi, K., Miyazaki, T., Takino, T. *et al.* (1995) Epidural pressure measurements: relationship between epidural pressure and posture in patients with with lumbar spinal stenosis. *Spine*, **20**, 650-653.

Waggener, J.D. and Beggs, J. (1967) The membraneous coverings of neural tissues: an electron microscopy study. *J. Neuropath.*, **26**, 412-426.

Waksman, B.H. (1961) Experimental studies of diphtheritic polyneuritis in the rabbit and guinea pig. III. The blood-nerve barrier in the rabbit. *J. Neuropath. Exp. Neurol.*, **20**, 35-77.

Yoshizawa, H., Kobayashi, S. and Hachiya, Y. (1991) Blood supply of nerve roots and dorsal root ganglia. *Orthop. Clin. North Am.*, **22**, 195-211.

□ **17** □

The pathoanatomic basis of somatic, autonomic and neurogenic syndromes originating in the lumbosacral spine

J. Randy Jinkins

Summary

Clinical manifestations engendered within the lumbosacral spine encompass both pain and disability. While present diagnostic imaging methods are excellent in their sensitivity to the detection of disease, they do not always clearly explain the specific origin or nature of patient signs and symptoms. Nevertheless, there are definite anatomically based neurogenic syndromes originating in the lumbosacral spine. These include local spinal, centripetally/centrifugally referred, and centripetally/centrifugally radiating syndromes that may be superimposed upon one another, thereby complicating precise clinical analysis. An in-depth review of the neuroanatomical and theoretical concepts associated with the syndromes of the lumbosacral spine provides a basis for the understanding of this complex, sometimes confounding area of clinicoradiological diagnosis.

Introduction

The clinical state of *neurogenic* spinal radiculopathy accompanying nerve root, spinal nerve, and dorsal root ganglion, injury, may be associated with definite *somatic* and *autonomic* syndromes. The combined clinical complex includes: 1) centripetally/centrifugally radiating radicular pain and paresthesias, 2) muscle strength and reflex dysfunction, 3) local and centripetally/centrifugally referred pain, 4) autonomic reflex dysfunction within the lumbosacral zones of Head, and 5) generalized alterations in autonomic viscerosomatic tone. These varied syndromes may be superimposed upon one another. The anatomical basis for the origin and mediation of clinical signs and symptoms related to the lumbo-

sacral neural plexus rests with: 1) afferent and efferent somatic neural branches emanating from the ventral and dorsal rami of the spinal nerve, 2) neural rami projecting directly to, and originating from, the paravertebral autonomical neural plexus, and 3) the dorsal and ventral spinal nerve roots and spinal nerves themselves. These fibres originate and terminate in the spinal column and related non-neural perispinal and intraspinal tissues, in the spinal nerves and their ramifications in regional neural tissue intimately related to the spinal elements, and in the peripheral neural and non-neural tissues. Thus, conscious perception, and unconscious effects originating from the vertebral column and its neural structures, although complex, have definite pathways represented in this network of innervation associated with intimately related and/or parallel peripheral and central nervous system (CNS) ramifications.

Anatomy of local spinal syndromes

Somatic innervation of ventral spinal elements

The anatomical basis for discogenic and, therefore, vertebrogenic pain, rests partially with afferent somatic fibres originating from the recurrent meningeal nerve (sinuvertebral nerve of Luschka). This nerve supplies the posterior longitudinal ligament, the meninges, the blood vessels, the posterior extent of the outermost fibres of the anulus fibrosus, a portion of the periosteum of the vertebral bodies, and the underlying bone. In addition, a variable small afferent branch from the ventral ramus of the somatic spinal nerve root may directly innervate the posterolateral

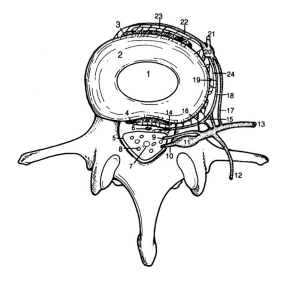

Figure 17.1. Schematic diagram of somatic and autonomic innervation of ventral spinal canal and structures of ventral aspect of spinal column: 1 = nucleus pulposus; 2 = anulus fibrosus; 3 = anterior longitudinal ligament/periosteum; 4 = posterior longitudinal ligament/periosteum; 5 = leptomeninges; 6 = epidural vasculature; 7 = filum terminale; 8 = intrathecal lumbosacral nerve root; 9 = ventral root; 10 = dorsal root; 11 = dorsal root ganglion; 12 = dorsal ramus of spinal nerve; 13 = ventral ramus of spinal nerve; 14 = recurrent meningeal nerve (sinuvertebral nerve of Luschka); 15 = autonomic (sympathetic) branch to recurrent meningeal nerve; 16 = direct somatic branch from ventral ramus of spinal nerve to lateral disk; 17 = white ramus communicans (not found, or found irregularly, caudal to L2); 18 = gray ramus communicans (multilevel irregular lumbosacral distribution); 19 = lateral sympathetic efferent branches projecting from gray ramus communicans; 20 = paraspinal sympathetic ganglion (PSG); 21 = craniocaudal extension of paraspinal sympathetic chain; 22 = anterior paraspinal afferent sympathetic ramus (i) projecting to PSG; 23 = anterior sympathetic efferent branches projecting from PSG; 24 = lateral paraspinal afferent sympathetic ramus projecting to PSG. (Note – afferent and efferent sympathetic paraspinous branches/rami may be partially combined *in vivo*) (Adapted from Jinkins, J.R., Whittemore, A.R. and Bradley, W.G. (1989) The anatomic basis of vertebrogenic pain and the autonomic syndrome associated with lumbar disk extrusion. *AJNR,* **10**, 219–231; *AJR,* **152**, 1277–1289; with permission.)

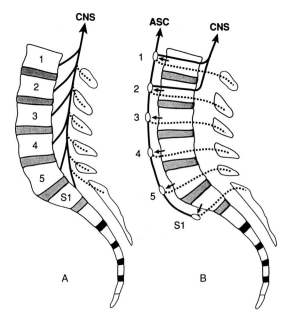

Figure 17.2 Schematic diagrams depicting lumbar afferent sensory patterns. A. Direct somatic afferent inflow into central nervous system (CNS) from branches of somatic spinal nerves at all levels. B. Ascending autonomic (sympathetic) afferent inflow diversion into CNS of lumbosacral sympathetic fibres. This inflow pattern is inconstant due to the absence, or irregular distribution, of white rami communicantes occurring between the L2 and S2 vertebral levels. ASC = ascending sympathetic chain; large diameter solid lines = afferent sympathetic network; short arrows = afferent sympathetic inflow from ventral spinal elements; dotted lines = afferent sympathetic inflow from dorsal spinal elements. (Adapted from Jinkins, J.R., Whittemore, A.R. and Bradley, W.G. (1989) The anatomic basis of vertebrogenic pain and the autonomic syndrome associated with lumbar disk extrusion. *AJNR,* **10**, 219–231; *AJR,* **152**, 1277–1289; with permission.)

aspect of the vertebral body and related tissues over an inconstant range. Irregular, unnamed afferent branches of the somatic nerves also likely contribute to direct spinal and perispinal soft tissue innervation. Any traumatic involvement of these neural and non-neural tissues may incite well-circumscribed local somatic pain because of this somatosensory innervation pattern (Figure 17.1), and because of the direct segmental nature of the afferent inflow from the segment or origin into the CNS via the somatic spinal nerves (Figure 17.2A) (Wiberg, 1949; Jackson *et al.*, 1966; Edgar and Ghadially, 1976; Bogduk *et al.*, 1981; Bogduk, 1983; Paris, 1983; Wyke, 1987; Lundborg and Dahlin, 1989; Groen *et al.*, 1990). This direct somatosensory afferent inflow seems to insure a relatively accurate spatial registration of impulses coming into the CNS with regard to stimulus origin. At the same time, injury to somatic efferent motor fibres contained in the ventral ramus of the spinal nerve, or the spinal nerve itself, might yield muscular weakness and muscle reflex dysfunction.

Somatic innervation of dorsal spinal elements

The posterior spinal zygapophysial (facet) joints, as well as the surrounding bone and posterior spinal muscular and ligamentous tissues, receive their innervation primarily, although not solely, from the dorsal rami of the spinal nerves. In total, there are potentially five main branches innervating these structures that are of somewhat irregular origin and number. These include neural fibres arising directly from the main trunk of the dorsal ramus of the spinal nerve, from the medial branch of the dorsal ramus, from the lateral branch of the dorsal ramus, from the main trunk of the ventral ramus, and from the combined spinal nerve itself before its bifurcation into the dorsal and ventral rami (Figure 17.3) (Bogduk and Long, 1979; Bogduk *et al.*, 1982; Auteroche, 1983). On careful anatomical study, the dorsal elements of the spinal column and surrounding tissues have been demonstrated to have remarkably variable fields of

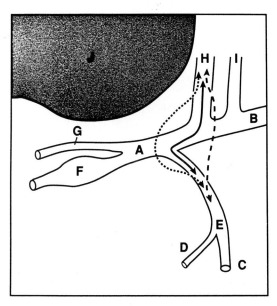

Figure 17.3 Schematic diagrams outlining innervation of structures of dorsal aspect of spinal column. A. Somatic-autonomic neural network innervating the dorsal spinal elements at or above the level of L2. (Adapted from Auteroche, P. (1983) Innervation of the zygapophysial joints of the lumbar spine. *Anat. Clin.*, **5**, 17–28, with permission). 1 = neural fibres from main trunk of spinal nerve (A); 2 = neural fibres from ventral ramus (B) of spinal nerve; 3 = neural fibres from lateral branch of dorsal ramus (C); 4 = neural fibres from medial branch of dorsal ramus (D); 5 = neural fibres from dorsal ramus (E) of spinal nerve; F = dorsal nerve root and ganglion; G = ventral nerve root; H = gray ramus communicans; I = white ramus communicans; J = intervertebral disc. B. Enlargement of neural interconnections between the autonomic nervous system (gray ramus communicans) and the dorsal spinal neural network (dorsal ramus of spinal nerve) at or above L2. Possible bidirectional routes of sympathetic fibres from the gray ramus communicans (H) to the dorsal ramus of the spinal nerve include pathways via the ventral ramus of the spinal nerve (solid line), via a direct branch of the gray ramus communicans (dashed line) by passing over the ventral ramus of the spinal nerve (B), or via a direct branch of the gray ramus communicans (dotted line) by passing over the main trunk of the spinal nerve (A). (A and B adapted from Auteroche, P. (1983) Innervation of the zygapophysial joints of the lumbar spine. *Anat. Clin.*, **5**, 17–28; with permission.)

innervation that are not confined to strict segmental patterns. This innervation shows bilateral asymmetry with intra- and interindividual variation in the craniocaudal extent of nerve supply.

Nevertheless, injury to these neural and non-neural structures would, in part, be expected to result in relatively well localized somatic pain because of the direct afferent somatosensory inflow into the CNS via the somatic spinal nerves. In general, this seems to occur in a manner similar to that outlined above for the ventral spinal elements (Figure 17.2A). Injury to somatic motor fibres contained in the dorsal ramus of the spinal nerve might yield muscular weakness and muscle reflex dysfunction.

Additional theoretical innervations of spinal elements

Local innervations at the level of the dorsal and ventral roots, spinal nerves, recurrent meningeal nerves, and other epidural structures, at the point of common expression of pathology (e.g. disc herniation), is an important consideration regarding the understanding of the manifestations of the lumbosacral syndromes. In addition to peripheral somatic afferent sensory and efferent motor nerves (Figures 4A,B), and the local somatic spinal afferent nerves (Figure 17.4C), there are nerve fibres innervating the nerves themselves, the *nervi nervorum* (Murphy, 1977).

These *nervi nervorum* are theoretically of three types. First, there are afferent sensory fibres to the nerve radicles in, traversing and around the spinal column (Figure 17.4D). These are responsible for local sensation and even pain when the nerve itself is injured. Second, there are local/radicular sympathetic afferent fibres which enter the paraspinal sympathetic chain via the gray rami communicantes and return to the CNS via the white rami communicantes (Figure 17.4E). These fibres relay afferent information from the spinal roots, nerves, and surrounding tissues, to the sympathetic nervous system. Third, there are local/radicular sympathetic efferent fibres which carry out sympathetic actions (e.g. vasoactive functions) upon the spinal roots, nerves and surrounding tissues (Figure 17.4F). This general format is probably replicated in its essential points in the posterior spinal elements, the autonomic fibres being initially transmitted via the dorsal roots of the spinal

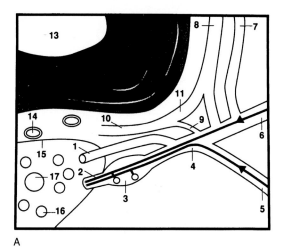
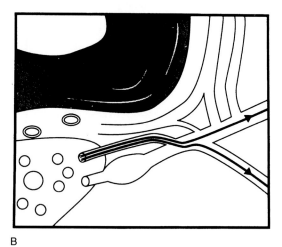

A   B

Figure 17.4 Schematic of somatic and autonomic innervation of spinal column and related structures. A: Peripheral somatic afferent sensory neural fibres from distant ventral and dorsal tissues. B. Peripheral somatic efferent motor neural fibres to ventral and dorsal tissues. C. Local somatic afferent sensory neural fibres from ventral (e.g. peripheral disk, epidural tisssues, dura, etc.) and dorsal tissues (e.g. facet joints, posterior spinal ligaments, etc.). D. Local/radicular afferent *nervi nervorum*. E. Local/radicular sympathetic afferent neural fibres from ventral spinal tissues (e.g. peripheral disk, epidural tissues, dura, etc.). F. Local/radicular sympathetic afferent neural fibres to ventral spinal tissues. G. Local/sympathetic afferent neural fibres from dorsal spinal tissues (e.g. facet joints, posterior spinal ligaments, etc.). H. Local/sympathetic efferent neural fibres to dorsal spinal and paraspinal tissues). 1 = ventral nerve root; 2 = dorsal nerve root; 3 = dorsal root ganglion; 4 = combined spinal nerve; 5 = dorsal ramus of spinal nerve; 6 = ventral ramus of spinal nerve; 7 = white ramus communicans (not found or irregularly found caudal to L2); 8 = gray ramus communicans (multilevel irregular lumbosacral distribution); 9 = branch to recurrent meningeal nerve from spinal nerve; 10 = recurrent meningeal nerve (sinuvertebral nerve of Luschka); 11 = autonomic (sympathetic) branch to recurrent meningeal nerve from gray ramus communicans; 12 = anulus fibrosus; 13 = nucleus pulposus; 14 = epidural vasculature; 15 = leptomeninges; 16 = intrathecal lumbosacral nerve root; 17 = filum terminale. (Reprinted with permission from Jinkins, J.R. (1993) The pathoanatomic basis of somatic and autonomic syndromes originating in the lumbosacral spine. *Neurol. Clin. North Am.,* **3**, 444-460.)

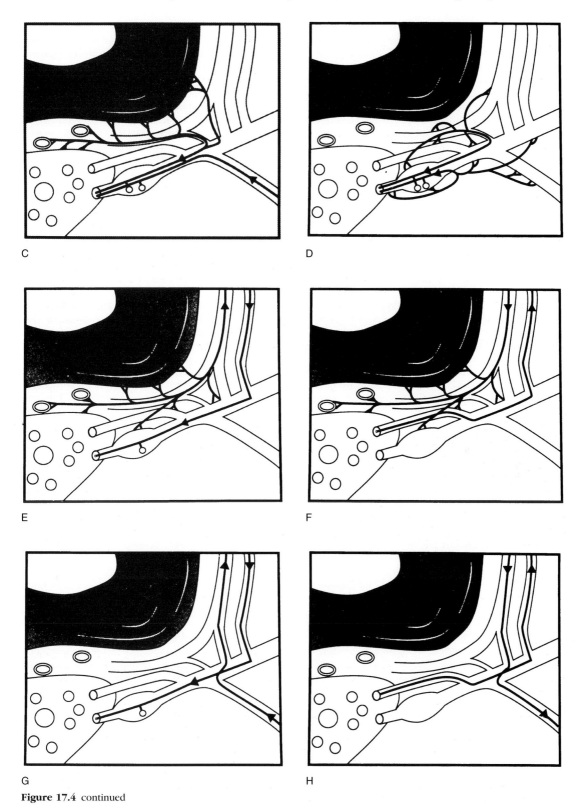

C

D

E

F

G

H

Figure 17.4 continued

nerves, and later accompanying the blood vessels supplying these tissues (Figures 17.4G,H) (Dass, 1952; Bogduk, 1980; Auteroche, 1983).

With this level of neuroanatomical complexity, it is not surprising that pathology affecting this particular region would be expected to potentially be somewhat confusing in its clinical manifestations. All possible somatoautonomic expressions (e.g. local pain, referred pain, autonomic dysfunction, etc.) could possibly emanate from this network of afferent and efferent fibres, that both traverse this area as well as originate and terminate here. This surely must be one of the more neurally labyrinthine regions in the entire peripheral nervous system. Why each patient might be expected to have a unique and compound-complex array of signs and symptoms can be easily appreciated if these intimately related anatomical ramifications are taken into account.

Anatomy of centripetally/ centrifugally referred spinal syndromes

As noted above, many afferent fibres from the spinal column project immediately to, and away from, the paraspinal sympathetic ganglia (Groen *et al.*, 1990). Afferent polymodal pain fibres traversing the sympathetic ganglia have been identified in all of the anterior vertebral structures except the nucleus pulposus. The tissues innervated include the anterior longitudinal ligament, the most peripheral laminae of the anulus fibrosus, the periosteum of the vertebral body, and the vertebral body itself (Pedersen *et al.*, 1956; Stilwell, 1956; Jackson *et al.*, 1966; Edgar and Ghadially, 1976; Paris, 1983). A major autonomic branch also extends posteriorly from either the sympathetic ganglion directly, or indirectly from gray ramus communicans to make up the bulk of the recurrent meningeal nerve (Figure 17.4E) (Kaplan, 1947; Wiberg, 1949; Pedersen *et al.*, 1956; Bogduk *et al.*, 1981; Jinkins *et al.*, 1989). Thus, afferent sympathetic fibres supply the whole of the disc periphery, and indeed the entire vertebral column (Jinkins *et al.*, 1989). This extensive network, known as the *paravertebral autonomic neural plexus*, was initially detailed by Stilwell (1956) (Figure 17.1).

Depending on the vertebral level, after traversing the sympathetic ganglia, many of these primary afferent fibres subsequently enter the ventral ramus of the somatic spinal nerve via the white ramus communicans. These axons then pass into the dorsal root ganglion, where the cell bodies lie (Figure 17.4E). Afterward, the dorsal nerve root carries the fibres until they penetrate the dorsolateral aspect of the spinal cord within the tract of Lissauer, adjacent to the dorsal-horn gray matter.

The anatomical path, and embryological origin, of these neural elements within the autonomic nervous system contribute, in part, to the imperfect conscious perception and somatic localization of many pain stimuli. Conscious somatotopic localization of pain is normally accomplished largely by the point of spatial entry of afferent impulses/axons into the CNS. Some pain-related impulses entering afferent sympathetic fibres may result in appropriately localized symptomatology, while other axons will be involved with important autonomic reflex functions. Impulses within different (or perhaps the same) afferent fibres, however, will result in the conscious picture of remote pain (i.e. perceived in the pelvis, buttocks, lower extremities). Such referred pain is projected to the region corresponding generally to the somatic distribution of the afferent fibres of the spinal nerve with which the afferent sympathetic fibres entered the spinal canal en route to the CNS.

A somatome is defined as a field of somatic and autonomic innervation that is based on the embryological segmental origin of the somatic tissues (Inman and Saunders, 1944). The complete somatome is composed of three basic elements: the cutaneous structures (dermatome), the skeletal musculature (myotome), and the bones, joints, and ligaments (sclerotome). The term 'somatic' indicates that these tissues originate embryonically from the precursor somites (Parke, 1982). Tissues originating from the same somite, therefore, will have a common neural circuitry and thus a common pathway of neural referral. Thus, distant pain referral is mentally 'projected' to these fields of innervation within the lumbosacral somatomes. The conscious somatic registration (or perhaps illusion) of referred pain is perceived by the brain within what have come to be known as the lumbosacral zones of Head. Unfortunately, these regions of pain referral are found in the same peripheral physical distribution as is the radiating pain seen in true neurogenic sciatica. Nevertheless, these zones of Head (as compared to the cutaneous dermatomes) are irregular, constricted, bilaterally asymmetric, and partially superimposed upon one another. Moreover, they are somewhat inconsistent from person to person (Figure 17.5) (Mooney and Robertson, 1976). Proof that the referred pain's origin is a process intimately involving an afferent limb of the peripheral nervous system, and that the illusory perception of distant referred pain is a mechanism of the CNS, is confirmed by the experimental finding that local anaesthesia of the actual region of impulse origin (spinal tissues), abolishes the pain referral, however, anaesthesia of the site of referral (the zone of Head) does not consistently ablate this referred pain (Groen *et al.*, 1988; Devor and Rappaport, 1990).

The referred nature and poor definition of the pain are potentially further complicated by the distribution patterns of the sympathetic afferent fibres of the

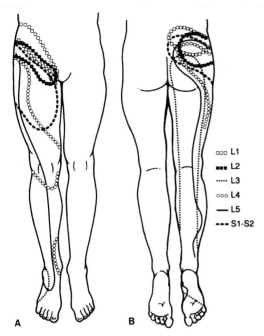

Figure 17.5 Right unilateral composite of lumbosacral Head zones of pain referral and proposed reflex autonomic dysfunction referral from segmental spinal levels. A: Anterior and B: posterior aspects. Note constricted, superimposed, and skipped regions. (Adapted from Jinkins, J.R., Whittemore, A.R. and Bradley, W.G. (1989) The anatomic basis of vertebrogenic pain and the autonomic syndrome associated with lumbar disk extrusion. *AJNR*, **10**, 219-231; *AJR*, **152**, 1277-1289; with permission.)

spine, which overlap craniocaudally as well as across the midline. In other words, there is no true anatomical midline, or accurate segmental nature, of the lumbosacral paravertebral autonomic (sympathetic) nervous system. In addition, after afferent sympathetic fibres enter the paraspinal sympathetic ganglia, they cannot always exit directly into the nearby somatic ventral or dorsal rami of the spinal root. These fibres instead may have to ascend to a more craniad level before entering the spine. In fact, afferent fibres can only join the spinal nerves, and subsequently the CNS, via the white rami communicantes. An important anatomical pattern illustrates that there are no, few, or irregularly distributed, white rami communicantes below the L2 vertebral level, or above the S2 level (Gray, 1985). Any sympathetic afferent fibres from the lower lumbar, and upper sacral region (L2-S2 levels), therefore, must ascend within the sympathetic chain before they are able to enter the spine at a level that has a white ramus communicans (Figure 17.2B). As a result of this *ascending sympathetic afferent diversion*, sympathetic pain impulses emanating from lumbosacral regions that do not have white rami communicantes

(L2-S2 levels) will be referred to the somatome corresponding to the final spinal entry level of the afferent fibre. Thus, the conscious perception of sympathetically mediated pain may be misregistered in the CNS, and pain referral may thereby occur to a somatome different from that which its origin would have indicated. This may also possibly result in summing of pain sensation due to the superimposition of afferent fibre input from several different levels (Groen *et al.*, 1988). These observations might explain the partial segmental superimposition, and irregular contracted nature, of the zones of Head in the lumbosacral region, as depicted in Figure 17.5. It should be noted that the overlapping areas of most common centrifugal pain referral from all lumbar levels, in fact, fall largely within the cutaneous dermatomes of the upper lumbar spinal nerves.

These unusual lumbosacral innervation patterns may also engender local referred pain to the spine itself and its surrounding tissues (Groen *et al.*, 1990). Conscious pain referral originating in the spinal column, and spinal neural tissue, and subsequently projected to the lumbosacral zones of Head, is linked with spinal nerves that coincidentally have afferent somatic projection fields within spinal and paraspinal structures. In other words, an integral component of the somatomes (e.g. myotomes, sclerotomes) of spinal nerves includes the spinal elements themselves. Thus, although the local referred pain is not perceived at the precise point of origin in the spine, it is still consciously imagined diffusely in the region of the low back. A combination of local referred, distant referred, and local somatic pain constitutes *vertebrogenic* pain, which, when combined with the sometimes concurrent radiating radicular neurogenic pain, seems partly to explain the parallel systems operating in the spinal column responsible for the complex and often superimposed syndromes of spinal pain (Dass, 1952; Groen *et al.*, 1988; Jinkins *et al.*, 1989).

Further inspection of Figure 17.5 reveals areas of unsuperimposed pain referral extending far distally into the lower extremities. This pattern may be explained by the fact that there is direct sympathetic afferent inflow into the S2-S4 pelvic somatic nerve roots, and also by the observation that the innervation of spinal structures may originate from as few as three, and as many as five, different adjacent spinal levels [9]. Hence, direct sacral inflow, and therefore direct pain referral, may occur over wide areas of the lower lumbosacral spine (Wyke, 1949; Ruch, 1982). There are gaps in somatic coverage within the zones of Head, perhaps because somatic tissues are not as densely populated with autonomic fibres as they are with afferent and efferent ramifications of native somatic nerves. Therefore, the autonomic projection fields may be somewhat functionally contracted. These general anatomical concepts help to clarify some of the mechanisms within the peripheral nervous system responsible for the rather nebulous fields characteristic of the zones of Head. As the foregoing seems to indicate, the entire network resulting in the perception of referred pain could be mediated within the autonomic (sympathetic) somatotopic organization of the CNS, running in parallel with somatic afferent systems. The peripheral neurological system follows two patterns during embryological development. The somatic nervous system has one distribution, which ramifies solely within the somatic tissues. However, the autonomic nervous system develops along two different pathways: 1) within visceral tissues, sometimes referred to as the visceral autonomic nervous system, and 2) within the somatic tissues in a distribution similar to that of the peripheral somatic nerves. There must also be parallel

sympathetic afferent links to the CNS in order to complete somatic tissue autonomic reflex arcs (Figure 17.6A). The presence of these peripheral autonomic afferent fibres within somatic tissues has been demonstrated clinically (Ruch, 1982). Because both visceral and somatic tissues are innervated by the sympathetic nervous system, and assuming that both tissues are served by afferent limbs, the CNS may then perceive an impulse origin within either tissue, on the basis of a central embryologically predetermined linkage. In actuality, however, the CNS may not be able accurately to discriminate spatially between the visceral and the somatic origin of a stimulus in certain circumstances. Thus, a visceral sympathetic afferent stimulus may erroneously be consciously perceived as arising within the somatic

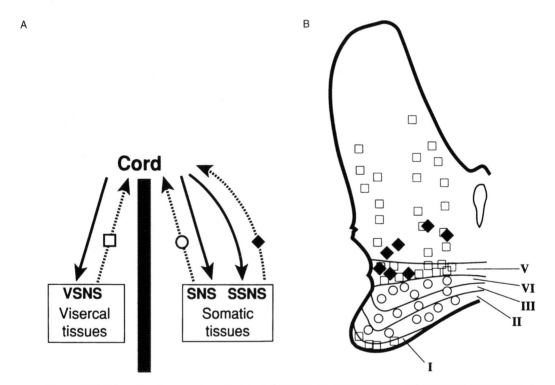

Figure 17.6 Schematic of proposed configuration of peripheral nervous system and its central terminations. A. Efferent pathways (solid arrows), afferent pathways (broken arrows), visceral tissue sympathetic afferent fibres (square), somatic tissue somatic afferent fibres (circle), and hypothesized somatic tissue sympathetic afferent fibres (diamond). VSNS = visceral sympathetic nervous system; SNS = somatic nervous system; SSNS = somatic sympathetic nervous system. Note: see use of same symbols and meanings in B. (Adapted from Jinkins, J.R., Whittemore, A.R. and Bradley, W.G. (1989) The anatomic basis of vertebrogenic pain and the autonomic syndrome associated with lumbar disk extrusion. *AJNR*, **10**, 219–231; *AJR*, **152**, 1277–1289; with permission.) B. Points of termination of visceral and somatic afferent fibres on cord neurons within dorsal and ventral gray matter of right spinal hemicord. I–V = laminae of dorsal horn; termination of somatic (somatic tissue somatic) afferent fibres on somatic cord neurons (circles); terminations of visceral (visceral tissue sympathetic) afferent fibres on visceral cord neurons (squares); terminations of somatic (proposed somatic tissue sympathetic) afferent fibres on viscerosomatic cord neurons (diamonds). Note overlapping regions covered by squares and diamonds resulting in a central nervous system convergence of afferent fibres from divergent origins. (Adapted from Jinkins, J.R., Whittemore, A.R. and Bradley, W.G. (1989) The anatomic basis of vertebrogenic pain and the autonomic syndrome associated with lumbar disk extrusion. *AJNR*, **10**, 219–231; *AJR*, **152**, 1277–1289; with permission.)

sector of the sympathetic afferent sensory projection field and, by definition, is thus referred to this location. The converse of this phenomenon might also be true, although perhaps more rarely perceived.

This explanation concisely fits the observation of referral of visceral sympathetic stimuli (e.g. cardiac pain) to the somatic sympathetic afferent projection field (e.g. left shoulder), thereby defining the zones of Head predominantly, or as a phenomenon of a developmentally dichotomous sympathetic nervous system ramifying within visceral and somatic tissues. Understood in this way, referred actions and conscious perceptions are an expected capacity of the autonomic (sympathetic) nervous system. Thus, the ascending afferent lumbar sympathetic diversion accounts for extrasegmental CNS misregistration and patterns of mismapped superimposition of pain within the lumbosacral zones of Head, but the actual primary referral seems to result from the mediation of the painful stimulus within the autonomic nervous system (Bogduk, 1983).

However, only so much can be understood within the framework of the peripheral nervous system and, thereafter, CNS mechanisms of pain referral must be considered. Anatomical data suggest that somatic and visceral autonomic afferents may have the same, or some of the same, central connections at the level of the spinal cord, thalamus, and sensory cortex (Willis and Grossman, 1973a,b; Ruch, 1982; Cervero, 1985; Wyke, 1987). The *convergence theory* for the occurrence of referred pain states that, because some of the same central pathways are shared by the converging visceral and somatic afferent systems, the CNS cannot precisely distinguish between the two origins of sensory input. An ancillary hypothesis indicates that, since the somatomes are normally continually relaying consciously noxious stimuli, as opposed to the viscera, through a process of *pattern recognition,* the CNS attributes most of the segmental afferent inflow to somatic origins regardless of the true site of the stimulus (Wills and Grossman, 1973a; Ruch, 1982). There is little doubt, however, that some degree of modulation of afferent input from any peripheral source occurs at the level of the spinal cord and above (Hannington-Kiff, 1978; Wyke, 1987).

Thus the mechanisms for somatotopic referral seem to lie at the level of the spinal cord and above. There seems to be a definite somatotopic organization of the spinal cord with regard to entering afferent fibres. The level of cord entry of afferent fibres is important, but of greater importance is the point of termination of the fibre spatially within the cord gray matter at any particular level. Somatic afferent fibres largely terminate on neurons ('somatic' neurons) within laminae II, III, and IV of the dorsal horn gray matter, while visceral afferent fibres terminate on neurons ('visceral' neurons) in laminae I and

V and within the ventral horn gray substance (Figure 17.6B). However, there is a third population of cells on which some afferents terminate known as 'viscerosomatic' neurons. The rationale for their terminology is that these latter neurons are driven by stimuli from both the somatic as well as the visceral tissues (Cervero, 1985). Some somatic afferents labelled 'indeterminate' terminate on these viscerosomatic neurons, which may indicate that these neural structures are in reality the postulated somatic tissue sympathetic afferent fibres (Cervero, 1985).

A complementary theory for referred pain considers the possibility of bifurcating peripheral sympathetic afferent fibres, with one limb entering the visceral tissues while the other ramifies within the somatic tissues (Figure 17.7) (Bahr *et al.*, 1981; Pierau *et al.*, 1984; Cervero, 1985; Dalsgaard and Ygge,

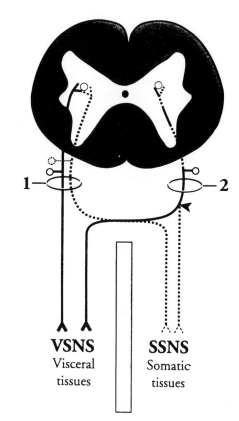

Figure 17.7 Schematic of proposed general organization of peripheral afferent sympathetic nervous system. 1 = dual afferent axon configuration; 2 = bifurcating (arrowhead) afferent axon pattern. Visceral sympathetic afferent fibres (solid axons); somatic sympathetic afferent fibres (dotted axons). VSNS = visceral sympathetic nervous system; SSNS = somatic sympathetic nervous system. (Adapted from Jinkins, J.R., Whittemore, A.R. and Bradley, W.G. (1989) The anatomic basis of vertebrogenic pain and the autonomic syndrome associated with lumbar disk extrusion. *AJNR,* **10**, 219-231; *AJR,* **152**, 1277-1289; with permission.)

1985). Nevertheless, the important concept is still that of convergence of multiple afferent axons on the same viscerosomatotopic registration region (or neuron) of the CNS, either primarily or via connecting interneurons. This may cause a false mental image of the localization of a sensory event. In context, therefore, referred pain to the peripheral tissues (e.g. zones of Head) from a stimulus source such as the spine, does not have its stimulus origin in the area of conscious perception in those peripheral tissues. This definition of central pain perception indicates that referred pain fields are thus 'illusory' or 'imagined' by the higher cognitive centres of the CNS because of afferent CNS convergence.

Autonomic nervous system function, however, is not confined to the conscious perception of painful stimuli. This network also has a major role in the mediation of unconscious normal autonomic function via autonomic reflex arcs occurring at the level of the spinal cord, which in turn are influenced by higher CNS levels (Willis and Grossman, 1973a; Jenkins, 1978; Cervero, 1985; Janig, 1985; Wyke, 1987). Just as the conscious perception of pain may be spatially misregistered, so too may various autonomic functions. Current understanding suggests that somatic, as well as autonomic fibres, both excite, or otherwise share, the same interneurons within the spinal cord (Wills and Grossman, 1973a). Aberrant autonomic reflex arcs resulting in referred autonomic dysfunction of spinal column origin might be represented in the form of aberrant centrifugal vasomotor, pilomotor, and sudomotor activity (Ruch, 1982). In addition to these positive sympathetic effects, reverse or paradoxic effects might be observed, presumably due to pre- and/or postsynaptic efferent inhibition by polysynaptic, polyaxonal afferent spinal cord input (Wyke, 1987; Willis and Grossman, 1973a).

However, these findings are seemingly minor, and are overshadowed by the manifestations of pain. Such autonomic dysfunction is often apparently disregarded. These phenomena may be more common than realized, and could be elicited with greater frequency if subjects were carefully scrutinized for such manifestations at the time of clinical examination.

Somatic muscle spasm is also associated with autonomic function/dysfunction (Feinstein *et al.*, 1954; Hockaday and Whitty, 1967; Ruch, 1982; Cervero, 1985; Wyke, 1987). Skeletal muscle spasm, which may become a painful process in and of itself, is theoretically accomplished by an aberrant reflex arc, similar to the autonomic reflex dysfunction discussed earlier. Thus, referred reflex somatic muscle spasm in the lumbosacral myotome, known as a viscerosomatic reflex, may account for clinically significant symptomatology (Janig, 1985). The spasm itself could be produced by an arrest of the usual negative feedback mechanisms that ordinarily affect muscular contraction, because the stimulus does not

originate within the area of the effect, the lumbosacral zone of Head, but instead from a distant referral source, the spine. Unopposed positive feedback mechanisms may be alternately responsible for the muscle spasm for similar reasons (Willis and Grossman, 1973a).

In all such autonomic reflex dysfunction, the afferent neural limb eventually enters the paraspinal sympathetic plexus. As previously discussed, largely because of the ascending sympathetic afferent inflow diversion (often entering at or above the L2 segmental level), and because of the peculiarities of the autonomic (sympathetic) nervous system (both in its central and peripheral ramifications), there may be a spatial mismapping of otherwise normal autonomic function, causing the efferent effector limb of the arc to occur in the peripheral somatome (Figure 17.8). This autonomic dysfunction, an aberrant somatosympathetic (or sympathosomatic) reflex, might include any one, or combination, of dermal blushing, pallor, pilo-erection, diaphoresis, or somatic muscle

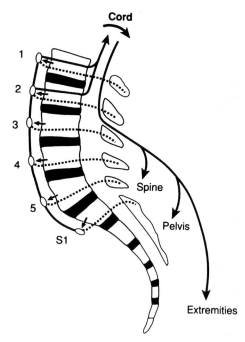

Figure 17.8 Aberrant autonomic reflex arc. Afferent limb is carried within ascending paraspinal sympathetic chain (open circles). After synapse in spinal cord, efferent limb is carried within peripheral ramifications (e.g. spine, pelvis, extremities) of somatic and/or sympathetic components of somatic spinal nerves (long multiheaded curved arrow). (Adapted from Jinkins, J.R., Whittemore, A.R. and Bradley, W.G. (1989) The anatomic basis of vertebrogenic pain and the autonomic syndrome associated with lumbar disk extrusion. *AJNR*, **10**, 219–231; *AJR*, **152**, 1277–1289; with permission.)

spasm, reflecting genuine peripheral signs and symptoms within the lumbosacral zones of Head (Ruch, 1982).

An additional possible referred phenomenon is the conscious perception of paraesthesias of the somatic tissues within the zones of Head (Ruch, 1982, Feinstein *et al.*, 1954). The mechanism for this is presumably located at the level of the cord, and/or above, which unpredictably facilitates (hyperaesthesia) or blocks (hypoaesthesia) somatic afferent activity within the somatome in response to elevated paraspinal sympathetic afferent inflow (Seltzer and Devor, 1979).

Finally, signs and symptoms of a general sympathetic outflow may occasionally play a role in the overall clinical complex during certain phases of spinal disease. For example, a general sympathetic outflow is occasionally seen clinically and experimentally in conjunction with acute traumatic stimulation of vertebral elements; it results in varied viscerosomatic reactions, including a change in blood pressure, heart rate, and respiratory rate, as well as elevations in alertness accompanied by nausea, all of which are *not* proportional to the severity and extent of the induced pain (Feinstein *et al.*, 1954; Pedersen *et al.*, 1956; Cervero, 1985).

Anatomy of centripetally/centrifugally radiating spinal syndromes

On a yet more elemental level, if, because of some pathological influence (Ochoa, 1980; Dahlin *et al.*, 1986; Lundborg and Dahlin, 1989; Jayson, 1992), the geometry of the cell membrane of the axon, and its sodium channels, changes so that the channel density increases, the ionic equilibrium across the membrane may be disrupted (Devor and Rappaport, 1990). The flow of normal ionic currents, and the maintenance of the normal axon membrane potential, are dependent upon this functional sodium channel density/membrane area relationship (Figure 17.9). Theoretically, if the functional sodium channel density per square area escalates, the influx of sodium ions into the cell cannot be offset, as it normally is by the sodium pump mechanism (Devor and Rappaport, 1990). The passive influx (by the sodium channels) out-paces the active efflux (by the sodium pump), and the cell membrane, in effect, autodepolarizes producing an ectopic bidirectional action potential radiating away from the site of origin of the initial membrane depolarization (Figure 17.10). The CNS interprets this potential (incoming within appropriate afferent fibres) as pain and paraesthesias, a sign for involuntary muscular activity, or as a signal for autonomic action. In this manner, axons in and of

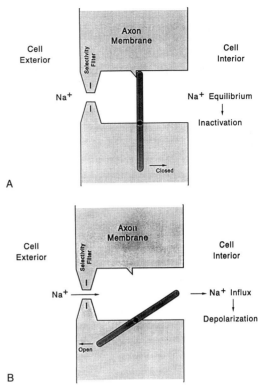

Figure 17.9 Schematic illustrating hypothetical mechanism of sodium channel function in axon membrane. (Adapted from Dudel, J. (1985) Excitation of nerve and muscle. In *Fundamentals of Neurophysiology* (R.F. Schmidt, ed.). Springer-Verlag, New York, pp. 19–68, with permission.) A. When sodium channel is closed, the passive influx of sodium ions does not occur, and no neuroelectrical activity along or across the axon membrane takes place. B. When sodium channel is open, as in normal longitudinal neuroelectrical axon conduction, the passive influx of sodium ions is facilitated resulting in depolarization across the axon membrane (NA^+ = sodium ions).

themselves may become ectopic sources of pathological neuroelectrical activity, resulting in abnormal clinical expression and conscious perception. This is the pathophysiological basis for the so-called *radiating radiculopathy*.

Because of the presence of this ectopic axonal pacemaker, the transmission of normal incoming or outgoing neuroelectrical impulses occurring in, and adjacent to, fibres with pathologically altered axon membranes, may also result in pain, paraesthesias and dysfunction that similarly originate at the level of the ectopic source of activity. This aberrant neuroelectrical coupling is believed to take place because of abnormal interaxonal 'cross-talk' based on chemical, neurochemical and/or *ephaptic* (neuroelectrical) factors (Gardner, 1966; Rasminsky, 1978a; Devor and Rappaport, 1990). Theoretically,

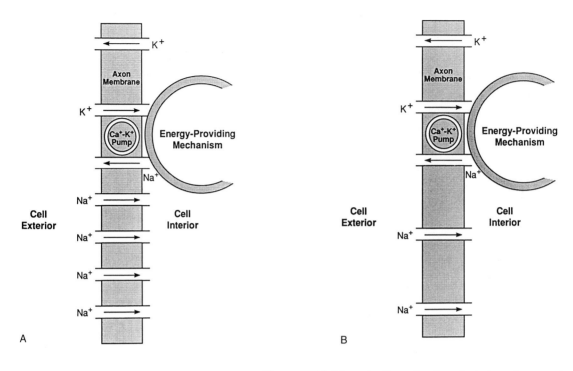

A

B

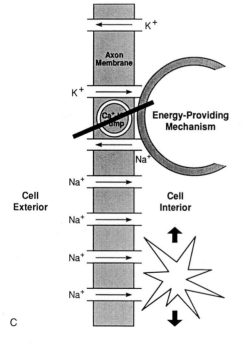

C

Figure 17.10 Schematic illustrating hypothetical mechanism of normal function and dysfunction in axon membrane resulting in axonal autodepolarization and ectopic axon impulse generation (i.e. radiating radiculopathy) (A) and (B). (Adapted from Dudel, J. (1985) Excitation of nerve and muscle. In *Fundamentals of Neurophysiology* (R.F. Schmidt, ed.), Springer-Verlag, New York, pp. 19–68, with permission.) A. Normal relationship between passive sodium channels in the axon membrane, and the active energy requiring sodium-potassium pump that maintains the neuroelectrical potential across the axon membrane during inactivity, and restores this potential after normal impulse transmission. (NA^+ = sodium ions, K^+ = potassium ions, arrows in conduits = flux in ion channels). B. Unbalanced relationship between the sodium channels and the potassium pump. In this circumstance, the functional sodium channel spatial density in the axon membrane has increased without a consonant increase in the potential of the sodium-potassium pump to balance this phenomenon. This abnormal relationship theoretically overwhelms the sodium-potassium pump's ability to maintain the neuroelectrical potential across the axon membrane, resulting in autodepolarization. C. The sodium-potassium pump itself may also be dysfunctional (bar). Such a functional defect in the axon membrane constitutes an ectopic source (star) of neuroelectrical activity (i.e. within the axon membrane). Because the resulting aberrant action impulse is transmitted in both directions along the axon, this phenomenon is theoretically, partly responsible for pathological efferent peripheral nervous system involuntary expression (e.g. muscle spasm, autonomic dysfunction) and central nervous system conscious perception (e.g. pain, paraesthesias).

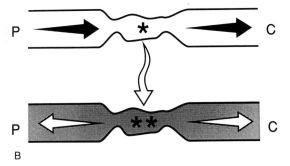

Figure 17.11 Spontaneous ectopic neuroelectrical activity resulting in central (C) and peripheral (P) aberrant impulse propagation in injured (wavy contoured channels) axons. These phenomena could, hypothetically, occur in spinal dorsal roots, ventral roots, or combined spinal nerves. A. Spontaneous ectopic neuroelectrical impulse (asterisk) originating in injured afferent axon (open channel: somatic or autonomic). The aberrant impulse (solid arrows) propagates away from the site of spontaneous depolarization. B. Spontaneous ectopic neuroelectrical impulse (asterisk) originating in injured efferent axon (shaded channel: somatic or autonomic). The aberrant impulse (open arrows) propagates away from the site of spontaneous depolarization.

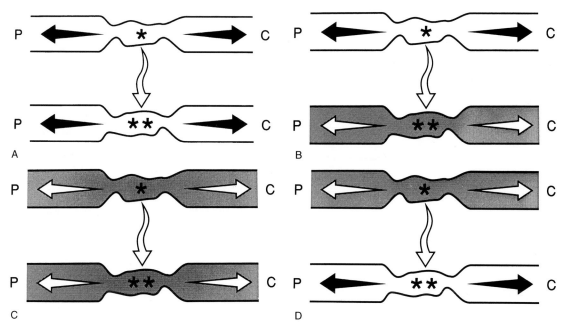

Figure 17.12 Spontaneous ectopic neuroelectrical activity resulting in ephaptic axo-axonal transmission–stimulation between adjacent injured axons (wavy contoured channels). These phenomena could hypothetically occur in spinal dorsal roots, ventral roots, or in combined spinal nerves. A. Spontaneous depolarization (single asterisk) originating in injured afferent axon (upper open channel: somatic or autonomic) results in neuroelectrical impulse (upper solid arrows) that propagates away from site of ectopic origin. At the same time, ephaptic transmission (open serpentine arrow) axo-axonally results in stimulation (double asterisk) of adjacent afferent axon (lower open channel: somatic or autonomic) acting as an ectopic receptor and effecting central (C) and peripheral (P) aberrant afferent axon impulse propagation (lower solid arrows). B. Spontaneous depolarization (single asterisk) originating in injured afferent axon (open channel: somatic or autonomic) results in neuroelectrical impulse (open straight arrows) that propagates away from the site of ectopic origin. At the same time, ephaptic transmission (open serpentine arrow) of electrical impulses axo-axonally results in stimulation (double asterisk) of adjacent efferent axon (shaded channel: somatic or autonomic) acting as an ectopic receptor and effecting central (C) and peripheral (P) aberrant efferent axon impulse propagation (open straight arrows). C. Spontaneous depolarization (single asterisk) originating in injured efferent axon (upper shaded channel: somatic or autonomic) results in neuroelectrical impulse (upper open straight arrows) that propagates away from the site of ectopic origin. At the same time, ephaptic transmission (open serpentine arrow) axo-axonally results in stimulation (double asterisk) of adjacent efferent axon (lower shaded channel: somatic or autonomic) acting as ectopic receptor and effecting central (C) and peripheral (P) aberrant afferent axon impulse propagation (lower open straight arrows). D. Spontaneous depolarization (single asterisk) originating in injured efferent axon (upper shaded channel: somatic or autonomic) results in neuroelectrical impulse (open straight arrows) that propagates away from the site of ectopic origin. At the same time, ephaptic transmission (open serpentine arrow) axo-axonally results in stimulation (double asterisk) of adjacent injured afferent axon (open channel: somatic or autonomic) acting as ectopic receptor and effecting central (C) and peripheral (P) aberrant afferent axon impulse propagation (solid straight arrows).

this cross-talk is responsible for abnormal links within the somatic and between the somatic and autonomic nervous systems. In this way, the resultant distant propagation may occur within axons that are anatomically unrelated to the origin of the neuroelectrical transmission.

Experiments support the concept that focal neural injury can act as both an ectopic stimulus as well as an ectopic receptor/transmitter (Lehmann and Ule, 1964; Gardner, 1966; Wallis *et al.*, 1970; Wall *et al.*, 1974; Howe *et al.*, 1976; Ramon *et al.*, 1976; Wettstein, 1977; Bostock and Sears, 1978; Rasminsky, 1978a,b; Seltzer and Devor, 1979; Calvin *et al.*, 1982; Rasminsky, 1989; Devor and Rappaport, 1990). First,

a chronically, repetitively injured afferent or efferent axon may act as a primary ectopic pacemaker, spontaneously discharging and initiating bidirectional axonal impulse transmission (Figure 17.11). Second, injured afferent or efferent axons acting as ectopic pacemakers may ephaptically (neuroelectrically) transmit neuroelectrical impulses to ectopic axonal receptors in adjacent injured afferent and/or efferent axons (Figure 17.12). This ephaptic transmission represents the type of interneural neuroelectrical 'cross-talk' referred to above (Gardner, 1966; Ramon *et al.*, 1976; Rasminsky, 1978a; Seltzer and Devor, 1979; Devor and Rappaport, 1990). Third, because of chronic injury, afferent or efferent axons acting as

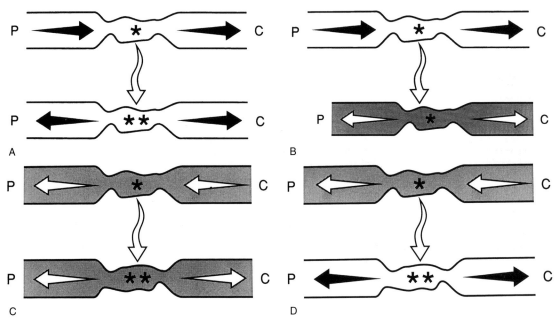

Figure 17.13 Aberrant neuroelectrical activity driven by incoming or outgoing axon impulses and resulting in ephaptic axo-axonal transmission–stimulation between adjacent injured axons (wavy contoured channels). These phenomena could hypothetically occur in spinal dorsal roots, ventral roots, or in combined spinal nerves. A. Incoming neuroelectrical impulse (upper open straight arrows) within afferent axon (upper open channel: somatic or autonomic) results in depolarization (single asterisk) at the site of axon injury. At the same time, ephaptic transmission (open serpentine arrow) axo-axonally results in stimulation (double asterisk) of adjacent injured afferent axon (lower open channel: somatic or autonomic) acting as ectopic receptor and effecting central (C) and peripheral (P) aberrant afferent axon impulse propagation (lower open straight arrows). B. Incoming neuroelectrical impulse (upper solid straight arrows) within afferent axon (upper open channel: somatic or autonomic) results in depolarization (single asterisk) at the site of axon injury. At the same time, ephaptic transmission (open serpentine arrow) of electrical impulse axo-axonally results in stimulation (double asterisk) of adjacent injured efferent axon (lower shaded channel: somatic or autonomic) acting as ectopic receptor and effecting central (C) and peripheral (P) aberrant afferent axon impulse propagation (lower open straight arrows). C. Outgoing neuroelectrical impulse (upper open straight arrows) within efferent axon (upper shaded channel: somatic or autonomic) results in depolarization (single asterisk) at the site of axon injury. At the same time, ephaptic transmission (open serpentine arrow) of electrical impulse axo-aonally causes stimulation (double asterisk) of adjacent injured efferent axon (lower shaded channel: somatic or autonomic) acting as ectopic receptor and effecting central (C) and peripheral (P) aberrant efferent axon impulse propagation (lower open straight arrows). D. Outgoing neuroelectrical impulse (upper straight arrows) within efferent axon (upper shaded channel: somatic or autonomic) results in depolarization (single asterisk) at the site of axon injury. At the same time, ephaptic transmission (open serpentine arrow) axo-axonally causes stimulation (double asterisk) of adjacent injured efferent axon (lower shaded channel: somatic or autonomic) acting as ectopic receptor and effecting central (C) and peripheral (P) aberrant efferent axon impulse propagation (lower solid straight arrows).

primary ectopic receptors may be driven by incoming peripheral afferent or outgoing central efferent somatic or autonomic impulses; they may then secondarily ephaptically transmit neuroelectrical impulses to ectopic receptors in adjacent injured afferent and/or efferent axons (Figure 17.13). Efferent autonomic fibres thus driving afferent pain fibres constitutes a relatively new theory of referred pain and dysfunction (Devor and Rappaport, 1990). Fourth, because neural injury may result in part in increased receptor sensitivity, afferent or efferent axons acting as ectopic pacemakers may ephaptically drive injured afferent fibre terminations on nerves, the afferent *nervi nervorum* (Figure 17.14) (Devor and Rappaport, 1990). Fifth, afferent or efferent axons acting as ectopic transmitters may be driven by incoming peripheral afferent, or outgoing central efferent, impulses and may secondarily transmit neuroelectrical impulses ephaptically to afferent somatic and autonomic fibre terminations on nerves, the afferent *nervi nervorum* (Figure 17.15). Sixth, autonomic efferent fibre terminations on nerves, the

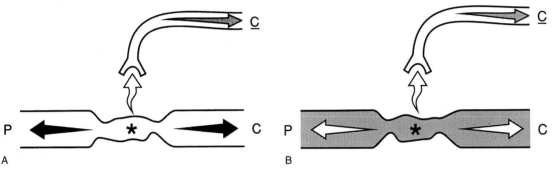

Figure 17.14 Spontaneous ectopic neuroelectrical activity resulting in ephaptic transmission between injured axons (wavy contoured channels) and afferent *nervi nervorum* (open bifid channels). These phenomena could hypothetically occur in spinal dorsal roots, ventral roots, or in combined spinal nerves. A. Spontaneous depolarization (single asterisk) originating in injured afferent axon (lower open channel: somatic or autonomic) results in neuroelectrical impulse (solid straight arrows) that propagates centrally (C) and peripherally (P) away from the site of ectopic origin. At the same time, ephaptic transmission (open serpentine arrow) axo-axonally causes stimulation of normal or injured (sensitized) receptor (open bifid channel: somatic or autonomic) of afferent *nervi nervorum*, effecting central (C) aberrant afferent axon impulse propagation (stippled arrow). B. Spontaneous depolarization (single asterisk) originating in injured efferent axon (lower shaded channel: somatic or autonomic) results in neuroelectrical impulse (open straight arrows) that propagates centrally (C) and peripherally (P) away from the site of ectopic origin. At the same time, ephaptic transmission (open serpentine arrow) axo-axonally causes stimulation of normal or injured (sensitized) receptor (open bifid channel: somatic or autonomic) of afferent *nervi nervorum* effecting central (C) aberrant afferent axon impulse propagation (stippled arrows).

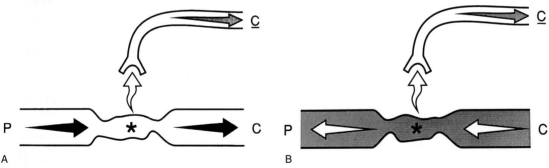

Figure 17.15 Ectopic neurogenic activity driven by incoming or outgoing somatic or autonomic axon impulses and resulting in ephaptic axo-axonal transmission–stimulation between injured axon (wavy contoured channels) and afferent somatic or autonomic *nervi nervorum* (open bifid channels). These phenomena could, hypothetically, occur in spinal dorsal roots, ventral roots, or in combined spinal nerves. A. Incoming neuroelectrical impulse (solid straight arrows) within afferent axon (open channel: somatic or autonomic) results in depolarization (asterisk) at the site of axon injury. At the same time, ephaptic transmission (open serpentine arrow) axo-axonally causes stimulation of normal or injured receptor (open bifid channel: somatic or autonomic) of afferent *nervi nervorum* and effects central (O aberrant afferent axon impulse propagation (stippled arrow). B. Outgoing neuroelectrical impulse (open straight arrows) within efferent axon (open channel: somatic or autonomic) results in depolarization (asterisk) at the site of injured axon. At the same time, ephaptic transmission (open serpentine arrow) axo-axonally causes stimulation of normal or injured receptor (open bifid channel: somatic or autonomic) of afferent *nervi nervorum* and effects central (O aberrant afferent axon impulse propagation (stippled arrow).

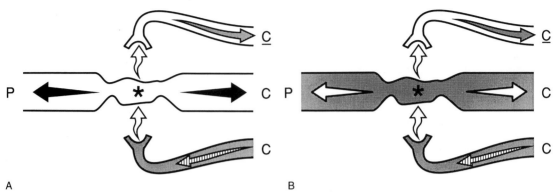

Figure 17.16 Aberrant neuroelectrical activity driven by outgoing autonomic efferent impulse resulting in ephaptic stimulation and transmission, respectively, between autonomic efferent *nervi nervorum* (shaded bifid channels), an injured adjacent axon (wavy contoured channels), and the afferent somatic or autonomic *nervi nervorum* (open bifid channels). These phenomena could hypothetically occur in spinal dorsal roots [A], ventral roots, or in combined spinal nerves. A. Incoming neuroelectrical impulse (hatched arrow) within efferent autonomic axon (shaded bifid channel) of the *nervi nervorum* results in ephaptic stimulation (lower open serpentine arrow) axo-axonally and depolarization (asterisk) at the site of injured afferent axon (wavy contour, open channel: somatic or autonomic) acting as ectopic receptor and effecting central (C) and peripheral (P) aberrant afferent axon impulse propagation (solid straight arrows). At the same time, ephaptic transmission (upper open serpentine arrow) axo-axonally causes stimulation of normal or injured (sensitized) receptor (open bifid channel: somatic or autonomic) of afferent *nervi nervorum* and effects central (C) aberrant afferent axon impulse propagation (stippled arrow). B. Incoming neuroelectrical impulse (hatched arrow) within normal or injured efferent autonomic axon (shaded bifid channel) of the *nervi nervorum* results in ephaptic stimulation (lower open serpentine arrow) axo-axonally and depolarization (asterisk) at the site of injured efferent axon (wavy contour, shaded channel: somatic or autonomic) acting as ectopic receptor and effecting central (C) and peripheral (P) aberrant efferent axon impulse propagation (open straight arrows) At the same time, ephaptic transmission (upper open serpentine arrow) axo-axonally causes stimulation of normal or injured (sensitized) receptor (open bifid channel: somatic or autonomic) of afferent *nervi nervorum* and effects central (5:) aberrant afferent axon impulse propagation (stippled arrow).

efferent *nervi nervorum,* may drive afferent or efferent axons acting as ectopic receptors, and at the same time transmit ephaptically to the afferent *nervi nervorum* (Figure 17.16). This is yet another possible mode of referred pain, muscular dysfunction, and aberrant autonomic activity. It is by these mechanisms that pathological peripherally driven, centrally driven, spontaneously generated, chemically stimulated and ephaptically transmitted neuroelectrical activity can hypothetically occur at and near, the site of neural injury. This thereby causes ectopic single fibre neuroelectrical phenomena and/or multifibre somatic-somatic, somatic-autonomic, autonomic-somatic or autonomic-autonomic aberrant neuroelectrical coupling (Devor and Rappaport, 1990). The expression of this abnormal neurogenic activity may potentially result in bizarre combinations of subjective symptoms (e.g. pain, paraesthesias) and objective signs (e.g. skeletal muscle spasm, sympathetic dysfunction). Thus, otherwise normal peripheral sensation, central voluntary muscle initiation, and somatic movements resulting in minor mechanical neural stimulation, might cause neuropathic phenomena: significant pain and paraesthesias, muscular dysfunction and autonomic derangement emanating from chronically injured spinal nerves/roots.

These manifestations are types of *neurogenic pathological pain* in that they are pain impulses that

are generated within axons which are hypermechanosensitive and perhaps chemosensitive, they are pain impulses that are ectopic in origin (the impulses are not initiated within a true pain receptor: other than the afferent, somatic *nervi nervorum*), and they are pain impulses that are far larger in proportion and duration than would be anticipated to originate from the mechanical perturbation of a normal, uninflamed or uninjured axon or neural termination (Smyth and Wright, 1958; Willis and Grossman, 1973a; Ochoa, 1980). Finally, because of acute and chronic mechanical compression, potentially the dorsal root ganglia have been shown to have a potentially significant role in the genesis of centripetally/centrifugally radiating lumbosacral pain syndromes (Howe *et al.*, 1977; Wall and Devor, 1983).

Conclusion

In common practice, a far-reaching, perplexing, combined somatic-autonomic neurogenic syndrome stems from spinal disease that includes varying degrees of 1) local somatic pain, 2) centripetally/centrifugally referred pain, 3) centripetally/centrifugally radiating pain, 4) local and referred sympathetic reflex dysfunction (diaphoresis, piloerection, vaso-motor changes, somatic muscle spasm), 5) somatic reflex dysfunction, 6) somatic muscle weakness, 7) peripheral somatic dysesthesias, and 8) generalized alterations in viscerosomatic tone (blood pressure, heart rate, respiratory rate, alertness).

Normal and pathological signs and symptoms originating from spinal pathology may be observed in an individual subject singly or in superimposed combinations. This range of manifestations may mis-lead both the patient and the physician as to the origin and the cause of the clinical problem. Such 'layering' of pain and disability chiefly occurs because of related patterns and distributions of sometimes intimately related peripheral nerve fibres, as well as their complex central connections. These networks consequently result in concurrent focal and diffuse, local and remote conscious perceptions and unconscious effects emanating from spinal disease (Jinkins *et al.*, 1989). An understanding of these anatomical and pathophysiological concepts should enable a clarification of the relationship between the clinical presentation of the patient and the roles, as well as the limitations, of medical imaging in the evaluation of the spine.

Acknowledgement

I thank J. Murray for preparation of the manuscript, C. Farias for the photographic reproductions, and G. Phan, N. Place, A. Pressley and C. Whitehead for the artwork.

References

Auteroch, P. (1983) Innervation of the zygapophysial joints of the lumbar spine. *Anat. Clin.*, **5**, 17-28.

Bahr, R., Blumberg, H. and Janig, W. (1981) Do dichotomiz-ing afferent fibers exist which supply visceral organs as well as somatic structures? A contribution to the problem of referred pain. *Neurosci. Lett.*, **24**, 25-28.

Bogduk, N. (1980) Lumbar dorsal ramus syndrome. *Med. J. Aust.*, **2**, 537-541.

Bogduk, N. (1983) The innervation of the lumbar spine. *Spine*, **8**, 286-293.

Bogduk, N. and Long, D.M. (1979) The anatomy of the so-called 'articular nerves' and their relationship to facet denervation in the treatment of low-back pain. *J. Neurosurg.*, **51**, 172-177.

Bogduk, N., Tynan, W. and Wilson, A.S. (1981) The nerve supply to the human lumbar intervertebral discs. *J. Anat.*, **132**, 39-56.

Bogduk, N., Wilson, A.S. and Tynan, W. (1982) The human lumbar dorsal rami. *J. Anat.*, **134**, 383-397.

Bostock, H. and Sears, T.A. (1978) The internodal axon membrane: electrical excitability and continuous conduc-tion in segmental demyelination. *J. Physiol.*, **280**, 273-301.

Calvin, W.H., Devor, M. and Howe, J.F. (1982) Can neuralgias arise from minor demyelination? Spontaneous firing, mechanosensitivity, and after discharge from conducting axons. *Exp. Neurol.*, **75**, 755-763.

Cervero, F. (1985) Visceral nociception: peripheral and central aspects of visceral nociceptive systems. *Philos. Trans. R. Soc. Lond.*, **8**, 325-337.

Dahlin, L.B., Rydevik, B. and Lundborg, G. (1986) Pathophy-siology of nerve entrapments and nerve compression injuries. In *Tissue Nutrition and Viability* (A.R. Hargens, ed.). Springer-Verlag, New York, pp. 135-160.

Dalsgaard, C.J. and Ygge, J. (1985) Separate populations of primary sensory neurons project to the splanchnic nerve and thoracic spinal nerve rami of the rat. *Med. Biol.*, **63**, 88-91.

Dass, R. (1952) Sympathetic components of the dorsal primary divisions of human spinal nerves. *Anat. Rec.*, **113**, 493-501.

Devor, M. and Rappaport, Z.H. (1990) Pain and the patho-physiology of damaged nerve. In *Pain Syndromes In Neu-rology* (H.L. Fields, ed.). Butterworths, Boston, pp. 47-83.

Edgar, M.A. and Ghadially, J.A. (1976) Innervation of the lumbar spine. *Clin. Orthop.*, **115**, 35-41.

Feinstein, B., Langton, J.N.K., Jameson, R.M. and Schiller, F. (1954) Experiments on pain referred from deep somatic tissues. *J. Bone Joint Surg.*, **36A**, 981-997.

Gardner, W.J. (1966) Cross talk – the paradoxical transmis-sion of a nerve impulse. *Arch. Neurol.*, **14**, 149-156.

Gray, H. (1985) *Anatomy of the Human Body*. Lea and Febiger, Philadelphia, pp. 1251-1254, 1264-1265.

Groen, G.J., Baljet, B. and Drukker, J. (1988) The innervation of the spinal dura mater: anatomy and clinical implica-tions. *Acta Neurochir. (Wien)*, **92**, 39-46.

Groen, G.J., Baljet, B. and Drukker, J. (1990) Nerves and nerve plexuses of the human vertebral column. *Am. J. Anat.*, **188**, 282-296.

Hannington-Kiff, J. (1978) The modulation of pain. In *Disorders of the Lumbar Spine* (A.J. Helfet and D.M.G. Lee, eds), J.B. Lippincott, Philadelphia, pp. 120-136.

Hockaday, J. M. and Whitty, C. W. (1967) Patterns of referred pain in the normal subject. *Brain*, **90**, 482-496.

Howe, J.F., Calvin, W.H. and Loeser, J.D. (1976) Impulses reflected from dorsal root ganglia and from focal nerve injuries. *Brain Res.*, **116**, 139-144.

Howe, J.F., Loeser, J.D. and Calvin, W.H. (1977) Mechano-sensitivity of dorsal root ganglia and chronically injured axons: a physiological basis for the radicular pain of nerve root compression. *Pain*, **3**, 25-41.

Inman, V.T. and Saunders, J.B de C. (1944) Referred pain from skeletal structures. *J. Nerv. Ment. Dis.*, **99**, 660-667.

Jackson, H.C., Winkelman, R.K. and Bickel, W.H. (1966) Nerve endings in the human lumbarspinal column and related structures. *J. Bone Joint Surg.*, **48A**, 1272-1281.

Janig, W. (1985) The autonomic nervous system. In *Funda-mentals of Neurophysiology*, (R.F. Schmidt, ed.). Springer-Verlag, New York, pp. 216-269.

Jayson, M.I.V. (1992) The role of vascular damage and fibrosis in the pathogenesis of nerve root damage. *Clin. Orthop. Rel. Res.*, **279**, 40-48.

Jenkins, T.W. (1978) Physiology of spinal nerves. In *Func-tional Mammalian Neuroanatomy*. Lea and Febiger, Philadelphia, pp. 107-133.

Jinkins, J.R., Whittemore, A.R. and Bradley, W.G. (1989) The anatomic basis of vertebrogenic pain and the autonomic syndrome associated with lumbar disk extrusion. *AJNR* **10**, 219-231, *AJR* **152**, 1277-1289.

Kaplan, E.B. (1947) Recurrent meningeal branch of the spinal nerves. *Bull. Hosp. Joint Dis. Orthop. Inst.,* **8**: 108-109.

Lehmann, H.J. and Ule, G. (1964) Electrophysiological findings and structural changes in circumspect inflammation of peripheral nerves. *Prog. Brain Res.,* **6**, 169-173.

Lundborg, G. and Dahlin, L.B. (1989) Pathophysiology of nerve compression. In *Nerve Compression Syndromes* (R.M. Szabo, ed.). Slack, Inc., Thorofare, NJ, p. 15

Mooney, V. and Robertson, J. (1976) The facet syndrome. *Clin. Orthop.,* **115**, 149-156.

Murphy, R.W. (1977) Nerve roots and spinal nerves in degenerative disk disease. *Clin. Orthop. Rel. Res.,* **129**, 46-60.

Ochoa, J. (1980) Nerve fiber pathology in acute and chronic compression. In *Management of Peripheral Nerve Problems* (G.E. Omer and M. Spinner, eds). W.B. Saunders, Philadelphia, p. 487.

Paris, S.V. (1983) Anatomy as related to function and pain. *Orthop. Clin. North Am.,* **14**, 475-489.

Parke, W.W. (1982) Development of the spine. In *The Spine* (R.H. Rothman and F.A. Simeone, eds). Saunders, Philadelphia, pp. 1-17.

Pedersen, H.E., Blunck, C.F.J. and Gardner, E. (1956) The anatomy of lumbosacral posterior rami and meningeal branches of spinal nerves (sinu-vertebral nerves) *J. Bone Joint Surg.,* **38A**, 377-391.

Pierau, F., Fellmer, G. and Taylor, D.C.M. (1984) Somatovisceral convergence in cat dorsal root ganglion neurones demonstrated by double-labelling with fluorescent tracers. *Brain Res.,* **321**, 63-70.

Ramon, F., Joyner, R.W. and Moore, J. W. (1976) Ephaptic transmission in squid giant axoms. *Biophys. J.,* **16**, 26a.

Rasminsky, M. (1978a) Ectopic generation of impulses and cross-talk in spinal nerve roots of 'dystrophic' mice. *Ann. Neurol.,* **3**, 351-357.

Rasminsky, M. (1978b) Physiology of conduction in demyelinated axons. In *The Physiology and Pathobiology of Axons* (S.G. Waxman, ed.). Raven Press, New York, pp. 361-376.

Rasminsky, M. (1989) Ectopic generation of impulses in pathological nerve fibers. In *Nerve Repair and Regeneration - Its Clinical and Experimental Basis* (D.L. Jewett and H.R. McCarroll, eds). Mosby, St Louis, pp. 178-195.

Ruch, T.C. (1982) Pathophysiology of pain. In *Physiology and Biophysics* (T.C. Ruch and H.D. Patton, eds). W.B. Saunders, Philadelphia, pp. 508-531.

Seltzer, Z. and Devor, M. (1979) Ephaptic transmission in chronically damaged peripheral nerves. *Neurology,* **29**, 1061-1064.

Smyth, M.J. and Wright, V.J. (1958) Sciatica and the intervertebral disk. An experimental study. *J. Bone Joint Surg.,* **40A**, 1401-1418.

Stilwell, D.L. (1956) The nerve supply of the vertebral column and its associated structures in the monkey. *Anat. Rec.,* **125**, 139-169.

Wall, P.D. and Devor, M. (1983) Sensory afferent impulses originate from dorsal root ganglia as well as from the periphery in normal and nerve injured rats. *Pain,* **17**, 321-339.

Wall, P.D., Waxman, S. and Basbaum, A.L. (1974) Ongoing activity in peripheral nerve injury discharge. *Exp. Neurol.,* **45**, 576-589.

Wallis, W.E., Van Poznak, A. and Plum, F. (1970) Generalized muscular stiffness, fasciculations and myokymia of peripheral nerve origin. *Arch. Neurol.,* **22**, 430-439.

Wettstein, A. (1977) The origins of fasciculations in motoneuron disease. *Neurology,* **27**, 357-358.

Wiberg, G. (1949) Back pain in relation to the nerve supply of the intervertebral disc. *Acta Orthop. Scand.,* **19**, 211-221.

Willis W.D. and Grossman R.G. (1973a) The spinal cord. In *Medical Neurobiology,* C.V. Mosby, St Louis, pp. 80-115.

Willis, W.D. and Grossman, R.G. (1973b) Sensory systems. In *Medical Neurobiology,* C.V. Mosby, St Louis, pp. 227-272.

Wyke, B. (1987) The neurology of low back pain. In *The Lumbar Spine and Back Pain* (M.I.V. Jayson, ed.). Churchill Livingstone, New York, pp. 56-99.

Section

IV

Diagnosis and Management

18

Imaging of mechanical and degenerative syndromes of the lumbar spine

Lindsay J. Rowe

Introduction

Imaging of the lumbar spine has undergone significant technological change in the last century since Roentgen's initial discovery in 1895 of the 'unknown ray' – the X-ray. A multitude of imaging modalities are available, each with its own advantages, limitations and applications (Table 18.1). To all clinicians involved in the diagnosis and management of lumbar spine disorders, the major difficulties with imaging arise from knowing which test to order for what clinical condition, understanding its limitations, and interpreting the findings in a clinical context (Modic and Herzog, 1994). This can be a bewildering and frustrating aspect of clinical spinal practice. It is the purpose of this chapter to clarify these issues and provide an imaging synthesis for degenerative disorders of the lumbar spine.

Imaging modalities

Conventional radiography

Since X-rays first came available in 1895, plain film radiography has been the mainstay of diagnostic investigation of skeletal and spinal disorders. With the advent of other, more sensitive, modalities the utilization of plain film lumbar spine imaging has come under increasing scrutiny.

Table 18.1 *Spinal imaging modalities*

Conventional radiography
   static; erect, recumbent
   dynamic; sagittal, coronal, longitudinal
Myelography
Discography
Facet arthrography
Computed tomography (CT)
   plain
      bone window
      soft tissue window
   reconstruction
   contrast (IV)
   myelography (CTM)
   discography (CTD)
Magnetic resonance imaging (MRI)
   T1
   T2
   proton density
   fat suppression
   others
   gadolinium enhancement
Nuclear medicine
   planar
      flow
      pool
      delayed
   SPECT
Videofluoroscopy
Ultrasound
Angiography

Indications

Consensus on clinical indicators to obtain lumbar spine radiographs has evolved (Deyo and Diel, 1986; Schultz *et al.*, 1992). These are factors which have medical implications such as tumours and fractures. A hierarchy of clinical indicators can be derived from a synthesis of the literature (Table 18.2). No such consensus has been developed for those involved in conservative care where structural details are therapeutically important such as in spinal manipulation, though chiropractors have published significant material in this area (Cox, 1989; Rowe, 1992; Haldeman, 1993) (Table 18.3).

Table 18.2 *Indicators for obtaining lumbar spine radiographs*

Probable indicators
>50 years of age
Trauma, recent and old
Neuromotor deficit
Unexplained weight loss
Night pain
Inflammatory arthritis
Drug or alcohol abuse
History of cancer
Use of corticosteroids
Fever of unknown origin (>100°F)
Abnormal blood finding (ESR, WBC)
Scoliosis or deformity
Previous surgery or invasive procedure
Failure to improve
Medicolegal implications

Possible indicators
Poor posture
Health policy
Unavailable alternative imaging
Unavailable previous imaging
Dated previous imaging
Patient reassurance
Recent immigrant
Manipulative therapy implications*
Athletes
Research

Non-indicators
Habit, routine, screening procedure
Postural analysis
Patient education
Financial gain
Assess post-discharge status
Frequent biomechanical analysis
Pre-employment screening
Non-licensed operator
Unfamiliarity with equipment
Pregnancy
Young patients
Poor equipment
Large patients
Inappropriate indicator

* See Table 18.3. Indications for obtaining lumbar spine radiographs in spinal manipulative therapy.

Table 18.3 *Indications for obtaining lumbar spine radiographs in spinal manipulative therapy*

Exclusion of significant pathology
bone: tumours, osteoporosis
joints: degenerative changes
soft tissues: aneurysms, calculi

Identification of structural malformations
congenital anomalies: transitional vertebrae, tropism
quantify leg length deficiency
identify scoliosis characteristics
spondylolisthesis

Determination of direction of thrust
curvature analysis
apex vertebrae
intersegmental displacements

Advantages

Conventional radiographic apparatus is readily available, reasonably priced and radiographs are quickly interpretable. Its main strengths are the depiction of bone morphology and that it can be performed in a weight-bearing position.

Limitations

There are two main limitations of plain films; failure to image soft tissues and relative insensitivity to bone destruction. No information is available on the status of the bone marrow, intraspinal neural elements and membranes (nerve roots, spinal cord), intervertebral disc, ligaments and paraspinal tissues. Up to 30–50% loss of bone density may be required in order to reliably depict it on plain radiographs (Rowe and Yochum, 1996a). Correlation of degenerative radiographic findings with pain syndromes is generally disappointing (Frymoyer *et al.*, 1984; Haldeman, 1993).

Technique

The standard lumbar study has been refined from a previous six-view study of AP, AP tilt, lateral, lateral lumbosacral spot, and two obliques. An absolute minimum are two views in the frontal and lateral planes (Scavone *et al.*, 1981; Rowe and Yochum, 1996a). Oblique and lumbosacral spot views are optional views only (Schultz *et al.*, 1992; Haldeman, 1993). The decision to obtain stress radiographs in the sagittal (flexion-extension) and coronal (lateral bending) planes remains still unresolved but are considered optional and not for routine use (Phillips *et al.*, 1990; Pope *et al.*, 1992). Upright views are preferred for frontal and lateral studies wherever possible for the study of degenerative syndromes. Depiction of bone pathology should be performed in the recumbent position. The use of balancing filtration improves image quality and reduces dose.

Complications

Radiographs of the lumbar spine are the largest single source of gonadal irradiation and add considerable financial burden to the health system (Deyo and Diel, 1986; Chisolm, 1991). This can be drastically reduced by proper patient selection, close collimation, reducing the number of views, high frequency generating or three-phase equipment and rare earth screens (Rueter *et al.*, 1992; Rowe and Yochum, 1996b). The average skin entrance dose is approximately 420 mRad (3.65 mGy) (Rueter *et al.*, 1992).

Myelography

In 1919, Dandy employed the procedure of introducing air into the subarachnoid space to examine the brain (Dandy, 1919). The use of positive contrast media was discovered by accident in 1922 by Sicard and Forrestier who inadvertently injected iodized poppy seed oil (Lipiodol) (Sicard and Forrestier, 1922). Myelography is being performed with far less frequency being replaced mainly by MRI.

Indications

Conventional myelography has few indications today unless CT and MRI are not readily available. In the past it has been useful in the investigation of spinal canal lesions (tumours, etc.), spinal stenosis, disc herniations and arachnoiditis. Other indications may include tears of the dura, nerve root avulsions and situations where MRI or CT cannot be performed.

Advantages

Myelography is readily available and generally can be performed on an outpatient basis which renders it relatively inexpensive (Boulay *et al.*, 1993). Non-ionic water-soluble contrast opacifies nerve roots and outlines individual nerves and the conus medullaris. It provides an overview of the entire lumbar spine and is useful for determining multilevel spinal stenosis.

Limitations

No information on bone marrow, paraspinal soft tissues, spinal cord, or disc pathology other than loss of height and showing some herniations. Limited knowledge is gained on nerve root disorders.

Technique

Water soluble contrast medium (10–12 ml) is instilled following lumbar puncture at the L2–L3 or L3–L4 level while in the prone position with the assistance of fluoroscopy. The table is tilted up to fill the caudal sac and a view taken from L1–S2. Right and left obliques, a cross-table lateral and PA view of the conus medullaris completes the examination. The caudal sac and individual nerve roots are examined for their size, shape and location.

Complications

The toxic effects of oil-based media (Pantopaque), specifically delayed onset of arachnoiditis from Pantopaque, are well documented (Burton, 1978). Non-ionic water-soluble contrast agents currently in use have rapidly gained acceptance due to their low meningeal reactions and toxic effects (MacPherson *et al.*, 1985). Meningeal irritation may account for headache (30–70%), nausea (30%), vomiting and dizziness (12–37%) (Hauge and Falkenburg, 1982). Spinoradicular symptoms are less common and consist of radicular pain, hyperaesthesia, hyper-reflexia and urinary retention. Cerebral symptoms such as seizures, visual and auditory disturbances, stroke and confusion, fever and leucocytosis are considered rare. Local problems from lumbar puncture may include intraspinal haematoma, abscess, or persistent dural tear with leakage of cerebrospinal fluid.

Discography

Schmorl and Junghanns introduced discography as an anatomic study to evaluate the internal structure of the cadaveric intervertebral disc (Schmorl and Junghanns, 1971). In 1948, Lindblom and Hirsch independently described the injection of a radiopaque contrast material into the lumbar intervertebral disc (Hirsch, 1948; Lindblom, 1948). In, 1968 Holt described a false positive rate of 37% on asymptomatic jail in-mates which has remained a contentious issue ever since (Holt, 1968; Simmons *et al.*, 1988). In the mid-1980s discography was combined with CT to provide greater detail of herniations and the patterns of internal disc disruption and their correlation with clinical manifestations (McCutcheon and Thompson, 1986).

Indications

Discography is largely reserved for those patients in whom MRI and CT have failed to determine a pathological cause or a site of discal disease and who are candidates for surgery (Colhoun *et al.*, 1988; Brightbill *et al.*, 1994).

Advantages

The procedure can be performed as an outpatient procedure similar to myelography and is reasonably available. It is the only imaging study of the disc that has the ability to provoke symptoms which can be correlated with any abnormality of structure.

Limitations

It is a test for only the intervertebral disc, though display of the bony anatomy is evident. Anular tears on conventional films can be obscured and requires CT-discography for full evaluation (Ninomiya and Muro, 1992). MRI similarly exquisitely demonstrates herniations but is not as sensitive as discography in the detection of internal disc disruptions with only two thirds identified (Yu *et al.*, 1989; Osti *et al.*, 1992). It is a relatively expensive, invasive and time-consuming procedure.

Technique

In the prone oblique position, with the non-painful side up, the needle is placed into the disc passing lateral to the pedicle (McFadden, 1988). Contrast medium is instilled while observing under fluoroscopy and monitoring the patient's response. A normal disc accepts 1–2.5 ml of contrast, pathological discs more. On filling, the normal opacified nucleus is oval in shape, located in the posterior two-thirds of the interspace and separated from the vertebral body end-plate by a 1–2 mm radiolucent zone. The disc space may be observed to widen with the injection. Changes in morphology occur with movement, traction reduces its circumference, and flexion-extension shows the nucleus to move in location (Brinkmann and Horst, 1985). A normal variant is a linear lucency in its midportion. There should be no escape of contrast into the spinal canal in a normal disc.

Complications

Radiation dose is relatively high due to the use of fluoroscopy for needle placement. The major complication is disc infection which is usually less than 1–2.3% (Wiley *et al.*, 1968; Fraser *et al.*, 1987). Contrary to belief there is no convincing evidence that discography injures the disc (Johnson, 1989), although occasional nerve injury may occur.

Facet arthrography

Facet joint injection was first attempted by Kellgren in 1939, then by Hirsch in 1963 and Mooney and Robertson in 1976, as pain provocational studies. Currently it is a commonly utilized procedure prior to placing anaesthetic facet blocks (Schwarzer *et al.*, 1994).

Indications

In unresponsive patients in whom a discogenic or other cause has not been delineated, facet arthrography followed by anaesthetic blocks may be of diagnostic and therapeutic value (Carrera and Williams, 1984; Schwartzer *et al.*, 1994). Continuity with an intraspinal soft tissue mass confirms the diagnosis of synovial cyst (Bjorkengren *et al.*, 1987; Abrahams *et al.*, 1988).

Advantages

Filling of the facet joint ensures the correct placement of an anaesthetic agent.

Limitations

Anaesthesia of the facet joints requires subjective interpretation by the patient which may be incorrect. To be sure of a truely positive response, a 'double block procedure' is mandatory (Schwartzer *et al.*, 1994). On the first visit a short-acting anaesthetic (lignocaine) is instilled into the facet joint. If there is a reported decrease in pain, 2 weeks later a second injection is performed with a longer acting agent such as bupivacaine. A positive response for asymptomatic joint is at least 50% decrease in pain with both injections which, following the second injection, lasts 3 hours or more (Schwartzer *et al.*, 1994).

Technique

The injection is performed as an outpatient procedure without pre-medication. In the prone oblique position, with fluoroscopic guidance, the needle is passed into the joint. Only 0.1–0.3 ml of contrast medium is then injected to confirm the intra-articular position. The capsular capacity of the upper lumbar facets is less than that of the lower facets, with the L5/S1 joint being the most capacious.

Complications

There has been little discussion or evidence published of problems arising secondary to facet arthrography. At least 4% of subjects may experience short term exacerbation of their symptoms (Destouet and Murphy, 1988). There is a hypothetical risk for infection, capsular or nerve injury. Arachnoiditis from the injection of steroids into the facets has been recorded (Tress and Lau, 1991).

Computed tomography

In 1973 Hounsfield first published details for obtaining axial images of the head for which he was awarded the Nobel prize in 1979 (Hounsfield, 1973). Significant advancements in hardware and computer technology rapidly transformed the technique into a highly sophisticated modality for body imaging. It is no longer referred to as 'CAT' scan (computed axial tomography), instead deriving the abbreviation 'CT' since images can be reformatted into many planes with computer technology (Multi-Planar Reconstructions, MPR).

Indications

CT has broad application to disorders of the lumbar spine including disc disease, spinal stenosis, bone and nerve tumours, infections, congenital, post-surgical, traumatic and paraspinal lesions. Paraspinal abnormalities may be identified in more than 1% of lumbar spine CT cases (Osborn *et al.*, 1982; Frager *et al.*, 1986).

Advantages

CT is now readily available and cost effective when patients are selected appropriately. It is non-invasive unless contrast is used, has excellent resolution, allows visualization of both soft tissue and bone details, and the information can be manipulated into different planes and densities.

Limitations

The correct levels for obtaining axial images is crucial to locating abnormalities. Reconstructed images in additional planes are prone to artefact, image degradation and loss of detail. Selection of the correct window setting is vitally important to isolating abnormalities. The spinal cord, its coverings and nerve roots require a myelogram to adequately demonstrate them (CT-myelography, CTM). Metallic implants, obese and restless patients suffer image degradation.

Technique

The study is performed supine with the knees flexed. Prone examinations are performed when combined with myelography (Tehranzadeh and Gabriele, 1984). Images are obtained in the axial plane from which additional planes can be derived and presented with varying contrast.

Initially a digital radiograph (scanogram, scout, pilot, localizer) is obtained in the lateral projection and, occasionally, other planes including frontal and obliques which often identify an abnormality (Nuri Sener *et al.*, 1993). On this scan the selection and angles of desired images can be localized. There is dispute as to whether selected angled gantry or sequential non-angled studies are better (Braun *et al.*, 1984). Sequential images at regular intervals allows for reformatting (reconstruction, multiplanar imaging) into additional planes (lateral, oblique, three-dimensional) (Rabassa *et al.*, 1993).

Most studies traverse the interval from the L3 pedicle to the sacral base, though some argue that inclusion of the L3-L4 disc without specific indication is unnecessary (de Vos Meiring *et al.*, 1994). These are performed at a slice thickness of 3–5 mm at 3–5 mm intervals, usually with overlapping (for example, 5 mm slices at 4 mm intervals) with a total of 25–30 slices (Braun *et al.*, 1984). Images should be displayed at 'soft tissue' and 'bone window' settings which enhance the visibility of the respective anatomical components. The addition of radiopaque contrast will allow improved visibility of some structures and improve diagnostic accuracy.

CT-myelography (CTM)

Water-soluble contrast is placed in the subarachnoid space by lumbar puncture in the conventional manner. Adequate mixing of contrast is necessary, and the patient may need to be rolled several times prior to CT scanning. CT should be performed within 6 hours of the introduction of intrathecal contrast with an optimum time of 2–3 hours. Prone positioning following intrathecal contrast may reduce lordosis and more satisfactorily outline the posterior disk margin with intrathecal contrast (Tehranzadeh and Gabriele, 1984).

CT-discography (CTD)

Discography is performed in the usual way. When combined with CT, greater detail on herniations and the patterns of internal disc disruption can be determined (McCutcheon and Thompson, 1986).

Intravenous injection

Conditions which are vascular and have permeable vessels such as intraspinal tumours, infections, and post-surgical fibrosis, will enhance with intravenous contrast. Normal vessels such as the epidural veins similarly will become more prominent.

Complications

Radiation dose varies considerably depending on the patient thickness, equipment and number of slices obtained ranging from 1–7 rads (average 3–5 rads) (Evens and Mettler, 1985). Contrast reactions, while less common, still occur, ranging from localized inflammation (arachnoiditis), infection (discitis), and mild to severe allergic reactions (urticaria, anaphylaxis).

Magnetic resonance imaging

The phenomenon of magnetic resonance (MR) was first reported in 1946 by Bloch and Purcell, for which they received the Nobel prize for physics in 1952 (Bloch, 1946; Purcell *et al.*, 1946). In July 1977, Damadian and Lauterbur utilized these principles to produce the first images of the chest which took 5 hours to complete (Lauterbur, 1973; Damadian, 1980; Vaughn, 1989). Rapid advancement in MR technology has made this modality the most significant contribution to the understanding of pathology, natural history, diagnosis and management of lumbar spine disorders.

MR availability is rapidly increasing, though cost containment issues have limited its general utilization (Rothschild *et al.*, 1990). The cost of a lumbar MRI study varies according to location, use of contrast and the number of images derived. A conservative estimate for MR of the lumbar spine may exceed $2 billion annually in the United States (Modic *et al.*, 1994).

Indications

As experience is gained and image quality improves the applications of MRI continue to expand. There are few conditions of the lumbar spine in which MRI is not the technique of choice following initial plain film radiographs. This includes disorders of the intervertebral disc, spinal ligaments, spinal cord and nerve roots, spinal canals (central and lateral), bone marrow and paraspinal soft tissues (Cotler, 1992; Holtas, 1993). It is especially useful in evaluation of failed back surgery syndrome in differentiating epidural fibrosis from recurrent disc herniation by demonstrating Gadolinium enhancement (Kormano, 1989). MRI should not be used as a screening test or done simultaneously with CT (Modic and Herzog, 1994).

Advantages

There are three primary advantages of spinal MRI – it does not use ionizing radiation, it is non-invasive, and it depicts soft tissues in exquisite detail (Cotler, 1992). No other non-invasive imaging modality has the ability to depict the internal structural and biochemical changes within the intervertebral disc and nerve elements. Because of its non-invasive nature, repetitive examinations can be conducted which allows many disease processes to be followed in response to treatment and aspects of its natural history elucidated (Dwyer, 1989).

It has largely replaced a number of other invasive investigative methods including myelography and discography. The major advantage of MRI over CT is that it doesn't require myelography to identify the neural elements adequately. MRI avoids the diagnostic errors made in CT by selecting inappropriate scanning levels, since sagittal images include at least the conus to the lower sacrum. MRI is also more sensitive than CT in the detection of degenerative disc disease (Modic *et al.*, 1984), metastatic or primary tumour (Colman *et al.*, 1988), and infections (Modic *et al.*, 1985).

Limitations

A major problem with spinal MR imaging is the high sensitivity for demonstrating disc disease. Up to 50% of asymptomatic lumbar spines will have disc abnormalities such as dehydration, bulging and herniation demonstrated on MRI, while CT can show the same abnormalities in around 35–50% (Wiesel *et al.*, 1984; Boden *et al.*, 1990; Jensen *et al.*, 1994). Gas, small deposits of calcium, osteophytes, bony stenosis and fractures are generally poorly seen on MRI (Resnick, 1985; Kormano, 1989; Cotler, 1992).

Restless and large patients may not be able to be scanned. Claustrophobia remains the single greatest problem, which can usually be alleviated by relaxation strategies, with sedation seldom required (Weinreb *et al.*, 1984; Quirk *et al.*, 1989). Certain ferromagnetic metallic implants will seriously malfunction within the magnetic field, including metallic intracranial clips, foreign bodies (soft tissue, eye), pacemakers, prosthetic heart valves, hearing aids, cochlear implants, some IUDs and TENS machines (Kelly *et al.*, 1986; Cotler, 1992). Teeth fillings, abdominal clips, joint prostheses and spinal instrumentation are not contraindications to MR scanning, though they do produce artefactual signal voids which can obscure anatomical details. MRI should be avoided in pregnancy.

Technique

A multitude of imaging formats can be employed by varying the planes imaged (coronal, axial, sagittal) and tissue density (pulse sequences, weighting). The usual lumbar spine protocols consist of sagittal and axial T1- and T2-weighted images and axial T1-weighted images with some variations (Herzog, 1991).

Planes

The basic study consists of a minimum of sagittal and axial images. This complements anatomical detail and provides a higher level of confidence for confirming and characterizing abnormalities.

1. Sagittal images. These should include the lower thoracic spine to the bottom of the sacrum and are the most useful diagnostic projections. Between 11 and 14 images are obtained sequentially, from right to left, at 3–5 mm thickness with 1–2 mm intervals (Heithoff and Amster, 1990). T1- and T2-weighted images are usually obtained in this plane.
2. Axial images. As in CT, 17–25 images are typically obtained from L3 pedicle to the upper sacrum, with selected images at upper levels as deemed clinically relevant (Heithoff and Amster, 1990). Bone detail is only fair in this plane, in contrast to the clarity of the intraspinal and paraspinal tissues. Usually, these are only obtained with T2-weighting unless gadolinium is used in which case T1-weighting is used. Slice thickness is 3–5 mm with 1–2 mm gaps between slices.
3. Coronal imaging. This is the least used spinal imaging plane. Effects of the lordosis and kyphosis make continuous imaging over multiple segments difficult, though oblique coronals will assist in minimizing sagittal curve effects. Coronal imaging is helpful in scoliosis and in demonstrating long lesions of the cord.

Pulse sequences

By varying the pulse sequences, the tissues will change in their relative contrast with some enhancing and some degrading (Table 18.4). The main parameters altered to derive the pulse sequences are the repetition time (TR) and echo time (TE). The main sequences used include T1, T2 and proton density. Where gadolinium is used, T1-weighted images are employed (Runge, 1983).

1. T1-weighted. The pulse parameters consist of short TR (400–600 ms) and short TE (15–30 ms). They are ideal for evaluating structures with fat, subacute or chronic haemorrhage, or proteinaceous materials. These are excellent images to show anatomic structures and delineate their interfaces (Herzog, 1991). T1 images provide morphological detail of the spinal cord, nerve roots, and surrounding tissues and spaces. Fat on these T1 images provides high signal to provide an excellent soft tissue interface for detecting these tissues. In the normal spine the signal intensity on T1 in descending order are fat, nucleus pulposus, bone marrow, cancellous bone, spinal cord, muscle, cerebrospinal fluid, anulus fibrosus, ligaments and compact cortical bone (Modic *et al.*, 1984).
2. T2-weighted. The pulse parameters consist of long TR (1500–3000 ms) and long TE (60–120 ms). The signal intensity is related to the amount of water within a tissue. High signal tissues ('white') include cerebrospinal fluid and intervertebral discs. Pathological conditions, including fluid collections, acute haemorrhage, infections, oedema, cysts, necrotic tumours, and neoplasms will elicit high signal (Herzog, 1991). T2 images produce an exquisite 'myelogram effect' of the cerebrospinal fluid and highlight the water content of the intervertebral disc. Bone has few mobile free protons and generates little signal ('black').
3. Proton density. The pulse parameters are long TR (1500–2000 ms) and short TE (15–30 ms). The signal intensity in the image reflects the total number of mobile hydrogen ions in the tissue. These images are particularly useful for evaluating tumours, oedema, ligamentous structures and articular cartilage (Grenier *et al.*, 1987a). The posterior anulus, ligamentum flavum, central and lateral canals, zygapophysial joints and posterior elements are most elegantly demonstrated (Herzog, 1991).

Contrast agents

The most common contrast agent is gadolinium DTPA (gadolinium, Magnevist) (Carr *et al.*, 1984; Runge, 1992). Gadolinium interacts with water protons to shorten their T1 relaxation time thus increasing the signal on T1-weighted images. It does not cross the normal blood–brain barrier but, when disrupted, will produce enhancement of the breach site making it especially useful in identifying tumours, infections, infarctions and inflammatory conditions of the spinal cord and meninges.

Complications

No known complications exist beyond the potential for injury from acknowledged contraindications for example critical metallic implants and foreign metallic bodies such as intracranial vascular clips, cardiac pacemakers and metal in the orbit (Kelly *et al.*, 1986; Cotler, 1992). The high level of noise generated during the examination may induce headache, temporary auditory deficits and disorientation (Rothschild *et al.*, 1990). Body temperature may rise less than one degree fahrenheit during the examination. Gadolinium may produce local pain, allergic reactions from hives to anaphylaxis, and some haemolysis (Salonen, 1990; Runge, 1992).

Nuclear medicine

In, 1919, Rutherford first demonstrated the emission of alpha particles from radium. The introduction of technetium in 1937 by Perrier and Segre, and later adapted in 1971 by Subramaniam and McAfee, revolutionized the medical applications of nuclear imaging to the skeletal system (Subramanian and McAfee, 1971; Holder, 1990). Improvements in isotope preparation and imaging hardware, such as in computer components, collimators and detectors, have improved image quality.

Table 18.4 *MRI signal intensity of tissues found in the lumbar spine*

Tissue	T1-weighted	T2-weighted
Epidural fat	High	High
Nucleus pulposus	Intermediate	High
Facet cartilage	Intermediate	Intermediate
Bone marrow	Intermediate	Intermediate
Cancellous bone	Intermediate	Low
Nerve, cord	Intermediate	Intermediate
Muscles	Low	Low
Thecal sac (CSF)	Low	High
Anulus fibrosus	Low	Low
Ligaments	Low	Low
Cortical bone	Low	Low
Gas	Low	Low
Blood vessels	Low	Low

Signal grading scale

Low:	black
Intermediate:	grey
High:	white

Indications

Increased bone uptake can be demonstrated with only a 3–5% change in bone activity and, therefore, has widespread applications in the diagnosis of spinal disease. It is especially useful in the early depiction and progress of infections, tumours, fractures, Paget's disease, articular disorders and bone pain of undetermined aetiology (Valdez and Johnson, 1994). It is as accurate in spinal osteomyelitis and metastatic disease as MRI (Modic *et al.*, 1985). Multiple myeloma can be normal on bone scan except for sites of pathological fracture. Unilateral pars defects which are symptomatic are frequently active on bone scan (Valdez and Johnson, 1994). Insufficiency fractures of the sacrum may only be found with bone scan with less than 5% being visible on plain films (Weber *et al.*, 1993).

Advantages

Nuclear medicine is readily available, in general, but usually requires specialized facilities. Nuclear imaging is an extremely sensitive marker of bone and joint disease for imaging the entire skeleton (Frank *et al.*, 1990). It has high sensitivity but relatively low specificity. Any disease process which disturbs the normal balance of bone production and resorption can be depicted on bone scan, usually as an increased uptake ('hot spot'), or occasionally decreased uptake ('cold spot').

Limitations

Specificity is generally low. Use of tomography (SPECT) enhances contrast and increases the sensitivity of the examination (Hellman *et al.*, 1986). In the degenerative spine, nuclear medicine has limited application (Valdez and Johnson, 1994). Herniated disc and spinal stenosis have normal scans. Some advanced degenerative discs with osteophytes, sclerosis and loss of height will show increased uptake. Similarly, facet arthrosis may be active on scan though the clinical utility of this finding is unclear (Valdez and Johnson, 1994). It is a relatively expensive examination.

Technique

The two most common agents employed are Technetium-99m and Galium-67. Essentially the radionuclide is injected intravenously and becomes protein bound where it perfuses into skeletal sites and binds to the bone crystal surface. Unbound radionuclide is renally excreted which may be as high as 50% 1 hour post injection. As the isotope undergoes degeneration, gamma rays are emitted which are detected by a scintillation camera. The greater the bone turnover, the higher the concentration of isotope and the greater the scintillation count which produces the 'hot spot' on the resultant image.

Three studies are usually obtained following injection ('three phase study'). One obtained immediately depicts the vascular tree distally and is called a 'flow' study. Within 5 minutes, images depict the capillary and venous phases of perfusion and this is called a 'blood pool' study. At around 2–3 hours there is significant bone uptake for 'bone image' study.

Complications

The whole body dose is approximately 0.13 rads (Maguire *et al.*, 1990). The organ receiving the highest radiation dose is the bladder due to renal excretion which can be minimized by pre-study hydration and post study frequent micturition. Bone scans should not be used during pregnancy. In lactating mothers isotope will be present in breast milk for several days (Maguire *et al.*, 1990).

Videofluoroscopy

Enthusiasm from early fluoroscopic investigations in the lumbar spine during the 1970s have since been tempered with the reality for rationalizing the high radiation doses and cost with the technical inherent inconsistencies in structural details, the wide range of normality, and the lack of clinical correlation (Howe, 1970, 1989).

Indications

The use of videofluoroscopy (VF) in the lumbar spine is not considered a standard diagnostic procedure and can only be regarded as a research investigative modality (Quebec Task Force, 1987; Haldeman *et al.*, 1993). Limited research investigations have provided some insight into lumbar kinematics, though these are few (Bronfort and Jochumsen, 1984; Breen *et al.*, 1989; Bell, 1990).

Advantages

The depiction of whole range mechanics is not demonstrated by any other method (Bronfort and Jochumsen, 1984). Utilization of computer digitizing techniques allows quantification of intersegmental kinematics (Breen *et al.*, 1989). Recording on videotape allows frame by frame analysis.

Limitations

Adequate equipment and its upkeep is exceptionally expensive. Depending on the jurisdiction, strict licence requirements usually preclude general usage outside qualified individuals. Normal motion patterns and methods of mensuration have not been established and to be accurate requires expensive and time-consuming computer digitization (Howe, 1970, 1989; Breen *et al.*, 1989; Cholewicki *et al.*, 1991). To digitize a single lateral flexion study may take at least 1 hour (Breen *et al.*, 1989). A wide variation in normal patterns has been observed which makes conclusions on observed findings difficult as there are no established norms (Bronfort and Jochumsen, 1984; Breen *et al.*, 1989). Poor structural detail disqualifies its use as a primary diagnostic modality with interobserver reliablity only around 50% (Bronfort and Jochumsen, 1984; Howe, 1989).

Technique

The lumbar spine is evaluated in the coronal (lateral flexion) and sagittal (flexion-extension) planes, beginning from the neutral position and progressively moving to the physiological end points possible.

Complications

The high radiation dose from the procedure is a major drawback. With strict guidelines such as proper patient selection, minimum screening times, short distances, and high quality equipment, this can be significantly reduced (Breen *et al.*, 1989).

Ultrasound

Diagnostic ultrasound (US) of the adult lumbar spine has received scant attention with a few notable exceptions (Porter *et al.*, 1980; Hammond, 1984; Portela, 1985; Tervonen and Koivukangas, 1989; Tervonen *et al.*, 1991). Ultrasound is freely available but is rarely performed for back pain having not gained general acceptance.

Indications

The most common application of sonography in the lumbar spine is in the diagnosis of spinal dysraphism (for example, spina bifida) *in utero* and in the neonate. Ultrasound has been used for the identification of paraspinal disease, spinal stenosis (Porter *et al.*, 1980), disc herniation (Portela, 1985), degenerative disc disease (Tervonen *et al.*, 1991) and spondylolisthesis (Hammond, 1984). It has also been used intra-operatively to assess the location and characteristics of tumours, syrinx, disc herniations and shunt placement (Rubin and Dohrmann, 1985). It is more readily performed following laminectomy and is useful in the diagnosis of post-operative complications such as pseudomeningocele.

Advantages

No ionizing radiation is used and, therefore it can be used more frequently and for screening such as in adolescent spondylolisthesis (Hammond, 1984). Identification of unsuspected paraspinal disease, such as aneurysm and lymphoma can be well demonstrated.

Limitations

No information is derived on bone or joint structure. The resolution within the canal and of its contents is not good enough to identify significant abnormalities reliably. Calcification of the ligamentum flavum, diminished interlaminar space (hyperlordosis, spurring, disc degeneration) and the presence of metallic implants impairs the examination. Image quality is limited by the calibre of the equipment and the skill of the operator and interpreter (Tervonen *et al.*, 1991).

Technique

To identify the spinal canal, spondylolisthesis, and some disc herniations, the transducer is placed on the back and directed through the interlaminar space and it is angled 15 degrees to each side. The beam deflects off the posterior borders of the disc and vertebral body and identifies the lamina. A transabdominal approach can be used with the beam directed through the plane of the intervertebral disc (Tervonen and Koivukangas, 1989).

Complications

No complications have been documented other than misdiagnosis of bone or intraspainal pathology.

Angiography

The study of the blood supply to the spine was originally based on the cadaveric works of Adamkiewicz and Kadyi in the 1880s (Smith and Cragg, 1991). Spinal angiography is a specialized procedure requiring specifically skilled operators and equipment.

Indications

The most common indication is to assist in identifying arteriovenous malformations, their arterial supply and venous drainage. Other rare indications include vascular tumours (haemangioblastomas), pre-scoliosis and occasionally pre-aortic aneurysm surgery. It may also be of assistance for possible pre-operative embolization such as in haemangiomas (Esparza *et al.*, 1978). Lumbar epidural venography has been previously used for diagnosing disc herniations but has been superseded by CT and MR imaging.

Limitations

The invasive and time-consuming nature of angiography has largely been replaced by CT and MR imaging. It is performed in a hospital setting with specialized equipment.

Technique

Initially the patient is sedated, some advocating general anaesthesia. A catheter is introduced through the femoral artery, and the segmental supply one level either side of the vertebral level involved selectively catheterized. The images are then digitally subtracted to enhance the vascular structures and diminish others.

Complications

The examination is invasive, time consuming, requires anaesthesia with its inherent risks, gives high radiation doses and does not demonstrate details of the cord itself. Neurological complications due to spasm, thrombosis or embolization occur in about 2.2% of spinal angiographies (Forbes *et al.*, 1993).

Posterior joint and neural arch syndromes

A number of conditions involving the posterior joints and neural arch are recognized (Table 18.5).

Table 18.5 *Posterior joint and neural arch syndromes*

Instability
Mechanical zygapophysial joint syndrome
Zygapophysial joint arthropathy
Synovial cyst
Degenerative spondylolisthesis
Baastrup's syndrome
Lumbosacral transitional vertebra
Spondylolisthesis
Retrolisthesis
Costotransverse arthropathy

Spinal instability

The definition of spinal instability remains enigmatic (Nachemson, 1985; Pope *et al.*, 1992). It is synonymous with a loss of motion segment stiffness such that, when forces are applied, exaggerated displacement occurs, i.e., greater than in a normal structure (Pope *et al.*, 1992). Such instability can result in pain, potential for progressive deformity, and places neurological structures at risk. There are many causes including fractures, dislocations, infections, tumours, spondylolisthesis, scoliosis, kyphosis and degenerative conditions.

Degenerative instabilities are those related to loss of joint stiffness, either from primary causes including disc and facet degeneration, or secondary to post-

treatment complications such as discectomy, laminectomy, fusion or chemonucleolysis (Frymoyer, 1991). Radiographic methods are the most consistently utilized means for detecting, quantifying and developing management strategies for instability. To date the clinical–radiological correlation between imaging findings of instability and their clinical significance remains largely unresolved (Boden *et al.*, 1990; Frymoyer, 1991).

Imaging features

Conventional radiography

This is the major method utilized for the study of instability and utilizes both static and dynamic studies.

Static findings

Those suggesting segmental instability include loss of disc height, traction osteophytes, facet arthrosis, translation and scoliosis (Frymoyer, 1991; Pope *et al.*, 1992). Scoliosis and translational displacements are best observed in upright weight-bearing studies (Friberg, 1987).

Progressive osteolysis of vertebral end-plates identical to that of a disc infection can occasionally be seen at a level of instability, especially following laminectomy (Bradford and Gotfreid, 1986).

Translations occur most commonly sagittally (anterolisthesis–retrolisthesis), laterally or into rotation.

Dynamic findings

Pivotal in these examinations is to subject the lumbar spine to forces that maximize the instability ('dynamic studies'). The most frequently employed studies utilize end points of physiological movements (flexion-extension, lateral bending) or axial loading (erect, weight bearing, distraction), or both (Dupuis *et al.*, 1985; Friberg, 1987).

Flexion–extension radiographs are the most commonly utilized studies. The two major intersegmental relationships evaluated are anteroposterior glide and angular separation (Sato and Kikuchi, 1993). A combined flexion–extension translation of more than 3 mm is considered to be evidence for instability, though some suggest 4–5 mm is more appropriate (Boden and Wiesel, 1990; Frymoyer, 1991). Increased retrolisthesis on extension occurs in approximately 30% of low back pain patients (Lehmann and Brand, 1983). Axial loading radiographs have demonstrated increasing symptoms correlating with an increase in the degree of spondylolisthesis (Friberg, 1987). Angular motion determined by end-plate parallelism should not exceed 7–9 degrees (Boden *et al.*, 1990).

The natural history of instability has not been fully elucidated, though there is evidence to suggest that at least 20% resolve the instability spontaneously, and those with purely increased posterior widening are self-limiting. The combination of posterior widening and forward translation is associated with a higher incidence of chronic disability (Sato and Kikuchi, 1993). Conversely hypomobility at all levels is found in low back pain with no single level showing a measurable difference in fixation (Pearcy, 1985; Dvorak *et al.*, 1991).

Despite these positive correlations with symptoms, dynamic studies of asymptomatic populations with measurable instability have cast considerable doubt on their validity (Phillips *et al.*, 1993). Additional detractions from the routine use of dynamic radiographs are the high levels of radiation, cost, observer errors, and lack of mid motion information (Pope, 1992).

Magnetic resonance imaging

MR imaging may be helpful in assessing functional stability after lumbar spinal fusion (Djukic *et al.*, 1990; Lang *et al.*, 1990). Stable fusions of greater than 12 months demonstrate sub-end-plate bands of high signal on T1 due to the conversion of red to yellow (fatty) marrow (Type 2). Conversely, unstable fusions due to inflammation, hyperaemia or granulation tissue exhibit sub-end-plate zones of low signal on T1 and high signal on T2 (Type 1).

Mechanical facet syndrome

The term 'facet syndrome' was first coined by Ghormley in 1933, characterized by back and leg pain emanating from mechanical irritation of a low lumbar zygapophysial joint (Ghormley, 1933). Traditionally, it has been a clinical diagnosis though there exist no reliable clinical or radiographic features. The facet syndrome may only account for around 15% of low back pain (Schwarzer *et al.*, 1994). The definitive diagnosis is confirmed with pain provocation with an intra-articular injection of saline or contrast media into the facet joint, and pain relief by injecting a solution of local anaesthetic (Jackson, 1992; Griffiths *et al.*, 1993).

Imaging features

Conventional radiography

Intersegmental disrelationships as depicted by conventional radiographs have been implicated as signs for facet syndrome (Peters, 1983). This includes named measurements including Hadley's 'S' curve, MacNab's line, sacral base angle, lumbosacral disc angle, retrolisthesis, anterolisthesis, Ferguson's gravity line and facet override. An isolated wide zygapophysial joint has been linked to the syndrome (unstable zygapophysial joint sign) (Abel, 1977).

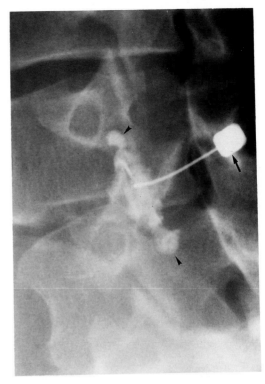

Figure 18.1 Facet arthrogram, L4–L5. A needle has been placed within the L4–L5 facet joint (arrow). A contrast agent has been placed into the joint which outlines the limits of the joint capsule (arrowheads). The injection of contrast is given prior to anaesthetic agents being placed into the joint to confirm the intra-articular position of the needle.

Facet arthrosis may occasionally be found in a symptomatic joint though this is an unreliable sign (Griffiths *et al.*, 1993). Facet arthrography is performed prior to the injection of anaesthetic to ensure proper placement (Figure 18.1). MRI and bone scanning have been unrewarding in the detection of symptomatic facet syndromes.

Facet arthropathy

Facet arthrosis is very common in the low lumbar spine. Histological evidence of facet arthrosis in the presence of normal radiographs approaches 20% of patients by 35 years of age (Giles and Taylor, 1985). Radiographic changes are visible in at least 65% by age 50–60 years (Pathria *et al.*, 1987).

Imaging features

Conventional radiography

Normal facets are only visible on approximately 40% of frontal films in contrast to almost 100% of oblique studies (Pathria *et al.*, 1987; Griffiths *et al.*, 1993).

Manifestations of facet arthrosis, best depicted on the oblique view consist of osteophytes, sclerosis and loss of joint space (see histological examples: Figures 6.8; 6.17).

Computed tomography

Axial CT bone window images demonstrate arthrosis accurately. As well as osteophytes, sclerosis and loss of joint space, subchondral cysts and the degree of stenosis can be assessed (Figure 18.2). Hypertrophy of the inferior facet tends to cause central stenosis, while involvement of the superior facet narrows the lateral canal (Dussault and Lander, 1990).

Magnetic resonance imaging

The joints can be seen on sagittal and axial images especially T2-weighted. Osteophytes, narrowing and sclerosis of the facet joint cannot be accurately assessed with MRI (Modic *et al.*, 1994). Fatty marrow within a degenerative articular process, most commonly the superior, shows increased signal on T1- and T2-weighted images (Grenier *et al.*, 1987). The major benefits derived from MRI is the assessment on adjacent lateral and central canals and their contained neural elements where they may be seen to be compressed, or displaced, frequently with a lack of surrounding epidural fat. Identification of accompanying synovial cysts can be easily made (Yuh *et al.*, 1991).

Synovial cysts

Synovial cysts represent either herniation of synovium beyond the confines of the joint capsule or mucinous degeneration of connective tissue adjacent to the joint (Abrahams *et al.*, 1988; Gorey *et al.*,

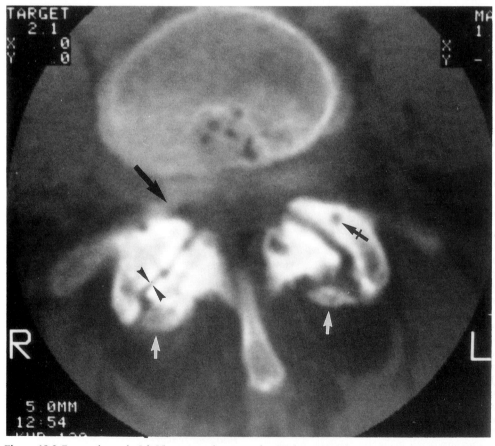

Figure 18.2 Facet arthropathy L4–L5, computed tomography. On this axial CT bone window image the presence of bilateral facet arthrosis is well demonstrated. Findings include osteophytes (arrows), sclerosis, loss of joint space (arrowheads) and subchondral cysts (crossed arrow). Evidence for anterolisthesis is provided by the 'double margin' sign at the posterior vertebral body margin (large arrow). The advantage of axial CT is the accurate depiction of these bony changes and assessment for the degree of stenosis. Hypertrophy of the inferior facet tends to cause central stenosis while involvement of the superior facet narrows the lateral canal.

1992). The most common level to be involved is the L4-L5 level where at least 75% occur, the remainder at L3–L4 and L5–S1, though rare cases may occur elsewhere (Hsu *et al.*, 1995). They invariably are found in conjunction with degenerative facet arthropathy (Jackson *et al.*, 1990).

Imaging features

Conventional radiography

Plain films are unlikely to elucidate the diagnosis unless the cyst is densely calcified or bone erosion is extensive. Degenerative facet arthropathy is usually the only finding with occasional coexisting degenerative spondylolisthesis (Hsu *et al.*, 1995). Myelography reveals an extradural filling defect.

Computed tomography

A smooth bordered extradural soft tissue mass lying near the facet joint-lamina region with extension into the lateral canal is the main feature (Hsu, 1995) (Figure 18.3A). Gas within the mass is a reliable sign for synovial cyst (Schultz *et al.*, 1984). The peripheral rim may be more prominent or even calcified with a more lucent central zone creating a characteristic 'target' appearance (Bjorkengren *et al.*, 1987). Injection of contrast into the cyst may demonstrate a central cavity and communication with the facet joint (Bjorkengren *et al.*, 1987; Abrahams *et al.*, 1988). Extrinsic bone pressure erosion with a smooth, sharply defined border most commonly into the inner surface of the lamina, can be observed (Gorey *et al.*, 1992).

Magnetic resonance imaging

A round, sometimes bilobed, dumb-bell-shaped well circumscribed mass 5–10 mm in diameter lies dorsally and in an extradural location (Hsu *et al.*, 1995) (Figure 18.3B). A high to intermediate signal on T1, and high to low signal on T2, is common. A peripheral rim of decreased signal on T2 is a consistent finding (Liu *et al.*, 1989; Rosenblum *et al.*, 1989). Calcification is not demonstrated on MRI (Hsu *et al.*, 1995). A high internal signal is found in the presence of haemorrhage which diminishes with time as the haematoma degrades with methaemoglobin formation (Jackson *et al.*, 1990). On Gadolinium-enhanced MR images there is early and persistent enhancement of the cyst wall and solid components, while there is delayed enhancement of the internal cavity (Yuh *et al.*, 1991).

Baastrup's disease

Approximation and contact between lumbar spinous processes with subsequent ligament degeneration and pseudojoint formation was first alluded to in 1834 by Meyer who referred to the condition as 'interspinous diarthroses' (Schmorl and Junghanns, 1971). In 1933 Baastrup recorded the first clinical observations in conjunction with the presence of these adventitious pseudojoints, a condition with which his name has become inexorably linked and the phrase 'kissing spinouses' has been coined (Baastrup, 1933) (see Figure 13.4).

Imaging features

Various associations have been recorded including hyperlordosis ('swayback'), degenerative spondylolisthesis, loss of disc space, advancing age, as well as congenital and acquired enlargement of the spinous processes (Jacobsen *et al.*, 1958; Cashley and Heyman, 1984; Resnick, 1985; Sartoris *et al.*, 1985).

Conventional radiography

On the frontal radiograph are seen the matching opposed cortices of the involved spinous processes exhibiting sclerosis, occasional cysts and osteophytes (Sandoz, 1960; Kattan and Pais, 1981; Resnick, 1985) (Figure 18.4). On lateral views in extension the spinous processes can be demonstrated to impact on each other (Resnick, 1985).

Three morphological types of interspinous neoarthroses are recognized: flat: the opposing surfaces lie in a predominantly horizontal plane; concave–convex: the contact surfaces are curved in a reciprocal, interlocking manner; and oblique: the plane is sloped away from the midline (Sandoz, 1960).

Magnetic resonance imaging

The supraspinous and interspinous ligaments may appear disrupted and exhibit irregular margins, and bursal cavities which contain fat may also be identified (Grenier *et al.*, 1987a). Sclerosis at the sites of impact on the spinous processes shows diminished signal.

Costotransverse arthropathy

Pain may be referred from the lower costal joints to the low lumbar spine (thoracolumbar syndrome, Maigne's syndrome) (Proctor *et al.*, 1985; Dreyfus *et al.*, 1994). These articulations have also been implicated in epigastric pain production, simulating upper gastrointestinal disease (Robert's syndrome) and other visceral conditions including pancreatitis and dissecting aortic aneurysm (Robert, 1980; Richards, 1987; Benhamou *et al.*, 1993). The most common levels are at T10–T11, though between T8 and T12 may be affected (Malmivaara *et al.*, 1987).

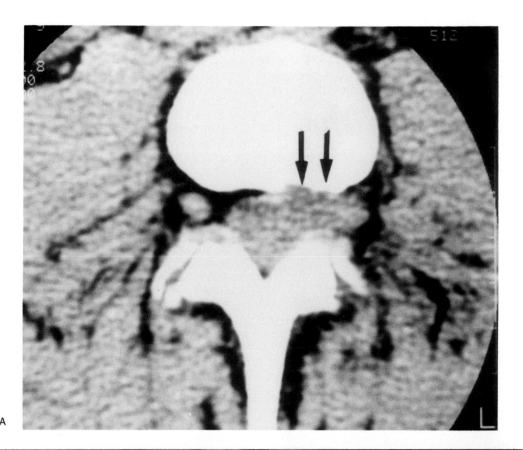

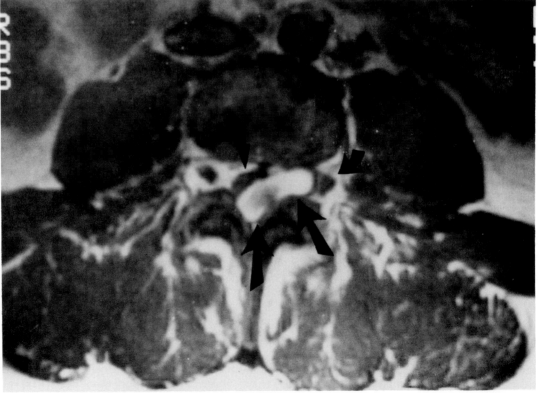

Figure 18.3 Synovial cyst, L3–L4. A. Computed tomography. A soft tissue density is seen to lie within the neural foramen (arrows). There is obliteration of the epidural fat and exiting nerve root. B. Magnetic resonance imaging, T2 weighted. A peripheral rim of decreased signal is apparent while the internal high signal of the lesion signifies its fluid content (large arrows). The thecal sac is compressed (small arrow) and the laterally displaced exiting nerve root identified (curved arrow). This bilobed dumb-bell-shaped mass lying dorsally in an extradural location is characteristic of a synovial cyst. The demonstration on MR imaging of its high fluid content confirms the diagnosis and strongly suggests the presence of haemorrhage. (Courtesy of Kenneth B. Heithoff MD, Minneapolis, USA.)

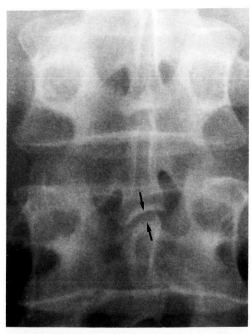

Figure 18.4 Baastrup's disease, L4–L5. Pseudoarthroses are apparent between the L4–L5 spinous processes (arrows). Note how the opposing spinous processes exhibit smooth, concave-convex cortical surfaces. The significance of the condition is probably overestimated. The most common level of involvement is the L4–L5 level. Three morphological types of interspinous neoarthroses are recognized; flat, concave-convex and oblique. (Courtesy of James R. Brandt DC, FACO, Minneapolis, USA.)

Imaging features

Conventional radiography

Frontal radiographs exhibit predominantly osteophytes at the joint margin in addition to sclerosis and articular narrowing (Benhamou *et al.*, 1993; Rowe and Yochum, 1996d).

Computed tomography

Such changes can also be demonstrated on axial CT images. Osteophytes, sclerosis, narrowing and fusion are clearly seen (Benhamou *et al.*, 1993).

Nuclear medicine

Focal tracer uptake ('hot spot') can be observed at these degenerative joints but is not an indicator of a symptomatic correlation (Benhamou *et al.*, 1993).

Intervertebral disc syndromes

Degenerative disc disease

Degenerative disc disease (DDD) is the most common pathology of the adult lumbar spine. The clinical significance for DDD is often indeterminate since at least 30–50% of asymptomatic lumbar spines demonstrate degenerative changes (Torgenson and Dotter, 1976; Wiesel *et al.*, 1984; Jensen *et al.*, 1994). Even in children under 15 years of age, 25% may have MRI evidence of DDD (Terrti *et al.*, 1991).

Table 18.6 *Imaging findings in degenerative disc disease*

Conventional radiography
  loss of disc height
  osteophytes
  vacuum phenomenon
  calcification
    annular, nuclear
  hemispherical spondylosclerosis
  subluxation
  facet arthropathy

Computed tomography
  disc bulge
  calcification
  vacuum phenomenon
    disc, canal
  osteophytes
    anterior, lateral, posterior
  canal stenosis
    central, lateral

Magnetic resonance imaging
  disc bulge
  reduced disc signal
  anular changes
    infolding, tears
  end-plate signal changes
    type I–III
  vacuum phenomenon
  calcification
  canal stenosis
    central, lateral

The pathophysiology of disc degeneration remains controversial. Anular tears, nuclear degradation and dessication, end-plate, bone marrow and ligamentous changes constitute the pathological basis for imaging findings (Ostrum *et al.*, 1993; Natarajan *et al.*, 1994) (Table 18.6).

Imaging features

Conventional radiography

The cardinal signs include loss of disc height, osteophytes, vacuum phenomenon, end-plate sclerosis, calcification and subluxation of paired facet surfaces (Rowe, 1989, 1996) (Figure 18.5) (see anatomical and histological examples: Figures 4.9 and 4.12, 4.17, 4.18, 4.22, 4.23, 6.5, 6.17).

Loss of disc height

A reduced L5 disc height in the absence of osteophytes, vacuum phenomenon or end-plate sclerosis is most likely developmentally small, rather than degenerative in nature such as with a lumbosacral transitional segment (lumbarization, sacralization). Loss of disc height is only a weak indicator of a pain producing level (Frymoyer *et al.*, 1984).

Osteophytes

Two basic morphological forms are described, 'claw' and 'traction', though intermediate conformations are found (Resnick, 1985). At least 75% of osteophytes coexist with a narrow disc height (Pate *et al.*, 1988).

Claw osteophytes are characterized by their triangular shape; a broad base with the distal tip curving vertically. These occur four times more commonly than other osteophytes, increase in frequency with age over 60 years, originate with equal frequency from the superior and inferior end-plates, and are evenly distributed throughout the lumbar spine (Pate *et al.*, 1988).

Traction osteophytes are thinner, originate 1–2 mm beyond the vertebral body margin, and project horizontally. These are more common under the age of

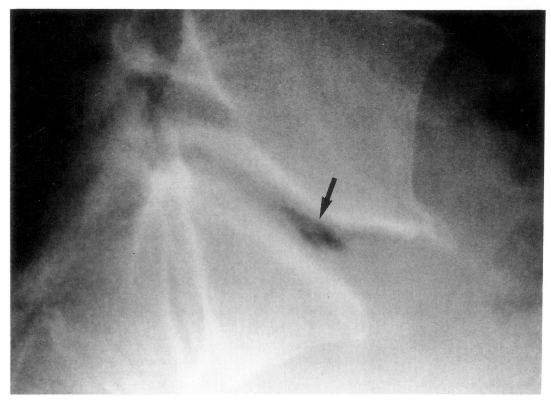

Figure 18.5 Degenerative disc disease, L5–S1. The disc space is narrowed in association with a vacuum phenomenon (arrow). An anterior traction osteophyte is present and retrolisthesis. These are the cardinal features of degenerative disc disease. The presence of intradiscal gas signifies the presence of fissures (degeneration), that physiological motion is still present and excludes infection as a cause for the diminution in disc height.

60 years with close to 70% arising from the superior end-plate between L3 and L5. It is the traction variety which is implicated as a sign of instability (Macnab, 1971; Dupuis *et al.*, 1985). Discography shows a marked correlation between loss in disc height and disc disruption with these osteophytes, though this does not correlate with the level of symptomatic disc pathology (Frymoyer, 1991).

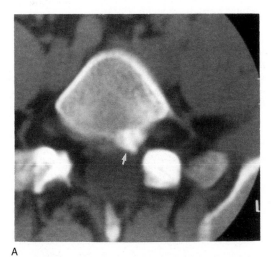

A

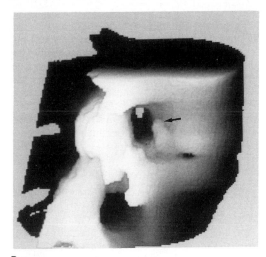

B

Figure 18.6 Posterior vertebral body osteophytes ('uncinate spurs'). A. Axial CT, bone window. A single posterior osteophyte is visible (arrow). B. Three-dimensional CT reconstruction. Graphic demonstration of the posterior osteophyte entering into the intervertebral foramen. Note its hook-like orientation extending upward to encroach directly onto the exiting nerve root (arrow). Posterior osteophytes are relatively uncommon in comparison to anterior and lateral osteophytes. Three-dimensional CT can be of considerable assistance in understanding the spatial relationships of structures affected by such abnormalities. (Courtesy of Kenneth B. Heithoff MD, Minneapolis, USA.)

Posterior body osteophyte formation is infrequent in the lumbar spine due to a less adherent posterior longitudinal ligament and anulus fibrosus (Eisenstein, 1977; Schmorl and Junghanns, 1971; Rowe, 1989). These have been referred to as 'uncinate spurs' due to the analogous location of similar posterolateral osteophytes in the cervical spine (Dupuis *et al.*, 1985) (Figure 18.6).

Vacuum phenomenon

Collections of nitrogen gas, derived from sub-end-plate tissues, can migrate into nuclear and anular fissures within a degenerative disc, producing a distinctive radiolucency referred to as the 'vacuum phenomenon (of Knuttson)' (Rowe, 1989). From 1 to 20% of the general population may exhibit this radiographic feature. The sign can be precipitated by hyperextension and abolished by flexion (Goobar *et al.*, 1987). Central vacuum phenomena correspond to fissuring of the nucleus pulposus, while peripheral lesions represent rim lesions where the anulus fibrosus has been disrupted from its attachment to the vertebral body margin (Resnick *et al.* 1981).

End-plate sclerosis

Two forms occur; localized and generalized. The local form characteristically lies on the anterior corner of a vertebral body immediately beneath an osteophyte. The more generalized form extends at least over two-thirds of the end-plate, beginning from the anterior vertebral surface, and is referred to as 'hemispherical spondylosclerosis' (HSS) (Dihlmann, 1981; Rowe and Yochum, 1988b). This most commonly involves the inferior end-plate of L4, exhibits a convex upper margin, and is homogenously sclerotic. The disc below is often narrowed with an anterior traction osteophyte commonly visible.

Subluxation

Vertebral displacement associated with disc degeneration is most commonly in a posterior direction (retrolisthesis, retrosubluxation, retroposition) and less often laterally (lateralisthesis). Anterolisthesis usually indicates facet arthropathy (degenerative spondylolisthesis).

Retroposition occurs due to the posterior orientation of the facet planes which draws the vertebra above posteriorly as disc height decreases (Smith, 1934; Fletcher, 1947; Resnick, 1985). (See histological example: Figure 6.5.) Other causes for retrolisthesis include disc infection, neoplasms and the level above spondylolisthesis (Haglestom, 1947; Henson, 1988). Retrolisthesis most commonly occurs at L5–S1 followed by L1–L2 and L2–L3. The average displacement is 3–9 mm. Anatomical variation of the lumbosacral junction where the sacrum is reduced in its sagittal dimension compared to that of the fifth lumbar, may account for up to two-thirds of these observed lumbosacral retropositions (Willis, 1935). Technical factors such as patient rotation and lateral flexion can simulate retrolisthesis, as do anatomical variations such as nuclear impressions (Melamed and Ansfield, 1947; Rowe, 1989). The majority of retro-positions are asymptomatic, though such a subluxa-tion tends to displace nerve roots cranially and predispose to lateral entrapment from the superior facet from the segment below (Johnson, 1934).

Calcification

Calcification within a degenerative disc is character-istically hydroxyapatite (Rowe and Yochum, 1996d). This may lie within the anulus fibrosus or nucleus pulposus, with or without an associated disc hernia-tion.

Anular calcification is the most common form and usually involves the outer anterior anular fibres (Schmorl and Junghanns, 1971). The radiographic appearance of anular calcification is distinctively located at the disc periphery as a thin, curvilinear density arching between two vertebral bodies.

Nucleus pulposus calcification will be visible as a homogenous round to oval radiopacity located cen-trally, but slightly posterior, in the disc space, simulating the appearance seen on a normal disco-gram. Histopathological examination reveals the cal-cium to be deposited within crevices of the nucleus pulposus (Schmorl and Junghanns, 1971).

Computed tomography

Signs of DDD on CT parallel those seen in plain films

Osteophytes   These are clearly seen on bone windows near the discovertebral junction as circumferential irregular bony excrescences. Claw osteophytes charac-teristically extend from a large part of the vertebral body. Posterior osteophyes extending into the inter-vertebral foramen ('uncinate spurs') are easily over-looked on axial images and are seen to advantage on sagittal re-constructions and 3D images (Figure 18.6B).

Vacuum phenomenon   Nitrogen gas accumulations are readily identified as radiolucent foci within the disc. Gas may also lie within a herniated disc and contribute to the space occupying effect of the lesion (Mortenson *et al.*, 1991). Gas within the spinal canal, without herniation, is a relatively uncommon finding and is indicative of disruption of the posterior anulus (Orrison and Lilleas, 1982). Disc infections other than rare peptococcus organisms do not demonstrate this sign due to fluid collections in the fissures (Resnick *et al.*, 1981; Rowe, 1988a).

Disc bulge   A consistent feature is circumferential bulging of the disc, beyond the vertebral bodies, which exhibits a convex posterior margin (Williams

et al., 1982). Additional features include vacuum phenomenon, osteophytes and annular calcification.

Calcification   Deposition of calcium can be identi-fied within the nucleus pulposus, anulus fibrosus, ligamentum flavum or posterior longitudinal liga-ment, as well as other pathological conditions such as arachnoiditis ossificans. A higher incidence of calcifi-cation is found within herniated discs treated with epidural steroids (Manelfe, 1992).

End-plate changes   Sclerosis is identified as increased density which may extend right across the end-plate or exist as a localized change often maximal near an osteophyte. Irregularity of the end-plate surface is common and can be due to Schmorl's nodes (see Figure 4.5) which may contain vacuum phenomena.

Stenosis   Encroachment of the spinal canals by osteophytes or soft tissue thickening is well seen on axial and sagittal reconstruction views.

Magnetic resonance imaging

The sensitivity of MRI in spinal imaging renders disc changes highly visible, though calcified tissue, gas and osteophytes are not well seen.

Reduced signal

Diminished signal intensity of the internal disc substance due to dehydration is the cardinal MRI sign of DDD (Modic *et al.*, 1994). Initially, this may be only slight but progresses in parallel with dessication (Tertti *et al.*, 1991). Loss of the normal horizontal low signal mid discal cleft is the earliest MRI sign of dehydration (Aguila *et al.*, 1985). With progressive dehydration, there is homogenous loss of disc signal best demonstrated on T2-weighted MRI sagittal images (Manelfe, 1992).

Vacuum phenomenon

A signal void occupies the vacuum site (Modic *et al.*, 1994). Gas collections as small as 0.1 ml can be detected (Berns *et al.*, 1991). MRI is not as sensitive in detecting intradiscal anatomy as plain films and CT (Grenier *et al.*, 1987b).

Anular infolding

With early dehydration, the innermost fibres of the outer anulus collapse centrally toward the inner nuclear complex (Scheibler *et al.*, 1991) (see histo-logical example: Figure 4.18).

Anular tears

This can be seen in two forms: disruption in the continuity of the anular fibres and a focal high intensity zone (HIZ) (Manelfe, 1992). The HIZ has attracted

Table 18.7 *Vertebral marrow changes in degenerative disc disease on MRI examination*

	T1-weighted	*T2-weighted*	*Marrow status*	*Significance*
Type 1	Low (Black)	High (White)	Fibrovascular	Back pain, hypermobility
Type 2	High (White)	High (White)	Fatty	Stability
Type 3	Low (Black)	Low (Black)	Fibrovascular	Back pain, hypermobility

considerable attention as it is considered by many to represent an area of inflammation from a tear within the pain sensitive outer anulus (internal disc disruption) (Yu *et al.*, 1988a; Aprill and Bogduk, 1992).

End-plate changes

Vertebral bone marrow changes are extremely common findings in concert with degenerative disc disease (de Roos *et al.*, 1987). Three patterns are recognized – Types 1, 2 and 3 (Modic *et al.*, 1988a,b).

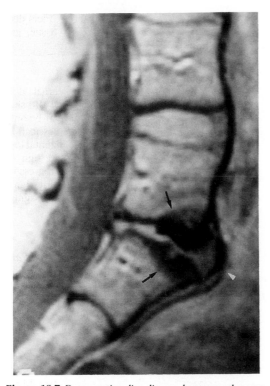

Figure 18.7 Degenerative disc disease, hypervascular marrow changes. On this sagittal T1-weighted image there is marked reduced signal of both end-plates (arrows). There is also anterior disc herniation (arrowhead). Low signal of the end-plates on T1 can correlate with inflammatory marrow and a higher incidence of back pain and segmental hypermobility. (Courtesy of Constance Gould DC, Pietermaritzburg, South Africa.)

Type 1 end-plate changes show decreased intensity on T1-weighted images and increased signal intensity on T2-weighted images (white–black). Type 2 end-plate changes show increased intensity on T1-weighted images and increased or isotintense signal intensity on T2-weighted images (white–white). Type 3 end-plate changes show decreased intensity on T1-weighted images and decreased signal intensity on T2-weighted images (black–black) (Table 18.7).

Low signal of the end-plates on T1 correlates with inflammatory marrow and a higher incidence of back pain and segmental hypermobility (Toyone *et al.*, 1994) (Figure 18.7). Conversely, high signal on T1 denotes the presence of fatty marrow as a sign of intersegmental stability, a useful sign in determining successful fusion (Lang *et al.*, 1990) (Figure 18.8). Type 1 changes tend to progress to Type 2 over time (hypervascular to fatty), whereas Type 2 remain stable (fatty) (Modic *et al.*, 1988a,b).

Bulging intervertebral disc

The phenomenon of a bulging intervertebral disc is a common imaging finding in the lumbar spine, usually of indeterminate significance (Boden *et al.*, 1990; Jensen *et al.*, 1994). In asymptomatic individuals between 20 and 39 years of age up to 35% and virtually 100% over age 60 years, will have at least one disc bulging on MRI (Wiesel *et al.*, 1984; Jensen *et al.*, 1994). When found in tandem with facet arthrosis a disc bulge contributes to both central and lateral stenosis.

Various terms include degenerative disc bulge, disc bulge, and non-herniating (self-contained) discal degeneration. The underlying pathology is loss of disc turgor due to degenerative changes within the nucleus producing concentric outward bulging of the anulus beyond the margin of the adjacent vertebral bodies (Williams *et al.*, 1982). Only 50% of all degenerative discs bulge. (Boden and Wiesel, 1990).

Imaging features

Conventional radiography

Plain films are frequently normal except for occasional loss of disc height, early osteophyte formation and a vacuum phenomenon. If the anulus calcifies the outline of the bulging disc may be seen.

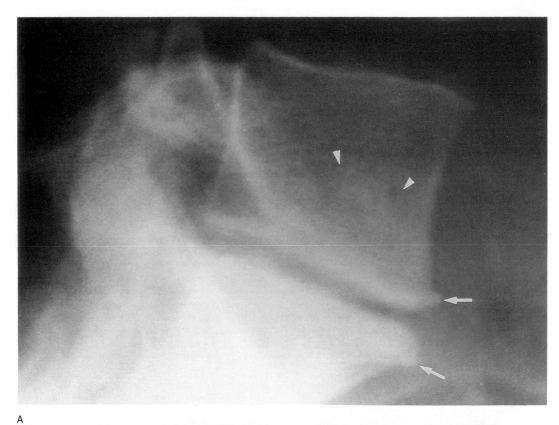

A

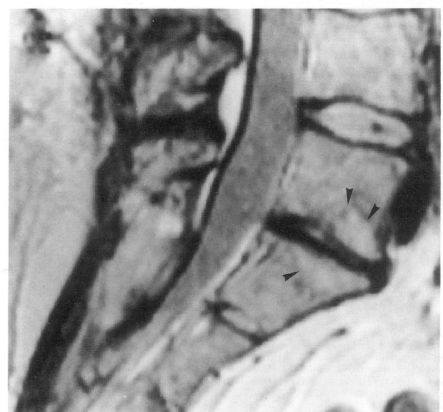

B

Figure 18.8 Degenerative disc disease, fatty marrow changes. A. Plain film. Observe the loss of disc height at the L5–S1 interspace and retrolisthesis. Small anterior osteophytes are present (arrows). There is evidence of hemispherical spondylosclerosis extending from the anteroinferior margin of the L5 end-plate (arrowheads). B. Magnetic resonance imaging, T1-weighted image. The area corresponding to the plain film L5 vertebral body sclerosis shows high signal with a similar change within the sacral base (arrowheads). The degenerative intervertebral disc lacks signal, consistent with dehydration. These are characteristic findings of degenerative disc disease. The high signal on T1 characterizes a fatty marrow replacement usually associated with a more clinially stable situation.

Computed tomography

CT demonstrates the bulging disc margin extending beyond the adjacent vertebral bodies creating a convex posterior disc margin (Williams *et al.*, 1982) (Figure 18.9). Typically there is no associated herniation. A bulge of more than 2.5 mm indicates tears are present within the anulus (Yu *et al.*, 1988b). A

vacuum phenomenon is a common finding. Bulging discs are often asymmetrical with scoliosis.

Magnetic resonance imaging

MRI depicts a diminished signal of the intervertebral disc space especially on T2-weighted images (Cotler, 1992). The convex contour of the bulging anulus is demonstrated and its integrity confirmed (Figure 18.10).

Internal disc disruption

Internal disc disruption (IDD) is a disorder characterized by tears of the anulus fibrosus which initiate a marked inflammatory reaction. The external shape is normal and there is no nerve compression. It was first alluded to by Dandy in 1941 who referred to 'concealed ruptured intervetebral discs' as the cause for back pain when a disc protrusion could not be demonstrated (Dandy, 1941). The entity was named, described and introduced by Crock (Crock, 1970). He

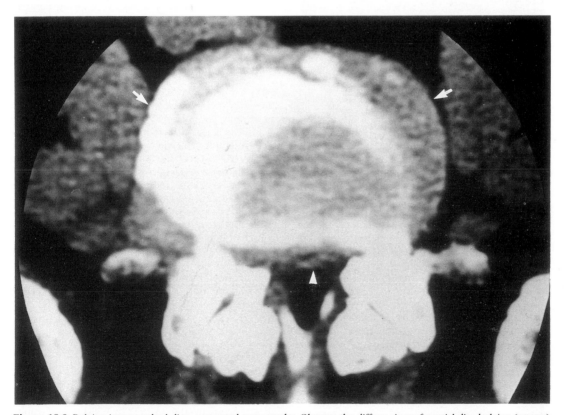

Figure 18.9 Bulging intervertebral disc, computed tomography. Observe the diffuse circumferential disc bulging (arrows). The posterior disc margin is characteristically convex (arrowhead). The phenomenon of a bulging intervertebral disc is a common imaging finding often of indeterminate significance. Up to 35% of 20–39 year olds, and virtually 100% over age 60 years, will have at least one disc bulging on MRI. When found in tandem with facet arthrosis a disc bulge contributes to both central and lateral stenosis.

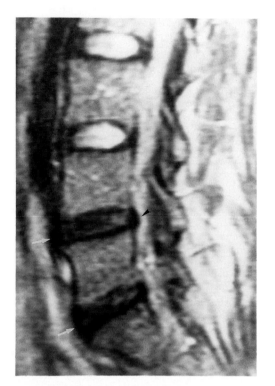

Figure 18.10 Degenerative disc disease L4–L5 and L5–S1, MRI. Diminished signal intensity of the internal disc substance due to dehydration can be seen at two levels (arrows). The L4–L5 disc exhibits posterior anular bulging (arrowhead). Compare this with the normal appearance at L3–L4. MRI is extremely sensitive in the depiction of disc degeneration. Up to 50% of asymptomatic lumbar spines will have disc abnormalities such as dehydration, bulging and herniation demonstrated on MRI, while CT can show the same abnormalities in around 35–50%.

identified a subset of low back and leg pain patients who, following spinal trauma, became incapacitated with pain and constitutional symptoms including malaise, lack of energy, depression and loss of weight (Crock, 1983, 1986, 1993).

The pathophysiology revolves around tears extending from the inner anulus to the pain sensitive outer anulus. Tears may be circumferential (Type 1), radial (Type 2), and disrupted from its attachment (Type 3) (Yu *et al.*, 1988a). This is postulated to initiate a strong autoimmune reaction resulting in progressive degradation of the disc (Crock, 1986; Gronblad *et al.*, 1994). Approximately 50% involve the L5 disc, 30% the L4 disc and 15% the L3 and L2 discs (Blumenthal *et al.*, 1988).

Imaging features

Findings are characteristically lacking on most modalities (Crock, 1970, 1991, 1993). Conventional radiographs, CT scan and myelograms all will appear normal. A traction osteophyte may occasionally be seen (Macnab, 1971). A peripherally placed vacuum phenomenon seen on CT may lie within an anular tear, a vacuum within the spinal canal denotes a communicating tear through the outer anulus (Orrison and Lilleas, 1982).

Computed tomography-discography

Combining CT with a discogram (CTD) can demonstrate internal tears which have been graded according to how far they extended peripherally (Vanharanta *et al.*, 1987) (Figure 18.11). Grade 0 are restricted to the nucleus pulposus; Grade 1 extend into the inner third of the anulus fibrosus; Grade 2 involve the middle third, and; Grade 3 continue into the outer one-third. Up to 70% of Grade 3 tears are symptomatic, correlating with the innervated anular component, while Grades 0 and 1 exist largely without clinical manifestations (Sachs *et al.*, 1987). Discography may be the imaging procedure of choice in IDD when MRI is normal but back pain remains unexplained and surgery is being contemplated (Colhoun *et al.*, 1988; Brightbill *et al.*, 1994).

Magnetic resonance imaging

MRI has demonstrated anular disruptions. These may be radial, circumferential or detachments at their insertions (rim lesions) (Yu *et al.*, 1988a, 1989). Localized anular tears can be identified on T2-weighted and proton density images as a high intensity zone (HIZ) (Aprill and Bogduk, 1992). Injection of gadolinium will identify these tears more readily (Ross *et al.*, 1989; Heithoff and Amster, 1990). The HIZ has attracted considerable attention as it is considered by many to represent an area of inflammation from a tear within the pain sensitive outer anulus (internal disc disruption) (Yu *et al.*, 1988b; Aprill and Bogduk, 1992). Despite these observed changes MRI of IDD has not been reliable in predicting symptomatic discs in comparison with discography (Simmons *et al.*, 1991; Osti *et al.*, 1992; Brightbill *et al.*, 1994).

Isolated disc resorption

The phenomenon of progressive loss of a single disc space over a number of years characterizes the lesion. It was first alluded to in 1932 by Williams and named in 1970 by Crock (Williams, 1932; Crock, 1970). The most common level is the L5 disc, occasionally L4 and rarely L3 (Crock, 1983). It is most likely due to an initial end-plate fracture or anular tear which begins a

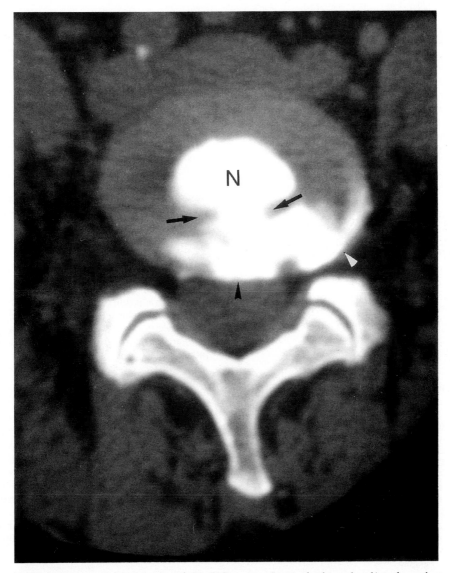

Figure 18.11 Internal disc disruption L4–L5, CT-discogram. Contrast has been placed into the nucleus pulposus (N) which has tracked posteriorly along a central radial tear (arrows) into circumferential tears of the peripheral anulus (arrowheads). There is no disc herniation present. Characteristically, without discogram the CT scan will appear normal. MRI may demonstrate a high signal intensity zone within the peripheral anulus. (Courtesy of Kenneth B. Heithoff MD, Minneapolis, USA.)

cascade of degenerative processes mediated largely by an aggressive immune system response (Venner and Crock, 1981; Crock, 1986).

Imaging features

Conventional radiography

The imaging findings consist of a diminished disc height, end-plate sclerosis, minimal osteophyte formation, vacuum phenomenon, and retrolisthesis.

Computed tomography

Evidence for minimal disc bulging, small peripheral osteophytes and vacuum phenomenon are the most consistent features.

Magnetic resonance imaging

Signs of dehydration may be the only sign with loss of height and low signal intensity. Marrow changes within the sub-end-plate zone are Modic type 2 (T1 white–T2 white), usually signifying stability due to fatty infiltration. Narrowing of the lateral canal may be observed.

Disc herniation

Nomenclature for disc disease is confusing and non-uniform (Yussen and Swartz, 1993). In this discussion the term 'herniation' means a movement of the nucleus pulposus material through the anulus fibrosus. Herniations are rare under the age of 20 and over age 65 with the peak age around 42 years (Weber, 1993). Approximately 47% of disc herniations occur at L4–L5, 43% at L5–S1, 7% at L3–L4, and 3% or less at L1–L2 or L2–L3 (Crock, 1986; Lukin *et al.*, 1988). Herniations occur posteriorly (56%), anteriorly (30%) and vertically into the vertebral bodies (14%) (Jinkins *et al.*, 1989). In posterior herniations approximately 60% are posterolateral, 30% central and 10% lateral (Lukin *et al.*, 1988). Asymptomatic disc herniations as high as 30–40% can be demonstrated by myelography, discography, CT and MRI (Wiesel *et al.*, 1984; Boden *et al.*, 1990; Jensen *et al.*, 1994).

Imaging features

Intervertebral disc herniations exhibit a number of imaging features (Table 18.8).

Table 18.8 *Imaging findings for lumbar disc herniation*

Conventional radiography
    antalgic scoliosis
    lateral flexion inhibition
    disc calcification in the canal
Myelography
    extradural filling defect
    non-filling of nerve root sheath
    elevation of nerve root sheath
Discography
    extravasation of contrast from anulus
Computed tomography
    deformity of the posterior disc margin
    mass soft tissue lesion
    displacement of epidural fat
    deformity of the thecal sac
    deformity of nerve roots
    calcification of the disc
    intraspinal vacuum phenomenon
Magnetic resonance imaging
    deformity of the posterior disc margin
    mass soft tissue lesion
    displacement of epidural fat
    deformity of the thecal sac
    deformity of nerve roots
    gadolinium enhancing nerve root
    calcification of the disc
    intraspinal vacuum phenomenon

Conventional radiography

Plain film radiography has generally little value in the detection of the presence, level and direction for lumbar disc herniation (Lukin *et al.*, 1988; Holtas, 1993). It is however a useful, cost-effective first line modality to identify anomalies and other bony abnormalities.

Calcification within a herniated disc is seen in less than 10% of cases on the lateral film (Smith, 1976; Rowe, 1988c). Additional features include loss of the lumbar lordosis, antalgic scoliosis with little intersegmental rotation above the herniation, and forward flexion of the segment above. On lateral flexion, there is a failure of the segment above the herniation to laterally flex ('lateral bending sign') (Weitz, 1981).

Myelography

Signs for disc herniation include a sharp, extradural impression adjacent to a disc space either ventrally or from one side. Non-visualization and/or elevation of a nerve root sleeve, and a displaced and swollen nerve root, are additional features (Figure 18.12). A major pitfall in missed disc herniations is at the L5–S1 level where the space between the disc and thecal sac may be large (Lukin *et al.*, 1988). When MRI is available, myelography should not be performed.

Discography

This provides a morphological and functional assessment. Combination with CT allows the recognition of the nature and location of anular tears with peripheral extensions more likely to be symptomatic (Sachs *et al.*, 1987; Vanharanta *et al.*, 1987; Greenspan, 1993). Provocation of pain assists in isolating an offending disc level, though there is a false positive rate of around 30% (Greenspan, 1993).

Computed tomography

Axial images graphically demonstrate disc herniations. Combining CT with myelography improves the diagnostic accuracy for identifying and quantifying thecal sac and nerve root compression (Lukin *et al.*, 1988; Yussen and Swartz, 1993). In post-surgical patients the differentiation between recurrent disc herniation and epidural fibrosis can be assisted by rapid infusion of contrast with the fibrosis uniformly enhancing (Schubiger and Valavanis, 1982).

CT signs for disc herniation include deformity of the posterior border of the disc, a protruding soft tissue mass, altered epidural fat visibility and location, neural element changes, vacuum phenomena, and calcification (Williams *et al.*, 1980) (Figure 18.12).

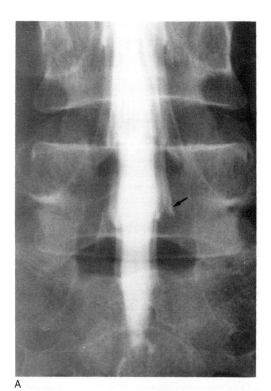

A

Figure 18.12 Intervertebral disc herniation L5–S1. A. Myelogram. On this frontal view the myelographic column appears largely normal, though the L5 nerve root on the right is elevated and displaced laterally (arrow). B. Computed tomography. On axial imaging the herniation is clearly evident as a focal convexity in the posterior disc margin (arrow). Note the asymmetry in the appearance of the epidural fat and S1 nerve roots. Myelograms should be used sparingly in the diagnosis of disc herniation. CT graphically demonstrates disc herniation as deformity of the posterior border of the disc, a protruding soft tissue mass, altered epidural fat visibility and location, neural element changes, vacuum phenomena and calcification. (Courtesy of Michael P. Buna DC, Victoria, Canada.)

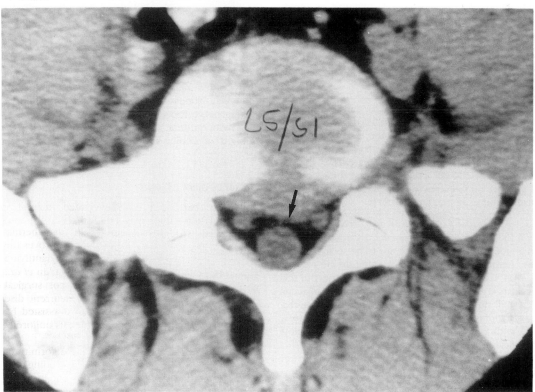

B

Deformity of the posterior border of the disc

Normally the posterior discal surface is slightly concave or straight. The L5–S1 disc is occasionally convex as a normal variant. In herniation there is a distinct alteration of this border which is convex and may be short based (focal) or broad based (diffuse).

Soft tissue mass

The attenuation value of a herniated disc (50–100 HU) is twice that of the thecal sac, though a large central herniation may be isodense and readily overlooked. Large herniations frequently migrate beneath the posterior longitudinal ligament (sub-ligamentous) above or below the disc of origin (see anatomical example: Figure 4.10).

Epidural fat

Bilateral symmetry of these tissues is striking on soft tissue windows. Three distinct areas can be seen; one posteriorly beneath the spinolaminar junction and one on each side at the lateral canal surrounding the exiting nerve root and adjacent thecal sac (see histological example: Figure 3.14). Asymmetry of the epidural fat is a reliable radiological marker of intraspinal disease which, in disc herniation, may be obliterated or displaced (see histological example: Figure 5.23).

Neural element changes

Individual nerve roots can be displaced, obliterated, flattened or enlarged. Alterations in the surrounding epidural fat may be the only clue to nerve root involvement. The thecal sac similarly can be displaced or altered in its shape. The ventral surface usually is separated by epidural fat from the disc margin with the contour of the disc–sac interface reflecting the status of the posterior disc–integrity. Disc hernia-tions, if large enough, contact the thecal sac causing a concave indentation on its ventral surface (see histological example: Figure 4.11).

Calcification

In about 10% of cases, calcium can be seen within a disc herniation (Rowe, 1988c). Typically the pattern is focal, tending to lie toward the outer aspect of the herniation and may bridge to attach to the adjacent vertebral rim. Such calcification is usually a sign of a long-standing herniation. Furthermore, patients trea-ted with epidural steroid injections may develop calcification in disc herniations (Manelfe, 1992).

Vacuum phenomenon

Gas may lie within a herniated disc and contribute to the space occupying effect of the lesion (Mortenson

et al., 1991). Occasionally, gas may also be present within the central canal signifying the presence of a communicating anular tear.

Magnetic resonance imaging

Some investigators advocate MRI as the initial method of choice in cases of suspected disc herniation as it is superior to all other imaging modalities (Takahashi *et al.*, 1993; Yussen and Swartz, 1993). Features include demonstration of the displaced mass, altered epidural fat, and deformed and displaced neural elements (Figure 18.13). It is extremely useful in the differ-ential diagnosis of intraspinal pathology. Post-surgical fibrosis can be accurately identified in almost 90% of cases by its poor margination, no mass effect, an intermediate signal on T1, and high signal on T2-weighted images and homogenous enhancement with gadolinium (Bundschuh *et al.*, 1988).

Mass

The majority of herniated fragments exhibit high signal on T2-weighted images (Czervionke, 1993). With time there may be a gradual loss of this high signal. On T1-weighted sagittal images the nuclear herniation is seen clearly contiguous between the disc of origin extending through a narrow neck at the normal disc margin and then expanding into the herniated component ('squeezed toothpaste sign') (Lukin *et al.*, 1988).

Epidural fat

T1-weighted images show these structures clearly as triangular zones of high signal surrounding the exiting nerve roots and thecal sac. Where there is a paucity of epidural fat, proton density images are the method of choice for demonstration (Czervionke, 1993).

Neural element changes

These are best seen on T1-weighted images. An individual nerve root may be displaced, flattened, enlarged and of higher signal intensity in response to

Figure 18.13 Intervetebral disc herniation L5–S1. A. Sagit-tal T1-weighted image. Herniation of the L5–S1 nucleus pulposus is dramatically demonstrated (arrow). The L4 disc demonstrates a degenerative disc bulge (arrowhead). B. Axial T1-weighted image. A left-sided paracentral herniation is present (arrow) which has created asymmetry to the appearance of the signal intense (white) epidural fat and impinged on the thecal sac. Epidural fat is prominent in this region and accounts for the false negative results from myelography, since no contact is made with the thecal sac unless there is a very large disc herniation. MRI is extremely useful in the differential diagnosis of intraspinal pathology.

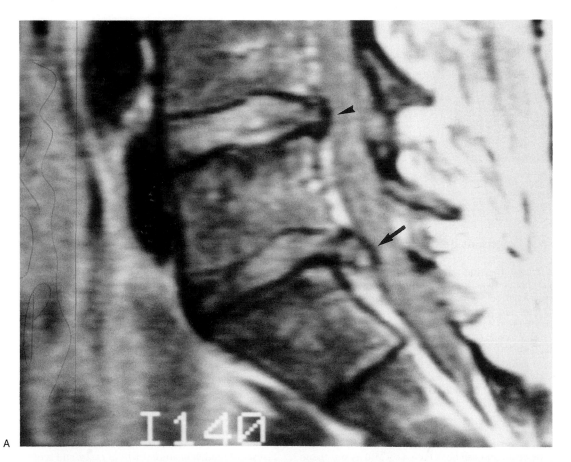

A

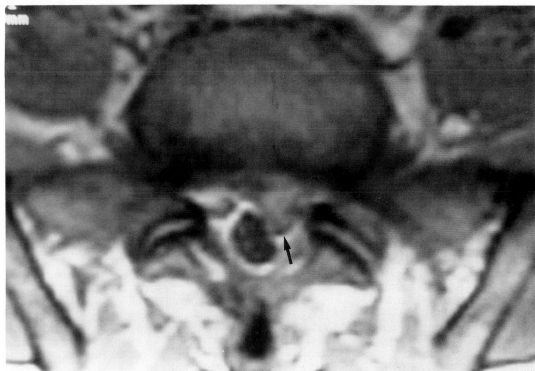

B

a herniation (Czervionke, 1993). Nerve root enhancement after the administration of gadolinium reflects breakdown of the blood–nerve barrier, a sign of nerve inflammation (Jinkins *et al.*, 1993). The thecal sac contour may be altered (effacement) on its ventral surface.

Calcification

A low signal within a herniated disc may signify calcification or a signal void from a collection of gas.

Free fragment disc herniation

A herniation which has disrupted the outer anulus may break away from its point of origin and move relatively freely within the epidural space. Synonyms include sequestration and sequestered or migrated fragment.

Once separated, the isolated fragment may move beneath the posterior longitudinal ligament (subligamentous) in a caudad or cephalad direction (dissection). If fragments lodge within the lateral canal the foramen may enlarge with time (Castillo, 1991). Occasional penetration of the posterior longitudinal ligament (transligamentous) results in a fragment either side of the ligament ('double fragment' sign) (Czervionke, 1993). Rare intradural penetrations occur and can be detected on MRI as soft tissue masses within the thecal sac (Czervionke, 1993). Embolization into the anterior spinal artery may infarct the cord, most commonly the conus (Toro *et al.*, 1994).

Imaging features

The same features for disc herniation may be observed on conventional radiographs and myelography.

Computed tomography

In non-sequential scanning techniques, free fragment herniations are readily overlooked. The disc of origin may show herniation or be relatively normal. The fragment lies 15–30 mm away from the disc within the spinal canal, lateral recess or intervertebral foramen. It characteristically gets larger in images away from the disc of origin and rarely midline due to a dividing septum connecting the vertebral body with the posterior longitudinal ligament (Schellinger *et al.*, 1990). It may be the same density as the disc or infrequently contains calcium. Its margins are usually irregular or polypoid (Williams *et al.*, 1980). At least 50% of fragments are separated from the disc of origin by epidural fat. A thin rim of enhancement with the administration of intravenous contrast due to encasement by ligament is rare (Witzmann *et al.*, 1991).

Magnetic resonance imaging

MRI is the method of choice in the detection of a migrated (sequestered) disc fragment (Jinkins *et al.*, 1993). MRI reveals a disc fragment remote from an adjacent disc with the optimum demonstration on sagittal MR images. Free fragments are rarely midline. The fragment may be hyperintense on T2-weighted images (Glickstein *et al.*, 1989). Gadolinium enhanced MRI frequently shows peripheral enhancement of the fragment due to a covering of granulation tissue (Yamashita *et al.*, 1994).

Posterior limbus bone

Herniation of the intervertebral disc into the posterior surface of the vertebral end-plate (Schmorl's node) may result in displacement of a discal bone fragment into the spinal canal which can produce nerve compression (Laredo *et al.*, 1986; Epstein and Epstein, 1991). This has been variously termed posterior limbus bone, posterior marginal intraosseous node, paradiscal defect, dislocated ring epiphysis, discovertebral rim lesion, apophysial ring fracture, and 'persistent epiphysis' (Goldman, 1990; Thiel *et al.*, 1992).

This most commonly involves adolescent and young adult males up to a ratio of 4:1, involves the posterior inferior end-plate of L4, has an associated history of trauma in around 10% of cases, and is often asymptomatic.

Imaging features

Conventional radiography

The lateral film is the most diagnostic where at the posterior body corner is seen a deflected flake of bone angling posteriorly into the spinal canal (Figure 18.14). A localized Schmorl's node may be determined beneath the bony fragment and the disc may be slightly narrowed (Laredo *et al.*, 1986; Gomori *et al.*, 1991). The plain film, however, may appear normal.

Computed tomography

CT examination clearly depicts the posterior limbus bone as a broad-based osseous density with roughened irregular margins lying within the canal. The underlying end-plate depression from the Schmorl's node can also be seen which may contain a vacuum phenomenon (Laredo *et al.*, 1986; Gomori *et al.*, 1991) (Figure 18.14). Lateral reconstructions assist in its depiction. Nerve root compression by the discal bony fragment can be assessed especially if combined with myelography.

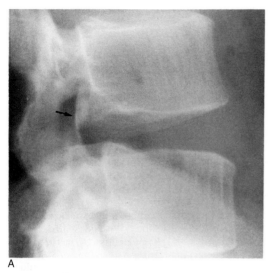

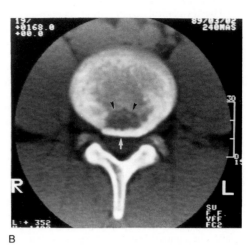

A   B

Figure 18.14 Posterior limbus bone, L4. A. Lateral lumbar radiograph. A linear bony flake is evident within the spinal canal (arrow). B. CT scan. On the axial image the lucent defect from a Schmorl's node can be seen (arrowheads) with the isolated bony flake displaced into the central canal (arrow). Posterior limbus bones are easily overlooked abnormalities on conventional radiographs but are seen well on CT scan. This most commonly occurs in adolescent and young adult males in a ratio of 4:1 involving the posterior inferior end-plate of L4.

Magnetic resonance imaging

MRI changes will consist of diminshed disc signal but the limbus bone itself may not be visible. A coexisting tandem lesion of disc herniation can be shown.

Epidural haematoma

Spontaneous spinal epidural haematomas have recently been described which can manifest symptoms indistinguishable from an acute or chronic disc herniation or spinal stenosis (Nehls *et al.*, 1984; Gundry and Heithoff, 1993; Kingery *et al.*, 1994). Males are affected in a ratio of at least 2:1, most commonly at L4, followed by L5 and the upper lumbar segments, respectively (Gundry and Heithoff, 1993).

These arise from bleeding vessels near the dorsal aspect of the mid-vertebral body near the exit point of the basivertebral vein (Gundry and Heithoff, 1993). In at least 50% of cases, they are associated with a coexisting disc herniation which is thought to initiate the bleed by tearing adjacent epidural veins. Symptoms generally diminish faster than due to disc herniation as the haematoma reduces in size. At operation, 50% are encapsulated as an isolated lesion, 40% are encapsulated in association with a disc herniation, and 10% remain unencapsulated (Gundry and Heithoff, 1993).

Imaging features

Computed tomography

A round ventral extradural mass is visualized extending from the level of the disc to the mid-vertebral body, simulating a sequestered disc fragment (Boyd and Pear, 1972; Levitan and Wiens, 1983). Characteristically, they are widest at the mid-vertebral body in contrast to a free fragment disc herniation. The attenuation values are similar to that of a herniated disc (60–70 HU) (Gundry and Heithoff, 1993).

Magnetic resonance imaging

Signal intensity is variable with only one-third suggestive of blood (increased signal on T2 and proton density) (Kingery *et al.*, 1994). They are, however, different in intensity from adjacent intervertebral discs. On sagittal images the haematoma lies interposed between the ventral aspect of the cord and dorsal surface of the vertebral body. It is often crescenteric in shape with the width greatest adjacent to the mid-vertebral body. The majority lie in a parasagittal location (Gundry and Heithoff, 1993). Gadolinium scans may show enhancement at its margins (Kingery *et al.*, 1994).

Degenerative spinal stenosis

Stenosis is the term applied to narrowing of the central or lateral spinal canals which produces compression of the contained neural elements. The entity of spinal stenosis was originally alluded to by Sapyener (1945), and later Verbiest (1949, 1954). Up to 28% of asymptomatic individuals may exhibit spinal stenosis on CT or MRI, emphasizing the need to carefully correlate the clinical and imaging findings (Kent *et al.*, 1992).

The key clinical manifestation is neurogenic claudication often reduced with lumbar flexion amongst other less significant findings (Pleatman and Lukin, 1988). The most common levels of involvement are L4–L5 and L5–S1. Isolating symptomatic nerve root involvement from lateral stenosis can be assisted by diagnostic nerve blocks (Rydevik, 1993).

The causes for canal narrowing are multiple, including congenital and acquired disorders such as ligament ossification, spondylolisthesis, Paget's disease, acromegaly, post-surgical callus, fluorosis, fracture and epidural lipomatosis (Pleatman and Lukin, 1988). However, the most common causes are degenerative in nature arising from the disc, facet joints and intraspinal ligaments, especially the ligamentum flavum (Yoshida *et al.*, 1992) (see Figure 13.11). Degenerative spondylolisthesis is a common cause of central and lateral stenosis. All of these disorders can be depicted by imaging modalities (Herzog, 1992).

The initial investigation should preferably be conventional lumbar spine radiographs, though some dispute this approach (Spengler, 1987). The modality of choice following these is MRI. CT is an adequate alternative and is improved with the addition of myelography to the study. CT bone windows provide the greatest accuracy for measuring bony canal dimensions. Myelography on its own is an out-dated procedure and should be avoided wherever possible (Kent *et al.*, 1992). Two types of lumbar stenosis are described, both of which are ammenable to imaging procedures: central and lateral.

Central canal stenosis

Decreased dimensions of the spinal canal which encases the thecal sac is a common sequel to degenerative changes. Central stenosis most commonly involves L3–L5 with generally more than one level involved. Minimum critical dimensions have been intensively investigated with normal ranges established. The accepted minimal sagittal dimension (anteroposterior) is 15 mm with a range down to 12 mm (Hinck *et al.*, 1965; Eisenstein 1977; Ullrich *et al.*, 1980). The lowest coronal measurement (interpediculate distance) is 25 mm (Hinck *et al.*, 1966), though some claim measurements of 16 mm or less (Ullrich *et al.*, 1988). The cross-sectional bony canal area minimum is 145 mm² (Ullrich *et al.*, 1988). A dural sac of 10 mm or less in sagittal dimension is usually associated with symptoms of spinal stenosis (Bolender *et al.*, 1985). The critical cross-sectional area of the dural sac at L3 is below 75 mm², and at L4 below 65 mm², when significant impediment of blood flow and nerve function will occur (Schonstrom *et al.*, 1984).

Imaging features

Conventional radiography

Plain films do not identify spinal stenosis due to soft tissue causes which make up at least 80% of cases (Schonstrom *et al.*, 1985). Large broad pedicles, flattened vertebral bodies, narrowed intervertebral discs and spondylolisthesis may be evident (Pleatman and Lukin, 1985). Forty per cent of bilateral claudication patients have degenerative spondylolisthesis. Measurement of the lateral projection from the spinolaminar junction or the line intersecting the tips of the articular processes, to the posterior surface of the vertebral body (Eisenstein method) should not be less than 12 mm (Eisenstein, 1977). The distance between the inner margins of the pedicles (interpediculate distance) should not be less than 25 mm (Hinck *et al.*, 1966). A 'spinal index' (canal: vertebral body diameter) may indicate stenosis at a ratio of less than 1:4.5 (Jones and Thompson, 1968).

Myelography

The major advantage of myelography is that it permits the demonstration of the upper and lower limits of the stenosis, though MRI can do the same (Pleatman and Lukin, 1988). It is the optimal procedure of choice for arachnoiditis which clinically can mimic stenosis and is more useful for central stenosis than lateral stenosis (Pleatman and Lukin, 1988). Evidence of spinal stenosis is a slow or blocked flow of the contrast column at an individual level, marked indentation of the contrast column usually in a symmetrical manner, and tortuous nerve roots.

Computed tomography

Axial images display the cross-sectional characteristics of the central canal and the contained neural elements (Figure 18.15). CT findings of spinal stenosis include a discal vacuum phenomenon, disc bulging, small canal, trefoil-shaped canal, facet arthrosis, ligamentum flavum hypertrophy greater than 4 mm, and a paucity of epidural fat (Pleatman and Lukin, 1988; Yoshida *et al.*, 1992) (Figure 18.16).

Magnetic resonance imaging

Sagittal images show the front-to-back compromise to advantage, axial images less so. The key features are the bulging discs, facet and ligamentum flavum hypertrophy. The compression on the thecal sac is best shown on T2-weighted sagittal images (Modic *et al.*, 1994). Central consolidation of nerve roots within the thecal sac produces an intermediate signal intensity which can be confused with arachnoiditis. Additionally, dampening of the CSF pulsations at the level of stenosis can increase the signal locally (Modic *et al.*, 1994). MRI has largely displaced the need to perform myelography.

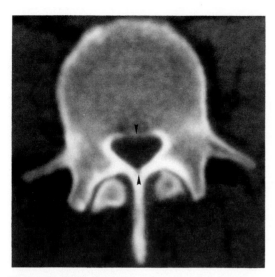

Figure 18.15 Congenital central canal stenosis, axial computed tomography. On this bone window image the pedicles are large, the interpediculate space is narrowed and there is a reduced sagittal dimension from the posterior surface of the vertebral body to the base of the spinous process (arrows). This is an example of a small canal secondary to large pedicles. The plain films on this patient were not helpful in its detection. (Courtesy of Geoffrey G. Rymer DC, Hornsby, Australia.)

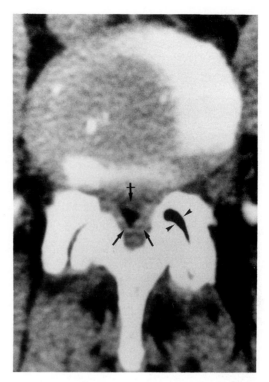

Figure 18.16 Degenerative central and lateral canal stenosis, axial computed tomography. Advanced facet arthrosis is evident on the right with osteophytes and a contained vacuum phenomenon in the joint cavity (arrowheads). Thickening of the ligamentum flavum (arrows) and posterior disc bulging (crossed arrow) contribute to produce central canal stenosis. The facet arthrosis has created the narrowed lateral canal. Centrally, the concentric stenosis is derived from the ligamentum flavum hypertorphy, bulging disc and loss of disc height.

Lateral canal stenosis

The lateral canal is a funnel-shaped tube which provides a path for the exit of a lumbar nerve from the thecal sac to beyond the pedicle. The most common cause for lateral stenosis is due to the degenerative triad of disc bulge, facet and ligamentum flavum hypertrophy. Divisions of the canal have been described with a plethora of terms and boundaries described. Four zones are conceptually evident from medial to lateral which can be imaged with CT and MRI: entrance zone (lateral recess, lateral gutter), mid-zone, exit zone (foraminal) and far lateral (Wiltse *et al.*, 1984; Lee *et al.*, 1988; Giles and Kaveri, 1990).

Entrance zone (lateral recess) stenosis

This contains the lumbar nerve root covered by dura and bathed in CSF with the disc anterior, the facet joint posterior and in its distal end a lateral wall formed by the pedicle (lateral recess). A lateral recess of less than 3 mm is stenotic, 3–5 mm borderline and above 5 mm normal (Ciric *et al.*, 1980; Dorwart *et al.*, 1983). The most common cause for narrowing of the entrance zone is facet hypertrophy, particularly the superior articular process (Lee *et al.*, 1988). A trefoil-shaped central canal occurs most commonly at L5

(15% of spines) and L4 (7% of spines) and has narrow lateral recesses which predispose to nerve compression (Eisenstein 1977, 1980).

Mid-zone stenosis

The ventral motor nerve root and dorsal root ganglion covered with dura and bathed in CSF lie beneath the pars interarticularis and below the pedicle. Causes for stenosis here are osteophytes from the insertion of the ligamentum flavum and the fibrocartilaginous bulge from a pars defect (Lee *et al.*, 1988) (Figure 18.17).

Exit zone (foraminal) stenosis

The peripheral lumbar nerve covered with perineurium traverses the intervertebral foramen beneath the pedicle, facet joint and posterior disc margin. Facet hypertrophy and osteophytes from the posterior vertebral body can compress the canal at this point.

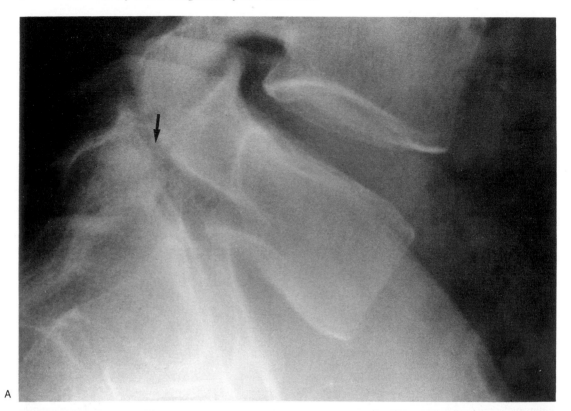

A

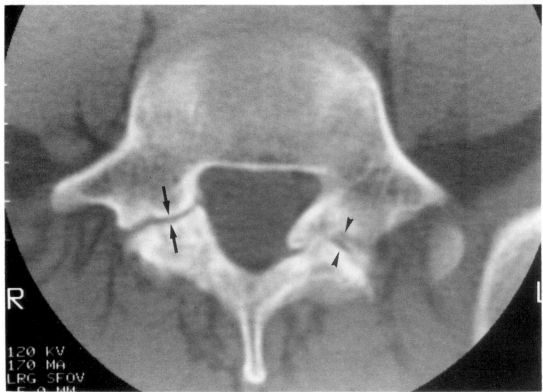

B

Far lateral stenosis

The L5 nerve root can be compressed between the L5 transverse process and sacral ala secondary to degenerative scoliosis or greater than grade 1 spondylolisthesis (Wiltse *et al.*, 1984).

Imaging features

Conventional radiography

Clues to lateral stenosis may include loss of disc height, facet arthrosis, scoliosis, spondylolisthesis, and reduced canal dimensions (Ben-Elijahu *et al.*, 1983; Porter, 1993). Identifying posterior body osteophytes is uncommon (Rowe, 1989). Flexion–extension films may show instability at the involved level giving rise to a dynamic element of the entrapment (Mior and Cassidy, 1982; Dupuis *et al.*, 1985).

Myelography

Generally this investigation is unhelpful, particularly when the exiting nerve root does not fill with contrast.

Computed tomography

The entire lateral canal can be evaluated on axial and reconstructed sagittal images. Axial images can show diminished dimensions, impinging osteophytes and disc bulging with a paucity of fat (Figure 18.16). On sagittal reconstructions canal narrowing and lack of perineural fat are the major features (Heithoff and Amster, 1990). Narrowing can be appreciated either from vertebral body osteophytes-facet hypertrophy ('front-to-back' stenosis), or from loss of disc height-displaced superior articular process ('up-down' stenosis), or from all directions (concentric stenosis) (Heithoff and Amster, 1990).

Magnetic resonance imaging

Foraminal stenosis is identified by an absence or paucity of perineural fat seen on sagittal and axial images (Osborne *et al.*, 1984).

Figure 18.17 Isthmic spondylolisthesis, L5–S1. A. Lateral lumbar radiography. The defect within the pars interarticularis is clearly visible (arrow). A small degree of anterolisthesis is apparent. B. CT scan. The axial bone window demonstrates the bilateral pars defects. Note the distinct asymmetry in the plane and margins of the defect, with the right cleft smooth and flat (arrows) while the left is irregular (arrowheads). The ventral motor nerve root and dorsal root ganglion, covered with dura and bathed in CSF, lie beneath the pars interarticularis and below the pedicle. Causes for mid-zone lateral stenosis here are osteophytes from the insertion of the ligamentum flavum and the fibrocartilaginous bulge from a pars defect.

References

Abel, M.S. (1977) The unstable apophyseal joint. An early sign of lumbar disc disease. *Skeletal Radiol.*, **2**, 31–37.

Abrahams, J.J., Wood, G.W., Eames, F.A. and Hicks, R.W. (1988) CT-guided needle aspiration biopsy of an intraspinal synovial cyst (ganglion), case report and review of the literature. *AJNR*, **9**, 398–400.

Aguila, L.A., Piraino, D.W., Modic, M.T. *et al.* (1985) Intranuclear cleft of the intervertebral disc. Magnetic resonance imaging. *Radiology*, **155**, 155–158.

Aprill, C. and Bogduk, N. (1992) High intensity zone: a diagnostic sign of painful lumbar disc on magnetic resonance imaging. *Br. J. Radiol.*, **65**, 361–369.

Baastrup, C.H. (1933) On the spinous processes of the lumbar vertebrae and the soft tissue changes between them, and on the pathological changes in that region. *Acta Radiol. (Stock.)*, **14**, 52–54.

Bell, G.D. (1990) Skeletal applications of videofluoroscopy. *J. Manipulative Physiol. Ther.*, **13**, 396–405.

Ben-Elijahu, D., Rutili, M. and Przybysz, J. (1983) Lateral recess syndrome; diagnosis and chiropractic management. *J. Manipulative Physiol. Ther.*, **6**, 25–31.

Benhamou, C.L., Roux, C., Tourliere, D. *et al.* (1993) Pseudovisceral pain referred from costovertebral arthropathies. *Spine*, **18**, 790–795.

Berns, D.H., Ross, J.S., Kormos, D. and Modic, M.T. (1991) The spinal vacuum phenomenon: evaluation by gradient echo MR imaging. *J. Comput. Assist. Tomogr.*, **15**, 233–236.

Bigos, S.J., Hansson, T., Castillo, R.N. *et al.* (1992) The value of pre-employment roentgenographs for predicting acute back injury claims and chronic back pain disability. *Clin. Orthop. Rel. Res.*, **283**, 124–129.

Bjorkengren, A.G., Kurz, L.T., Sartoris, D.J. and Griffiths, S.R. (1987) Symptomatic intraspinal synovial cysts, opacification and treatment by percutaneous injection. *AJR*, **149**, 105–107.

Bloch, F. (1946) Nuclear induction. *Phys. Rev.*, **70**, 460–474.

Blumenthal, S.L., Baker, J., Dossett, A. and Selby, D.K. (1988) The role of anterior fusion for internal disc disruption. *Spine*, **13**, 566–569.

Boden, S.D. and Wiesel, S.W. (1990) Lumbosacral segmental motion in normal individuals. *Spine*, **15**, 571–576.

Boden, S.D., Davis, D.O., Dina, T.S. *et al.* (1990) Abnormal magnetic-resonance scans of the lumbar spine in asymptomatic subjects. *J. Bone Joint Surg.*, **72A**, 403–408.

Bolender, N.F., Schonstrom, N.S.R. and Spengler, D.M. (1985) Role of computed tomography and myelography in the diagnosis of central spinal stenosis. *J. Bone Joint Surg.*, **67A**, 240–246.

Boulay, G.H., Hawks, S., Lee, C.C. *et al.* (1990) Comparing the cost of spinal MR with conventional radiography and radiculography. *Neuroradiology*, **32**, 124–136.

Boyd, H.R. and Pear, H.L. (1972) Chronic spontaneous epidural hematoma. Report of two cases. *J. Neurosurg.*, **36**, 239–242.

Bradford, D.S. and Gotfreid, Y. (1986) Lumbar spine osteolysis; an entity caused by spinal instability. *Spine*, **11**, 1013–1019.

Braun, I.F., Lin, J.P., George, A.E. *et al.* (1984) Pitfalls in the computed tomographic evaluation of the lumbar spine in disc disease. *Neuroradiology*, **26**, 15–20.

Breen, A., Allen, R. and Morris, A. (1989) Spine kinematics: a digital videofluoroscopic technique. *J. Med. Eng. Technol.*, **11**, 224-228.

Brightbill, T.C., Pile, N., Eichekberger, R.P. and Whitman, M. (1994) Normal magnetic resonance imaging and abnormal discography in lumbar disc disruption. *Spine*, **19**, 1075-1077.

Brinckmann, P.H. and Horst, M. (1985) The influence of vertebral body fracture, intradiscal injection, and partial discectomy on the radial bulge and height of human lumbar discs. *Spine*, **10**, 138-145.

Bronfort, G. and Jochumsen, O.H. (1984) The functional radiographic examination of patients with low back pain: a study of different forms of variations. *J. Manipulative Physiol. Ther.*, **7**, 89-97.

Bundschuh, C.V., Modic, M.T., Ross, J.S. *et al.* (1988) Epidural fibrosis and recurrent disk herniation in the lumbar spine; MR imaging assessment. *AJR*, **150**, 923-932.

Burton, C.V. (1978) Lumbosacral arachnoiditis. *Spine*, **2**, 24-30.

Carr, D.H., Brown, J., Bydder, G.M. *et al.* (1984) Gadolinium-DTPA as a contrast agent in MRI: initial experience in 20 patients. *AJR*, **143**, 215-224.

Carrera, G.F. and Williams, A.L. (1984) Current concepts in evaluation of the lumbar facet joints. *CRC Crit. Rev. Diagn. Imaging*, **21**, 85-104.

Cashley, M. and Heyman, K. (1984) Radiological incidence of inter-spinal osteo-arthrosis (Baastrup's disease) ('Kissing spine). *Anglo-European Chiropractic College*.

Castillo. M. (1991) Neural foramen remodelling caused by a sequestered disk fragment. *AJNR*, **12**, 566.

Chisolm. R. (1991) Guidelines for radiological investigations. *Br. Med. J.*, **303**, 811.

Cholewicki, J., McGill, S.M., Wells, R.P. and Vernon, H. (1991) Method for measuring vertebral kinematics from fluoroscopy. *Clin. Biomech.*, **6**, 73-78.

Ciric, I., Mikhael, M.A., Tarkington, J.A. *et al.* (1980) The lateral recess syndrome. A variant of spinal stenosis. *J. Neurosurg.*, **53**, 433-443.

Colhoun, E., McCall, I.W., Williams, L. *et al.* (1988) Provocation discography as a guide to planning operations on the spine. *J. Bone Joint Surg.*, **70B**, 267-271.

Colman, R.K., Porter, B.A., Redmond, J. III, *et al.* (1988) Early diagnosis of spinal metastases by CT and MR studies. *J. Comput. Assist. Tomogr.*, **12**, 423-426.

Cotler, H.B. (1992) Clinical applications for magnetic resonance imaging of the spine. *Am. Acad. Orthop. Surg. (Instructional. Course. Lectures)*, **XLI**, 257-264.

Cox, J. (1989) *Low Back Pain*, 4th edn. Williams and Wilkins, Baltimore.

Crock, H.V. (1970) A reappraisal of intervertebral disc lesions. *Med. J. Aust.*, **1**, 983-989.

Crock, H.V. (1983) *Practice of Spinal Surgery.* Springer Verlag, Berlin, Heidelberg, New York.

Crock, H.V. (1986) Internal disc disruption. *Spine*, **11**, 650-653.

Crock, H.V. (1991) Internal disc disruption. In *The Adult Spine. Principles and Practice* (J.W. Frymoyer, ed.). Raven Press, New York, pp. 2015-2025.

Crock, H.V. (1993) Applied anatomy of the spine. *Acta. Orthop. Scand. (Suppl)*, **251**, 56-58.

Czervionke, L.F. (1993) Lumbar intervertebral disc disease. *Neuroimag. Clin. North Am.*, **3**, 465-485.

Damadian, R. (1980) Field focusing NMR (FONAR) and the formation of chemical images in man. *Philos. Trans. R. Soc. Lond. B*, **289**, 503-510.

Dandy, W.E. (1919) Roentgenography of the brain after injection of air into the spinal canal. *Ann. Surg.*, **70**, 397-403.

Dandy, W.E. (1941) Concealed ruptured intervertebral disks. Plea for elimination of contrast mediums in diagnosis. *JAMA*, **117**, 821-823.

de Roos, A., Kressel, H., Spritzer, C. and Dalinka, M. (1987) MR imaging of marrow changes adjacent to end plates in degenerative lumbar disk disease. *AJR*, **149**, 531-534.

de Vos Meiring, P., Gandhi, M. and Nakielny, R.A. (1994) Computed tomographic scanning of L3/L4 in suspected disc prolapse: is it necessary? *Br. J. Radiol.*, **67**, 323-324.

Destouet, J.M. and Murphy, W.A. (1988) Arthrography and the facet syndrome. Chapter 16. In *Imaging Modalities in. Spinal. Disorders* (M.E. Kricun, ed.) W.B. Saunders, Philadelphia.

Deyo, R. and Diel, A. (1986) Lumbar spine films in primary care: current use and effects of selective ordering criteria. *J. Gen. Intern. Med.*, **1**, 20-25.

Dilhuran, W. (1981) Hemispherical spondylosclerosis-a polyetiologic syndrome. *Skeletal Radiol.*, **7**, 99-106.

Djukic, S., Lang, P., Morris, J. *et al.* (1990) The postoperative spine. Magnetic resonance imaging. Radiographic imaging in orthopedics. *Orthop. Clin. North Am.*, **21**, 603-624.

Dorwart, R.H., Vogler, J.B. and Helms, C.A. (1983) Spinal stenosis. *Radiol. Clin. North Am.*, 301-325.

Dreyfus, P., Tibliletti ,C. and Dreyer, S.J. (1994) Thoracic zygapophysial joint pain patterns. *Spine*, **19**, 807-811.

Dupuis, P.R., Yong-Hing, K., Cassidy, J.D. and Kirkaldy-Willis, W.H. (1985) Radiologic diagnosis of degenerative spinal instability. *Spine*, **10**, 262-276.

Dussault, R.G. and Lander, P.H. (1990) Imaging of the facet joints. *Radiol. Clin. North Am.*, **28**, 1033-1053.

Dvorak, J., Panjabi, M.M., Novotny, J.E. *et al.* (1991) Clinical validation of functional flexion-extension roentgenograms of the lumbar spine. *Spine*, **16**, 943-950.

Dwyer, A.J. (1989) Time and disease: the fourth dimension of radiology. *Radiology*, **173**, 17-21.

Eisenstein, S. (1977) The morphometry and pathological anatomy of the lumbar spine in South African negroes and caucasoids with specific reference to spinal stenosis. *J. Bone. Joint. Surg.*, **59B**, 173-180.

Eisenstein, S. (1980) The trefoil configuration of the lumbar vertebral canal. *J. Bone. Joint. Surg.*, **62B**, 73-77.

Epstein, N.E. and Epstein, J.A. (1991) Limbus lumbar vertebral fractures in 27 adolescents and adults. *Spine*, **16**, 962-966.

Esparza, J., Castro, S., Portillo, J.M. and Roger, R. (1978) Vertebral hemangiomas. Spinal arteriography and preoperative embolization. *Surg. Neurol.*, **10**, 171-173.

Evens, R.J. and Mettler, F.A. (1985) National CT use and radiation exposure, United States 1983. *AJR*, **144**, 1077-1081.

Fletcher, G.H. (1947) Backward displacement of fifth lumbar vertebra in degenerative disc disease. *J. Bone Joint Surg.*, **29**, 1019-1026.

Forbes, G., Nichols, D.A., Jack, C.R. Jr *et al.* (1988) Complications of spinal arteriography. Prospective assessment of risk for diagnostic procedures. *Radiology*, **169**, 479-484.

Frager, D.H., Elkin, C.M., Kansler, F. *et al.* (1986) Extraspinal abnormalities identified on lumbar CT. *Neuroradiology,* **28**, 58–60.

Frank, J.A., Ling, A., Patronas, N. *et al.* (1990) Detection of malignant bone tumors, MR imaging vs scintigraphy. *AJR,* **155**, 1043–1048.

Fraser, R.D., Osti, O.L. and Vernon-Roberts, B. (1987) Discitis after discography. *J. Bone Joint Surg.,* **69B**, 26–35.

Friberg, O. (1987) Lumbar instability: a dynamic approach by traction–compression radiography. *Spine,* **12**, 119–129.

Frymoyer, J.W. (1991) Segmental instability. Overview and classification. In *The. Adult Spine, Principles and Practice* (J.W. Frymoyer, ed.). Raven Press, New York, pp. 1873–1891.

Frymoyer, J.W., Newberg, A., Pope, M.H. *et al.* (1984) Spine radiographs in patients with low-back pain. *J. Bone Joint Surg.,* **66A**, 1048–1055.

Ghormley, R.K. (1933) Low back pain with special reference to the articular facets, with presentation of an operative procedure. *JAMA,* **101**, 1773–1777.

Giles, L.G.F. and Kaveri, M.J.P. (1990) Some osseous and soft tissue causes of human intervertebral canal (foramen) stenosis. *J. Rheumatol.,* **17**, 1474–1481.

Giles, L.G.F. and Taylor, J.R. (1985) Osteoarthrosis in human cadaveric lumbosacral zygapophysial joints. *J. Manipulative Physiol. Ther.,* **8**, 239–243.

Glickstein, M.F., Burke, D.L. and Kressel, H.Y. (1989) Magnetic resonance demonstration of hyperintense herniated discs and extruded disc fragments. *Skeletal. Radiol.,* **18**, 527–530.

Goldman, A.B., Ghelman, B. and Doherty, J. (1990) Posterior limbus vertebrae: a cause of radiating back pain in adolescents and young adults. *Skeletal Radiol.,* **19**, 501–507.

Gomori, J.M., Floman, Y. and Liebergall, M. (1991) CT of adult lumbar disc herniations mimicking posterior apophyseal ring fractures. *Neuroradiology,* **33**, 414–418.

Goobar, J.E., Pate, D., Resnick, D. and Sartoris, D.J. (1987) Radiography of the hyperextended lumbar spine: an effective technique for the demonstration of discal vacuum phenomena. *J. Can. Assoc. Radiol.,* **38**, 271–274.

Gorey, M.T., Hyman, R.A., Black, K.S. *et al.* (1992) Lumbar synovial cysts eroding bone. *AJNR,* **13**, 161–163.

Greenspan, A. (1993) CT-discography vs MRI in intervertebral disc herniation. *Appl. Radiol.,* **22**, 34–40.

Grenier, R., Kressel, H.Y., Schiebler, M.L. *et al.* (1987a) Normal and degenerative posterior spinal structures, MR imaging. *Radiology,* **165**, 517–525.

Grenier, N., Grossman, R.I., Scheibler, M.L. *et al.* (1987b) Degenerative lumbar disk disease: pitfalls and usefulness of MR imaging in detection of vacuum phenomenon. *Radiology,* **164**, 861–865.

Griffiths, H.J., Parantainen, H. and Olsen, P.N. (1993) Disease of the lumbosacral facet joints. *Neuroimaging Clin. North Am.,* **3**, 567–575.

Gronblad, M., Virri, J., Tolonen, J. *et al.* (1994) A controlled immunohistochemical study of inflammatory cells in disc herniation. *Spine,* **19**, 2744–2751.

Gundry, C.R. and Heithoff, K.B. (1993) Epidural hematoma. *Radiology,* **187**, 427–431.

Hagelstam, L. (1947) Retroposition of vertebrae as an early sign of tuberculous spondylitis of the lumbar spine. *Acta. Orthop. Scand.,* **17**, 31.

Haldeman, S, Chapman-Smith, D. and Petersen, D.M. (1993) *Guidelines for Chiropractic Quality Assurance and Practice Parameters.* Aspen Publishers. 's location

Hammond, B.R. (1984) *The Detection of Spondylolysis Using Lumbar Sonography.* Doctor of Philosophy Thesis, University of Surrey, Guildford.

Hansen, D.T. (1988) *Chiropractic Standard. of Practice and Utilization Guidelines in the Care and Treatment of Injured Workers.* Department of Labor and Industries, State of Washington.

Hauge, O. and Falkenburg, H. (1982) Neuropsychologic reactions and other side effects after metrizamide myelography. *AJNR,* **3**, 229–232.

Heithoff, K.B. and Amster, J.L. (1990) The Spine. In *MRI. of. the Musculoskeletal System* (J.H. Mink and A.L. Deutsch, eds). Raven Press, New York, pp. 117–191.

Heithoff, K.B., Gundry, C.R., Burton, C.V. and Winter, R.B. (1994) Juvenile discogenic disease. *Spine,* **19**, 335–340.

Hellman, R.S., Nowak, D., Collier, R.D. *et al.* (1986) Evaluation of distance-weighted SPECT reconstruction for skeletal scintigraphy. *Radiology,* **159**, 473–475.

Henson, J., McCall, I.W. and O'Brien, J.P. (1987) Disc damage above a spondylolisthesis. *Br. J. Radiol.,* **60**, 69–72.

Herzog, R.J. (1991) Magnetic resonance imaging of the Spine. In *The Adult Spine: Principles and Practice* (J.W. Frymoyer, ed.). Raven Press, New York, pp. 457–510.

Herzog, R.J. (1992) The radiologic evaluation of lumbar degenerative disk disease and spinal stenosis in patients with back or radicular symptoms. *Am. Acad. Orthop. Surg. (Instructional. Course. Lectures),* **XLI**, 193–203.

Hinck, V.C., Hopkins, C.E. and Clark, W.M. (1965) Sagittal diameter of the lumbar spinal canal in children and adults. *Radiology,* **85**, 929–937.

Hinck, V.C., Clark, W.M. and Hopkins, C.E. (1966) Normal interpediculate distances (minimum and maximum) in children and adults. *AJR,* **97**, 141–153.

Hirsch, C. (1948) Attempt to diagnose the level of disc lesion clinically by disc puncture. *Acta Orthop. Scand.,* **18**, 132.

Holder, L.E. (1990) Clinical radionuclide bone imaging. *Radiology,* **176**, 607.

Holt, E.P. (1968) The question of lumbar discography. *J. Bone Joint Surg.,* **50A**, 720.

Holtas, S. (1993) Radiology of the degenerative lumbar spine. *Acta. Orthop. Scand. (Suppl.),* **251**, 16–18.

Hounsfield, G.N. (1973) Computerized transverse axial scanning (tomography) I. Description of a system. *Br. J. Radiol.,* **46**, 1016.

Howe, J.W. (1970) Preliminary observations from cineroentgenological studies of the spinal column. *Am. Chiro. Assoc. J. Chiro.,* **October**, 65–70.

Howe, J.W. (1989) Caution must be exercised in use of video fluoroscopy. *Am. Chiro. Assoc. J. Chiro.,* **June**, 38–41.

Hsu, K.Y., Zucherman, J.F., Shea, W.J. and Jeffrey, R.A. (1995) Lumbar intraspinal synovial and ganglion cysts (facet cysts). *Spine,* **20**, 80–89.

Jackson, D.E., Atlas, S.W., Mani, J.R. and Norman, D. (1990) Intraspinal synovial cysts, MR imaging. *Radiology,* **170**, 527–530.

Jackson, R.P. (1992) The facet syndrome. Myth or reality? *Clin. Orthop. Rel. Res.,* **279**, 110–121.

Jacobsen, H.G., Tausend, M.E., Shapiro, J.H. and Poppel, M.H. (1958) The 'swayback' syndrome. *AJR,* **79**, 677–683.

Jensen, M.C., Brant-Zawadzki, M.N., Obuchowski, N. *et al.* (1994) Magnetic resonance imaging of the lumbar spine in people without back pain. *N. Engl. J. Med.*, **331**, 69–73.

Jinkins, J.R., Roeder, M.B. (1993) MRI of benign lumbosacral nerve root enhancement. *Semin. Ultrasound CT MRI*, **14**, 446–454.

Jinkins, J.R., Whitemore, A.R. and Bradley, W.G. (1989) The anatomic basis of vertebrogenic pain and the autonomic syndrome associated with lumbar disc extrusion. *AJR*, **152**, 1277–1289.

Johnson, D.W., Farnum, G.N., Latchaw, R.E. and Erba, S.M. (1988) MR imaging of the pars interarticularis. *AJNR*, **9**, 1215–1220.

Johnson, R.G. (1989) Does discography injure normal discs? An analysis of repeat discograms. *Spine*, **14**, 424–426.

Johnson, R.W. (1934) Posterior luxations of the lumbosacral joint. *J. Bone Joint Surg.*, **16**, 867–876.

Jones, R.A.C. and Thomson, J.L.G. (1968) The narrow lumbar canal. *J. Bone Joint Surg.*, **50B**, 595–605.

Kattan, K.R. and Pais, M.J. (1981) The spinous process: the forgotten appendage. *Skeletal Radiol.*, **6**, 199–204.

Kelly, W.M., Paglen, P.G., Pearson, J.A. *et al.* (1986) Ferromagnetism of intra ocular foreign body causes unilateral blindness after MR study. *AJNR*, **7**, 243–245.

Kent, D.L., Haynor, D.R., Larson, E.B. and Deyo, R.A. (1992) Diagnosis of lumbar spinal stenosis in adults. A meta analysis of the accuracy of CT, MR and myelography. *AJR*, **158**, 1135–1144.

Kingery, W.S., Seibel, M., Date, E.S. and Marks, M.P. (1994) The natural resolution of a lumbar spontaneous epidural hematoma and associated radiculopathy. *Spine*, **19**, 67–69.

Kormano, M. (1989) Imaging methods in examining the anatomy and function of the lumbar spine. *Ann. Med.*, **21**(5), 335–340.

Lang, P., Chafetz, N., Genant, H.K. and Morris, J.M. (1990) Lumbar spinal fusion. Assessment of functional stability with magnetic resonance imaging. *Spine*, **15**, 581–588.

Laredo, J.D., Bard, M., Chretien, J. and Kahn, M.F. (1986) Lumbar posterior marginal intraosseous node. *Skeletal Radiol.*, **15**, 201–208.

Lauterbur, P.C. (1973) Image formation by induced local interactions: examples employing nuclear magnetic resonance. *Nature*, **242**, 190–191.

Lee, C.K., Rauschning, W. and Glenn, W. (1988) Lateral lumbar spinal canal stenosis. Classification, pathologic anatomy and surgical decompression. *Spine*, **13**, 313–320.

Lehmann, T. and Brand, R. (1983) Instability of the lower lumbar spine. *Orthop. Trans.*, **7**, 97.

Levitan, L.H. and Wiens, C.W. (1983) Chronic lumbar epidural hematoma: CT findings. *Radiology*, **148**, 707–708.

Lindblom, K. (1948) Diagnostic puncture of intervertebral discs in sciatica. *Acta. Orthop. Scand.*, **17**, 231.

Liu, S.S., Williams, K.D., Drayer, B.P. *et al.* (1989) Synovial cysts of the lumbar spine: diagnosis by MR imaging. *AJNR*, **10**, 1239–1242.

Lukin, R.R., Gaskill, M.F. and Wiot, J.G. (1988) Lumbar herniated disk and related topics. *Semin. Roentgenol.*, **XXIII**, 100–105.

Macnab, I. (1971) The traction spur, An indicator of segmental instability. *J. Bone Joint Surg.*, **33A**, 663–670.

MacPherson, P., Teasdale, E., Coutinho, C. and McGeorge, A. (1985) Iohexol versus Iopamidol for cervical myelography: a randomised double blind study. *Br. J. Radiol.*, **58**, 849–851.

Maguire, C., Florence, S., Powe, J.E. *et al.* (1990) Hepatic uptake of technetium-99m HM-PAO in a fetus. *J. Nucl. Med.*, **31**, 237.

Malmivaara, A., Videman, T., Juosma, E. and Troup, J.D.G. (1987) Facet joint orientation, facet and costovertebral joint osteoarthrosis, disc degeneration, vertebral osteophytosis, and Schmorl's nodes in the thoracolumbar junctional region of cadaveric spines. *Spine*, **12**, 458–461.

Manelfe, C. (1992) Imaging of degenerative processes of the spine. *Current Opinions Radiol.*, **4**, 63–70.

McCutcheon, M.E. and Thompson, W.C. (1986) CT scanning of lumbar discography. A useful adjunct. *Spine*, **11**, 257–259.

McFadden, J.W. (1988) The stress lumbar discogram. *Spine*, **13**, 931–933.

Melamed, A. and Ansfield, D.J. (1947) Posterior displacement of lumbar vertebrae. *AJR*, **58**, 307–328.

Mior, S.A. and Cassidy, J.D. (1982) Lateral nerve entrapment: pathological, clinical and manipulative considerations. *J. Can. Chiro. Assoc.*, **26**, 13–20.

Modic, M.T. and Herzog, R.J. (1994) Spinal imaging modalities. What's available and who should order them? *Spine*, **19**, 1764–1765.

Modic, M.T., Pavlicek, W., Weinstein, M.A. *et al.* (1984) Magnetic resonance imaging of intervertebral disc disease: clinical and pulse sequence considerations. *Radiology*, **152**, 103–111.

Modic, M.T., Feiglin, D.H., Piraino, D.W. *et al.* (1985) Vertebral osteomyelitis. Assessment using MR imaging. *Radiology*, **157**, 157–166.

Modic, M.T., Steinberg, P.M., Ross, J.S. *et al.* (1988a) Degenerative disk disease. Assessment of changes in the vertebral body marrow with MR imaging. *Radiology*, **166**, 193–199.

Modic, M.T., Masaryk, T.J., Ross, J.S. and Carter, J.R. (1988b) Imaging of degenerative disk disease. *Radiology*, **168**, 177–186.

Modic, M.T., Masaryk, T.J. and Ross, J.S. (1994) *Magnetic Resonance Imaging of the Spine*. C.V. Mosby, New York.

Mortensen, W.W., Thorne, R.P. and Donaldson, W.F. (1991) Symptomatic gas-containing disc herniation. *Spine*, **16**, 190–192.

Nachemson, A. (1985) Lumbar spine instability. A critical update and symposium summary. *Spine*, **10**, 290–291.

Natarajan, R.N., Ke, J.H. and Andersson, G.B.J. (1994) A model to study the disc degeneration process. *Spine*, **19**, 259–265.

Nehls, D.G., Shetter, A.G., Hodak, J.A. and Waggner, J.D. (1984) Chronic spinal epidural hematoma presenting as lumbar stenosis: clinical, myelographic, and computed tomographic features; a case report. *Neurosurgery*, **14**, 230–233.

Ninomiya, M. and Muro, T. (1992) Pathoanatomy of lumbar disc herniation as demonstrated by computed tomography/discography. *Spine*, **17**, 1316–1320.

Nuri Sener, R., Ripeckyj, G.T., Otto, P.M. *et al.* (1993) Recognition of abnormalities on computed scout images in CT examinations of the head and spine. *Neuroradiology*, **35**, 229–231.

Orrison, W.W. and Lilleas, F.G. (1982) CT demonstration of gas in a herniated nucleus pulposus. *J. Comput. Assist. Tomogr.*, **6**, 807–808.

Osborn, A.G., Koehler, P.R. *et al.* (1982) Computed tomography of the paraspinal musculature: normal and pathologic anatomy. *AJR,* **138,** 93–98.

Osborne, D.R., Heinz, E.R., Bullard, D. *et al.* (1984) Role of computed tomography in the radiological evaluation of painful radiculopathy after negative myelography. Foraminal neural entrapment. *Neurosurgery,* **14,** 147–153.

Osti, O.L. and Fraser, R.D. (1992) MRI and discography of annular tears and intervertebral disc degeneration. *J. Bone Joint Surg.,* **74B,** 431–435.

Ostrum, B.J., Romy, M. and Swartz, J.D. (1993) Pathophysiological basis of lumbar disc degeneration. Imaging analysis. *Semin. Ultrasound CT MRI,* **14,** 399–403.

Paajanen, H., Alanen, A., Erkintalo, M. *et al.* (1989) Disc degeneration in Scheuermann disease. *Skeletal Radiol.,* **18,** 523–526.

Pate, D., Goobar, J., Resnick, D. *et al.* (1988) Traction osteophytes of the lumbar spine: radiographic–pathologic correlation. *Radiology,* **166,** 843–846.

Pathria, M., Sartoris, D.J. and Resnick, D. (1987) Osteoarthritis of the facet joints: accuracy of oblique radiographic assessment. *Radiology,* **164,** 227–230.

Pearcy, M.J. (1985) Stereoradiography of lumbar spine motion. *Acta. Orthop. Scand. (Suppl),* 212.

Peters, R.E. (1983) The facet syndrome. *J. Austr. Chiro. Assoc.,* **13**(3), 15–27.

Phillips, R.B., Howe, J.W., Bustin, G. *et al.* (1990) Stress X-rays and the low back pain patient. *J. Manipulative Physiol. Ther.,* **13,** 127–133.

Pleatman, C.W. and Lukin, R.R. (1988) Lumbar spinal stenosis. *Semin. Roentgenol.,* **XXIII,** 106–110.

Pope, M.H., Frymoyer, J.W. and Krag, M.H. (1992) Diagnosing instability. *Clin. Orthop. Rel. Res.,* **279,** 60–67.

Portela, L. (1985) Sonography of the normal and abnormal intact lumbar spinal canal. *AJR,* **144,** 386–390.

Porter, R.W. (1993) Central spinal stenosis. Classification and pathogenesis. *Acta Orthop. Scand. (Suppl),* **251,** 64–68.

Porter, R.W., Hibbert, C. and Wellman, P. (1980) Backache and the spinal canal. *Spine,* **5,** 99–105.

Proctor, D., Dupuis, P. and Cassidy, J.D. (1985) Thoracolumbar syndrome as a cause of low-back pain: a report of two cases. *J. Can. Chiro. Assoc.,* **29,** 71–73.

Purcell, E.M., Torrey, H.C. and Pound, R.V. (1946) Resonance absorption by nuclear magnetic moments in solids. *Phys. Rev.,* **69,** 37–38.

Quebec Task Force on Spinal Disorders (1987) Scientific approach to the assessment and management of activity related spinal disorders: a monograph for clinicians. *Spine,* **12**(7-S), 3–59.

Quirk, M.E., Letendre, A.J., Ciottone, R.A. and Lingley, J.F. (1989) Evaluation of three psychologic interventions to reduce anxiety during MR imaging. *Radiology,* **173,** 759–762.

Rabassa, A.E., Guinto, F.C., Crow, W.N. *et al.* (1993) CT of the spine: value of reformatted images. *AJR,* **161,** 1223–1227.

Resnick, D. (1985) Degenerative diseases of the vertebral column. *Radiology,* **156,** 3–14.

Resnick, D., Niwayama, G., Guerra, J. *et al.* (1981) Spinal vacuum phenomena: anatomical study and review. *Radiology,* **139,** 341–348.

Richards, A.J. (1987) Abdominal pain of spinal origin. *Clin. Exp. Rheumatol (Suppl),* **5,** 517.

Robert, F.W. (1980) Costotransverse arthrosis of the tenth dorsal vertebra (D10) (Abstract). *AJR,* **134,** 423.

Rosenblum, J., Mojtahedi, S. and Foust, R.J. (1989) Synovial cysts in the lumbar spine: MR characteristics. *AJNR,* **10,** 94.

Ross, J.S., Modic, M.T. and Masaryk, T.J. (1989) Tears of the anulus fibrosus: assessment with Gd-DTPA-enhanced MR imaging. *AJNR,* **10,** 1251–1254.

Rothschild, P.A., Crooks, L.E. and Margulis, A.R. (1990) Direction of MR imaging. *Invest. Radiol.,* **25,** 275–281.

Rowe, L.J. (1988a) Vacuum phenomenon. *J. Austral. Chiro. Assoc.,* **18,** 125.

Rowe, L.J. (1988b) Hemispherical spondylosclerosis: a case report. *J. Austral. Chiro. Assoc.,* **18,** 55–56.

Rowe, L.J. (1988c) Images, Intervertebral disc calcification. *J. Austral. Chiro. Assoc.,* **18,** 31–32.

Rowe, L.J. (1989) Degenerative disc space narrowing – differential considerations. *J. Austral. Chiro. Assoc.,* **19,** 60–61.

Rowe, L.J. (1992) *Skeletal Radiology and its Applications to the Practice of Chiropractic.* Thesis, Master of Applied Science. Royal Melbourne Institute of Technology University.

Rowe, L.J. and Yochum, T.R. (1996a) Principles of radiological interpretation. In *Essentials of Skeletal Radiology,* 2nd edn, Chapter 7 (T.R. Yochum and L.J. Roux, eds). Williams and Wilkins, Baltimore.

Rowe, L.J. and Yochum, T.R. (1996b) Radiographic positioning and normal anatomy. In *Essentials of Skeletal Radiology,* 2nd edn, Chapter 1 (T.R. Yochum and L.J. Rowe, eds). Williams and Wilkins, Baltimore.

Rowe, L.J. and Yochum, T.R. (1996c) Measurements in skeletal radiology. In *Essentials of Skeletal Radiology,* 2nd edn, Chapter 3 (T.R. Yochum and L.J. Rowe, eds). Williams and Wilkins, Baltimore.

Rowe, L.J. and Yochum, T.R. (1996d) Arthritis. In *Essentials of Skeletal Radiology,* 2nd edn, Chapter 10 (T.R. Yochum and L.J. Rowe, eds). Williams and Wilkins, Baltimore.

Rowe, L.J. and Yochum, T.R. (1996e) Scheuermann's disease. In *Essentials of Skeletal Radiology,* 2nd edn, Chapter 13 (T.R. Yochum and L.J. Rowe, eds), Williams and Wilkins, Baltimore.

Rubin, J.M. and Dohrmann, G.J. (1985) The spine and spinal cord during neurosurgical operations: real-time ultrasonography. *Radiology,* **155,** 197–200.

Rueter, F.G., Conway, B.J., McCrohan, J.L. *et al.* (1992) Radiography of the lumbosacral spine: characteristics of examinations performed in hospitals and other facilities. *Radiology,* **185,** 43–46.

Runge, V.M. (1992) Magnetic resonance imaging contrast agents. *Curr. Opin. Radiol.,* **4,** 3–12.

Rydevik, B. (1993) Spinal stenosis – conclusions. *Acta. Orthop. Scand. (Suppl),* **251,** 81–82.

Sachs, B.L., Vanharnta, H., Spivey, M.A. *et al.* (1987) Dallas discogram description. A new classification of CT/discography in low back disorders. *Spine,* **12,** 287–294.

Salonen, O.L. (1990) Case of anaphylaxis and four cases of allergic reaction following Gd-DTPA administration. *J. Comput. Assist. Tomogr.,* **14,** 912–913.

Sandoz, R. (1960) Degenerative conditions of the lumbosacral spine. *Ann. Swiss. Chiro.,* **77,** 101.

Sarpyener, M.A. (1945) Congenital stricture of the spinal canal. *J. Bone Joint Surg.,* **27,** 70–79.

Sartoris, D.J., Resnik, D., Tyson, R. and Haghighi, P. (1985) Age-related alterations in the vertebral spinous processes and intervening soft tissues, Radiologic–pathologic correlation. *Radiology,* **145,** 1025–1030.

Sato, H. and Kikuchi, S. (1993) The natural history of radiographic instability of the lumbar spine. *Spine*, **18**, 2075–2079.

Scavone, J.G., Latshaw, R.F. and Weidner, W.A. (1981) Anteroposterior and lateral radiographs: an adequate lumbar spine examination. *AJR*, **136**, 715–717.

Scheibler, M.L., Camerino, V.J., Fallon, M.D. *et al.* (1991) In vivo and ex vivo magnetic resonance imaging evaluation of early disc degeneration with histopathologic correlation. *Spine*, **16**, 635–640.

Schellinger, D., Manz, H.J., Vidic, B. *et al.* (1990) Disk fragment migration. *Radiology*, **175**, 831–836.

Schmorl, G. and Junghanns, H. (1971) *The Human Spine in Health and Disease*, 2nd edn. Translated by E.F. Besermann. Grune and Stratton, New York.

Schonstrom, N.S.R., Bolender, N.F., Spengler, D.M. and Hansson, J. (1984) Pressure changes within the cauda equina following constriction of the dural sac. *Spine*, **9**, 604–607.

Schubiger, O. and Valavanis, A. (1982) CT differentiation between recurrent disc herniation and post-operative scar formation: the value of contrast enhancement. *Neuroradiology*, **22**, 251–255.

Schulz, E.E., West, W.L., Hinshaw, D.B. *et al.* (1984) Gas in a lumbar extradural juxtaarticular cyst, a sign of synovial origin. *AJR*, **143**, 875.

Schultz, G., Phillips, R.B., Cooley, J. *et al.* (1992) Diagnostic imaging of the spine in chiropractic practice: recommendations for utilisation. *Chiro. J. Austr.*, **22**, 141–152.

Schwarzer, A.C., Aprill, C.N., Derby, R. *et al.* (1994) Clinical features of patients stemming from the lumbar zygapophysial joints. *Spine*, **19**, 1132–1137.

Sicard, J.A. and Forrestier, J.E. (1922) Methode general d'exploration radiologique par l'huile iodee (Lipiodol) *Bull. Mem. Soc. Med. Hop. Paris*, **46**, 463–469.

Simmons, J.W., Emery, S.F., McMillin, N.J. *et al.* (1991) Awake discography: a comparison study with magnetic resonance imaging. *Spine*, **16**, 216–221.

Simmons, W., Aprill, C.N., Dwyer, A.P. and Brodsky, A.E. (1988) A reassessment of Holt's data: the question of lumbar discography. *Clin. Orthop. Rel. Res.*, **237**, 120–124.

Smith, A.D. (1934) Posterior displacement of the fifth lumbar vertebra. *J. Bone Joint Surg.*, **16**, 877–888.

Smith, D.M. (1976) Acute back pain associated with a calcified Schmorl's node. A case report. *Clin. Orthop.*, **117**, 193.

Smith, T.P. and Cragg, A.H. (1991) Angiography of the spine, Chapter 24. In *The Adult Spine, Principles and Practice*. Raven Press, New York.

Spengler, D.M. (1987) Degenerative stenosis of the lumbar spine. *J. Bone Joint Surg.*, **69A**, 305–308.

Subramanian, G. and McAfee, J.G. (1971) A new complex of 99m-Tc for skeletal imaging. *Radiology*, **99**, 192.

Takahashi, M., Shimomura, O. and Sakae, T. (1993) Comparison of magnetic resonance imaging with myelography and computed tomography–myelography in the diagnosis of lumbar disc herniation. *Neuroimaging. Clin. North Am.*, **3**, 487.

Tallroth, K. and Schlenzka, D. (1990) Spinal stenosis subsequent to juvenile lumbar osteochondrosis. *Skeletal Radiol.*, **19**, 203–205.

Tehranzadeh, J. and Gabriele, O.F. (1984) The prone position for CT of the lumbar spine. *Radiology*, **152**, 817–818.

Tertti, M., Paajanen, H., Laato, M. *et al.* (1991) Disc degeneration in magnetic resonance imaging: a comparative biochemical, histologic and radiologic study in cadaver spines. *Spine*, **16**, 629–634.

Tervonen, O. and Koivukangas, J. (1989) Transabdominal ultrasound measurement of the lumbar spinal canal: its value for evaluation of lumbar spinal stenosis. *Spine*, **14**, 232–235.

Tervonen, O., Lahde, S. and Vanharanta, H. (1991) Ultrasound diagnosis of lumbar disc degeneration. *Spine*, **16**, 951–954.

Thiel, H.W., Clements, D.S. and Cassidy, J.D. (1992) Lumbar apophyseal ring fractures in adolescents. *J. Manipulative Physiol. Ther.*, **15**, 250–254.

Torgerson, W.R. and Dotter, W.E. (1976) Comparative roentgenographic study of the asymptomatic and symptomatic lumbar spine. *J. Bone Joint Surg.*, **58A**, 850–853.

Toro, G., Roman, G.C., Navarro-Roman, L. *et al.* (1994) Natural history of spinal cord infarction caused by nucleus pulposus embolism. *Spine*, **19**, 360–366.

Toyone, T., Takahashi, K., Kitahara, H. *et al.* (1994) Vertebral bone-marrow changes in degenerative lumbar disc disease. *J. Bone Joint Surg.*, **76B**, 757–764.

Tress, B. and Lau, L. (1991) Depomedrol and facet joint injections. (Letter) *Australas. Radiol.*, **35**(3), 291.

Ullrich, C.G., Binet, E.F., Sanecki, M.G. and Kieffer, S.A. (1980) Quantative assessment of the lumbar spinal canal by computed tomography. *Radiology*, **134**, 137–143.

Valdez, D.C. and Johnson, R.G. (1994) Role of technetium-99m planar bone scanning in the evaluation of low back pain. *Skeletal Radiol.*, **23**, 91–97.

Vanharanta, H., Sachs, B.L., Spivey, M.A. *et al.* (1987) The relationship of pain provocation to lumbar disc deterioration as seen by CT/discography. *Spine*, **12**, 295–298.

Vaughan, B. (1989) A short illustrated history of magnetic resonance imaging. *Australas. Radiol.*, **33**, 390–398.

Venner, R.M. and Crock, H.V. (1981) Clinical studies of isolated disc resorption in the lumbar spine. *J. Bone Joint Surg.*, **63B**, 491–494.

Verbiest, H. (1949) Sur certaines formes rares de compression de la queue de cheval. Les stenoses osseuses du canal vertébral. In *Hommages à Clovis Vincent*. Paris, Maloine.

Verbiest, H. (1954) A radicular syndrome from developmental narrowing of the lumbar vertebral canal. *J. Bone. Joint. Surg.*, **36B**, 230–237.

Weber, H. (1993) The natural course of disc herniation. *Acta. Orthop. Scand. (Suppl)*, **251**, 19–20.

Weber, M., Hasler, P. and Gerber, H. (1993) Insufficiency fractures of the sacrum. Twenty cases and review of the literature. *Spine*, **18**, 2507.

Weinreb, J.C., Maravilla, K.R., Peshock. R. *et al.* (1984) Magnetic resonance imaging. Improving patient tolerance and safety. *AJR*, **143**, 1285.

Weitz, E.M. (1981) The lateral bending sign. *Spine*, **6**, 388.

Wiesel, S.W., Tsourmas, N., Feffer, H.L. *et al.* (1984) A study of computer–assisted tomography. I. The incidence of positive CAT scans in an asymptomatic group of patients. *Spine*, **9**, 549.

Wiley, J., McNab, I. and Wortzman, G. (1968) Lumbar discography and its clinical applications. *Can. J. Surg.*, **11**, 280–289.

Williams, A.L., Haughton, V.M., Daniels, D.L. *et al.* (1980) Differential diagnosis of extruded nucleus pulposus. *Radiology*, **148**, 141–148.

Williams, A.L., Haughton, V.M., Meyer, G.A. and Ho, K.C. (1982) Computed tomographic appearance of the bulging anulus. *Radiology,* **142**, 403–408.

Williams, P.C. (1932) Reduced lumbosacral joint space, its relation to sciatic irritation. *JAMA,* **99**, 1677–1682.

Willis, T.A. (1935) Backward displacement of 5th lumbar vertebra. *J. Bone Joint Surg.,* **17**, 347–352.

Wiltse, L.L., Guyer, R.D., Spencer, C.W. *et al.* (1984) Alar transverse impingement of the L5 nerve, The far-out syndrome. *Spine,* **9**, 31–41.

Witzmann, A., Hammer, B. and Fischer, J. (1991) Free sequestered disc herniation at the S2 level misdiagnosed as neuroma. *Neuroradiology,* **33**, 92–93.

Yamashita, K., Hiroshima, K. and Kurata, A. (1994) Gadolinium-DTPA-enhanced magnetic resonance imaging of a sequestered lumbar intervertebral disc and its correlation with pathologic findings. *Spine,* **19**, 479–482.

Yoshida, M., Shima, K., Taniguchi, Y. *et al.* (1992) Hypertrophied ligamentum flavum in lumbar spinal canal stenosis. *Spine,* **17**, 1353–1360.

Yu, S.W., Sether, L.A., Ho, P.S. *et al.* (1988a) Tears of the anulus fibrosus. Correlation between MR and pathologic findings in cadavers. *AJN,* **9**, 367–370.

Yu, S., Haughton, V.M., Sether, L.A. and Wagner, M. (1988b) Tears of the anulus fibrosus in bulging intervertebral discs. *Radiology,* **169**, 761–763.

Yu, S., Haughton, V.M., Sether, L.A. *et al.* (1989) Comparison of MR and discography in detecting radial tears of the anulus. A postmortem study. *AJNR,* **10**, 1071–1077.

Yuh, W., Drew, J., Weinstein, J. *et al.* (1991) Intraspinal synovial cysts, magnetic resonance evaluation. *Spine,* **16**, 740–745.

Yussen, P.S. and Swartz, J.D. (1993) The acute lumbar disc herniation. Imaging diagnosis. *Semin. Ultrasound CT MRI,* **14**, 389–398.

19

Psychosocial aspects of back pain

Basil James and Frank McDonald

There is now general and increasing recognition of:

1. the essential subjectivity of the pain experience, no matter what the cause or causes;
2. the contribution of factors other than physical lesions to the experience of pain, to its expression and its communication and its impact on quality of life; and
3. the consequential need to evaluate and respond to the subjective experience and the other relevant factors as part of the overall treatment of patients with pain.

None of these is an easy matter to address, and the present chapter sets out:

1. to clarify the difficulties; and
2. to suggest strategies of assessment and treatment likely to enhance the therapeutic endeavour.

In doing so, it introduces the important influence of the treating person as an integral part of the patient's experience – a phenomenon given only very limited attention in most texts on pain.

The implications of the subjectivity of pain

Most current definitions of pain have their basis in that of Mersky (1975): 'an unpleasant experience which we primarily associate with tissue damage or describe in terms of such damage or both'.

As such, it is clear that whilst any associated tissue damage may or may not be directly observable, the subjective experience is conveyed indirectly through the words or behaviour of the sufferer. It falls into the category of 'private data', and can be felt by the sufferer as exquisitely lonely. Lasagna (1960) put it eloquently: '. . . the investigator . . . is at the mercy of the patient, upon whose ability and willingness to communicate he is dependent'.

The implications of the variety of human experience

Notwithstanding its distressing and unpleasant nature, and the dedication of health professionals to eradicate it or minimize its impact, it is sometimes helpful and illuminating to recall that pain has purpose and value. It is, of course, informative with respect to noxious environmental agents and processes both within and without the organism; and it acts to motivate or drive behaviour likely to lessen the threat to the organism's integrity and function. The human organism, however, is distinguished among others by its self-consciousness, its inner, abstract and conceptual world, and its capacity for the attribution of meaning. Pain itself thus often acquires meaning, sometimes of a very idiosyncratic kind, as the nature of the world in which we live is construed not only abstractly, but very individually (e.g. Kelly, 1955). Lastly, the important social or interpersonal nature of the human environment inevitably incorporates persons or human institutions into the framework by which the origin of the pain is understood, or through which the essential suffering may be relieved. Thus the health care system provides an important setting for what Mechanic (1962) termed 'illness behaviour' – the (usually socially sanctioned) (see Parsons, 1964) action taken by an individual in response to his/her non-perception of signs of illness. Pilowsky (1969, 1990) described such behaviour which was apparently pathological or unadaptive as 'abnormal illness behaviour'. However, given further information about the details of the patient's psychological and social status, the behaviour may seem less unadaptive.

Thus, without knowledge of the individual person, information about pain is incomplete; and although in many instances this may not greatly affect outcome, it inevitably plays some part in optimizing therapeutic success; and in some, the consequences of such ignorance can result in failure, chronicity, exasperation for patient, family, insurers and treaters, and be enormously expensive in time and money.

Questions therefore arise immediately regarding the use of screening procedures, the nature of any further investigations, and the range of treatments or treatment adjuncts which might be available.

Screening instruments

The use, routinely, of a preliminary screening questionnaire has much to commend it, provided it is presented in such a way that the patient can perceive it neither as intrusive nor as indicative of any preconception that he/she is 'imagining' the pain, or 'putting it on'. Indeed, from the very first contact that the patient has with the clinic or its staff, thought must be given to the possible interpretations which may be placed on each approach or communication. It is wise to remember that, whilst we as professionals are conducting a psychological evaluation of patients, patients are, in their own way, conducting psychological evaluations of professionals! (Questions arise with regard to the professionals' trustworthiness, especially concerning private and personal feeling issues, the willingness and ability to understand, etc.)

The advantages of routine screenings include:

- The fact that it is routine and thus no patient can feel singled out.
- It is a useful and quick way of gathering information.
- It conveys to the patient the 'person' orientation of the clinic, and an interest in related factors that may already be perceived by him/her as important.
- It can provide the opportunity for the subsequent examiner to seek to amplify at an early stage or subsequently, the significance of some of the responses of the patient.
- The possibility of the use of the results for monitoring progress, or for research.

It is, however, important that the questionnaire does not replace, nor is perceived by the patient as replacing, the interpersonal aspects of the clinical transaction.

One commonly used questionnaire, very suitable for the purposes described, is the Oswestry Back Pain Disability Questionnaire (Fairbank *et al.*, 1980).

It is relatively brief, and thus not overly demanding on the patient's time; the questions are easily understood as relevant to back pain disability, and although widening the sphere of inquiry to include social life, travelling and sexual activity, it is unlikely to be seen as intrusive.

The Psychological Assessment Questionnaire of Main and Waddell (1984) is also suitable for similar reasons, and although its focus is more on emotion and on the physical symptoms characteristic of anxiety, thus yielding valuable data on affective status, the format of the questions is such that they are unlikely to alienate the subjects in the ways described.

The clinical interview

The ordinary initial clinical interview provides considerable opportunity for arriving at some conclusions, albeit tentative, regarding psychological or social factors. Even without the advantage of a preliminary screening questionnaire, and without extensive questioning with respect to psychosocial details, multiple relevant cues are available from a carefully elicited history of the complaint through noting the patient's dress and appearance, posture, eye contact, facial expression and body movements, as well as the language the patient uses, the allusions, the emphases, the repetitions or omissions, etc. Although it is beyond the scope of this present chapter to explore the detailed possibilities of such examinations, the clinician unused to interpreting the possible significance of the data, or who may sense some cynicism regarding it, may recall the guided practice necessary, for example, for learning to hear and interpret heart sounds or expertly to read X-ray plates.

It is also important, at this early stage, to exhibit and convey to the patient one's own attitude of non-judgmental concern and empathy. The correct use of the self as an investigating instrument is as important as the correct positioning of the patient in the use of the stethoscope, or the manoeuvres necessary for eliciting an ankle jerk. Although self-evident, and barely arguable, unfortunately it cannot go without saying, and most case notes of patients of any chronicity will contain at least some pejorative comment, confirming the not infrequent perception of patients regarding the disparaging language or incredulous facial expressions or manner of examiners. Some conditions and some patients are undoubtedly exasperating, but the capacity to respond empathically to the complicating psychological and social variables, and to view them as professionally interesting issues which themselves may require attention, assists not only in achieving the alliance with the patient which is the essential platform for all further therapeutic work, but also helps change a long and frustrating clinical session into an intriguing puzzle.

These comments regarding the initial interview are not intended either to suggest that the majority of patients with back pain need specialized psychological/psychiatric treatment, nor to urge clinicians of all kinds to be specialists in these areas. What is necessary, however, is to avoid if at all possible making a bad situation worse; and to recognize the kinds of alerting signals which may at least at some stage lead to more specialized referral, and which are comparable to signs in the physical arena such as pallor or an upgoing toe. Certainly, in ascertaining early indications of the importance of psychological issues, it is of course necessary to bear in mind that these issues may no less frequently be the consequence of pain as they are contributing factors.

One particularly important goal in the initial assessment of the patient with back pain is the inquiry regarding depression. A review by Sullivan (1992) suggests that the prevalence of depression among chronic low back pain patients is three to four times that of the general population. As indicated, a preliminary questionnaire screening may already provide an early indication, and depressed patients are often relieved to be able to share the problem with a sympathetic examiner. Sleep disturbance, especially early morning waking, loss of interest, energy and concentration, inability to experience pleasure or joy, and a mood of dejection (which may be expressed very variously) are important diagnostic clues. Not only does depression commonly lead to an amplification of the pain experience, but it is a highly treatable syndrome, either by psychological strategies or by antidepressant medication, depending on its nature.

Further psychological/psychiatric investigation

The need for further evaluation is signalled either by evidence elicited at the initial examination as above, or by continued failure of the patient's condition to respond as expected to the usual treatments. It is very important to note, however, that such non-response does not, *per se*, necessarily indicate psychopathology.

The decision to recommend more intensive psychological/psychiatric evaluation is one which needs to be conveyed with tact and empathy. The routine use of a screening questionnaire, and the demonstrated concern of the first examining clinician for the patient as a person, will have paved the way for easy referral. Emphasis should continue to be clearly on the patient's quality of life, on the inseparability of this from the pain, and of the pain experience from the person. The maintenance of judgement-free language and attitude remains paramount.

Further investigation of the psychological/psychiatric dimension

As the evaluation becomes more specialized and detailed, the focus moves more towards the person with the symptom rather than the symptom itself, though the latter remains importantly linked with the other variables.

Different clinicians will use different methods of exploring the personal domain. Generally speaking, psychologists will tend to use structured interviews in conjunction with established instruments such as questionnaires, and some advantages may be claimed in terms of their uniformity and standardization; on the other hand, psychiatrists are more likely to use the clinical interview with the claimed advantages here of greater opportunities for the development of the therapeutic relationship, and paradoxically, the lack of uniformity or standardization, with a consequently greater opportunity to explore the subjective response.

Whichever route is used, however, the aims will be to explore a large number of variables which together may help in the drawing, metaphorically, of a 'map' which will help make sense of the clinical presentation, progress and responses of the patient. Upon the 'contours' of this 'map' will then be constructed individually based therapeutic strategies designed to assist the patient to move from his/her present status to a mutually negotiated 'destination' or improved clinical/social/existential state.

Practically, the emerging 'map' is examined for several possible features. As already indicated, specific psychiatric disorders are sought, such as a major depressive disorder, any of the anxiety disorders, or substance abuse disorder, and specific treatments provided as appropriate.

Beyond these syndromes, however, are issues of past experience, personality and current stressors which form an amalgam in the inner world of the patient, colour perceptions and generate a wide variety of emotions and behaviours. Many of these may, individually or together, affect either the pain experience itself, or the impact the pain has on the patient's life, as well as attitudes to treatment and to the desired or expected outcomes. None of these may have been clearly formulated in the patient's mind, and the desired treatment outcome in particular needs to be clarified very carefully and tactfully.

If the outcome desired by the patient is not understood, and if it is at variance with that towards which the treating team is working, lack of success and mutual frustration is inevitable. Any discovered dissonance between these goals should be used to trigger a discussion, the outcome of which should be mutually agreed, and acceptable, treatment targets.

Among the important personal variables which require understanding are the following:

- Past experience, specifically of others, and most especially of others early in developmental life; the way past needs seem to have been understood or not, and have been met or ignored or frustrated; the degree to which others might be trusted; and, often particularly relevant to the present dilemma, how the patient has, in the past, experienced and dealt with helplessness and dependency.
- The stage of psychological development of the patient (not always correlating with chronological age) and the stage of development of his/her family, together with past memories of family affairs stirred by present events.
- What current stressors may be at play – interpersonal, financial, etc.; and what events, such as bereavements, etc. have been experienced in recent times.
- From what activities/roles has the patient habitually derived his/her fulfilment and life satisfaction, and how has the pain influenced those.
- The meaning of the pain to the individual patient, and of the injury or other condition which may underlie it. To what extent, for instance, may it be seen as attributable to indifference or neglect by self or others, as a providential 'test', as a punishment, etc.
- What has been lost or gained by the back pain problem, and what would be lost or gained by improvement or cure. The influence, for example, of the nature of the patient's work, is illustrated by the report by Bigos *et al.* (1991) that a mean of 250% higher incidence of reports of back injury are made by persons with poor job satisfaction compared to those who enjoy their work.
- What are, if any, the strongly held principles and philosophies which guide the patient's life, how were they formed, and how may they be relevant to the present circumstances.
- What are the predominant emotions of the patient with regards to his/her pain, and how do they relate to the patient's underlying thoughts and perspectives.

In the above illustrated list of important psychological issues, some emphasis has been given to those which may have a bearing on the experience of pain, or on the reaction to it. It is important to note, however, that many stressors may have no discernible relationship with pain *per se*, but may serve, together with the pain, to summate and exceed the capacity of the person to cope overall, each by itself being, in the individual case, a necessary but insufficient factor to cause psychological decompensation. The pain then serves as the legitimate vehicle or 'the offering' (Balint, 1964) by which the patient seeks medical or related help. Turner *et al.* (1987) found that amongst volunteers for cognitive-behavioural treatment of chronic low back pain, only 43% ranked pain or its limitations as their primary stressor. Other stressors rated as primary were work and finance (34%) and family problems (23%). Schwartz *et al.* (1994) provide good experimental evidence that subjects complained significantly more of pain and showed less persistence with a physical task following discussion of a stressful life issue than they did following a neutral communication topic. In many cases, of course, the pain precipitates compounding social consequences, so that a complex of problems is added to those existing – not just one straw breaking the camel's back.

As the clinical assessment unfolds, often over several appointments, the patient's progressive clarification of some of the contributing factors can itself be therapeutic, as their stressfulness becomes less, simply by being seen to be finite rather than amorphously and darkly oppressive; moreover, as they become identified, it often becomes possible to design remedial strategies. The act of sharing problems with a supportive professional also has some heartening and strengthening effect. Such changes for the better comprise some of the processes involved in psychotherapy of the so-called 'dynamic' kind.

An alternative approach (often seen in some professional circles as somewhat in competition with the 'dynamic' approach, though in the present authors' views, each complements the other, and is likely to be helpful at various stages of the patient's progress), is the set of 'cognitive-behavioural' therapies. The fundamental underpinnings of such treatments are that individuals tend to develop assumptions about, and consequent perceptions and expectations of, their world, and to codify these as their own (again often poorly articulated) individualized set of cognitions. They are used to generate, and are themselves perpetuated by, the ongoing silent commentary or inner dialogue we know as thoughts. With respect to pain, for instance, ongoing cognitions may generate destructive or complicating attitudes to the pain, to the setting of realistic goals or to the acceptance of recommended treatment strategies.

In the cognitive-behavioural approach, the interview techniques are somewhat more structured and focused, seeking to identify both the relevant (internal) cognitions, and the external environmental factors which serve to increase or decrease the tolerance of pain (not the pain itself). Examples of the latter would be worry, tension, work, alcohol, relaxation, interpersonal conflict, weekends, positive emotional states, study, physical and sexual activity, application of heat or cold, and responses from family or work colleagues that may be solicitous, overprotective, indifferent or punitive.

Two major foci are common to all psychosocial assessment protocols derived from this cognitive behavioural approach; cognitive/affective responses and behaviour patterns.

The currently predominant cognitive-behavioural view of chronic pain pays special attention to those attributed meanings which have implications for patients' perception of having or not having power to manage their pain; whether or not they take appropriate action to reduce their pain; their actual activity patterns and the reciprocal psychological effects; the nature and level of their mood and self perceptions and whether or not they continue their search for explanations and treatment from health services. In patients for whom avoidance has evolved as their main coping strategy, clinicians might uncover escalating self-demeaning soliloquies such as 'it hurts if I try to exercise or become active . . . I'm only doing more damage . . . I must be making my spine crumble even faster . . . I'm helpless . . . I'm a useless person . . . I can never be relied upon . . . I've lost my old place in the family, the workforce and society'. The inner search for explanation can lead to a belief of being punished for past misdeeds, with erosion of self-image, consequent depression and demoralization, and progressively lowered resistance to this style of coping. The 'personal, permanent and pervasive' cognitive attributions relating to misfortune that accompany learned helplessness (Peterson and Seligman, 1984) can easily be seen in this group.

Coping mechanisms of relentless confrontive denial of the need to make adjustments and the absence of a problem-solving stance characterize patients at the other end of the spectrum. Pain episodes in these patients trigger internal dialogues that are very different in content, but which can have the same ultimate effect on mood, motivation and self-perception. Thus: 'I'm not going to let this pain beat me . . . I can handle it . . . if I stay active and busy I can keep my mind off this pain . . . that's the only way . . . I can't stand feeling useless . . . I hate it when anyone thinks I'm not pulling my weight' etc. The end result of this stoic minimization of their condition may be an increase in the average intensity of pain, physical collapse or exhaustion. A sense of failure and helplessness can set in as such patients achieve less and less over the long term.

Compensation factors may influence the cognitions of those awaiting the outcome of litigation. Concerns may be felt that significant improvement may jeopardize the chance of what they perceive as a just settlement, and that they will be seen as having been malingerers and liars. Further, the perception by

patients of clinicians as sceptical or incredulous may lead to desperate attempts to convince the examiners of their true suffering, with the apparent 'exaggerations' serving to confirm the clinician's sceptical stance. Adversarial legal systems and compensation schemes which provide pain-contingent payments risk putting patients in a powerful bind, conditioning pain complaints (Mills and Horne, 1986).

Cognitive assessment seeks to discover the particular idiosyncratic variations on such attributional themes. The patient is asked to describe his/her thoughts or images at times of peaks in pain. Initially, patients are seldom fully aware of their internal dialogues, which have often become submerged beneath the more conspicuous feeling states. Requests to visualize a recent episode accompanied by moment to moment 'thinking aloud' strategy may help to recapture such barely conscious and largely automatic thoughts. The thought may be accompanied by fantasies such as further physical damage to the spine and soft tissues. The use of individually designed diaries and questionnaires, maintained by patients on a daily basis, helps capture these experiences which are otherwise rapidly forgotten.

The minor proportion of angry and demanding patients who cause major difficulties often require special strategies such as clearly stated treatment agreements. However, the most commonly experienced negative emotion in clinical populations of chronic low back pain patients is frustration (Wade *et al.*, 1990). Frustration has been described (Selye, 1979) as one of the most harmful psychogenic stressors. The examiner might inquire about how frustration is managed, or the patient's habitual response of frustration may be apparent from his/her history, including examples of the way the patient has met insoluble problems. If deficiencies in skills are detected, such as the employment of a futile or persistent search for a solution rather than an attempt at pacifying the emotion, the so-called 'emotion defusion' techniques involving imagery and relaxation may be indicated as part of treatment.

Behavioural assessment of the psychosocial aspects of pain may incorporate an informal analysis of the externally applied rewards, such as solicitous spouses (Block, *et al.*, 1980) and punishments that can modulate its characteristics. Whilst the behavioural approach has had only modest (20–30%) long-term effects on pain intensity reports (Keefe and Lefebvre, 1993) it has yielded some clinically useful strategies.

Personality typing alone has not been shown to be more predictive of pain chronicity, or to predict responsiveness to cognitive behavioural treatments (Turk and Rudy, 1987; Phillips, 1988). Traditional psychopathologically orientated measuring instruments are therefore of little value in evaluation. However, two overlapping measures of specific intrapersonal characteristics are shown to co-vary with tolerance of chronic pain and the attainment of treatment goals – perception of 'self-efficacy' or personal effectiveness, reflected in ratings of perceived personal control over pain; and the more general construct of 'internal locus of control'. This latter characteristic is the sense that events are under personal control rather than due to circumstances, fate or luck (Council *et al.*, 1988; Crisson and Keefe, 1988; Jensen and Karoly, 1991; Jensen *et al.*, 1991). These can change with standard cognitive-behavioural treatments which aim to extend the individual's range of practical response to pain. Interview assessment of these variables may be informally quantified on a ten point rating scale to aid pre-selection and treatment evaluation.

Specific behavioural and cognitive therapies

The behavioural paradigm is based on observable behaviours and the influence of associations, rewards and punishment that come from the environment. Behaviourists maintain that a patient is best understood and described by what he/she does in a particular situation. No inquiry is made into inner events. Treatment aims at changing specific behaviours measured by observation and rating which in turn improve thoughts and feelings.

Behavioural strategies require behavioural or environmental change as a first step, maintaining that changes in thoughts and feelings will follow. Examples of treatment targets of this approach include reducing medication usage, improving exercise tolerance and raising activity level. Graded reduction of analgesics involves changes to how patients schedule their medication intake. A key feature of any behavioural plan is to move from an 'as needed' or p.r.n. basis to a predetermined schedule, e.g. 4- or 6-hourly time intervals (Fordyce, 1976; Sternbach, 1982). Some empirical support for the superiority of such time-contingent over on-demand schedules comes from studies by White and Sanders (1985) and Berntzen and Gotestam (1987). In addition to lower levels of pain, mood levels were found to be significantly improved in both groups of chronic pain patients.

A second application of behavioural principles is described as 'activity pacing', in which the patients are encouraged to extend their range of activities such as standing, walking and sitting, including such behaviours as gardening, housework, performance of a hobby, socializing, sex, working, playing with children, exercise and driving. Instruction in the principles of pacing is popularly regarded by chronic patients as one of the more useful strategies learned in pain control programmes. Patients record how long an activity may comfortably last before they notice an increase in their pain. It is then suggested that upon the next attempt they stop at a half-way point and then switch to a different physical position and engage in an alternative, usually lighter, activity. Relaxation and other strategies are applied during a 15-minute break before recommencing. Over a number of weeks, at their own pace and rate, patients increase their activity by small amounts. A guiding principle is to never allow the pain to rise above tolerance levels. The result is usually a very welcome increase in overall activity levels with significantly less pain. Endurances have been reported to be extended up to 2- to 5-fold (Sternbach, 1987).

Social reinforcement techniques require the involvement of persons such as family members who have most contact with the patient, and teaching them to distinguish pain behaviours (e.g. complaints of pain or related issues such as medication) from healthy behaviours. Patients and family members separately tally these behaviours to increase reliability of measures. Family members are trained in how to give praise and attention for healthy behaviours (e.g. during exercise) and how to minimize attention and ignore pain behaviours.

Progressive muscle relaxation training also comes into the category of behavioural therapies, and appears to be an effective adjunct for most, though not all, patients with chronic low back pain (Jessup and Gallegos, 1993). This skill is best used preventively but if it is well practised it can be helpful in the event of spasms that might occur after sudden twisting and turning.

The concept of pain behaviour has drawn its fair share of criticism, including allegations that the theoretical basis is too simplistic, and that the wrong variables (i.e. behaviour) are being measured because they can be measured accurately, and that the more important issues of subjective experience are being ignored. Keefe and Lefebre (1994) list six such controversial areas, and provide their refutations. The latter are not entirely convincing, and Merskey (1995) cites the experience of patients being pushed repeatedly to do things which are increasingly difficult and painful for them, describing such techniques as 'not a pretty matter'. He takes issue with Fordyce's (1976) view that the subjective state of the patient is not a matter of concern to him, provided behaviour can change; and claims that the notion of treating the pain behaviour involves some denial of the patient's experience. A further criticism by Merskey that such treatments may be more in the interests of insurance companies than of patients may also be seen to be understandable in the light of Keefe and Lefebre's (1994) account of Caudill's (1991) cost-benefit analysis of an outpatient behavioural pain management programme which revealed a 36% reduction in total clinic visits over the course of treatment and a saving to the HMO (Health Maintenance Organization) of $35 000 over 2 years.

The cognitive-behavioural paradigm, as indicated above, has as its rationale that patients respond primarily to their cognitive representation of their environment rather than to the environment *per se*. It incorporates the action strategies and conditioning approaches of the behavioural model but largely as a means of testing and modifying maladaptive cognitions. Its main emphasis has been on developing strategies that seek to directly modify negative thoughts and images.

Specific strategies include 'imaginal rehearsal' in which the principles of systematic desensitization are used. The patient induces relaxation and is then asked to recall a relatively low stress situation or emotional reaction that lowered pain tolerance, and to note the earliest physical changes. Maintaining the relaxed state in the presence of progressively more stressful imagery aims to counter-condition the links between emotional states and higher pain levels.

The strategy of distraction redirects attention of patients during periods of intense pain, particularly at times such as night, when the competing stimulation of daily activity is absent. These include such every-day activities as getting out of bed, reading or watching television. Giving this example may stimulate patients to discover other ways which are particularly helpful to them as individuals to bring about distraction. The general principle is that the strategy is required to divert attention away from the body to outside stimuli.

Lastly, the cognitive therapeutic approach addresses some of the revealed 'self-talk' described earlier in this chapter. The assumptions underlying phrases indicative of helplessness and self-recrimination are challenged in therapy, and identified distortions or over-generalizations are replaced with thoughts that are more realistic, positive and accurate. 'Re-labelling' seeks to replace words and phrases carrying negative, defeating or self-denegratory implications, with other words which, although equally accurate, bear with them connotations of hope, encouragement and support.

In practice, many of the strategies referred to have behavioural and cognitive components, well illustrated by the multidimensional treatment package of Philips (1987). The 40 patients described had a mean chronicity of 8.6 years, but over nine weekly group sessions each of 90 minutes, 70% reported pain ratings which were 'improved' or 'much improved', with an additional 13% rating themselves 'pain free' or 'virtually pain free'. A 12-month follow-up was said to have yielded reports of exercise capacity improvements of 87% and elimination of drugs in 63%. Details of the programme, which include activity pacing, mood control techniques and anxiety management/relaxation training, graded increases in exercise and physical fitness and a range of cognitive and behavioural strategies increasing control over pain episodes, are published in a treatment manual (Philips, 1988).

Conclusion

The most important step in the management of chronic pain is assessment. The inclusion from the outset of an approach which acknowledges the contributions of psychological/psychiatric and social factors, as well as physical, facilitates the identification of the major importance of these factors in some patients, and facilitates the subsequent incorporation into the assessment and treatment programme, where indicated, of the psychological/psychiatric dimension.

The person, style and behaviour of the examining clinician is an integral part of the total setting in which the examination takes place, and can significantly influence the patient's own behaviour and subsequent outcome. Psychotropic medication, and therapies based on relationship, behavioural and cognitive approaches all appear to have important places. Which particular technique, or combination of techniques, may be most suitable for each type of patient has been to date insufficiently explored, and remains an important research goal. The availability in a particular setting, however, of as full a range of treatment options as possible seems highly desirable, and care should be taken to avoid, as far as possible, the prescription of treatment based on the theoretical orientation and ideology of the clinic rather than on the need of the patient.

References

Balint, M. (1964) *The Doctor, his Patient and the Disease*, 2nd edn. Churchill Livingstone, Edinburgh.

Berntzen, D. and Gotestam, K.G. (1987) Effects of on-demand versus fixed interval schedules in the treatment of chronic pain with analgesic compounds. *J. Consult. Clin. Psychol.*, **55**, 213-217

Bigos, S.J., Battie, M.C., Spangler, D.M. *et al.* (1991) A prospective study of work perceptions and psychosocial factors affecting the reporting of back injury. *Spine*, **16**, 1-6.

Block A.R., Kramer E.F. and Gaylor, M. (1980) Behavioural treatment of chronic pain: the spouse as a discriminant cue for pain behaviour. *Pain*, **9**, 243-252.

Brown, G.K.A. (1990) Causal analysis of chronic pain and depression. *J. Abnorm. Psychol.*, **99**, 127-137.

Caudill, M., Schnable, R., Zuttermeister, P. *et al.* (1994) In: Keefe F.J. and Lefebvre J., *Proceedings of the Seventh World Congress on Pain - Progress in Pain Research and Management* Vol. 2 (G.F. Gebhart, D.L. Hammond and T.S. Jensen, eds). IASP Press, Seattle.

Council, J.R., Ahern, D.K., Follick, M.J. *et al.* (1988) Expectancies and functional impairment in chronic low back pain. *Pain*, **33**, 323-331.

Crisson J.E. and Keefe F.J. (1988) The relationship of locus of control to pain coping strategies and psychological distress in chronic pain patients. *Pain*, **35**, 147-154.

Fairbank, J., Davies, J., Coupar, J. and O'Brian, J.P. (1980) The Oswestry Low Back Pain Disability Questionnaire. *Physiotherapy*, **66**, 271-273.

Fordyce, W.E. (1976) *Behavioural Methods for Chronic Pain and Illness*. C.V. Mosby, St Louis, Missouri.

Jensen, M.P. and Karoly, P. (1991) Control beliefs, coping efforts and adjustment to chronic pain. *J. Consult. Clin. Psychol.*, **59**, 431-438.

Jensen M.P., Turner, J.A. and Romano, J.M. (1991) Self-efficacy and outcome expectancies. relationship to chronic pain coping strategies and adjustment. *Pain*, **44**, 263-269.

Jessup, B.A. and Gallegos, X. (1993) Relaxation and biofeedback. In: *Textbook of Pain*, 3rd edn (P.D. Wall and R. Melzack, eds). Churchill Livingstone, Edinburgh.

Keefe, F.J. and Lefebvre, J.C. (1993) Behaviour therapy. In: *Textbook of Pain*, 3rd edn (P.D. Wall and R. Melzack, eds). Churchill Livingstone, Edinburgh.

Keefe F.J. and Lefebvre, J. (1994) *Proceedings of the Seventh World Congress on Pain - Progress in Pain Research and Management*. Volume 2 (G.F. Gebhart, D.L. Hammond and T.S. Jensen, eds), IASP Press, Seattle.

Kelly, G.A. (1955) *The Psychology of Personal Constructs* Volumes 1 and 2. Norton: New York.

Lasagna, L. (1960) Clinical measurement of pain. *Ann. N. Y. Acad. Sci.*, **86**, 28-37.

Main, J.C. and Waddell G. (1984) The detection of psychological abnormality in chronic low back pain using four simple scales. *Curr. Concept. Pain*, **2**, 10-15.

Mechanic, D. (1962) The concept of illness behaviour. *J. Chron. Dis.*, **156**, 189-194.

Merskey, H. (1975) Psychological aspects of pain. In *Pain. Clinical and Experimental Perspectives* (M. Weisenberg, ed.). C.V. Mosby, St Louis, p. 21.

Mills, H. and Horne, G. (1986) Whiplash - manmade disease? *N. Z. Med. J.*, **99**, 373-374.

Parsons, T. (1964) *Social Structure and Personality*. Collier Macmillan, London.

Peterson, C. and Seligman, M.E.P. (1984) Causal explanations as a risk factor for depression. Theory and evidence. *Psychol. Rev.*, **91**, 347-374.

Philips, H.C. (1987) The effects of behavioural treatment on chronic pain. *Behav. Res. Ther.*, **25**, 365-377.

Philips, H.C. (1988) *The Psychological Management of Chronic Pain: A Treatment Manual*. Springer, New York.

Pilowski, I. (1969) Abnormal illness behaviour. *Br. J. Psychol.*, **42**, 347-351.

Pilowski, I. (1990) The concept of abnormal illness behaviour. *Psychosomatics*, **31**, 207-213.

Schwartz, L. Slater, M.A. and Birchley, G.R. (1994) Interpersonal stress and pain behaviors in patients with chronic pain. *J. Consult. Clin. Psychol.*, **62**, 861-864.

Selye, H. (1979) *The Stress of My Life. A Scientist's Memoirs*, 2nd edn. Van Nostrand Reinhold, New York.

Sternbach, R.A. (1982) The psychologist's role in the diagnosis and treatment of pain patients. In *Psychological Approaches to the Management of Pain* (J. Barber and C. Adrian, eds). Brunner Mazel, New York.

Sternbach, R.A. (1987) *Mastering Pain*. Arlington Books, London.

Turk, D.C. and Rudy, T.E. (1987) Towards a comprehensive assessment of chronic pain patients. *Behav. Res. Ther.*, **25**, 237-249.

Turner, J.A., Clancy, S. and Vitaliano, P.P. (1987) Relationships of stress, appraisal and coping, to chronic low back pain. *Behav. Res. Ther.*, **25**, 281-288.

Wade, J.B., Price, D.D., Hamer, R.M. *et al* (1990) An emotional component analysis of chronic pain. *Pain*, **40**, 303-310.

White, B. and Sanders, S.H, (1985) Differential effects on pain and mood in chronic pain patients with time versus pain - contingent medication delivery. *Behav. Ther.*, **16**, 28-38.

20

Diagnosis of mechanical low back pain with or without referred leg pain

L.G.F. Giles

Introduction

An overview of diagnostic procedures for the management of low back pain of mechanical origin, with or without leg pain, by specific disciplines, i.e. medicine and surgery, chiropractic, osteopathy and physiotherapy will be described, respectively, in the four chapters which follow. This brief introductory chapter sets the scene for the following discipline specific chapters and places mechanical low back pain, with or without referred leg pain, in the overall topic of spinal pain. Low back pain must be viewed in the context of (i) clearly defined pathological conditions, and (ii) the less well defined, but much more prevalent, condition of spinal pain of mechanical origin (Beaumont and Paice, 1992). It is vital to distinguish mechanical causes of back pain from other causes as patients with mechanical causes are likely to respond to physical forms of treatment (Jenner and Barry, 1995).

One of the major difficulties involved in evaluating a patient with low back pain of mechanical origin, with or without root symptoms, is that multifactorial aetiologies are possible (Haldeman, 1977; Gross, 1979) for this multidimensional problem that can affect every aspect of an individual's life (Bowman, 1994). The painful structure, or structures, are not amenable to direct scrutiny. Therefore, a tentative diagnosis is usually arrived at for an individual case by taking a careful case history and employing a thorough physical examination, with imaging and laboratory procedures as indicated (Bigos *et al.*, 1994a). In this context, it should be noted that there are three main approaches to patient evaluation, i.e. (i) assessment of pain (using subjective self-report measures estimating pain severity, quality and location), (ii) investigation of personality structure, and

(iii) clinical identification of signs and symptoms deemed excessively, or inappropriately, abnormal (Main and Waddell, 1982).

Nontheless, there is still little consensus, either within or among specialties, on the use of diagnostic tests for patients with low back pain (Cherkin *et al.*, 1994). Furthermore, in spite of following a thorough examination procedure, one often merely eliminates frank pathologies and the precise cause of low back pain of mechanical origin, with or without referred leg pain, often remains obscure (Riihimaki, 1991; Margo, 1994), especially when dysfunction and degenerative pathology of spinal and sacroiliac joints co-exists.

Specifically, diagnostic problems relate to (a) the limitations of many diagnostic procedures, including plain film radiography, myelography, computerized tomography (CT), magnetic resonance imaging (MRI), and bone scans, (b) inadequacies in the precise anatomical knowledge of the spine, and (c) there sometimes being multifactorial causes of pain at a given level of the spine. Also, there is often disagreement on which imaging procedures have diagnostic validity for mechanical back pain, with or without referred leg pain, for example in the use of flexion–extension plain film radiography (Dvorak *et al.*, 1991; Knight, 1993; Sato and Kikuchi, 1993). In addition, Buirski and Silberstein (1993) found that MRI can only be used as an assessment of nuclear anatomy and not for symptomatology. Furthermore, roentgenographic diagnosis often proves difficult because of the anatomical complexity of the spine (Le-Breton *et al.*, 1993).

Additionally, some diagnostic and therapeutic chemical agents may be harmful, as can be the case when such chemicals injected into intervertebral discs extravasate into the epidural space (Weitz, 1984; Adams *et al.*, 1986; MacMillan *et al.*, 1991), causing complications due to contact between them and neural structures (Dyck, 1985; Merz, 1986; Watts and Dickhaus, 1986).

That low back pain with or without sciatica is not a diagnostic end-point, but rather a label for a pain syndrome that encompasses a long differential diagnosis, should always be remembered (Young, 1993; Herr and Williams, 1994), even though the most common cause of this syndrome is dysfunction and degeneration of spinal intervertebral joints (mechanical back pain) (McCowin *et al.*, 1991; Murtagh, 1991, 1994; Day *et al.*, 1994). Mechanical back pain is due to injury, accounting for approximately 72% of back pain, while lumbar spondylosis accounts for approximately 10% of painful backs (Murtagh, 1991, 1994). Root compression due to *mechanical dysfunction*, with resulting radiculopathy, has to be differentiated from *frank pathological* conditions causing radiculopathy; both conditions may result in signs and symptoms such as pain, paraesthesia, sensory disturbance, loss or weakness of tendon reflexes, and muscular weakness (Benini, 1987).

It is still only rarely possible to validate a diagnosis in cases where pain arises from the spine (White and Gordon, 1982) and, because it is not possible to establish the pathological basis of back pain in 80–90% of cases (Chila *et al.*, 1990; Spratt *et al.*, 1990; Pope and Novotny, 1993), this leads to diagnostic uncertainty and suspicion that some patients have a 'compensation neurosis' or other psychological problem. It is also appropriate at this time to recognize the role of psychological factors which are discussed in detail in Chapter 19. Although the complex interaction of psyche and soma in the aetiology of back pain is not well understood, a psychogenic component may be primary (conversion disorder), secondary (depression caused by chronic pain), contributory (myofascial cycle dysfunction), or absent (Keim and Kirkaldy-Willis, 1987).

In previous chapters, the anatomy of the lumbosacral spine has been given in considerable detail. Therefore, it is not necessary to reiterate it here, other than to highlight clinically important aspects, under the following subheadings, and to emphasize that it is mandatory for low back pain patients, with or without leg pain, to undergo a comprehensive case history interview, followed by a thorough and careful physical examination and, when necessary, laboratory procedures, in order to make a differential diagnosis.

Nerve roots

The relationship of the lumbosacral roots of the spinal nerves to the vertebrae and intervertebral discs is of major clinical significance (Figure 20.1). In this

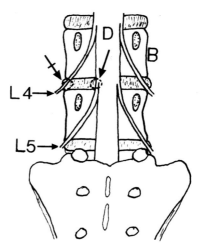

Figure 20.1 Schematic relationship of spinal nerve roots, in their respective root sleeves, to the vertebral bodies (B) and intervertebral discs. The L4 and L5 posterior spinal elements have been removed. A fourth lumbar disc *medial* herniation (arrow) will affect the L5 nerve roots and can also affect some of the sacral nerve roots. A fourth lumbar disc *lateral* herniation (tailed arrow) may affect the L4 nerve and its spinal ganglion at this level, depending on the location of the ganglion, but not the L5 neural structures. B = body of fourth lumbar vertebra; D = dural tube.

context, it is important to note that the termination of the spinal cord (conus medullaris) is normally at the lower border of the first lumbar vertebra by 12 years of age, due to the cephalad migration of the spinal cord as skeletal growth is more rapid than neural growth (Keim and Kirkaldy-Willis, 1987). In adults, the conus medullaris is usually at the level of the first lumbar intervertebral disc (between L1 and L2) (see Figure 20.6) (Wilkinson, 1986) but may vary its position between the T12 and L2 intervertebral discs (see Figures 3.5 and 13.5).

The position of an intervertebral disc herniation is of great significance in correlating symptoms with signs, as well as with various imaging procedures. For example, a *midline* herniation posteriorly of the L4–L5 intervertebral disc may affect the L5–S5 nerves, depending on the size of the herniation, but not the L4 nerve. A posterolateral herniation of the L5–S1 intervertebral disc may affect the L4 nerve (Figure 20.1) but not the L5 nerve. A clear understanding of this concept is essential for localizing the possible level of spinal involvement.

Two other important neurological concepts have been recognized for anatomically normal spines. First of all, the distribution of cutaneous areas supplied with afferent nerve fibres by single posterior spinal nerve roots, i.e. dermatomes of the human body (Dorland, 1974; Barr and Kiernan, 1983), have been

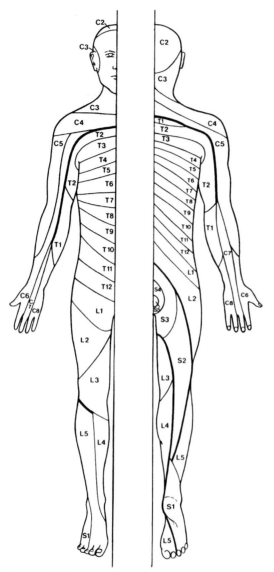

Figure 20.2 Sensory (dermatomes) on the anterior and posterior surfaces of the body. Axial lines, where there is numerical discontinuity, are drawn thickly. (Modified from Wilkinson, J. L. (1986) *Neuroanatomy for Medical Students*. John Wright and Sons, Bristol, p. 29.)

ment. Secondly, careful examination of motor innervation of limb musculature also allows the nerve roots causing a specific motor deficit to be identified (Figure 20.3).

In general, nerves from two adjoining spinal segments govern a specific joint movement. In the lower limbs, joint innervation is segmental, with each joint innervated by nerves arising one segment lower in the spinal cord than those that innervate the next proximal joint. Thus, a total of three to five spinal segments controls the following, i.e. hip, knee, and ankle, as shown in Figure 20.3 (Quiring and Warfel, 1960; Hoppenfeld, 1976, 1977; Keim and Kirkaldy-Willis, 1987; Moore, 1992).

History of low back pain

The importance of an exhaustive case history cannot be overemphasized, and it should take into account facts such as the patient's age, occupation, medication, previous injuries, onset of pain, recreational activities and frequency thereof, pain aggravation and characteristics, location distribution, and any related neurological symptoms (numbness, paraesthesia, weakness). Some conditions provide reasonably characteristic patterns, while others do not. For example, morning stiffness may be associated with ankylosing spondylitis, or with mechanical degenerative changes such as discogenic low back pain, although it may be more prolonged in the former. If walking or standing cause low back pain, spinal stenosis may be the aetiology. Standing may aggravate pain due to disc herniation while walking may lessen the pain. Pain which occurs at night, and which is relieved by aspirin may be associated with an osteoid osteoma which is a benign tumour of bone (Keim and Kirkaldy-Willis, 1987).

Pain diagrams which have been designed to give a patient's subjective interpretation of pain, its location, its characteristics, its frequency and its intensity, should be used to complete the history (Huskisson, 1974, Mooney and Robertson, 1976, Chan *et al.*, 1993) (Figure 20.4).

Until a thorough history has been taken and a thorough examination performed, to rule out organic disease, it is not wise to label a patient as being neurotic or a malingerer. It should be remembered that it is thought that such patients form only a small minority of cases (approximately 0.1%) (Ghormley, 1958). Furthermore, some studies comparing compensation and non-compensation patients show no difference (Leavitt *et al.*, 1982; Pelz and Merskey, 1982; Melzack *et al.*, 1985; Mendelson, 1987), and the stereotype describing migrant workers as malingerers cannot be supported (Hewson *et al.*, 1987).

fairly well established (Figure 20.2). According to Keim and Kirkaldy-Willis (1987), this enables deficits of a specific nerve root to be accurately localized during sensory examination although Jinkins (1993) suggests that there is some overlap of sensation (see Chapter 17 for details). When spinal and or neural anomalies are present, Wigh (1980) warns of the difficulty of correctly localizing the level of involve-

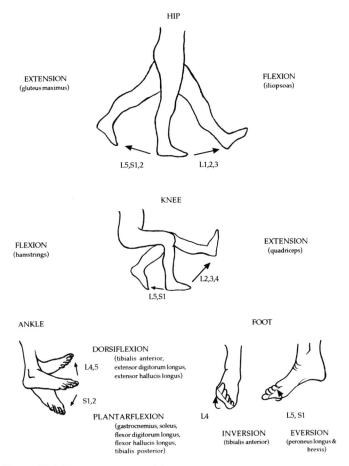

Figure 20.3 Motor innervation of the lower limb. (Modified from: Hoppenfeld, S. (1977) *Orthopaedic Neurology. A Diagnostic Guide to Neurologic Levels.* J.B. Lippincott, Philadelphia; Keim, H.A. and Kirkaldy-Willis, W.H. (1987) *Clinical Symposia. Low Back Pain.* **39**. Ciba-Geigy, Jersey; Moore, K.L. (1992) *Clinically Oriented Anatomy,* 3rd edn. Williams and Wilkins, Baltimore.)

Physical examination

The physical examination should be orderly and systematic and should include the following (Table 20.1)

Low back pain of mechanical origin occurs most commonly in the 25- to 40-year age group (Weinstein *et al.*, 1990); thus, in older patients, the possibility of spinal disease must be considered, although it should not be presumed absent in younger patients. With increasing age, the importance of rectal, or rectal and vaginal, examination should be stressed so that local lesions and involvement of accessible lumbodorsal plexuses can be ruled out if possible, as low back pain can be referred from various palpable visceral

structures (Chusid, 1985). The possibility of reflex sympathetic dystrophy should not be overlooked (Tierney, 1992).

Some possible causes of low back pain

Some possible causes of acute and chronic low back pain, which should be considered in the differential diagnosis, are summarized in Table 20.2.

Definitions vary for the time factor associated with acute and chronic low back pain depending on the viewpoint of authors (Nachemson and Andersson, 1982; Deyo, 1988; Bigos *et al.*, 1994; Henderson *et*

<u>PAIN ASSESSMENT</u>

NAME...AGE..............MALE / FEMALE

OCCUPATION..........................

----

1.   PLEASE MARK WHERE YOU FEEL PAIN AT THIS MOMENT USING
     THESE CODES:

STABBING PAIN ↓↓↓

DEEP PAIN   >>>>

BURNING PAIN   X X

PINS & NEEDLES / / /

NUMBNESS   OOO

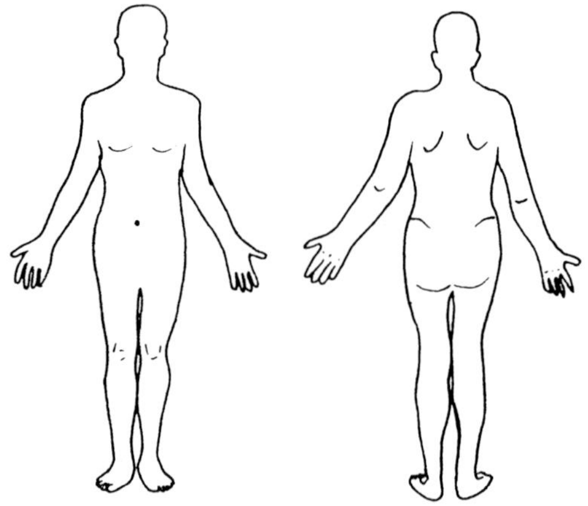

----

2.   <u>PAIN FREQUENCY</u> *(PLEASE TICK <u>ONE</u> BOX ONLY)*

ONCE PER MONTH

ONCE PER WEEK

ONCE PER DAY

FREQUENT

CONSTANT

----

3.   <u>PAIN SCALE</u> *(PLEASE PLACE A MARK ON THE FOLLOWING LINE TO
     INDICATE YOUR PAIN AT THIS MOMENT)*

NO   PAIN AS BAD AS
PAIN   ├──────────────────────────────────────┤   IT COULD BE

Figure 20.4 Subjective pain assessment: pain diagram, pain frequency, and visual analogue
scale.

al., 1994). However, it is reasonable to broadly classify acute low back pain as being of 7 days or less duration, which may be followed by a sub-acute stage of up to 12 weeks; after this the pain can be considered chronic (Deyo, 1988).

Deep tenderness of the spine, with or without cutaneous hyperalgesia, is usually due to local dis-

ease of, or injury to, the tissues at the site of tenderness; almost entirely cutaneous tenderness is a referred phenomenon found in visceral disease (Mackenzie, 1985). It is necessary to differentiate between cutaneous and deep tenderness and, in the case of the latter, between tenderness elicited by pressing upon the spinous processes and tenderness

Table 20.1 *Elements of the physical examination (adapted from Hoppenfeld, 1976; Mackenzie, 1985; Keim and Kirkaldy-Willis, 1987)*

Erect posture examination	

Observe for:

fluidity of movement
body build
skin markings - café-au-lait spots, lipomata, & hairy
    patches often denote underlying neurologic or bone
    pathology
posture
deformities
pelvic obliquity
spine alignment

Sacroiliac joint:

examine for joint motion

Test spinal column motion for:

flexion
extension
side bending
rotation

Palpate for:

iliac crest levels
anterior and posterior superior iliac spine levels
any break in contour of spinous processes -
    (spondylolisthesis - Figure 13.16)
muscle spasm
trigger zones
myofascial nodes
supraspinous and interspinous ligament tenderness
adjacent muscle tenderness
sciatic nerve tenderness
posterior aspect of coccyx
relative motion between adjacent vertebrae (by motion
    palpation)

Observe gait:

Walking on heels (tests foot and great toe dorsiflexion)
Walking on toes (tests calf muscles)

Kneeling	*Seated*

Ankle jerk
Sensation on calf and sole

Straight leg raising; slump test
Knee jerk
Calf circumference measurement

Supine	

Straight leg raising
Flex thigh on pelvis then extend knee with foot
    dorsiflexed (sciatic nerve stretch)
Hoover test *
Kernig test (spinal cord stretch) *

Tests to increase intrathecal pressure
  Milgram test *
  Naffziger test *
  Valsalva manoeuvre *
Sacroiliac joint
  compression test
  pelvic rock test
  Gaenslen's sign *
  Fabere/Patrick test *
Hip joint
  Fabere/Patrick test
  hip flexion

Palpate abdomen:
  listen for bruit (abdominal and inguinal)
Palpate for peripheral pulses and skin temperature

Palpate for flattening of lumbar lordosis during leg raising

Measure
  thigh circumference bilaterally
  leg lengths (anterior superior iliac spine to medial
    malleolus) for an *approximate* clinical impression of
    leg lengths

Test sensation and motor power

Prone	

Palpate
  sciatic nerve between ischial tuberosity and greater
    trochanter
  ischial bursa
  cluneal nerves crossing the iliac crest for renal
    tenderness and local tenderness or spasm

Palpate trochanteric bursa
Spine extension

Femur extension test for hip extension

* See Abbreviations and Definitions chapter.

Table 20.2 *Possible causes of low back pain. (Reproduced with permission from Hart, F.D. (1985) Back, pain in. In French's Index of Differential Diagnosis (F.D. Hart, ed.), 12th edn. Butterworth, Oxford, pp 72–73.)*

Acute back pain

- febrile disorders
- injury

Chronic back pain

1. *Traumatic, mechanical or degenerative:*
   (a) Low back strain; fatigue, obesity; pregnancy. (b) Injuries of bone, joint or ligaments. (c) Degenerative disease of the spine (osteoarthrosis) including ankylosing hyperostosis. (d) Intervertebral disc lesions. (e) Lumbar instability syndromes, e.g. spondylolisthesis. (f) Scoliosis: primary and secondary. (g) Spinal stenosis.

2. *Metabolic:*
   Osteoporosis. Osteomalacia. Hyper- and hypoparathyroidism. Ochronosis. Fluorosis. Hypophosphataemic rickets.

3. *Unknown causes:*
   Inflammatory arthropathies of the spine, such as ankylosing spondylitis and the spondylitis of Reiter's (Brodie's) disease, psoriasis, ulcerative colitis, Whipple's and Crohn's diseases. Rarely polymyositis and polymyalgia rheumatica. Paget's disease of bone. Scheuermann's disease.

4. *Infective conditions of bone, joint and theca of spine:*
   Osteomyelitis. Tuberculosis. Undulant fever (abortus and melitensis). Typhoid and paratyphoid fever and other *Salmonella* infections. Syphilis. Yaws. Very rarely Weil's disease (leptospirosis icterohaemorrhagica). Spinal pachymeningitis. Chronic meningitis. Subarachnoid or spinal abscess.

5. *Psychogenic:*
   Anxiety. Depression. Hysteria. Compensation neurosis. Malingering.

6. *Neoplastic – benign or malignant, primary or secondary:*
   Osteoid osteoma. Eosinophilic granuloma. Metastatic carcinomatosis. Bronchial carcinoma. Oesophageal carcinoma. Sarcoma. Myeloma. Primary and secondary tumours of spinal canal and nerve roots: ependymoma; neurofibroma; glioma; angioma; meningioma; lipoma; rarely cordoma. Reticuloses, e.g. Hodgkin's disease.

7. *Cardiac and vascular:*
   Subarachnoid or spinal haemorrhage. Luetic or dissecting aneurysm. Grossly enlarged left atrium in mitral valve disease. Rarely myocardial infarction.

8. *Gynaecological conditions:*
   Tuberculous disease. Rarely prolapse or retroversion of uterus. Dysmenorrhoea. Chronic salpingitis. Pelvic abscess or chronic cervicitis. Tumours.

9. *Gastrointestinal conditions:*
   Peptic ulcers. Cholelithiasis. Pancreatitis. Rarely appendicitis, or from new growth of intra-abdominal viscus (colon, stomach, pancreas), or from retroperitoneal structures.

10. *Renal and genitourinary causes:*
    Carcinoma of kidney. Calculus. Hydronephrosis. Polycystic kidney. Necrotizing papillitis. Pyelitis and pyelonephritis. Perinephric abscess. Infection or new growth of prostate.

11. *Blood disorders:*
    Sickle-cell crises. Acute haemolytic states.

12. *Drugs:*
    Corticosteroids. Methysergide. Compound analgesic tablets.

13. *Normality:*
    (Non-disease).

---

in the adjacent muscles (Mackenzie, 1985). Spinal disease is usually accompanied by local muscular spasm, and the muscles thus affected become tender, although they are not themselves the site of the disease (Mackenzie, 1985). This is important in the differential diagnosis as local spasm can be a response to disease of the vertebrae, intervertebral discs, or to the spinal cord and its membranes (Mackenzie, 1985). The chief morbid conditions causing spinal tenderness are summarized by Mackenzie (1985) in Table 20.3.

Mechanical low back pain

As low back pain, with or without referred leg pain, of mechanical origin is the most common form of this condition, it deserves special mention. Poor muscle tone and posture are important factors in the aetiology of back pain of mechanical origin and can lead to hyperlordosis with, for example, narrowing of

the intervertebral canal, especially in the lateral recesses (via impingement by the superior articular process of the inferior lumbar vertebra) (Keim and Kirkaldy-Willis, 1987).

The intervertebral and zygapophysial joints at each spinal level can be affected by postural deficiencies and injury, causing mechanical degenerative changes which can lead to zygapophysial joint and nerve root syndromes, the pathogenesis of which has been described by Keim and Kirkaldy-Willis (1987) and Kirkaldy-Willis (1988). Figure 20.5 summarizes the pathogenesis of these degenerative changes.

The following diagrammatic summary of clinical features of a herniated lumbar intervertebral disc indicate how the level of herniation can result in buttock and leg pain, numbness, weakness, atrophy and abnormal reflexes (Figure 20.6).

Spontaneous recovery from disc herniation is well known and is an important aspect of treatment strategy (Fager, 1994). Furthermore, Saal and Saal (1989) reported 90% good or excellent outcome with 'aggressive' non-operative treatment in a selective

Table 20.3 *Summary of chief conditions causing spinal tenderness. (Reproduced with permission from Mackenzie, I. (1985) Spine, tenderness of. In French's Index of Differential Diagnosis (F.D. Hart, ed.), 12th edn. Butterworth, Oxford, p. 788.)*

1. Diseases of the overlying skin and subcutaneous tissue

These are rare and clinically obvious

2. Diseases of the vertebral column

    a. INFLAMMATORY

Pott's disease	Spondylitis ankylopoietica
Staphylococcal spondylitis	Actinomycosis
Typhoid spine	Hydatid cyst
	Paget's disease

    b. DEGENERATIVE

Spondylosis	Nucleus pulposus herniation
Osteochondritis (rare)	

    c. NEOPLASTIC

Secondary deposit	Myelomatosis
Sarcoma	Leukaemic deposits

    d. TRAUMATIC

Fracture	Nucleus pulposus herniation
Dislocation	Spondylolisthesis

    e. EROSION BY AORTIC ANEURYSM

3. Diseases of the spinal cord and meninges

Metastatic epidural abscess or tumour	Herpes zoster
Meningioma	Meningitis serosa circumscripta
Neurofibroma	Tumour of the spinal cord
	Syringomyelia

4. Hysteria and malingering: compensation neurosis

5. Metabolic disorders: osteoporosis, osteomalacia, hyperparathyroidism

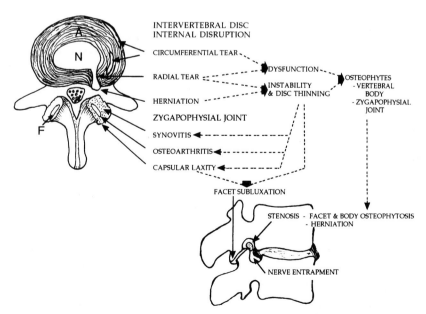

Figure 20.5 This figure summarizes the pathogenesis of intervertebral disc and zygapophysial joint functional and degenerative changes, as well as the development of nerve root entrapment syndromes.

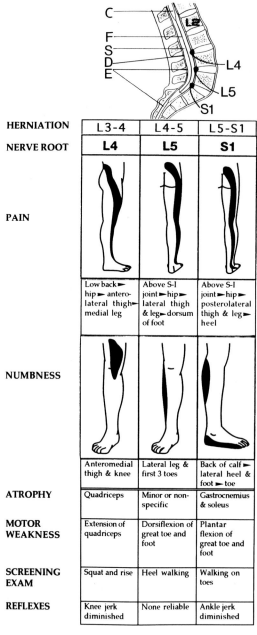

HERNIATION	L3-4	L4-5	L5-S1
NERVE ROOT	**L4**	**L5**	**S1**
PAIN			
	Low back ► hip ► antero-lateral thigh ► medial leg	Above S-I joint ► hip ► lateral thigh & leg ► dorsum of foot	Above S-I joint ► hip ► posterolateral thigh & leg ► heel
NUMBNESS			
	Anteromedial thigh & knee	Lateral leg & first 3 toes	Back of calf ► lateral heel & foot ► toe
ATROPHY	Quadriceps	Minor or non-specific	Gastrocnemius & soleus
MOTOR WEAKNESS	Extension of quadriceps	Dorsiflexion of great toe and foot	Plantar flexion of great toe and foot
SCREENING EXAM	Squat and rise	Heel walking	Walking on toes
REFLEXES	Knee jerk diminished	None reliable	Ankle jerk diminished

Figure 20.6 Clinical features of a posterolateral lumbar intervertebral disc herniation. C = conus medullaris; D = dural tube; E = epidural space; F = filum terminale; S = subarachnoid space. (Modified from Wilkinson, J.L. (1986) *Neuroanatomy for Medical Students.* John Wright and Sons, Bristol, p. 46; Keim, H.A. and Kirkaldy-Willis, W.H. (1987) Low back pain. *Clinical Symposia,* **39**, 18, Ciba-Geigy; Bigos, S., Bowyer, O., Braen, G. *et al.* (1994) *Acute Low Back Problems in Adults.* Practice Guideline, Quick Reference Guide Number 14. US Department of Health and Human Services, Public Health Service, Agency for Health Care Policy and Research, Rockville, MD, AHCPR Pub. No. 95-0643.)

group of patients with confirmed disc herniation and radiculopathy. Also, lumbar intervertebral disc extrusions can morphologically change in a manner consistent with resorption when treated non-surgically (Saal *et al.*, 1990). However, the indications for surgery will be discussed in Chapter 21.

Although the zygapophysial joint is now universally accepted as an important source of back pain (Mooney and Robertson, 1976; Schwarzer *et al.*, 1994a,b; Stolker *et al.*, 1994), and its neurology is more accurately understood (Giles, 1989; Gronblad *et al.*, 1991a,b), the existence of the 'facet syndrome' (Ghormley, 1958) as a clinical entity is still questioned by some (Kuslich *et al.*, 1991; Jackson, 1992; Schwarzer *et al.*, 1994a,b). However, it is well accepted and supported by others (Kirkaldy-Willis and Tchang, 1988; Weinstein, 1988; Yong-Hing, 1988; Empting-Koschorke *et al.*, 1990; El-Khoury and Renfrew, 1991; Goupille *et al.*, 1993).

Imaging

Routine radiographs of the lumbosacral spine and pelvis, as well as the thoracic spine, should be taken to establish a baseline and to rule out metabolic, inflammatory, and malignant conditions (Keim and Kirkaldy-Willis, 1987). These radiographs should be taken in the erect posture, using carefully standardized procedures, to determine accurately whether possibly significant leg length inequality is present with corresponding pelvic obliquity (Giles and Taylor, 1981; Giles, 1984, 1989). In some cases, left and right lateral bending radiographs can be helpful in localizing a motion segment problem, e.g. due to intervertebral disc herniation (Duncan and Hoen, 1942; Sandoz, 1971; Weitz, 1981; Giles, 1989). Also, instability at given spinal levels can be demonstrated using dynamic radiography in some conditions (Morgan and King, 1957; Boden and Wiesel, 1990; Shaffer *et al.*, 1990; Sato and Kikuchi, 1993; Toyone *et al.*, 1994). These conditions include isolated posterior slippage in extension, combined posterior opening and forward translation in flexion (Sato and Kikuchi, 1993). However, an unequivocal definition of instability in lumbar disease has yet to be established, as does the relationship between radiologically demonstrable lumbar instability and clinical symptoms (Sato and Kikuchi, 1993; Frymoyer and Krag, 1986).

Further imaging procedures may be necessary such as (i) magnetic resonance imaging, which can provide very good detail of soft tissue structures in and about the spinal column and pelvis without the need of contrast, (ii) computed tomography scans which are particularly good at showing bony structures and are useful for some neural problems, (iii) myelography which, although invasive, is a further possibility if necessary, especially when surgery is contemplated, and (iv) bone scans when tumour, infection or small fracture(s) are suspected.

Unfortunately, all the above procedures have some limitations, for example plain film radiographs will not show an osseous erosion until approximately 40% decrease in bone density has occurred (Michel *et al.*, 1990). In addition, MRI may not show signs of traumatic lumbar disc herniation until some months later (Ando and Mimatsu, 1993). Furthermore, it is well known that there is a high rate of false positive findings as a result of asymptomatic degenerative changes. Therefore, these several limitations show that imaging procedures may only give a 'shadow of the truth' and this important fact should be remembered. This is particularly true when a patient's physical examination and imaging studies are not remarkable and do not pinpoint the cause of symptoms. The limitations of present diagnostic imaging procedures in not being able to show all soft tissue lesions, such as some of those shown histologically in Chapters 3, 4, 5, 6, 12, 13 and 14 is a serious shortcoming. In Chapter 18, advantages and limitations of imaging procedures are explained in great detail.

When nerve root dysfunction is suspected, electromyography (EMG) and nerve root conduction studies can be helpful (Hoppenfeld, 1977; Chusid, 1985).

Laboratory tests

When bony pathology is suspected, serum (i) calcium, (ii) phosphorus, (iii) alkaline phosphatase (particularly alkaline phosphatase isoenzyme determination by electrophoresis, which differentiates alkaline phosphatase of osteoblastic origin from alkaline phosphatase from other sources (Brown, 1975)), and (iv) prostate-specific antigen (for males over 40 years of age) may be helpful in detecting bone disease. Early inflammatory changes may be detected by an increase in C-reactive protein and in the erythrocyte sedimentation rate (ESR). An abnormal full blood count can be helpful, for example, in cases where there is suspicion of primary haematological disorders and for some infections (Henderson *et al.*, 1994). Serum immunoelectrophoresis of serum and urinary proteins may also be useful diagnostic procedures, in the diagnosis of multiple myeloma (Brown, 1975). Other tests which should be considered, when indicated, are urine culture and sensitivity for infection in genitourinary tract infections as well as latex flocculation for rheumatoid spondylitis, serum and urine amylase and lipase for chronic pancreatitis (Collins, 1968; Schroeder *et al.*, 1992).

In this chapter it is not necessary to list every spine-related condition with its possible abnormalities in serology, haematology, urinalysis and other laboratory tests, as these have been well documented in numerous clinical diagnosis texts, including illustrated versions (Collins, 1968). In some cases, particular reference to painful syndromes associated with the spine have been summarized (Haldeman *et al.*, 1993; Henderson *et al.*, 1994).

Laboratory evaluations are important when the clinician suspects metabolic disturbance, malignancy, infection or one of the arthritides such as ankylosing spondylitis or rheumatoid arthritis. Nonetheless, it should be noted that various tests have different levels of *accuracy* which is calculated from the *sensitivity* (proportion of individuals with the condition whose tests are positive), and the *specificity* (proportion of individuals without the condition whose tests are negative (Bloch, 1987; Nachemson, 1992; Henderson *et al.*, 1994)).

Physical examination

In many cases, the shortcomings of physical examination and imaging procedures are recognized. However, the value of subjective pain diagrams (Figure 20.4), including the visual analogue scale, and simple psychological questionnaires, for example, Oswestry Back Pain Disability Questionnaire (Fairbank *et al.*, 1980), Neck Disability Index Questionnaire (Vernon and Mior, 1991), Psychosocial Assessment Questionnaire (Main and Waddell, 1984) are accepted for their valuable role in helping the clinician to come to a probable diagnosis.

Treatment

It is important to realize that effective treatment must be based on an accurate exclusion diagnosis of the aetiology of back pain, with or without referred leg pain, bearing in mind that, in the majority of cases of back pain with or without referred leg pain of mechanical origin, a precise diagnosis cannot be made (Margo, 1994). However, it is essential to exclude disease processes and psychological conditions which should be treated by a medical or surgical approach, rather than by spinal mechanical therapy. In the preceeding chapter, psychosocial and psychiatric approaches were described, and in Chapter 21, medical and surgical approaches to the problem of low back pain with or without referred leg pain of mechanical origin are presented. This is followed by chiropractic (Chapter 22), osteopathy (Chapter 23) and physiotherapy (Chapter 24) approaches to mechanical spinal pain with or without referred leg pain. In some instances, particularly chronic pain syndromes, patients would obviously benefit from a multidisciplinary team approach.

References

Adams, M.A., Dolan, P. and Hutton, W.C. (1986) The stages of disc degeneration as revealed by discogram. *J. Bone Joint Surg.*, **68B**, 36.

Ando, T. and Mimatsu, K. (1993) Traumatic lumbar disc herniation. A case report. *Spine*, **18**, 2355-2357.

Barr, M.L. and Kiernan, J.A. (1983) *The Human Nervous System. An Anatomical Viewpoint*, 4th edn. Harper and Row, Philadelphia.

Beaumont, B. and Paice, E. (1992) Back pain. *O..cas. Pap. R. Coll. Gen. Pract.*, **58**, 36-38.

Benini, A. (1987) Clinical features of cervical root compression C5-C8 and their variations. *Neuro-Orthop.*, **4**, 74-88.

Bigos, S., Bowyer, O., Braen, G. *et al.* (1994) *Acute Low Back Problems in Adults: Assessment and Treatment.* Quick reference guide for clinicians Number 14. US Department of Health and Human Services, Public Health Service, Agency for Health Care Policy and Research, Rockville, Maryland: AHCPR Pub. No. 95-0643.

Bloch, R. (1987) Methodology in clinical back pain trials. *Spine*, **12**, 430.

Boden, S.D. and Wiesel, S.W. (1990) Lumbosacral segmental motion in normal individuals. *Spine*, **15**, 571-576.

Bowman, J.M. (1994) Experiencing the chronic pain phenomenon: a study. *Rehabil. Nurs.*, **19**, 91-95.

Brown, M.D. (1975) Diagnosis of pain syndromes of the spine. *Orthop. Clin. North Am.*, **6**, 233-248.

Buirski, G. and Silberstein, M. (1993) The symptomatic lumbar disc in patients with low back pain: magnetic resonance imaging appearances in both a symptomatic and control population. *Spine*, **18**, 1808-1811.

Chan, C.W., Goldman, S. and Ilstrup, D.M. (1993) The pain drawing and Waddell's nonorganic physical signs in chronic low-back pain. *Spine*, **18**, 1717-1722.

Cherkin, D.C., Deyo, R.A. and Wheeler, K. (1994) Physician variation in diagnostic testing for low back pain. Who you see is what you get. *Arthritis Rheum.*, **37**, 15-22.

Chila, A.G., Jeffries, R.R. and Levin, S.M. (1990) Is manipulation for your practice? *Patient Care*, **May 15**, 77-92.

Chusid, J.G. (1985) *Correlative Neuroanatomy and Functional Neurology*, 19th edn. Lange Medical Publications, Los Altos, CA, p. 376.

Collins, R.D. (1968) *Illustrated Manual of Laboratory Diagnosis.* J.B. Lippincott, Philadelphia.

Day, L.J., Bovill, E.G., Trafton, P.G. *et al.* (1994) Orthopedics. In *Current Surgical Diagnosis and Treatment* (L.W. Way, ed.). Prentice-Hall, New York, p. 1101.

Deyo, R.A., Bass, J.E., Walsh, N.E. *et al.* (1988) Prognostic variability among chronic pain patients: implications for study design, interpretation, and reporting. *Arch. Phys. Med. Rehabil.*, **69**, 174-178.

Dorland's Illustrated Medical Dictionary. 25th edn. W.B. Saunders, Philadelphia.

Duncan, W. and Hoen, T.I. (1942) A new approach to the diagnosis of herniation of the intervertebral disc. *Surg. Gynecol. Obstet.*, **75**, 257-267.

Dvorak, J., Panjabi, M.M. and Novotny, J.E. (1991) Clinical validation of functional flexion-extension roentgenograms of the lumbar spine. *Spine*, **16**, 943-945.

Dyck, P. (1985) Paraplegia following chemonucleolysis. *Spine*, **10**, 359.

El-Khoury, G.Y. and Renfrew, D.L. (1991) Percutaneous procedures for the diagnosis and treatment of lower back pain: discography, facet-joint injection and epidural injection. *Am. J. Roentgenol.*, **157**, 685-691.

Empting-Koschorke, L.D., Hendler, N., Kolodny, A.L. *et al.* (1990) Tips on hard-to-manage pain syndromes. *Patient Care*, **April 30**, pp. 26-46.

Fager, C.A. (1994) Observations on spontaneous recovery from intervertebral disc herniation. *Surg. Neurol.*, **42**, 282-286.

Fairbank, J., Davies, J. and Coupar, J. (1980) The Oswestry low back pain disability questionnaire. *Physiotherapy*, **66**, 271-273.

Ghormley, R.K. (1933) Low back pain with special reference to the articular facets with presentation of an operative procedure. *J. Am. Med. Assoc.*, **101**, 1773-1777.

Ghormley, R.K. (1958) An etiologic study of back pain. *Radiology*, **70**, 649-652.

Giles, L.G.F. (1984) Letter to the Editor. *Spine*, **8**, 842.

Giles, L.G.F. (1989) *Anatomical Basis of Low Back Pain.* Williams and Wilkins, Baltimore.

Giles, L.G.F. and Taylor, J.R. (1981) Low back pain associated with leg length inequality. *Spine*, **6**, 510-521.

Goupille, P., Fitoussi, V., Cotty, P. *et al.* (1993) Arthro-infiltrations des articulaires posterieures lombaires dans les lombalgies chroniques. Resultats chez 206 patients. *Rev. Rheum. Ed. Fr.*, **60**, 797-801.

Grönblad, M., Weinstein, J.N. and Santavirta, S. (1991a) Immunohistochemical observations on spinal tissue innervation. *Acta Orthop. Scand.*, **62**, 614-622.

Grönblad, M., Korkala, O., Konttinen, Y.T. *et al.* (1991b) Silver impregnation and immunohistochemical study of nerves in lumbar facet joint plical tissue. *Spine*, **16**, 34-38.

Gross, D. (1979) Multifactorial diagnosis and therapy for low back pain. In *Advances in Pain Research and Therapy*, Vol. 3. Raven Press, New York, pp. 671-683.

Haldeman, S. (1977) Why one cause of back pain? In *Approaches to the Validation of Manipulation Therapy* (A.A. Buerger and T.S. Tobis, eds), Charles C. Thomas, Springfield, IL, pp. 187-197.

Haldeman, S., Chapman-Smith, D. and Paterson, D.M. (1993) *Guidelines for Chiropractic Quality Assurance and Practice Parameters.* Aspen, Gaithersburg, pp. 55-80.

Hart, F.D. (1985) Back, pain in. In *French's Index of Differential Diagnosis* (F.D. Hart, ed.), 12th edn. Butterworth, Oxford, pp. 72-73.

Henderson, D., Chapman-Smith, D., Mior, S. *et al.* (1994) Clinical guidelines for chiropractic practice in Canada. *J. Can. Chioprac. Assoc. (Suppl.)*, **38**.

Herr, C.H. and Williams, J.C. (1994) Supralevator anorectal abscess presenting as acute low back pain and sciatica. *Ann. Emerg. Med.*, **23**, 132-135.

Hoppenfeld, S. (1976) *Physical Examination of the Spine and Extremities.* Appleton-Century-Crofts, New York.

Hoppenfeld, S. (1977) *Orthopaedic Neurology: A Diagnostic Guide to Neurologic Levels.* J. B. Lippincott, Philadelphia.

Huskisson, E.C. (1974) Measurement of pain. *Lancet*, **2**, 1127-1131.

Jackson, R.P. (1992) The facet syndome. Myth or reality? *Clin. Orthop. Rel. Res.*, **279**, 110-121.

Jenner, J.R. and Barry, M. (1995) Low back pain. *BMJ*, **310**, 929-932.

Jinkins, J.R. (1993) The pathoanatomic basis of somatic and autonomic syndromes originating in the lumbosacral spine. *Neuroimag. Clin. North Am.*, **3**, 443-463.

Keim, H.A. and Kirkaldy-Willis, W.H. (1987) *Clinical Symposia. Low Back Pain.* **39**. Ciba-Geigy, Jersey.

Kirkaldy-Willis, W.H. and Tchang, S. (1988) Diagnostic techniques. In *Managing Low Back Pain* (W.H. Kirkaldy-Willis, ed.), 2nd edn. Churchill Livingstone, New York, pp. 155-181.

Knight, R.Q. (1993) Complementary angles. A simplification of sagittal plane rotational assessment in cervical instability. *Spine*, **18**, 755-758.

Kuslich, S.D., Ulstrom, C.L. and Michael, E.J. (1991) The tissue origin of low back pain and sciatica: a report of pain response to tissue stimulation during operations on the lumbar spine using local anesthesia. *Orthop. Clin. North Am.*, **22**, 181-187.

Le-Breton, C., Meziou, M. and Laredo, J.D. (1993) Sarcomes pagetiques rechidiens. A propos de huit observations. *Rev. Rhum. Ed. Fr.*, **60**, 16-22.

Mackenzie, I. (1985) Spine, tenderness of. In *French's Index of Differential Diagnosis* (F.D. Hart, ed.), 12th edn. Butterworth, Oxford, p. 788.

MacMillan, J., Schaffer, J.L. and Kambin, P. (1991) Routes and incidence of communication of lumbar discs with surrounding neural structures. *Spine*, **16**, 167-171.

Main, C.J. and Waddell, G. (1982) Chronic pain, distress and illness behaviour. In *Clinical Psychology and Medicine: A Behavioural Perspective* (C.J. Main, ed.). Plenum, New York, pp. 1-62.

Main, C.J. and Waddell, G. (1984) The detection of psychological abnormality in chronic low back pain using four simple scales. *Curr. Concep. Pain*, **2**, 10-15.

Margo, K. (1994) Diagnosis, treatment and prognosis in patients with low back pain. *Am. Fam. Phys.*, **49**, 171-179.

McCowin, P.R., Borenstein, D. and Wiesel, S.W. (1991) The current approach to the medical diagnosis of low back pain. *Orthop. Clin. North Am.*, **22**, 325-325.

Merz, B. (1986) The honeymoon is over: spinal surgeons begin to divorce themselves from chemonucleolysis. *JAMA*, **256**, 317.

Michel, B.A., Lane, N.E., Jones, H.H., *et al.* (1990) Plain radiographs can be used in estimating lumbar bone density. *J. Rheumatol.*, **17**, 528-531.

Mooney, V. and Robertson, J. (1976) The facet syndrome. *Clin. Orthop. Rel. Res.*, **115**, 149-156.

Moore, K.L. (1992) *Clinically Oriented Anatomy*, 3rd edn. Williams and Wilkins, Baltimore.

Morgan, F.P. and King, T. (1957) Primary instability of lumbar vertebrae as a common cause of low back pain. *J. Bone Joint Surg.*, **39B**, 6-22.

Murtagh, J. (1991) Low back pain. *Aust. Fam. Phys.*, **20**, 320-326.

Murtagh, J.E. (1994) The non pharmacological treatment of back pain. *Aust. Prescrib.*, **17**, 9-12.

Nachemson, A.L. (1992) Newest knowledge of low back pain. A critical look. *Clin. Orthop. Rel. Res.*, **279**, 8-20.

Nachemson, A.L. and Andersson, G.B.J. (1982) Classification of low-back pain. *Scand. J. Work Environ. Health*, **8**, 134-136.

O'Reilly, S. (1994) Treatment of chronic non malignant pain in general practice. *Aust. Fam. Phys.*, **23**, 2274-2283.

Pope, M.H. and Novotny, J.E. (1993) Spinal biomechanics. *J. Biomech. Eng.*, **115**, 569-574.

Quiring, D.P. and Warfel, J.H. (1960) *The Extremities*, 2nd edn. Kimpton, London.

Riihimaki, H. (1991) Low-back pain, its origin and risk indicators. *Scand. J. Work Environ. Health*, **17**, 81-90.

Saal, J.A., Saal, J.S. and Herzog, R.J. (1990) The natural history of lumbar intervertebral disc extrusions treated nonoperatively. *Spine*, **15**, 683-686.

Sandoz, R. (1971) Newer trends in the pathogenesis of spinal disorders. In *Annals of the Swiss Chiropractors' Association* (E. Valentine, ed.), vol. V. Imprimeries Populairesm, Geneva.

Sato, H. and Kikuchi, S. (1993) The natural history of radiographic instability of lumbar spine. *Spine*, **18**, 2075-2079.

Schroeder, S.A., Tierney, L.M., McPhee, S.J. *et al.* (1992) *Current Medical Diagnosis and Treatment*. Appleton and Lange, Connecticut.

Schwarzer, A.C., Aprill, C.N., Derby, R. *et al.* (1994a) Zygapophysial joint in chronic low back pain. *Spine*, **19**, 801-806.

Schwarzer, A.C., Aprill, C.N., Derby, R. *et al.* (1994b) Clinical features of patients with pain stemming from the lumbar zygapophysial joints. Is the lumbar facet syndrome a clinical entity? *Spine*, **19**, 1132-1137.

Shaffer, W.O., Spratt, K.F., Weinstein, J. *et al.* (1990) The consistency and accuracy of roentgenograms for measuring sagittal translation in the lumbar vertebral motion segment: an experimental model. *Spine*, **15**, 741-750.

Spratt, K.F., Lehmann, T.R. and Weinstein, J.N. (1990) A new approach to the low-back physical examination. Behavioural assessment of mechanical signs. *Spine*, **15**, 96-102.

Stolker, R.J., Vervest, A.C.M. and Goren, G.J. (1994) The management of chronic spinal pain by blockades; a review. *Pain*, **58**, 1-20.

Tierney, L.M. (1992) Blood vessels and lymphatics. In *Current Medical Diagnosis and Treatment* (S.A. Schroeder, L.M. Tierney, S.J. McPhee *et al.* eds), Appleton and Lange, Connecticut, pp. 373.

Toyone, T., Takahashi, K., Kitahara, H. *et al.* (1994) Vertebral bone-marrow changes in degenerative lumbar disc disease. An MRI study of 74 patients with low back pain. *J. Bone Joint Surg.*, **76B**, 757-764.

Vernon, H. and Mior, S. (1991) The neck disability index: a study of reliability and validity. *J. Manipulative Physiol. Ther.*, **14**, 409-415.

Watts, C. and Dickhaus, E. (1986) Chemonucleolysis: a note of caution. *Surg. Neurol.*, **26**, 236.

Weinstein, J.N. (1988) The perception of pain. In *Managing Low Back Pain* (W.H. Kirkaldy-Willis, ed.), 2nd edn. Churchill Livingstone, New York, pp. 83-90.

Weinstein, S.M., Herring, S.A. and Shelton, J.L. (1990) Injured worker: assessment and treatment. *Phys. Med. Rehabil.: State of the Art Reviews*, **4**, 361-377.

Weitz, E.M. (1981) The lateral bending sign. *Spine*, **6**, 388-397.

Weitz, E.M. (1984) Paraplegia following chymopapain injection. *J. Bone Joint Surg.*, **66A**, 1131.

White, A.A. and Gordon, S.L. (1982) Synopsis: workshop on idiopathic low back pain. *Spine*, 7, 141-149.

Wigh, R. (1980) The thoracolumbar and lumbosacral transitional junctions. *Spine*, **5**, 215-222.

Yong-Hing, K. (1988) Surgical techniques. In *Managing Low Back Pain* (W.H. Kirkaldy-Willis, ed.), 2nd edn. Churchill Livingstone, New York, pp. 315-343.

Young, W.B. (1993) The clinical diagnosis of lumbar radiculopathy. *Semin. Ultrasound CT MRI*, **14**, 385-388.

21

Medical and surgical management of low back pain of mechanical origin

Bruce R. Knolmayer, Robert McAlindon and Sam W. Wiesel

Introduction

Mechanical disorders of the lumbosacral spine are the most common cause of low back pain. Mechanical back pain may be defined as pain secondary to overuse, injury, or deformity of a structure. These disorders are generally quite specific and local in nature, affecting a specific anatomic location or relationship. Systemic illness plays no role in the aetiology of mechanical low back pain. The presence of systemic complaints should alert the clinician that the cause of pain may not be lumbosacral in nature. Mechanical disorders often have cyclical periods of pain followed by periods of partial resolution. They often are exacerbated by specific activities and relieved by others. Both the medical history and physical examination can help localize the disorder to specific locations within the lumbosacral spine. A good history and physical examination along with the proper imaging studies should suffice in formulating a working diagnosis of the mechanical pathology. This chapter will review the five most common mechanical disorders that cause symptoms: back strain, herniated disc, spinal stenosis, and spondylolisthesis (Table 21.1). Each will be addressed with regard to history, physical, diagnostic studies, prognosis, and treatment.

Table 21.1 *Comparison of the mechanical causes of low back pain*

	Muscle strain	Herniated nucleus pulposus	Osteoarthritis	Spinal stenosis	Spondylolisthesis
Age (years)	20–40	30–50	>50	>60	20
Pain pattern Location	Back (unilateral)	Back (unilateral)	Back (unilateral)	Leg (unilateral)	Back
Onset	Acute	Acute (prior episodes)			
Standing	↑	↓	↑	↑	↑
Sitting	↓	↑	↓	↓	↓
Bending	↑	↑	↓	↓	↑
Straight leg	–	+	–	+ (stress)	–
Plain X-ray	–	–	+	+	+

From Borenstein, Wiesel and Boden, 1995

Back strain

Definition

Back strain is defined as a non-radiating low back pain associated with a mechanical stress to the lumbosacral spine. Most people with low back pain actually have an underlying mechanical cause (Nachemson, 1976). Furthermore, 60–70% will have back strain as a common cause among those with mechanical low back pain.

Pathophysiology

Back strain may result from a variety of underlying conditions with several different causes. These include damage to muscle and ligaments, microtears in the anulus fibrosus, or an anatomic abnormality. Muscle strain leading to symptoms may occur by several different mechanisms. Direct or indirect trauma may cause muscle fibre damage. This damage to the muscle unit may be a simple stretching of the myofibrils, or a complete disruption of the musculo-tendinous unit. Muscle fatigue and overuse may also lead to muscle strain. As a muscle fatigues, it depletes its natural aerobic energy sources and must depend on anaerobic mechanisms for fuel. The byproduct of anaerobic mechanisms, lactic acid, tends to accumulate in these circumstances. If lactate levels reach a high enough concentration, crystallization may occur. These lactate crystals, and indeed the lactate itself, act to mechanically irritate, inflame, and damage the muscle–ligamentous unit. Inflammation of the muscle fibres initiates a complex cascade which, itself, leads to further accumulation of acute phase reactants and which may perpetuate the inflammatory response. Pain and oedema ensue, and the patient experiences low back pain. Furthermore, muscle spasm may also lead to muscle strain. Prolonged contraction will, eventually, lead to impaired blood flow to the muscle itself. If the contraction persists, transient ischaemia results which can lead to pain. Paraspinous muscles may become deconditioned after injury. This diminution of muscle mass is observed clinically as a decrease in muscle power. Both fatiguability and strength may be compromised in an individual who is then at risk for further muscle injury, and pain, as a result of any physical activity.

Low back pain due to muscle strain may also be seen in individuals who undertake activity in excess of the support provided by the muscular–ligamentous–bony axis. The force placed on the lumbosacral spine cannot be resisted by the musculature or, if the muscle is fatigued by the force, the force eventually becomes transmitted to the ligaments, zygapophysial (facet) joints, and eventually the disc. Disruption of annular fibres may occur, which can generate pain (Farfan *et al.*, 1970). The facet joints then become subjected to increased weight-bearing. This may lead to premature wear on the articulations, as well as arthritic symptomatology. Both the anular fibre fissuring, as well as the facet joint becoming a load bearing structure, may lead to back strain.

If the lumbosacral spine or surrounding structures are anatomically abnormal, 'normal motion' may result in strain pain (Borenstein *et al.*, 1995). Patients with abnormal or asymmetric facet joints have restriction of motion. With this in mind, joint surfaces may receive different amounts of load as compared to normal individuals. A greater degree in orientation, or abnormality in orientation of the facet joints, as compared to those in a normal spine, will suggest a differing amount of load transferred across their surfaces. Supporting structures around the facet joints may then be forced to bear a greater burden of load as a compensatory mechanism. In this instance, normal motions are gained only through abnormal mechanisms. This may lead to damage in the compensatory structures including the muscles, ligaments, discs, and some bony structures. This anatomic variation may be located anywhere within the postural axis from the thorax to the lower back/pelvis to the legs. An example of this process may be the low back pain found in the patient with tight hamstrings. Tight hamstrings limit full extension of the lumbar spine, resulting in greater stretching forces being placed on the interspinous ligaments. This continuous stress on the ligaments may eventually lend itself to strain and pain.

History, physical examination and diagnostic studies

When questioning patients about their back pain, they often complain of low back pain which does not radiate. The pain may be limited to a small focal area, or it may involve a wide diffuse area, of the lumbosacral spine. There may be referred-type pain to the buttocks or the posterior thigh, since both lower back and posterior thigh structures originate from the same embryonic origin. This pain never radiates below the knee, and should not be confused with true radiculopathy. If the low back pain is sudden in onset, and follows a known injury, it will worsen in both intensity and size of distribution over a few hours. This change in pain characteristic probably represents an inflammatory oedema in the injured structure, with a concomitant reflex contraction of the surrounding musculature. Flexion and/or extension of the spine during this period may also exacerbate the pain.

The usual physical findings are limited to local tenderness over the involved area with limited motion. Patients with low back pain often have painful attacks that will vary and may be stratified into three levels. Mild back pain is associated with subjective pain without objective findings. Patients are frequently able to return to their usual activities in less than a week. Moderate back strain is characterized by pain as well as a physical objective finding, such as decreased range of spinal motion or palpable muscle spasm. Activity is generally limited for 2 weeks. Severe back strain may cause patients to tilt toward one side when ambulating. Ambulation itself becomes difficult, and full recovery may take as long as 6–8 weeks. The patient with back strain has no neurological deficits. Both radiographic and laboratory findings in patients with back strain are normal. If the clinician is confident in his diagnosis of back strain, then no radiographic examination is necessary (Deyo and Diehl, 1986).

Treatment and prognosis

Therapy for patients with low back strain includes controlled physical activity, non-steroidal anti-inflammatory medications, muscle relaxants, and physical therapy. A short period of bed rest, generally less than 2 days, should be sufficient to allow the pain to subside. Bed rest of 7 or more days has been shown to be of no additional benefit to the patient with back strain (Deyo *et al.*, 1986). Initially, limited physical activity allows the injured tissues to rest, permitting a greater opportunity for healing without re-injury.

Non-steroidal anti-inflammatory medications are helpful in making patients comfortable while their injury heals. Rapid onset medications are recommended and must be continued until the patient's symptoms have resolved. Muscle relaxants are helpful in patients with palpable spasm or muscle pain which either limits daily activities or inhibits normal sleeping patterns. The combination of non-steroidal anti-inflammatory medication, and muscle relaxant therapy, is quite effective at blunting the acute pain and allowing early mobilization of the lower spine in patients with back strain. Furthermore, physical therapy modalities may help to decrease pain and spasm. As soon as the very acute pain is diminished, patients are encouraged to increase their physical activity. A physical therapist may be of benefit in encouraging mobility and helping to maintain range of motion in the patient. A local injection of anaesthetic may help relieve muscle spasm in patients refractory to the NSAID/muscle relaxant protocol. The injection provides an anaesthetic relief to the local pain, and may also block the reflex spasm which may occur with back strain. Braces are reserved only for those patients who must remain active during the healing phase. The braces help to limit the amount of motion that may lead to impairment of healing and may also add an element of support to the damaged musculoskeletal bony axis.

Patients with back strain generally improve over a 2-week period. About 90% of patients are free of back strain symptoms by 2 months (Dillane *et al.*, 1966). Recovery can be expected to be complete and without lasting impairment. Ten percent of patients, however, may continue to experience low back pain. The pain may continue for months or years. These individuals who develop a chronic pain after back strain must be evaluated and treated in a manner that takes into account the specific difficulties of individuals with chronic low back pain. A more extensive protocol including psychiatric support, vocational rehabilitation, and physical therapy may be necessary.

The vast majority of patients with an episode of low back strain are at risk for future episodes which are more severe and of greater duration (Troup *et al.*, 1981). The risk for an additional episode of back pain lessens after 2 years. About one-half of all patients can expect a second episode of back strain within 5 years.

Acute herniated nucleus pulposus

Definition

A herniated disc can be defined as a protrusion of the nucleus pulposus through the fibres of the anulus fibrosus (Mixter and Barr, 1934). Most disc ruptures occur in the third or fourth decade of life, while the nucleus is still gelatinous. The herniation usually protrudes in a posterolateral direction, tending to compress the adjacent nerve root. Herniation can be classified as bulging, protruding, extruding, or sequestered (American Academy of Orthopaedic Surgeons, 1987). In the bulging and protruding types, the posterior longitudinal ligament remains intact although the nucleus pulposus impinges on the anulus fibrosus. In the extruding type, the nucleus pulposus is emerging through the anulus fibrosus but is confined by the posterior longitudinal ligament. On the other hand, in the sequestered type, the ligament has been disrupted and a portion of the disc has protruded into the epidural space.

Pathophysiology

Intervertebral discs protrude because of attritional and degenerative changes. Disc degeneration itself may play a role in low back pain but it also is very important in herniation of the intervertebral discs. The intervertebral discs themselves are composed primarily of collagen and mucopolysaccharides. Beginning early in the third decade of life, the collagenous bundles begin to show signs of deterioration, which progresses throughout life.

The mechanism by which disc herniation causes irritation of the nerve root is not fully understood, but is believed to be a result of mechanical and chemical factors. A mechanical compression can be expected to cause ischaemia and ipsilateral neurologic dysfunction, with inflammation of the compressed root. An injured disc may also result in production of irritant substances which can leak into the spinal canal, causing irritation of the nerve roots.

The most likely time of day for disc herniation is in the morning. This probably represents an optimal opportunity for herniation when such factors as disc height, disc water content, and spinal position are considered. The herniation usually occurs through a defect just lateral to the midline posteriorly, where the posterior longitudinal ligament is weakest. The most common levels of herniation are L5–S1 and L4–L5 which account for about 90% of all herniations (Sprangforth, 1972). Only 35% of all patients with a herniated disc will develop radiculopathy. The development of radiculopathy depends on the size of the individual's canal, the location of the herniation, and the extent to which the herniation occurs. Patients with very capacious spinal canals may have no impingement of the spinal root by the nucleus pulposus. As a result, radiculopathy may be totally absent, and back pain may be minimal. Patients with smaller canals have no room for the protruding nucleus, and impingement of the neural elements will occur. As expected, the greater the amount of nucleus that protrudes, the greater the chance for neural compromise, while bulging discs in which the nucleus does not completely penetrate the anulus may produce minimal symptoms. Central protrusions may affect neural elements at lower levels. Discs which protrude in an extremely lateral position may affect the nerve root at that level. The common location of a mid-lateral herniation will affect the inferior nerve root. An L5–S1 mid-lateral herniation, for example, primarily involves the S1 nerve root.

History, physical examination and diagnostic studies

The patient typically presents with a sharp, excruciating pain. It may not only present in the lower back, but may also radiate down the leg in the anatomic distribution of the affected nerve root. In many cases, there may be a prior history of intermittent episodes of low back pain. These episodes may represent fissuring or tearing of the anulus and subsequent inflammation of the sinuvertebral nerve. The disc herniation itself occurs with a sudden physical effort when the trunk is flexed, or rotated. The radiculopathy may vary in intensity. Some patients are unable to ambulate because of pain and may feel as though their back is locked. Other individuals may only experience a dull ache which increases in intensity with ambulation. In general, the radiculopathy is worsened when the spine is flexed and relieved when the spine is extended. Those with herniated discs may have increased pain with sitting, driving, walking, coughing, or performing a Valsalva-type manoeuvre.

Patients with herniated discs either may have no objective physical findings or may exhibit a large variety of them. Many of the physical examination findings depend on the amount of neural involvement, and the irritation of the sinuvertebral nerve, with its subsequent back pain symptomatology. Many patients will demonstrate a decrease in the range of motion of the lumbosacral spine. Patients may list to one side as they bend forward. When ambulating, patients may exhibit an antalgic gait, or hold the involved leg flexed, in order to minimize the weight bearing on the affected side.

The neurological examination can be quite variable. Objective evidence of nerve root compression may, or may not, be present. It is possible to have mild nerve root impingement that causes pain yet leaves enough room for the nerve root to function normally. In this example, no motor abnormality would be seen. The neurological examination may also help to localize the level of nerve root impairment. A mid-lateral L5–S1 disc herniation will affect the S1 nerve root, as mentioned above. The patient may display gastrocnemius or soleus weakness, and posterior calf sensory changes. The patient found to have weakness in great toe extension, and a sensory deficit over the anterior leg, would most likely have herniation at the L4–L5 level with compression of the L5 root. Nerve root sensitivity can be demonstrated by manoeuvres that place the root under tension. The straight leg raising test is probably the most common. This test is considered positive if pain develops below the knee, or if the patient's radicular symptomatology is reproduced, when the leg on the affected side is flexed at the hip. This places that nerve on stretch, thereby exacerbating the radicular-type symptoms. Back pain and/or buttock pain alone does not indicate a positive test in this instance.

Plain X-rays may be entirely normal in patients with herniated discs. CT scan, myelography, and MRI are helpful in discovering the pathology and determining the exact level. The CT scan may demonstrate a disc bulge but may not be sensitive enough to determine the exact level of neural compromise. Myelography is good in identifying the affected level but is invasive and has the potential risks of dye toxicity and dural pathology. As a result, MRI has become the gold standard for clinical diagnosis (Figure 21.1). Both posterior and far lateral herniations can be detected with this imaging modality. Migratory fragments may also be discovered. It is important to remember that the radiographic finding of herniation becomes important only in the clinical setting of a patient who demonstrates historical and physical findings of radiculopathy.

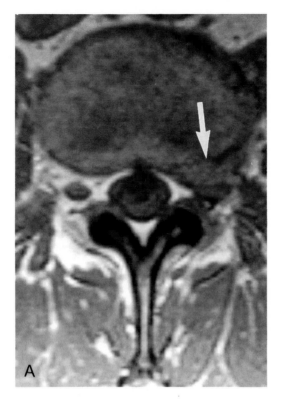
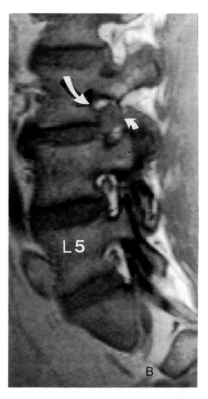

Figure 21.1 MRI of the lumbar spine. Transverse (A) and sagittal (B) views of a 53-year-old man with chronic low back pain, associated with radicular symptoms. This MRI in the transverse view reveals a large herniated disc at the L3–L4 intervertebral level (arrow). The sagittal view demonstrates this herniation (white arrows) (courtesy of Dr L.G.F. Giles).

Treatment and prognosis

Eighty percent of patients with herniated discs will respond to non-operative treatment (Weber, 1978). In the majority of cases, this is sufficient to allow return to normal daily function. If patients have insight into the rationale for treatment, the chances for success are very good. The primary element for non-operative management is controlled physical activity. For the first few days, bed rest may be necessary in acute herniation. The semi-Fowler position, in which the hips and knees are flexed, minimizes intradiscal pressure and decreases nerve root tension (Boren-stein *et al.*, 1995). Once the acute pain has subsided, the patient is gently mobilized. Sitting is minimized because it causes increased pressure on the nerve root. Ambulation is increased as tolerated, while exercises, which increase back and abdominal strength as supportive measure are undertaken.

Drug therapy, including muscle relaxants and non-steroidal anti-inflammatory medication, may also be used. The symptoms of low back pain and radiculo-pathy are influenced by a large inflammatory response to the herniation itself. The patient's pain will generally be relieved once the inflammation is controlled. There may be a small amount of residual numbness or tingling in the involved extremity, but this is usually tolerable to the patient. If an adequate course of non-steroidal anti-inflammatory medication has proven unsuccessful, a short course of steroidal medication may be attempted. Muscle relaxants are used in patients with uncontrollable muscle con-tracture associated with nerve root compression. The majority of these medications provide a tranquillizing effect which may be beneficial in the acute phase of herniation as well.

The next alternative in treatment is an epidural steroid injection. This medication is injected directly into the epidural space, near the area of the nerve root compression. Epidural injections have been shown to be 40% effective in actually relieving radicular pain. The maximum benefit is usually achieved within 2 weeks. These injections may be repeated another one or two times if some benefit has been observed.

Surgical intervention is reserved for patients in whom conservative measures have failed. Patients who have persistent pain, radicular symptomatology, and abnormal physical findings, as well as radiographic evidence of pathology, are candidates for surgical intervention. If the frequency and intensity of attacks are severe enough to interfere with the individual's ability to pursue employment and enjoy normal activities of daily living, surgery may be necessary.

Spinal stenosis

Definition

Spinal stenosis can be defined as narrowing of the spinal canal. The actual mechanical pressure exhibited on the contained neural structures will determine the degree of narrowing. The classification of spinal stenosis includes developmental and acquired forms. Degenerative causes are responsible for the vast majority of individuals with lumbar spinal stenosis.

Pathophysiology

Spinal stenosis represents an end point of the long-term arthritic process. Osteoarthritis is nearly universally present in individuals over 75 years of age (Lawrence *et al.*, 1966). This osteoarthritis, which commonly affects the lumbosacral spine, is a slowly progressive disorder which will lead to eventual narrowing of the spinal canal or frank spinal stenosis. The aetiology of osteoarthritis is multifactorial and implicated are genetic, biomechanical, and biochemical factors. Major changes occur in the lumbar spine between the third and fifth decades of life. The earliest changes are seen in the intervertebral discs. The nucleus pulposus loses water content and becomes firm. The anulus also fissures and begins to degenerate. As the disc loses height, stress is transmitted to the posterior elements including the ligaments and facet joints. These structures are ill-suited to sustain compressive, tensile, and shear loads. Capsular strain, hypermobility, and degenerative changes develop around the facet joints and osteophyte formation occurs both along the endplates and the neural foramina.

Biochemical and metabolic alterations in articular cartilage herald the onset of facet joint disease. The normal proteoglycan content present in articular cartilage changes over time and, with it, its mechanical properties. The shock absorbency of the cartilage is proportional to the proteoglycan content and its ability to bind water. The normal amount of proteoglycan diminishes with age and the glycosaminoglycan composition also changes. Chondroitin sulphate is reduced and eventually replaced with keratin

sulphate (Mankin, 1974). The result of these alterations lead to an excess amount of water retention by the cartilage itself. The shock absorbency is altered and the normal collagen matrix is disrupted (Mankin and Thrasher, 1975).

Biomechanical factors also alter cartilage which further leads to cartilage destruction. Coincidentally, along with the disc and facet joint cartilage changes, the ligamentum flavum also changes in response to abnormal stress. The ligament is compelled to assume variable tensile loads, brought on by the loss of disc height, and may undergo hypertrophy.

The osteophytic spurring, the cartilaginous loss, the facet hypermobility, and the hypertrophied ligamentum flavum all act to diminish the spinal canal size. Disc degeneration, the earliest manifestation of this process, may be painless. Once facet joint dysfunction occurs, pain may result. This stage of disease may have pain limited to a very local area directly over the joint itself. Extension of the spine will exacerbate symptoms at this time.

Symptoms of neural compromise, including radiculopathy and pseudoclaudication only occur when the disease process causes mechanical compression of the nerve root. The degree of symptomatology depends on the extent of the disease, the capacity of the spinal canal, and the shape of the canal. Patients with trefoil-shaped canals have been found to have greater susceptibility to spinal stenotic syndromes. As the spine ages, postural alterations (mainly increased lordosis) occur. These postural changes can lead to chronic muscle tension, back strain, and further worsening of low back pain symptoms.

The pathogenesis of symptoms of spinal stenosis remain unclear. Pseudoclaudication symptoms may stem from compression of vascular structures which result in diminished blood flow to the nerve root (Jellinger and Neumayer, 1972). This compression may affect arteries, capillaries, or veins. Another theory suggests that direct mechanical pressure on the nerve root leads to pseudoclaudication symptoms as well. Radicular symptoms in spinal stenosis closely mimic those seen with a herniated disc. Direct mechanical compression on the nerve root, either from the ligamentum flavum, an osteophyte, or an inflamed facet joint capsule, can cause sensory or motor impairment as well as pseudoclaudication.

History, physical examination, and diagnostic studies

Patients with osteoarthritis and spinal stenosis of the spine may complain of a broad range of symptoms. Patients with degenerative arthritis of the facet joints develop midline pain in the back, directly over those joints. Any body motion that compresses these joints, such as extension, worsens symptomatology. As the degenerative process continues, symptoms of canal compromise and neural impairment surface. Pseudoclaudication is associated with pain in the buttock, thigh, or leg that develops with standing or walking in the presence of normal blood flow. Walking distance may be curtailed. The majority of patients have both back and leg pain, and it is not unusual to have both legs affected at the same time. Any position that flexes the lumbar spine will be associated with some resolution of symptoms, while spinal extension worsens symptomatology. The physical findings in those patients with osteoarthritis and/or spinal stenosis can be variable. The patients may have a mild decrease in range of motion of the spine, or mild pain over specific facet joints. With more extensive disease, nerve impingement becomes a concern. Pseudoclaudication can be variable, from mild pain at the ends of long walks to severe pain simply with standing. Objective signs of muscle weakness, atrophy, and asymmetry of reflexes, may be noted. The patient's symptoms can often be reproduced on walking and positive neurological findings can be observed. This exercise trial may be referred to as a 'stress test' because it elicits the patient's symptoms, and aids in the diagnosis. In many cases, however, no objective clinical findings can be found on physical examination.

Plain radiographs are very helpful in visualizing osteophytic changes of the spine. Intervertebral disc degeneration is seen by narrowing of disc height. Traction osteophytes, decreased interpedicular distance, decreased sagittal diameter, and facet degeneration may be evident on plain radiographs. CT scan can help determine the shape and size of the canal and also the amount of canal impingement. Myelography will demonstrate subtotal or total obstruction of the canal by demonstrating inhibition of dye column flow down the spinal canal (Figure 21.2). A combined CT-myelogram is an excellent study, since it is dynamic and allows clear documentation of locations which are severely compressed. The role of MRI continues to be developed but at present is still limited because it is a static examination. With newer three-dimensional and contrast-imaging techniques, the MRI will increase in effectiveness for diagnosis of this disorder.

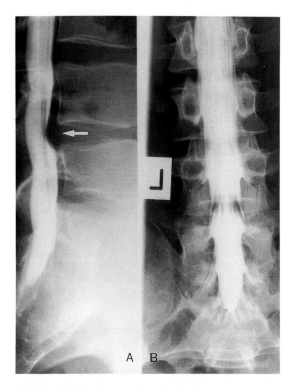

Figure 21.2 Myelogram of a 30-year-old man with significant stenosis at the L4–L5 region of the spine (arrow). This represents lateral (A) and postero-anterior (B) radiographs taken during the dynamic study (courtesy of Dr L.G.F. Giles).

Treatment and prognosis

The majority of patients with spinal stenosis or osteoarthritis of the spine can be treated non-surgically. Non-steroidal anti-inflammatory agents help control symptoms. Lumbosacral corsets are helpful in reminding the patient to avoid excessive spinal movement. Short courses of oral steroids are used in patients with extreme symptoms refractory to non-steroidal medication. Epidural steroids may be introduced, and have a direct effect on blunting the inflammatory response at the nerve root level. These non-surgical modalities may be repeated as necessary. Physical therapy, including deep heat, ultrasonography, and massage, may help to alleviate some of the low back symptoms associated with spinal stenosis and osteoarthritis. Although these modalities may provide short-term relief, it rarely provides long-term relief. Unfortunately, no cure exists for osteoarthritis, and as such, most patients with spinal stenosis have a relapsing in course with recurrent episodes of pain. Through modification of activities, and treatment of recurrences, however, most are able to avoid operative intervention.

Operative therapy requiring laminectomy to free the nerve root may be necessary in patients refractory to non-operative measures. Although the symptoms may be unilateral, a complete bilateral laminectomy to prevent future contralateral symptomatology is recommended. When the operation has been completed, all residual mechanical pressure on the nerve roots should have been eradicated by the procedure.

Spondylolisthesis

Definition

Spondylolisthesis is a condition in which all or part of the vertebral body has translated forward on another. The posterior elements, which include the facet joints, pedicles and lamina, and the pars interarticularis, are responsible for maintenance of the normal vertebral alignment. Without these structures, the remaining support of the column, including the anterior and posterior ligaments in the vertebral disc axis, is ill-suited to maintain normal spinal alignment. Should any disruption occur in any or all of these posterior supporting structures, translocation of one vertebral body forward on top of an adjacent vertebral body may occur.

Pathophysiology

The underlying defect in most cases of spondylolisthesis is a defect in the pars interarticularis. There also appears to be an underlying genetic component in many cases. Five types of spondylolisthesis are commonly recognized, types I–V (Wiltse *et al.*, 1976).

Type I, or dysplastic spinal listhesis is secondary to a congenital defect of either the superior sacral, or inferior L5, facets with slipping of the L5 body anteriorly on S1. The dysplastic spondylolisthetic patient has the defect present at birth. Usually, only a short period is needed until translation occurs.

Type II, or isthmic, represents the most common form of spondylolisthesis and may be secondary to a fracture or defect in the pars interarticularis, termed spondylolysis (Figure 21.3). The defect, if bilateral, will allow the eventual forward translation to occur. The actual pars defect may be an elongation which may represent a repaired fracture, a healing fracture, or a subacute fracture. The exact etiology of this defect in the spondylolytic patient is not clear. The lesion is rarely seen in children less than 5 years old. The most popular explanation is that the defect occurs in genetically predisposed individuals. The fracture eventually occurs through this weakened segment. The fracture itself is generally thought to be a fatigue-type fracture caused by repetitive continued subacute stresses. In the end, predisposed individuals who participate in sporting activities become more susceptible to this translation. Gymnasts and wrestlers may develop the condition early in life. Spondylolisthesis is a common cause of back pain in young individuals and is actually the most common cause of back pain in patients under the age of 26 years old.

Type III, or degenerative spondylolisthesis, occurs secondary to degeneration of the lumbar facet joints, with alteration of joint anatomy. There is no pars defect present in such a situation. The facet orienta-

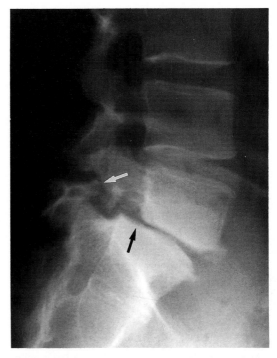

Figure 21.3 Lateral spot view of the lumbosacral junction demonstrating a type I spondylolisthesis with 25% slippage of the vertebral body (black arrow). Note also the pars defect as shown by the white arrow. This radiograph represents a Type II or isthmic spondylolisthesis (courtesy of Dr L.G.F. Giles).

tion, through a degenerative and remodelling process, takes on a more horizontal position which allows eventual movement of the vertebral bodies. As expected, degenerative spondylolisthesis occurs in the older patient, generally greater than 40 years old and evolves over a long period of time. The degenerative spondylolisthesis is most common at the L4–L5 level. Strong lumbosacral ligaments which connect the iliac wings to the L5 body predisposes the higher unprotected L4–L5 region to degenerative changes. The L4 vertebra has a relatively small transverse process, less ligamentous support, and more mobility. The facet joints at this L4–L5 level are also directed more sagittally than those at the lower L5–S1 vertebral area. This allows for more anterior motion. The excess stress results in advanced degenerative changes occurring at this level. Slippage is never greater than 30% of the body diameter of L5 because the spinous processes of L4 actually impact on this body. Facet joint arthritis, and disc space narrowing, are also commonly seen in this clinical setting as well.

The final two types are due to either trauma or an underlying pathologic process. Type IV, or traumatic spondylolisthesis, represents an acute fracture of a posterior element, either the pedicle, the lamina, or the facets. The pars interarticularis is not involved in this type of injury. The most common site is L4–L5. Type V, or pathologic spondylolisthesis, represents a structural weakness in the posterior elements due to a disease process.

History, physical examination and diagnostic studies

Pain is the most common symptom of spondylolisthesis and spondylolysis. In adolescents, the most common pain pattern associated with low-grade spondylolisthesis is a dull, aching pain in the back, buttocks, and posterior thigh. The cause of back pain presenting after age 30 in a patient with spondylolisthesis may not be due to a pars defect or slippage and other reasons for the back pain should be explored. Those older patients with symptomatology may complain of low back pain or leg pain which is posterolateral, going down the leg or up into the hip. The pain may increase with activity and decrease with rest.

On physical examination, patients may have an actual palpable step-off of the lumbar spine. This slip is recognized when the translation has reached 75% of the vertebral body inferior to it. The typical patient exhibits no scoliosis. Range of motion is generally normal. The neurological examination also is usually normal. If nerve root irritation is present, hamstring tightness may be elicited. Patients with this condition may waddle as they walk, and also exhibit flexion of the hips and knees with flattening of the lumbar lordosis, in an attempt to ease the low back pain.

Plain lateral radiographs of the lumbar spine will show translation of vertebral bodies. Oblique views may demonstrate pars interarticularis fractures if no frank translation is seen on lateral views. The actual amount of slippage is graded by the system of Meyerding: Grades 0–IV (Figure 3.16) (Meyerding, 1941). The top of the inferior vertebral body upon which the translation is occurring is divided into parallel quarters. A slip of 25% or less is Grade I, while the translation of 75% or more is considered Grade IV. Dynamic translation, defined as the change in position as the spine moves from extension to flexion, is also performed. Normal lumbar vertebral levels should have less than 3 mm of dynamic translation. X-rays taken in both flexion and extension can help the clinician determine the extent of dynamic translation. Other imaging modalities also may be useful. Bone scintigraphy may help define stress fractures of the pars interarticularis which may otherwise be difficult to diagnose. The MRI also plays a role when radiculopathy is present. The exact location and degree of neural impingement may be determined by MRI methods.

Treatment and prognosis

Non-operative treatment of spondylolisthesis is effective in the majority of patients with low back pain. Rest, anti-inflammatory medications, and protected activity will aid in the resolution of acute symptoms. Back and abdominal strengthening exercises are recommended to help support this area of the spine. Brace therapy may also be of benefit. Bracing in a younger patient may provide immediate symptomatic relief in a combination with flexion type exercises. It may also reduce the amount of lumbar lordosis and possibly the propensity to translate. Surgical fusion of the unstable segment is indicated only to relieve pain, not correct the translocation. Surgery may include spinal fusion for patients with low back pain symptoms and decompression for patients who also have nerve root irritation.

Conclusion

Mechanical disorders of the lumbosacral spine are the most common causes of low back pain. The most common include muscle strain, acute herniated nucleus pulposus, spinal stenosis, and spondylolisthesis. Although the pathophysiologies may differ, each has low back pain as a common complaint. Treatment modalities consist of both conservative and surgical means. Fortunately, most patients can be treated successfully with non-operative intervention including NSAIDs, rest, and/or physical therapy. However, when these measures fail, operative therapy may then be indicated.

References

American Academy of Orthopaedic Surgeons (1987) *A Glossary on Spinal Terminology*. American Academy of Orthopaedic Surgery, Chicago, pp. 34–35.

Borenstein, D., Wiesel, S. and Boden, S. (1995) *Low Back Pain: Medical Diagnosis and Comprehensive Management*, 2nd edn. W.B. Saunders, Philadelphia, pp. 183–217.

Deyo, R.A. and Diehl, A.K. (1986) Lumbar spine films in primary care: current use and selective ordering criteria. *J. Gen. Intern. Med.,* **1**, 20.

Deyo, R.A., Diehl, A.K. and Rosenthal, M. (1986) How many days of bed rest for acute low back pain? *N. Engl. J. Med.,* **315**, 1064.

Dillane, J.B., Fry, J. and Kalton, G. (1966) Acute back pain syndrome: a study from general practice. *Br. Med. J.,* **3**, 82.

Farfan, H.F., Cossette, J.W., Robertson, G.W. *et al.* (1970) Effects of torsion on lumbar intervertebral joints: the role of torsion in the production of disc degeneration. *J. Bone Joint Surg.,* **52A**, 468.

Jellinger, K. and Neumayer, E. (1972) Claudication of the spinal canal and cauda equina. In *Handbook of Clinical Neurology*, (P.J. Vinken and G.W. Bruyn, eds), Vol 12. Vascular Diseases of the Nervous System. North-Holland Publishing Company, Amsterdam, pp. 507–547.

Lawrence, J.S., Bremner, J.M. and Bier, F. (1966) Osteoarthrosis. Prevalence in the population and relationship between symptoms and X-ray changes. *Ann. Rheum. Dis.*, **25**, 1.

Mankin, H.J. (1974) The reaction of articular cartilage to injury and osteoarthritis. *N. Engl. J. Med.*, **291**, 1285, 1335.

Mankin, H.J. and Thrasher, Z.A. (1975) Water content and binding in normal and osteoarthritic human cartilage. *J. Bone Joint Surg.*, **57A**, 76.

Meyerding, H.W. (1941) Low backache and sciatic pain associated with spondylolisthesis and protruded intervertebral disc. *J. Bone Joint Surg.*, **23**, 461.

Mixter, W.J. and Barr, J.S. (1934) Rupture of the intervertebral disc with involvement of the spinal canal. *N. Engl. J. Med.*, **211**, 210.

Nachemson, A. (1976) The lumbar spine – an orthopedic challenge. *Spine*, **1**, 59.

Sprangforth, E.V. (1972) The lumbar disc herniation: a computer-aided analysis of 2,504 operations. *Acta Orthop. Scand. (Suppl.)*, **142**, 1.

Troup, J.D.G., Martin, J.W. and Lloyd, D.C.E.F. (1981) Backpain in industry: a prospective study. *Spine*, **6**, 61.

Weber, H. (1978) Lumbar disc herniation: a prospective study of prognostic factors including a controlled trial. *J. Oslo City Hosp.*, **28**, 36.

Wiltse, L.L., Newman, P.H. and Macnab, L. (1976) Classification of spondylolisthesis. *Clin. Orthop.*, **117**, 23.

22

Chiropractic management of low back pain of mechanical origin

S.H. Burns and D.R. Mierau

Introduction

This chapter deals with chiropractic assessment and treatment of patients with mechanical low back pain (LBP). For many years, chiropractors and their methods of treatment were viewed with curiosity and scepticism by allopathic medicine. Reasons for this included the cult-like reputation of chiropractic beliefs and practices, terminology used by practitioners that was meaningless or confusing to others, the training of chiropractors in private institutions, and the profession's poorly defined scope of practice.

In recent years there has been a shift in interest from philosophical dogma to scientific evaluation of the treatment, effects, and cost-effectiveness of spinal manipulation therapy (SMT). In fact, SMT is now the most studied form of treatment for back pain, supported by a considerable body of clinical research.

Although many original theories have proven to be inaccurate, it is notable that some early principles of the chiropractic paradigm are now well accepted within mainstream medicine. Early chiropractic doctrines are categorized below.

Principles that have become widely accepted:

- That *dysfunction* rather than *disease* is the main cause of backache in society.
- That the posterior joints are more commonly involved in back pain syndromes than is the intervertebral disc.
- That prolonged rest is not beneficial, but exercise and early return to activity are important in recovery from back injuries.

Beliefs that have largely been abandoned:

- 'The bone out of place theory' (that manipulation or adjustments change the position of vertebral alignment).
- That chiropractic treatment can change the morphological shape of the spine (e.g. change structural scoliosis).
- That the nervous system rather than the immune system is central to disease resistance.

Included in this chapter are the salient features of the typical history, examination and treatment of low back pain patients as performed in a chiropractic clinical setting. Clinical trials of efficacy and cost-effectiveness of chiropractic manipulation treatment for low back pain are also discussed.

Patient history

The nature of most back pain is such that an in-depth analysis of a patient's medical history is likely to reveal more about the diagnosis than is the physical examination. With a well documented and structured history the purpose of further testing is often to confirm an already suspected diagnosis. This can result in reduced costs and patient exposure, through the selective use of diagnostic tests, without increasing the risk of missing serious pathology (Deyo, 1986a; Deyo *et al.*, 1992).

In a chiropractic setting, the first purpose of the history should be to determine whether the patient's back pain is of mechanical or non-mechanical origin.

Table 22.1 *Patient history with various causes of low back pain*

Cancer	Infection	Fracture	Mechanical
Patient older than 50 years	IV drug abuse	Recent trauma	Often has associated injury
Previous history of cancer	Recent urinary tract infection	Patient is older than 50 years	Pain intensity affected by position
Patient has night pain	Recent skin infection	Long-term corticosteroid use	Rest brings relief
Unexplained weight loss	Unexplained fever	Osteoporosis	Responds to manual treatment
Failed physical treatment			Pain is recurrent in nature
Unremitting pain greater than 1 month			Pain improves with time

It is therefore more important to place the patient's problem into a diagnostic *category* than to determine its precise aetiology. The line of questioning, then, will initially focus on ruling out underlying pathology while considering mechanical causes. Table 22.1 summarizes typical historical aspects of various diagnostic categories of back pain.

Table 22.2 *Common low back pain syndromes*

Syndrome	Characteristic features
Posterior joint	Pain often sharp, with sclerotomal pattern referral to leg, usually above knee. Limitation in ROM is in extension/ipsilateral side-bending. Stiffness/tenderness to pressure over posterior joints.
Sacroiliac joint	Usually dull ache over SI/buttock. Worse with forward bending or contralateral side-bending. Pain when seated or rising. Referral into anterior thigh/groin. Some hip joint stress tests positive for SI joint pain.
Discogenic	Deep, dull, poorly localized pain. Not reproduced by palpation. Flattened lordosis. Limitation in forward bending.
Myofascial	Usually dull, unilateral pain. Myotomal referral pattern to leg, rarely below knee. Pain/limitation of motion when bending *away* from side of pain or forward.
Nerve root irritation/ entrapment	A sharp 'burning' pain with dermatomal/radicular pattern into leg. Leg pain may be worse than LBP. Pain/restriction on forward bending, contralateral side-bending. Positive nerve root tension signs (SLR, femoral stretch).

When it seems certain that pain is likely to be mechanical in nature, a more precise anatomical origin should be sought. Practitioners tend to think of back pain in terms of clinical syndromes. By definition, syndromes comprise a predictable set of signs and symptoms which, when taken together, implicate an anatomical source of pain. For LBP, these include posterior joint syndromes, sacroiliac joint syndrome, discogenic back pain, myofascial syndromes, thoracolumbar syndrome (including irritation of the cluneal nerve) and spinal joint dysfunction with nerve root irritation. Table 22.2 outlines features suggestive of various low back pain syndromes.

Examination

The typical chiropractic low back examination entails:

1. Inspection
2. Range-of-motion
3. Provocation (stress) tests
4. Neurological examination
5. Palpation
6. Specialized tests – when appropriate
7. Ancillary tests (usually radiographic or laboratory)
8. Questionnaires

These steps are discussed in further detail below.

1. Inspection

Inspection typically includes observation of the patient's general posture, gait, spinal curvatures, presence or absence of antalgia, or, in cases of trauma, spinal deformities suggestive of fracture. Practitioners have traditionally placed considerable emphasis on the role of posture and spinal morphology in the development of back pain. However, research evidence indicates that factors such as increased lumbar lordosis or small scoliotic curves are not in fact significant risk factors for LBP (Nilsonne and Lundgren, 1968; Collis and Ponseti, 1969; Rowe, 1969; Pope *et al.*, 1985; Battie *et al.*, 1990; Bigos *et al.*, 1992).

2. Range-of-motion

Range-of-motion testing can be important for several reasons and when taken into account can supply considerable information. In a condition notorious for its lack of objective or reproducible signs (Nelson *et al.*, 1979), range-of-motion testing is noteworthy for being at least moderately reproducible and reliable (McCombe *et al.*, 1989; Hyytiainen *et al.*, 1991). Therefore, limitations in spinal movement can be critical for documenting impairment or patient progress (Triano and Schultz, 1987). In addition, restriction of movement in various directions can implicate the anatomical structures responsible. For example, back pain from posterior joints may cause painful limitation of extension and lateral bending to the involved side. However, when soft tissue structures such as muscles and tendons are the primary cause of pain, the deficit may be in forward flexion or contralateral side-bending (Lewit, 1985). Albeit this is over-simplified, range-of-motion testing does have anatomically interpretative value. Conversely, full and pain-free range-of-motion in the presence of significant back pain should raise the suspicion of a non-mechanical cause.

Lumbar mobility can be assessed in a variety of ways; from simple but crude visual estimates to sophisticated computer goniometry. Lumbar movement is a function of combined spinal joint and hip joint movements. Although 'eyeballing' range-of-motion may be appropriate for everyday clinical purposes, it is not very precise, nor does it isolate the lumbar component from the combined total. Neither will using a tape measure for fingertip-to-floor distance, but it is more precise. However, using a tape measure and the modified Schober's test will give an estimate of true lumbar motion (Macrae and Wright, 1969). Goniometers, which may be gravity or computer-based give a more accurate measure yet (Gill *et al.*, 1988). Whether or not a device measures isolated lumbar motion or combined hip/back motion is a function of the instrument's design. Goniometers are more commonly used in cases with medical/legal issues (e.g. assessment of impairment) or for the purposes of clinical research.

3. Pain provocation tests

These tests are designed to isolate and stress specific anatomical structures and when painful, implicate them as the source of back pain. Although the validity

and reproducibility of these tests have rarely been examined (LaBoeuf, 1990), they are commonly used in both chiropractic and orthopaedic low back examinations. For the lumbar spine, these may include repeated springing pressure across the spinous processes, combining extension and lateral bending pressure on the facet joints (Kemp's test), or mechanically stressing the sacroiliac (SI) joints. SI joint stress tests are actually adaptations of orthopaedic hip tests including Faber-Patrick, Gaenslen's and Yeoman's tests. Therefore, it is important to identify the precise anatomical site of pain in a positive test (e.g. hip or SI joint) to avoid misinterpretation. Mierau (1991) has shown that in subjects with sacroiliac joint pain, scintigraphic bone scanning commonly shows increased radionuclide uptake at the symptomatic joint when two of the three above tests are positive. In general, stress tests are more useful for acute back pain where a specific structure may have been injured. In chronic cases, where pain becomes diffuse and generalized, the specificity of tests decreases (Waddell *et al.*, 1991).

4. Neurological examination

The main purpose of neurological testing in a chiropractic setting is to screen for nerve root involvement and to distinguish referred leg pain from true radiculopathy. The distinction is important because the treatment and prognosis are different for patients with radiculopathy than they are for patients with mechanical back pain referring to the leg (Cassidy and Kirkaldy-Willis, 1988). Cases of severe nerve root compression are not common in most chiropractic offices. Practitioners are more likely to encounter what might be termed nerve root 'irritation', resulting in sciatica but not frank neurological deficit. Nerve root irritation may be thought of as *symptoms* from inflamed nerve roots. This gives pain in the distribution of the sciatic (or femoral) nerve and positive dural tension signs, but does not result in severe loss of sensation, motor power or deep tendon reflexes. A basic neurological examination would involve the following:

Sensory, motor power and reflex testing of the lower limb

These properties can be screened for the L4, L5 and S1 nerve roots. Because chiropractors are more likely to see subtle rather than severe cases, procedures may need to be modified to elicit a mildly positive test. For instance, muscle testing by having the patient perform a single, maximal contraction against the examiner's hands may indicate normal strength. However, having the patient repeatedly rise on the heels and toes could reveal early fatiguing on the involved side, suggesting mild nerve root comprise.

Nerve root tension tests

These include the straight leg raising (SLR) test for the sciatic (L5/S1) nerve roots and the heel-to-buttock test for the femoral (L4) nerve. Restriction in either of these is often interpreted as proof of a disc herniation. However, it is important to note that although SLR is a sensitive test in the presence of disc herniation, the test has low specificity (Deyo and Diehl, 1986). Hip joint pathology, sacroiliac joint dysfunction or hamstring tightness are among other common causes of SLR restriction. Therefore, improvement in SLR following manual therapy must not be misinterpreted as having affected a disc herniation. The test is also subject to diurnal fluctuations (Porter and Trailescu, 1990). Therefore, changes in SLR may have more to do with the time of day the test is done than with effects of treatment.

Unlike the SLR test, the crossed leg or 'well leg' raise test has poor sensitivity but good specificity with respect to disc herniation (Anderrson, 1991). This means that, although false negatives are common, reproduction of sciatic leg pain when the opposite leg is raised is a strong indication of disc prolapse (Kosteljanetz *et al.*, 1988).

Other neurological tests are used selectively and when appropriate. With claudicant patients in whom spinal stenosis is suspected, tests for long tract signs, including Babinski's response and ankle clonus, should be done. A specialized test, such as the Herron–Pheasant test where prolonged lumbar extension is thought to decrease the volume of the lateral nerve root canal, may show reflex or other changes only after the position has been held for some time (Kirkaldy-Willis, 1988). In patients complaining of thoracolumbar pain, the skin rolling test done along the course of the cluneal (sensory) nerve may cause pain, as does pressure over the nerve where it crosses the iliac crest (Bernard and Kirkaldy-Willis, 1987).

5. Palpation

Too much credence is placed in the interpretive value of spinal palpation. Often much more than can be justified is read into palpating small irregularities in spinal contours or subtle changes in joint movement. Because practitioners tend to rely heavily on these 'listings' when determining which segments to manipulate (Schafer and Faye, 1989), several studies have looked at the reliability of spinal palpation. In general, these studies show poor inter-examiner reliability and only moderate intra-examiner reliability (Keating, 1989, 1990; Haas, 1991; Panzer, 1991). Although this raises serious questions about the importance attributable to palpation, most practitioners still consider it an indispensable clinical skill. The technique primarily involves assessing zygapo-

physial joint motion, usually by passive challenging of the joints. Normally mobile joints have a springy end feel described by Mennel (1949) as 'joint play'. In mechanical back pain, this quality is often reduced or lost. Joint challenge then becomes painful to the patient. With experience and practice, a reasonable goal of palpation would be to determine whether or not the facet joints are causing pain and, if so, identify the side and level of vertebral involvement.

While spinal palpation may be over-emphasized in the average chiropractic low back examination, other areas of palpation are sometimes neglected. A thorough low back examination should include palpation of the abdomen, the inguinal lymph nodes, and peripheral pulses in the limb, especially if the patient has claudicant symptoms. Although palpation of the prostate gland is taught at college, it would be rare to find it done in private practice. This is unfortunate given the prevalence of prostatic cancer with metastasis to the spine as a cause of back pain (Schaberg and Gainor, 1985; Deyo and Diehl, 1988).

6. Specialized tests

Most specialized clinical testing is done when an underlying, non-mechanical cause is suspected. For instance, in patients suspected of a having rheumatological component to their back pain – such as ankylosing spondylitis – chest expansion or occiput-to-wall test may be appropriate. Spinous percussion is sometimes useful when lumbar compression fracture is suspected. The distracted leg raise or 'flip test' may be used if patients with sciatic complaints are suspected of malingering. Because psychosocial problems may accompany chronic back pain syndromes, Waddell's tests for non-anatomical back pain are often used (Waddell *et al.*, 1980). These tests include simulated lumbar spine loading (axial and rotational) and observing for descriptors and distributions of the pain that do not correspond to known anatomical patterns. Inappropriately extreme reactions to lumbar examination, such as excessive grimacing and withdrawal, are also considered positive Waddell's signs (Waddell *et al.*, 1984). It is important to note that the Waddell's tests of non-anatomical pain are just that – a means to measure indicators – they are not meant to imply malingering or deliberate symptom magnification. The tests are often interpreted as suggesting significant psychological overlay but, in themselves, are not confirmatory.

7. Ancillary tests

The accessibility to ancillary testing – including diagnostic imaging, electro-diagnostics and laboratory analysis – depends on local jurisdiction. However, all practitioners do use X-rays and are trained to read them. They are also trained in the indications for basic laboratory tests and how to interpret them.

Radiographs

Practitioners tend to over-utilize X-rays, especially full spine studies. Fortunately this practice is in decline as the profession moves toward adherence to more standardized indications for radiography. Table 22.3 summarizes the historical and physical indications justifying lumbar radiographs. Other important considerations regarding lumbar radiographs are:

i) *Low diagnostic yield.* For instance, it has been shown that unsuspected pathological findings seen on lumbar radiographs may occur as infrequently as 1 in 2500 studies (Brolin, 1975).

ii) *High gonadal radiation.* The gonadal radiation from one unshielded lumbar series has been estimated to be equivalent to the gonadal radiation from one chest radiograph per day, for 6 years (Penfil and Brown, 1968).

iii) *Poor correlation to symptoms.* There is a tendency to over-interpret radiographs. This includes attributing significance to small vertebral displacements (Bronfort, 1984; Owens, 1991) or malalignments, as well as the practice of making various measurements (roentgenometrics) which have no proven significance. Dynamic (i.e. flexion–extension, lateral flexion) studies are also commonly used but have yet to be proven valuable (Henley *et al.*, 1976; Penning *et al.*, 1984; Haas *et al.*, 1990,1991; Dvorak *et al.*, 1991). There is very little clinically relevant biomechanical information obtainable from plain film X-rays (Nachemson, 1975; DuPuis *et al.*, 1985; Frymoyer *et al.*, 1986). Especially disturbing is the practice among some practitioners of taking pre and post-treatment films in an attempt to assess clinical improvement. This has no value but does expose patients to considerable unnecessary radiation.

In modern chiropractic practice, radiographs are used to rule out pathology or significant spinal deformity in suspected cases. It should be remembered, however, that plain film radiographs are not sensitive for exposing early stages of pathology, since a significant degree of bone destruction is required before it becomes appreciable on plain film. Radiographs are useful in suspected cases of cancer, infection, fracture or dislocation, severe osteoarthrosis, spondylolisthesis or clinically important spinal deformities. If, based on the history, there is no suspicion of these, then radiographs are not usually necessary. Deyo *et al.* (1986, 1987) have shown that by using selective criteria, the use of lumbar X-rays can be significantly reduced without reducing diagnostic accuracy.

Table 22.3 *Grounds for radiography in low back pain*

History	Physical
Age over 50	Significant spinal deformity
Severe, or night pain	Neurological deficit
Significant trauma	Marked loss of flexibility
Unexplained weight loss	Unexplained fever
Past history of significant disease	Lymphadenopathy
No response to treatment	Swelling, heat or redness
History of drug or alcohol abuse	
×Litigation or compensation	

(adapted from Deyo, Diehl, 1986)

Laboratory tests

A good argument can be made for the use of simple laboratory tests over X-rays in ruling out pathology as a cause of back pain. For instance, erythrocyte sedimentation rate (ESR) is highly sensitive in the presence of many serious diseases, although it is not specific. When screening for pathology, sensitivity is more important than specificity. Fernbach (1976) demonstrated that in patients with spinal malignancy as a cause of back pain, 94% had elevated ESR. Other tests that are inexpensive and occasionally useful include serum alkaline phosphatase and serum calcium levels. Urinalysis is sometimes useful in suspected cases of back pain from urinary tract infections.

Questionnaires

Standardized questionnaires are being used increasingly in all areas of back pain assessment, including chiropractic. They may be used to describe and quantify pain, impairment (physical limitation), or disability (the functional consequences of physical impairment). Also, as it becomes increasingly clear that chronic back pain is strongly linked to psychosocial factors, many questionnaires target these issues. These may include general psychological profiles, coping strategies, measures of depression, motivation, job satisfaction, etc. Table 22.4 summarizes some commonly used questionnaires and their design purpose.

Treatment methods

Various methods and modalities - including massage, electrotherapy, ultrasound, heat/cold and exercise - are used in a typical chiropractic office. However, spinal manipulation is the cornerstone of almost all

Table 22.4 *Common questionnaires in the assessment of low back pain*

Variable	Methods of assessment
Pain	Visual analog scale, (Huskisson, 1974) McGill Pain Score, (Melzak, 1987) Pain Drawing, (Ransford, 1976)
Coping abilities	Pain Management Inventory (Brown and Nicassio, 1987)
Disability	Oswestry Disability Score, (Fairbanks *et al.*, 1980) Sickness Impact Profile, (Deyo *et al.*, 1986) Roland–Morris Disability Score, (Roland and Morris, 1983) Pain Disability Index, (Tait *et al.*, 1990)
Psychological profiles	Minnesota Multiphasic Personality Inventory (MMPI), (Sternbach *et al.*, 1973) Million Behavioral Health Inventory, (Million *et al.*, 1982) Beck Depression Inventory, (Beck, 1972)

chiropractic treatment. Dysfunction of these joints, particularly the zygapophysial joints, is central to the chiropractic model of mechanical LBP and research evidence, such as diagnostic facet injection blocks, support this concept (McCall *et al.*, 1979; Fairbanks *et al.*, 1981). Chiropractors are well trained and experienced in manipulative techniques and provide about 90% of spinal manipulations performed in the United States (Shekelle and Adams, 1992; Shekelle *et al.*, 1992). Therefore, a discussion of chiropractic management of back pain is largely a discussion of SMT.

Manipulation defined

In manual medicine there are two commonly used modalities; *mobilization* and *manipulation*. The terms are often used interchangeably, but they are different and have different effects. Part of the distinction can be appreciated if joint motion is thought of as a continuum from ankylosed to unstable (Figure 22.1). In this model, mobilization occurs within the passive range of motion. Manipulation, however, takes the joint slightly past the passive range of motion and into what has been termed the 'paraphysiological space' (Sandoz, 1976). Forcing a joint beyond this space, past the limit of anatomical integrity, would result in capsular sprain and finally ligamentous disruption with instability. Much of the art of manipulation lies in the ability to work within the narrow zone between passive mobilization and joint sprain.

Performed on spinal joints, mobilization and manipulation look and feel different (Figure 22.2). Mobilization is typically described as a gentle, oscillatory, high amplitude, low velocity manoeuvre which gives the patient a feeling of stretching. Manipulation, by contrast, is a quick, forceful but controlled thrust which usually yields the cracking

noise associated with SMT. The procedure requires considerable practice and expertise. The force must be calculated and precise. Too little will not have the desired therapeutic effect, while too much force will injure the patient.

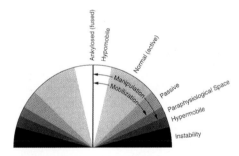

Figure 22.1 Model of possible motion in any synovial joint. The joint surfaces are separated further in manipulation than in mobilization. The 'paraphysiological space' is more conceptual than actual. (Adapted from Sandoz, 1976.)

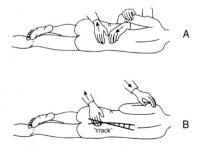

Figure 22.2 Lumbar spine mobilization vs. manipulation. (A) Mobilization is typically a slow, repeated stretching manoeuvre within the passive ROM. (B) Manipulation is a rapid, single thrust which forces the joint slightly beyond the passive ROM. The accompanying cracking sound indicates joint cavitation.

Effects of manipulation

The effects of SMT can be categorized as *physiological* or *neurological* (reflexogenic). Some of the proposed effects are speculative and are the topic of research investigation.

Physiological effects

Much of what is known about the physiological effects of spinal joint manipulation is extrapolated from studies of the metacarpophalangeal (MCP) joint. The joint is well suited for study because it is easy to manipulate and radiograph. The first study of MCP joint manipulation was published by two anatomists (Roston and Wheeler-Haines, 1947). They showed that after a critical degree of tension the joint surfaces would suddenly spring apart and a cracking sound would be heard. The phenomenon, known as joint 'cavitation', results in an increase in joint space (about 25%) and the formation of a carbon dioxide gas bubble within the synovial fluid (Unsworth *et al.*, 1971). Both result from the rapid drop in intra-articular pressure as the elastic barrier of resistance is

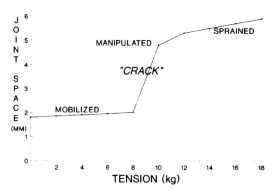

Figure 22.4 The load-separation curve for a normal metacarpophalangeal joint. At a critical distraction force (about 9 kg), the joint surfaces spring apart and the cracking noise associated with cavitation is heard. These properties define a *manipulated* joint. (Modified from Unsworth *et al.*, 1947.)

overcome. The widened joint space and gas bubble are both radiographically demonstrable in a manipulated – but not mobilized – joint (Figure 22.3). The cracking sound is thought to occur as the gas bubble collapses; this occurs almost as quickly as it is formed. Figure 22.4 shows the load-separation curve for the MCP joint and distinguishes manipulation from mobilization based on width of the joint space. After the joint has been cavitated, there is a refractory period of 15–20 minutes during which a crack cannot be produced again. This is likely the time required for the carbon dioxide gas to be resorbed into the synovial fluid. During this period the joint surfaces re-approximate but the inter-articular space does remain greater than before manipulation.

The functional effect of joint cavitation is increased freedom of movement. Mierau *et al.* (1988) have demonstrated a significant increase in passive MCP joint flexion in manipulated versus mobilized subjects. The results indicate that manipulation and mobilization are distinct therapies and have different effects on joint function. Practitioners look for increased range of spinal motion following manipulation and consider it an important determinant of a successful treatment.

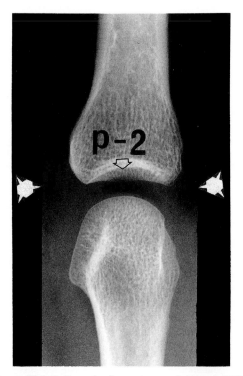

Figure 22.3 Radiograph of a metacarpophalangeal (MCP) joint following manipulation. There is an increase in the joint space and a gas bubble (arrow) - the result of intra-articular pressure changes.

Neurological effects

Patients often report immediate and significant pain relief following spinal joint manipulation. Several neurological mechanisms have been proposed to explain this. Korr (1975) developed a model of back pain caused by paraspinal muscle spasm secondary to aberrant proprioceptive input from the muscle spindle cells. This results in fixation of the underlying spinal joints. He believed that manipulation produces a barrage of neural output from the spindle cells and

Table 22.5 *Effects of spinal manipulation*

Known	Probable	Possible
Joint cavitation	Joint capsule neuro-stimulation which could lead to:	Breaking of articular adhesions
Increased range of movement	• inhibition of pain • paraspinal muscle relaxation • autonomic nervous system stimulation	Release of entrapped joint capsular structures

resets the firing rate or *gain*. The muscle relaxes and joint movement is possible again.

Melzak and Wall (1965) developed the Gate Control theory of pain, providing a model whereby increased afferent input to the spine would result in reflex inhibition of pain transmission. Several studies examining spinal pain tolerance following manipulation appear to support this as a tenable model (Terret and Vernon, 1984; Vernon, 1988; Vernon *et al.*, 1990).

Wyke (1985) proposed that manipulation creates rapid bursts of transmission in afferent nerve fibres of the spinal joint capsules, ligaments and surrounding musculature. These signals are thought to affect both the dorsal root ganglion and spinal cord (substantia gelatinosa) to reduce muscle hypertonicity and decrease pain transmission, respectively. There may be some truth in this; studies using electromyography of paraspinal muscles show a change in activity following manipulation (Grise, 1974; Herzog *et al.*, 1995). These EMG changes are a function of the speed of the thrust, not the force. When mobilization (a much slower modality) is used, there is no change in myoelectric activity (Herzog *et al.*, 1995).

There may even be effects at the autonomic nervous system level. The sympathetic chain that runs along the lumbar spine does communicate with the spinal nerve through the grey ramus communicans. Therefore the possibility exists of a link between mechanical stimulation of the joints and an autonomic nervous system response. Some of these proposed effects include vasomotor activity (Yates *et al.*, 1988), the release of endorphins (Vernon *et al.*, 1986) and enhanced phagocytic and neutrophil cell activity following manipulation (Brennan *et al.*, 1991, 1992). However, the degree of these effects is unknown and it is doubtful that they are of any clinically practical importance.

Other speculation about the possible effects of joint manipulation often reflect the proponents' opinion regarding the underlying cause of mechanical back pain. Cyriax (1974), for example, proposed that manipulation tore interarticular facet joint adhesions. These adhesions do exist and are demonstrable histologically. They appear to be part of the normal ageing process in many people. However, there is no direct evidence that manipulating spinal joints will break these adhesions.

Giles (1986, 1987) has demonstrated that synovial folds are innervated and that they may become entrapped between zygapophysial joint surfaces, possibly producing pain. Again, it is not known how commonly this occurs, whether or not it is a significant cause of back pain, or whether or not manipulation frees these entrapped synovial folds. Bogduk and Engel (1984) have also suggested that meniscoids may play a role in facet joint pain.

For many years, it was believed that the main effect of vertebral 'adjusting' was to reposition subluxated vertebrae. Herzog (1994) has demonstrated small vertebral movements during manipulation but the movement does not result in a repositioning of vertebrae. Table 22.5 reviews the proposed effects of SMT.

How chiropractors manipulate the lumbar spine

Practitioners become adept at spinal manipulation through training and practice. The most common method, called side posture manipulation, is shown in Figure 22.5. The procedure can be outlined as follows:

1. The patient is positioned so that they are lying comfortably on their side, with the painful side of the spine up.
2. The spinal level requiring treatment is located with the chiropractor's hand.
3. A moment of force is created at that spinal level by counter-rotation of the pelvis and torso. The degree of flexion at the hip and pelvis opens the facets at a desired spinal level. The amount of rotation at the torso then determines where the moment of force will lie along the lumbar spine. With practice, a torsional moment can be created precisely at a stiff segment, facilitating the procedure considerably.

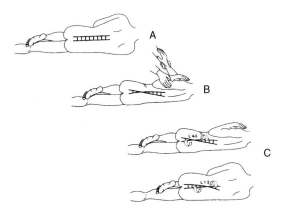

Figure 22.5 Patient positioning for typical side posture spinal joint manipulation. (A) The neutral position; no rotational force in spine. (B) Counter-rotation of pelvis and torso creates a moment of force. (C) Location of turning moment can be controlled by the amount of pelvic flexion\upper body rotation.

4. A quick thrust is applied, often using the spinous process as a lever. Studies have demonstrated that the peak force required to cavitate facet joints in the thoracic spine is 400–600 newtons (Conway *et al.*, 1993). It is likely similar for the lumbar spine. The amplitude, velocity and direction are all critical. Because the axis of rotation lies anterior to the facet joints, a torquing force is created, opening (cavitating) the joint on the up side.

Indications and contraindications for SMT

This form of therapy is useful for several low back syndromes with varying degrees of effectiveness (Cassidy *et al.*, 1985). In general the indications are mechanical back pain in the absence of serious or surgically amenable pathology. If demonstrable pathology and mechanical back pain coexist the treatment addresses the mechanical portion of the problem. Contraindications may be absolute or relative. Certainly conditions such as tumours, infections or acute fractures constitute absolute contraindications. However, a condition such as spondyloarthropathy may be a relative contraindication because patients do poorly if manipulated during arthritic flare-ups. However, they may respond well during quiescent phases of their disorder. Table 22.6 outlines the indications and contraindications for manipulation therapy.

Other treatment methods

Although manipulation is the mainstay of almost all chiropractic treatment for back pain, other treatments are added for various patient needs. Therapeutic choices are often determined by the length of time the patient has been suffering with backache. In acute back pain, the goals of treatment are decreased pain and increased range of motion; both of which can be achieved with SMT. However, in chronic cases there may be a variety of physical and psychosocial problems which are not amenable to manual therapy of any kind. These issues must be addressed as part of the treatment plan if success is to be achieved. Practitioners must be cognisant of this and recognize the limitations of passive therapy to help patients who have a multitude of complicating problems. Therefore the types of treatment and goals of therapy may be quite different for chronic versus acute patients. These are contrasted in Table 22.7.

Most practitioners prescribe some form of exercise for low back pain (Christensen and Morgal, 1993). The spectrum of exercise therapy extends from simple stretching routines to rigorous fitness and work-hardening programmes. Practitioners usually favour lumbar flexion exercises, as described by Williams (1974), rather than the McKenzie style extension exercises (see Chapter 24). This is in keeping with the chiropractic model of back pain in which the facet joint plays a critical role; lumbar

Table 22.6 *The indications and contraindications for manipulative therapy*

Indications	Contraindications
Mechanical low back pain (joint dysfunction)	Cancer or other destructive lesions of the spine
Intervertebral disc disease (HNP)	Severe osteopenia
Spinal stenosis (central or lateral)	Active spondyloarthropathies
LBP with spondylolisthesis	Cauda equina syndrome
Post-operative LBP	Referred pain from visceral disease
LBP in pregnancy and postpartum LBP	Significant psychological overlay

Table 22.7 *Goals of treatment: acute vs. chronic low back pain*

Goals of treatment		Types of treatment	
Acute	*Chronic*	*Acute*	*Chronic*
Decrease pain	Return-to-work	NSAIDs	Conditioning exercise
Increase mobility	Increase functional capacity	Rest	Work hardening
	A.D.L.	Modalities	Counselling
	Resolution of psychosocial issues	Manipulation/mobilization	Functional restoration programmes
	Develop coping strategies		
	Deal with legal issues		

flexion stretches facet joints while extension approximates them. In fact, it is likely that patient compliance with stretching exercises is more crucial than the type of stretching programme (Kendall and Jenkins, 1968; Buswell, 1982). Regardless, stretching exercises are designed to increase lumbar range of motion. Back and trunk strengthening exercises are usually prescribed for patients who are deconditioned due to the prolonged inactivity that accompanies chronic back pain syndromes. There is some evidence that increased fitness has a protective effect against future back injuries (Cady *et al.*, 1979).

Many practitioners utilize back schools. These have been in existence since the late 1960s and may be used for patients with acute back pain, chronic back pain, or as a prevention measure in high risk occupation groups. The effectiveness of back school alone is questionable (Linton and Kamwendo, 1987; Cohen *et al.*, 1994); although, from an empirical standpoint, many practitioners find that patients appreciate the material and that they cope better with their back conditions afterwards. Back school is best used when combined with a more active form of therapy such as fitness training and does appear to enhance its effects (Kohles *et al.*, 1990).

It is well accepted that patients with chronic back pain syndromes develop psychosocial problems associated with their condition. Some practitioners utilize the services of pain management clinics or psychotherapy services specializing in chronic pain syndromes, for appropriately selected patients.

Regimens of therapy

There has been wide variation among practitioners regarding the appropriate protocol for treatment of various back conditions (Shekelle and Brook, 1991). Variations include frequency and duration of treat-

ment as well as the indications for referral or additional testing. Consensus documents in North America have been developed to provide guidelines in these areas (Haldeman *et al.*, 1993; Henderson *et al.*, 1994). Hopefully this will lead to a more consistent delivery of treatment and decrease the widely varying practice habits among practitioners – a problem that leads to confusion and frustration for the patient, insurance carriers and governments.

Both American and Canadian guideline documents recommend no more than 10 treatments in a 2-week period for acute, uncomplicated LBP before seeking a second opinion or ordering additional diagnostic tests. Chronic LBP syndromes (i.e. 12 weeks or more duration) or back pain accompanied by sciatica are recognized as requiring a considerably longer period of treatment before improvement can be expected.

Trials of SMT and chiropractic management

There is a common misconception that chiropractic manipulative therapy is an unstudied and unscientific discipline. In fact, there are more than 50 clinical trials using SMT for low back pain. In many (but not all) trials the treatment is delivered by chiropractors. Unfortunately, many of these studies contain methodological or statistical errors. Difficulties include: lack of controls, inadequately described treatment, poorly defined inclusion/exclusion criteria, improper sample size, lack of randomization, failure to account for drop-outs, improper statistical analysis and inappropriate extrapolation of results. Despite the various shortcomings and pitfalls, there is a sufficient body of evidence to warrant the use of SMT for mechanical low back pain. These studies can be divided into those that examine *effectiveness* (or efficacy) and those that assess *cost-effectiveness* of treatment.

Effectiveness trials

Of the 50 or so studies of manipulation for LBP, almost half lack a control group. Because the natural history of back pain is generally favourable and spontaneous remission is common, little can be concluded when studies lack control groups. In studies which use controls or comparison groups, alternate treatments include sham manipulation, mobilization, modalities (e.g. ultrasound, electrotherapy, heat), analgesics, traction, exercise, back school, bed rest or surgery. Outcome measures also vary widely and have included: pain, range of motion, disability, return to work, use of pain medication, patient satisfaction and health care utilization. Detailed analysis of these studies is beyond the scope of this chapter, except to say the large majority favour manipulation over other forms of treatment. The interested reader should refer to an in-depth review by Bronfort (1992). Based on approximately 30 studies using controls and randomization, the following conclusions can be made:

a) Spinal manipulation is the most studied form of treatment to date for low back pain.
b) There is more evidence to support the use of manipulation therapy for back pain than any other treatment.
c) The effects of manipulation therapy are time dependent (as with all other treatments).
d) Manipulation is most effective for uncomplicated mechanical LBP of short duration and is less effective in chronic cases.
e) There is no evidence that manipulation therapy *prevents* back pain or any other disorder.

The substantial and favourable body of evidence supporting the use of SMT in low back pain conditions has lead to its recommendation as a first line of treatment in recently published multidisciplinary guideline documents in the United States and Britain (Bigos *et al.*, 1994; Rosen *et al.*, 1994). The American-based Agency for Health Care Policy and Research (AHCPR) recommends only manipulation or non-prescription medications in the treatment of acute back pain (Bigos *et al.*, 1994). These guidelines also advise against many traditional but unproven treatments including most prescription drugs, various physical modalities (massage, TENS, ultrasound, etc.), injections, acupuncture, and prolonged bed rest.

Cost-effectiveness studies

Cost-effectiveness studies have become more common in recent years because of rising health care costs and budgetary restraints. The cost-effectiveness of chiropractic treatment in particular is being studied because of public pressure to have it included in government-sponsored health care plans. These studies are often culled from Workers' Compensation Board or insurance company data, which is collected for bureaucratic purposes rather than scientific scrutiny. This can make statistical analysis difficult. However, enough information has been accumulated to make several valid comparisons of chiropractic treatment to traditional medical management. ·

Johnson *et al.* (1989) reviewed 17 cost-comparison studies, done in the United States between 1940 and 1981, in which chiropractic treatment was compared to other, more traditional treatment for low back injuries. The review concludes that in 14 of 17 studies, chiropractic treatment was less costly and in all but one study resulted in decreased work loss. Other studies show that, in general, chiropractic management of back pain results in more office visits than medical treatment, comparable treatment costs, but significantly decreased absenteeism and shorter disability (Manga *et al.*, 1993). The net result is significant cost savings in most cases. This occurs because the majority of costs associated with low back pain are for disability payments and lost productivity, not treatment (Cats-Baril and Frymoyer, 1991). Unnecessary hospitalization and sophisticated and expensive (but usually unwarranted) diagnostic testing drives the costs of this mostly benign condition further yet. Dillon (1981) has shown that these spin-off costs are 16–20 times less when patients are managed by chiropractors rather than medically. The conclusions of approximately 20 studies looking at cost-effectiveness of various treatments for low back pain can be summarized as follows:

a) Chiropractic is the most cost-effective treatment for LBP studied to date. The lower cost of chiropractic treatment results from:
  ● fewer auxiliary tests/services;
  ● reduced length of LBP disability;
  ● reduced rates of chronicity.
b) Budgetary issues support the use of chiropractic as a first line treatment for most back pain conditions.
c) Hospital treatment for low back pain is almost always economically wasteful.

As health care financial restrictions continue, the main challenge to all professions may be to show that their treatment is more effective and less costly than no treatment at all. Recent studies show promise for approaching most low back injuries as self-limiting; requiring little or no treatment (Malmivaara *et al.*, 1995). Simple reassurance and timely return to activity may be superior to either chiropractic or medical/physiotherapy treatment (Indahl *et al.*, 1995).

Summary

Despite a colourful and controversial history, practitioners have gained recognition as being well trained in the assessment and treatment of mechanical back pain. The mainstay of chiropractic management, spinal manipulation, has been studied from the physiological, clinical efficacy and cost-containment standpoints. The challenge for the profession now is to standardize and improve professional training (preferably in university settings), establish a clearly defined scope of practice and improve relations with other health care professionals. The result will be better quality management of mechanical back pain.

References

Andersson, G.B. (1991) Sensitivity, specificity and predictive value. A general issue in the screening for disease and in the interpretation of diagnostic studies in spinal disorders. In *The Adult Spine: Principles and Practice* (J.W. Frymoyer, ed.). Raven Press, New York, pp. 277-287.

Battie, M., Bigos, S.J., Fisher, L.D. *et al.* (1990) Anthropometric and clinical measurements as predictors of industrial back pain complaints: a prospective study. *J. Spinal Disord.*, **3**, 195-204.

Beck, A.T. (1972) *Depression: Causes and Treatment.* University of Pennsylvania Press, Pennsylvania.

Bernard, T.N. and Kirkaldy-Willis, W.H. (1987) Recognizing specific characteristics of nonspecific low back pain. *Clin. Orthop. Rel. Res.*, **217**, 96.

Bigos, S.J., Battie, M.C., Fisher, L.D. *et al.* (1992) A prospective evaluation of pre-employment screening methods for acute industrial back pain. *Spine*, **17**, 922-926.

Bigos, S., Bowyer, O., Braen, G. *et al.* (1994) *Acute Low Back Problems in Adults. Clinical Practice Guideline No. 14.* AHCPR Publication No. 95-0642. Agency for Health Care Policy and Research, Public Health Service, US Dept. of Health and Human Services, Rockville, MD.

Brennan, P., Kokjohn, K., Kaltinger, C. *et al.* (1991) Enhanced phagocytic cell respiratory burst induced by spinal manipulation. *J Manipulative Physiol. Ther.*, **14**, 399-408.

Brennan, P., Triano, J., McGregor, M. *et al.* (1992) Enhanced neutrophil respiratory burst as a biological marker for manipulation forces: duration of the effect and association with substance P and tumour necrosis factor. *J Manipulative Physiol. Ther.*, **15**, 83-89.

Bogduk, N. and Engel, R. (1984) The menisci of the lumbar zygapophysial joints: a review of their anatomy and clinical significance. *Spine*, **9**, 454-460.

Brolin, I. (1975) Product control of lumbar films. *Läkartidningen*, **72**, 1793-1795 (in Swedish).

Bronfort, G. (1992) Effectiveness of spinal manipulation and adjustments. In *Principles and Practice of Chiropractic* (S. Haldeman, ed.). Appleton and Lange, Norwalk. pp. 415-441.

Bronfort, G. and Jochumsen, (1984) The functional radiographic examination of patients with low back pain: a study of different forms of variation. *J Manipulative Physiol. Ther.*, **7**, 89.

Brown, G. and Nicassio, P. (1987) Development of a questionnaire for the assessment of active and passive coping stratagies in chronic pain patients. *Pain*, **31**, 53-64.

Buswell, J. (1982) Low back pain: a comparison of two treatment programmes. *N.Z.J. Physiother.*, **10**, 13-17.

Cady, L.D., Bischoff, D.P., O'Connell, E.R. *et al.* (1979) Strength and fitness and subsequent back injuries in firefighters. *J. Occup. Med.*, **21**, 269-272.

Cassidy, J.D. and Kirkaldy-Willis, W.H. (1988) Manipulation. In *Managing Low Back Pain*, 2nd edn (W.H. Kirkaldy-Willis, ed.). Churchill Livingstone, pp. 287-296.

Cassidy, J.D., Kirkaldy-Willis, W.H. and McGregor, M. (1985) Spinal manipulation for the treatment of chronic low back and leg pain: an observational trial. In *Empirical Approaches to the Validation of Manipulative Therapy* (A.A. Buerger and P.E. Greenman, eds). Charles C Thomas, Springfield, IL.

Cats-Baril, W.L. and Frymoyer, J.W. (1991) The economics of spinal disorders. In *The Adult Spine: Principles and Practice* (J.W. Frymoyer, ed.). Raven Press, New York, pp. 85-105.

Christensen, M.G. and Morgal, D.D. (eds) (1993) *Job Analysis of Chiropractic in Canada*. National Board of Chiropractic Examiners, Greeley, Colorado.

Cohen, J., Goel, V., Frank, J.W. *et al.* (1994) Group education interventions for people with low back pain: an overview of the literature. *Spine*, **19**, 1214-1222.

Collis, D.K. and Ponseti, I.V. (1969) Long term follow-up of patients with idiopathic scoliosis not treated surgically. *J. Bone Joint Surg.*, **51**, 425.

Conway, P.W.J., Herzog, W., Zhang, Y.-T. *et al.* (1993) Forces required to cause cavitation during spinal manipulation in the thoracic spine. *Clin. Biomech.*, **8**, 210-214.

Cyriax, J. (1974) *Textbook of Orthopaedic Medicine*, Vol 2. 9th edn. Baillière Tindall, London.

Deyo, R.A. (1986a) Early diagnostic evaluation of low back pain. *J. Gen. Int. Med.*, **1**, 328-338.

Deyo, R.A. (1986b) Comparative validity of the sickness impact profile and shorter scales of functional assessment in low-back pain. *Spine*, **11**, 951-954.

Deyo, R.A. and Diehl, A. (1986) Lumbar spine films in primary care: current use and effects of selective ordering criteria. *J. Gen. Int. Med.*, **1**, 20-25.

Deyo, R.A. and Diehl, A. (1988) Cancer as a cause of back pain. *J. Gen. Int. Med.*, **3**, 230-238.

Deyo, R.A., Diehl, A. and Rosenthal, M. (1987) Reducing roentgenography use. Can patient expectations be altered? *Arch. Int. Med.*, **147**, 141-145.

Deyo, A., Rainville, J. and Kent, D.L. (1992) What can the history and physical examination tell us about low back pain? *JAMA*, **268**, 760-765.

Dillon, J.L. (1981) Health economics and chiropractic. *Ann. Swiss Chiro. Assoc.*, **7**, 7-17.

DuPuis, P.R., Yong-Hing, K., Cassidy, J.D. and Kirkaldy-Willis, W.H. (1985) Radiologic diagnosis of degenerative lumbar spinal instability. *Spine*, **10**, 262-276.

Dvorak, J., Panjabi, M.M., Novotny, J.E. *et al.* (1991) Clinical validation of functional flexion-extension roentgenograms of the lumbar spine. *Spine*, **16**, 943-950.

Fairbanks, J.C.T., Davies, J.B., Mbaot, J.C. and O'Brien, J.P. (1980) The Oswestry low back pain disability questionnaire. *Physiotherapy*, **66**, 271-273.

Fairbanks, J.C.T., Park, W.M., McCall, I.W. and O'Brian, J.P. (1981) Apophyseal injection of local anaesthetic as a diagnostic aid in primary low-back pain syndrome. *Spine*, **6**, 598-605.

Fernbach, J.C., Langer, F. and Gross, A.E. (1976) The significance of low back pain in older adults. *Can. Med. Assoc. J.*, **115**, 898-900.

Frymoyer, J.W., Phillips, R., Newberg, A. and MacPherson, M.S. (1986) A comparative analysis of the interpretations of lumbar spine radiographs by chiropractors and medical doctors. *Spine*, **11**, 1020-1023.

Giles, L.G.F. (1986) Lumbosacral and cervical zygapophysial joint inclusions. *Manual Med.*, **2**, 89-92.

Giles, L.G.F. and Taylor, J.R. (1987) Human zygapophysial joint capsule and synovial fold innervation. *Br. J. Rheumatol.*, **26**, 993-998.

Gill, K., Krag, M.H., Johnson, G.B. *et al.* (1988) Repeatability of four clinical methods of assessment of lumbar spinal motion. *Spine*, **13**, 50-53.

Grice, A.S. (1974) Muscle tonus change following manipulation. *J. Can. Chiro. Assoc.*, **74**, 29-31.

Haas, M. (1991) The reliability of reliability. *J. Manipulative Physiol. Ther.*, **14**, 199-208.

Haas, M., Nyiendo, J., Peterson, C. *et al.* (1990) Inter-rater reliability of roentgenological evaluation of the lumbar spine in lateral bending. *J. Manipulative Physiol. Ther.*, **13**, 179-189.

Haas, M. and Nyiendo, J. (1991) Lumbar motion trends and correlation with low back pain. A roentgenological evaluation of quatitative segmental motion in lateral bending. In

Haldeman, S. (1991) *Proceedings of the Scientific Symposium of the 1991 World Chiropractic Congress.* World Federation of Chiropractic, Toronto, May 4-5.

Haldeman, S., Chapman-Smith, D. and Petersen, D.M. (eds) (1993) *Guidelines for Chiropractic Quality Assurance and Practice Parameters*. Aspen.

Henderson, D., Chapman-Smith, D., Mior, S. and Vernon, H. (eds) (1994) Clinical Guidelines for Chiropractic Practice in Canada (Suppl). *J. Can. Chiro. Assoc.*, 38.

Henly, E.N., Matteri, R.E. and Frymoyer, J.W. (1976) Accurate roentgenographic determination of lumbar flexion-extension. *Clin. Orthop.*, **115**, 145-148.

Herzog, W. (1994) The biomechanics of spinal manipulative treatments. *J. Can. Chiro. Assoc.*, **38**, 216-222.

Herzog, W., Conway, P.J., Zhang, Y.T. *et al.* (1995) Reflex responses associated with manipulative treatments on the thoracic spine: a pilot study. *J. Manipulative Physiol. Ther.*, **18**, 233-236.

Huskisson, E.C. (1974) Measurement of pain. *Lancet*, **2**, 1127.

Hyytiainen, K., Salminen, J.K., Suvitie, T. *et al.* (1991) Reproducibility of nine tests to measure spinal mobility and trunk muscle strength. *Scand. J. Rehab. Med.*, **23**, 3-10.

Indahl, A., Velund, L. and Reikeraas, O. (1995) Good prognosis for low back pain when left untampered. *Spine*, **20**, 473-447.

Johnson, M.R., Schultz, M.K. and Ferguson, A.C. (1989) A comparison of chiropractic, medical, and osteopathic care for work-related sprains and strains. *J. Manipulative Physiol. Ther.*, **12**, 335-344.

Keating, J.C. (1989) Inter-examiner reliability of motion palpation of the lumbar spine: a review of quantitative literature. *AJCM*, **2**, 107-110.

Keating, J.C., Giljium, K., Menke, M. *et al.* (1990) Inter-examiner reliability of eight evaluative dimensions of

lumbar segmental abnormality. *J. Manipulative Physiol. Ther.*, **13**, 463-468.

Kendall, P.H. and Jenkins, J.M. (1968) Exercises for backache: a double blind controlled trial. *Physiotherapy*, **54**, 154-157.

Kirkaldy-Willis, W.H. (1988) The site and nature of the lesion. In *Managing Low Back Pain,* 2nd edn. (W.H. Kirkaldy-Willis, ed.). Churchill Livingstone, pp. 133-154.

Kohles, S., Barnes, D., Gatchel, R.J. and Mayer, T.G. (1990) Improved physical performance outcomes after functional restoration treatment in patients with chronic low back pain. Early versus recent training results. *Spine*, **15**, 1321-1324.

Korr, I.M. (1975) Proprioceptor and somatic dysfunction. *J. Am. Osteopath. Assoc.*, **74**, 638-650.

Kosteljanetz, U., Bang, F. and Schmidt-Olsen, S. (1988) The clinical significance of straight leg raising (Lasegue's sign) in the diagnosis of prolapsed lumbar disc. *Spine*, **13**, 393-395.

LaBoeuf, C. The sensitivity of seven lumbo-pelvic orthopaedic tests and the arm-fossa test. *J. Manipulative Physiol. Ther.*, **13**, 138-143.

Lewit, K. (1985) The muscular and articular factor in movement restriction. *Man. Med.*, **1**, 83-85.

Linton, E.J. and Kamwendo, G.K. (1987) Low back schools: a critical review. *Physiotherapy*, **67**, 1375-1383.

Macrae, I.F. and Wright, V. (1969) Measurements of back movement. *Ann. Rheum. Dis.*, **28**, 584-589.

Malmivaara, A., Hakkinen, U., Aro, T. *et al.* (1995) The treatment of acute low back pain – bed rest, exercises, or ordinary activity? *N. Engl. J. Med.*, **332**, 351-355.

Manga, P., Angus, D., Papadopoulos, C. and Swan, W. (1993) *The Effectiveness and Cost-Effectiveness of Chiropractic Management of Low-Back Pain.* Kenilworth Publishing, Ontario, Canada.

McCall, I., Park, W.M. and O'Brien, J.D. (1979) Induced pain referral from posterior lumbar elements in normal subjects. *Spine*, **4**, 441-446.

McCombe, P.G., Fairbanks, J.C.T., Cockersole, B.C. and Pynsent, P.B. (1989) Reproducibility of physical signs in low-back pain. *Spine*, **14**, 908-918.

Melzack, R. (1975) The short-form McGill Pain Questionnaire. *Pain*, **30**, 191-197.

Melzack, R. and Wall, P.D. (1965) Pain mechanisms: a new theory. *Science*, **150**, 971.

Mennel, J. (1949) *The Science and Art of Joint Manipulation,* 2nd edn. Churchill, London

Mierau, D.R. (1991) Scintigraphic analysis of idiopathic sacroiliac joint pain. In *Proceedings of the Scientific Symposium of the 1991 World Chiropractic Congress* (S. Haldemann, Chairman), World Federation of Chiropractic, Toronto, May 4-5.

Mierau, D.R., Cassidy, J.D., Bowen, V. *et al.* (1988) Manipulation and mobilization of the third metacarpophalangeal joint. A quantitative radiographic and range of motion study. *Man. Med.*, **3**, 135-140.

Million, R., Hall, W., Nilsen, K.H. *et al.* (1982) Assessment of the progress of the back-pain patient. *Spine*, **7**, 204-212.

Nachemson, A. (1975) Toward a better understanding of low-back pain: a review of the mechanics of the lumbar disc. *Rheumatol. Rehabil.*, **14**, 129-143.

Nelson, M.A., Allen, P., Clamp, S. *et al.* (1979) Reliability and reproductivity of clinical findings in low back pain. *Spine*, **4**, 97-101.

Nilsonne, V. and Lundgren, K.D. (1968) Long-term prognosis in idiopathic scoliosis. *Acta Orthop. Scand.*, **39**, 456.

Owens, E. (1991) Line drawing analyses of static cervical X-ray used in chiropractic. *Proceedings of the Sixth Annual Conference on Research and Education;* June 21-23; Consortium for Chiropractic Research, Monterey.

Panzer, D. (1991) Lumbar motion palpation: a literature review. *Proceedings of the Sixth Annual Conference on Research and Education*, June 21-23, Consortium for Chiropractic Research, Monterey.

Penfil, R.L. and Brown, M.L. (1968) Genetically significant dose to the United States population from diagnostic medical roentgenology. *Radiology*, **90**, 209-216.

Penning, L., Wilmink, J.T. and van Woerden, H.H. (1984) Inability to prove instability. A critical appraisal of clinical-radiological flexion-extension studies in lumbar disc degeneration. *Diagn. Imaging Clin. Med.*, **53**, 186-192.

Pope, M.H., Bevins, T., Wilder, D.G. *et al.* (1985) The relationship between anthropometric, postural, muscular, and mobility characteristics of males, age 18-55. *Spine*, **10**, 644.

Porter, R.W. and Trailescu, I.F. (1990) Diurnal changes in straight leg raising. *Spine*, **15**, 103-106.

Ransford, A.O., Cairns, D. and Mooney, V. (1976) The pain drawing as an aid to the psychological evaluation of patients with low back pain. *Spine*, **1**, 127-134.

Roberts, F., Roberts, E., Lloyd, K. *et al.* (1978) Lumbar spinal manipulation on trial. Part II. Radiological assessment. *Rheumatol. Rehabil.*, **17**, 54.

Roland, M. and Morris, R. (1983) A study of the natural history of back pain, Part I: Development of a reliable a sensitive measure of disability in low-back pain. *Spine*, **8**, 141-144.

Rosen, M., Breen, A. *et al.* (1994) *Report of a Clinical Standards Advisory Group Committee on Back Pain.* HMSO, London.

Roston, J.B. and Wheeler-Haines, R. (1947) Cracking in the metacarpophalangeal joint. *J. Anat.*, **81**, 165-173.

Rowe, M.L. (1969) Low back pain disability in industry: a position paper. *J. Occup. Med.*, **11**, 161-169.

Sandoz, R. (1976) Some physical mechanisms and effects of spinal adjustments. *Ann. Swiss Chiropract. Assoc.*, **6**, 91-141.

Schaberg, J. and Gainor, B.J. (1985) A profile of metastatic carcinoma of the spine. *Spine*, **10**, 19-20.

Schafer, R. and Faye, L. (1989) *Motion Palpation and Chiropractic Technic: Principles of Dynamic Chiropractic.* The Motion Palpation Institute, Huntington Beach.

Shekelle, P. and Brook, R. (1991) A community-based study of the use of chiropractic services. *Am. J. Public Health*, **81**, 439 - 442.

Shekelle, P. and Adams, A. (1992) Spinal manipulation for low back pain. *Ann. Int. Med.*, **117**, 590-598.

Shekelle, P., Adams, A., Chassin, M. *et al.* (1992b) The appropriateness of spinal manipulation for low back pain. *Ann. Int. Med.*, **117**, 590-598.

Sternbach, R.A., Wolff, S.R., Murphy, R.W. and Akeson, W.H. (1973) Aspects of chronic low back pain. *Psychosomatics*, **14**, 52-56.

Tait, R.C., Chinall, J.T. and Krause, S. (1990) The Pain Disability Index; psychometric properties. *Pain*, **40**, 171-182.

Terret, A.C.J. and Vernon, H. (1984) Manipulation and pain tolerance: a controlled study of the effect of spinal manipulation on paraspinal cutaneous pain tolerance levels. *Am. J. Phys. Med.*, **63**, 217.

Triano, J. and Schultz, A. (1987) Correlation of objective measures of trunk motion and muscle function with low-back disability ratings. *Spine*, **12**, 561.

Unsworth, A., Dawson, D. and Wright, V. (1971) Cracking joints. *Ann. Rheum. Dis.*, **30**, 348-358.

Vernon, H. (1988) Pressure pain threshold and manipulation - a single case study. *J. Can. Chiro. Assoc.*, **32**, 17-22.

Vernon, H., Dhami, I., Howley, T. and Annett, R. (1986) Spinal manipulation and beta-endorphin: a controlled study of the effect of a spinal manipulation on plasma beta-endorphin levels in normal males. *J. Manipulative Physiol. Ther.*, **9**, 115-123.

Vernon, H., Aker, P.D., Burns, S.H. *et al.* (1990) Pressure pain threshold evaluation of the effect of spinal manipulation in the treatment of chronic neck pain: a pilot study. *J. Manipulative Physiol. Ther.*, **13**, 13-16.

Waddell, G., McCulloch, J.A., Kummel, E. and Venner, R.M. (1980) Nonorganic physical signs in low-back pain. *Spine*, **5**, 117-125.

Waddell, G., Main, C.J., Morris, E.W. *et al.* (1984) Chronic low-back pain, psychologic distress and illness behaviour. *Spine*, **9**, 209-213.

Waddell, G., Allen, D.B. and Newton, M. (1991) Clinical evaluation of disability on back pain. In *The Adult Spine: Principles and Practice* (J.W. Frymoyer, ed.). Raven Press, New York, pp. 155-168.

Williams, P (1974) *Low Back and Neck Pain: Causes and Conservative Treatment*. Charles C. Thomas, Springfield, IL.

Wyke, B.D. (1985) Articular neurology and manipulative therapy. In *Aspects of Manipulation Therapy* (E.F. Glasgow, L.T. Twomey, E.R. Scull and A.M. Kleynhams, eds). Churchill Livingston, Edinburgh, pp. 72-77.

Yates, R.G., Lamping, D.L., Abram, N.L. and Wright, C. (1988) Effects of chiropractic treatment on blood pressure and anxiety: a randomized, controlled trial. *J. Manipulative Physiol. Ther.*, **11**, 484-488.

23

Osteopathic management of mechanical low back pain

Tim McClune, Robert Clarke, Charlotte Walker and Kim Burton

Introduction

Low back trouble is, for something so prevalent, a surprisingly ill-understood disorder. Whilst the previous chapters in this book have attempted to unravel the current knowledge of the epidemiology, pathology, biomechanics and the like in order to provide a useful framework for clinical management, this chapter aims to set out an approach to management adopted by the typical osteopath. However, as with the other 'manipulative' professions (and arguably most of clinical medicine), osteopaths vary dramatically in their beliefs and methods, so what follows is distilled from a mixture of traditional practice and contemporary research findings; the intention is to provide a rational framework for the assessment, treatment and rehabilitation of low back pain patients in the setting of an osteopathic clinic. Inevitably there will be considerable overlap with the chapters from the other therapies which use physical modes of therapy, and doubtless there will be osteopaths (and scientists) who will disagree with what follows.

Clinicians traditionally use three main sources for their choice of treatment (Weber and Burton, 1986): their own experience, what they learn from colleagues, and reports from investigations. The first two are empirical and unreliable, but are the most frequently used sources; the third, whilst being the most rational basis of the three, suffers from the problem of dissemination – it follows that, at best, the resultant therapy will be suboptimal. In describing the osteopathic approach we are aware that we are only offering a part of an overall management strategy, a part that is underdeveloped yet offers the possibility of considerable help for a proportion of the patients. Demands for strict scientific proof of the efficacy of any treatment, though absolutely essential,

must not be confused with the duty to comfort the patient in all ways (Weber and Burton, 1986).

Low back pain is experienced by most people, at some stage in their lives, to some extent. The clinical challenge is arguably not so much the resolution of immediate symptoms (the natural history is believed to take care of that for many), rather it is the reduction of recurrence rates and the prevention of progression to chronicity. That medical (and other) management has failed is evident from the rising tide of back pain disability which is increasing exponentially in all industrialized societies; it might be argued that the majority of current intervention achieves little.

The recent publication of two major documents, one in the USA (Agency for Health Policy and Research, 1994) and one in the UK (Clinical Standards Advisory Group, 1994) have addressed this problem and are likely to have a significant influence on back pain management. These documents are clinical guidelines for the primary care management of back pain patients. The essential message is that for the vast majority of back pain, the approach should be one of early positive management, promoting early return to normal activity (including work) along with a reduction of passive (rest and avoidance) approaches. The guidelines stress the need to consider the psychosocial as well as physical aspects of management. Included as an early therapeutic option is the use of manipulative treatment, assuming that serious spinal pathology has been eliminated in a diagnostic triage.

That osteopathy, or indeed any other manipulative therapy, should not be considered a sole solution is evidenced from a recent report on a 1-year prospective investigation in osteopathic practice (Burton et al., 1995). Typically half the patients attending for back pain were still disabled to some extent 12 months after consultation; it was a combination of psychosocial variables, rather than physical findings, which best predicted outcome. In another study, some 10% of patients had an increased level of pain at 1 year and, of those who improved, a sizeable number did so whilst getting stiffer, despite manipulative treatment (Burton *et al.*, 1990). Osteopathy, then, is not a panacea for back pain and will not be considered here as such, rather it will be presented in a manner which owes something to traditional beliefs, yet complements the philosophy embodied in the American and British clinical guidelines, and is offered as one component of the primary care strategy for reducing both symptoms and the risk of chronicity.

Assessment

Interview

Introduction

Assessment of the patient is seen as being fundamental to the choice of management strategy; this goes beyond allocation of a diagnostic label. A case history is taken in a structured fashion, followed by a detailed physical examination. The function of the case history is to enable the practitioner to obtain information which, when combined with the physical findings, can be used to fully evaluate the patient's needs. It is also the starting point of the establishment of a therapeutic relationship with the patient, allowing the development of trust and confidence.

The main objectives are:

1. to identify the presenting symptoms;
2. to identify any possible cause;
3. to establish the start point and progression of the presenting symptoms;
4. to obtain details of any previous history (of low back pain);
5. to determine the symptom modifying factors (aggravating and relieving postures or activities);
6. to identify any diurnal pattern of symptoms;
7. to obtain information on any other relevant medical problems;
8. to permit some insight into occupation, general lifestyle and relevant psychosocial issues.

Presenting symptoms

Fifty-two percent of patients seen by osteopaths in the UK present with low back pain; the general characteristics are similar to those found in general medical practice (Burton, 1981). It is reasonable to suppose that this situation is typical for other countries. The osteopath believes that the characteristics and certain aspects of pain are of great value in aiding the practitioner in the evaluation. The description of pain quality, and intensity, can give insight into the tissues involved and the ongoing pathological processes. Damage to, and inflammation of, the joint capsule, muscles and ligaments is said to produce a dull, deep, nagging or burning ache. A throbbing, beating, pounding pain suggests inflammation with vascular congestion. A throbbing pain that is excruciating, rather than a mere ache, is more indicative of a serious pathology. A transient catch or jab may be due to a functional defect of a joint segment, resulting in a disturbance of joint mechanics. Any involvement of a spinal nerve root can excite a severe, sickening toothache type of pain, which may also be described as shooting and associated with paraesthesia or anaesthesia. However, the above must be considered as 'traditional concepts'; they have, in general, not been confirmed by scientific research. Although pain *quality* cannot be measured quantitatively, pain *intensity* can be, to some extent, using the visual analogue scale which at the moment appears to be the most suitable and reliable method available (Bolton and Christensen, 1994). The location and pattern of pain, although essential to identify, can be misleading because the site of the pain does not necessarily correspond to the area of abnormality. Low back trouble may present with pain in the back with, or without, associated referral to the lower extremities; occasionally, there may be leg symptoms only, or the leg pain may be more severe than the back pain. The various pain sensitive structures of the low back can give rise to pain anywhere in the distribution of their segmental somatic or autonomic innovation in the corresponding dermatome, myotome or sclerotome. This can be of a radicular or non-radicular pattern. Radicular pain has been defined as pain resulting from a lesion of a spinal nerve root, radiating from the back into the dermatome of that nerve root; however, there is a large degree of overlap between areas, as no one area is exclusively innovated by one nerve root. Non-radicular pain is that radiating to the buttock and leg in a non-dermatomal pattern. It can be located around the sacroiliac joint, gluteus medius origin, posterior iliac crest, anterior superior iliac spine, greater trochanter, postero- or anterolateral thigh or the calf.

Associated symptoms

The patient is asked about the nature and site of any associated symptoms, such as paraesthesia, numbness or weakness. The presence of any of these in a dermatomal or myotomal distribution may indicate the possibility of a nerve root irritation; a more generalized distribution may be an accompaniment of non-radicular pain. It is important to pay special attention to evidence of saddle anaesthesia and alteration in micturition or anal sphincter control to exclude cauda equina involvement.

Onset and temporal pattern

The apparent causative action, if any, is important to determine. This, together with knowledge of subsequent events, can aid diagnosis and treatment selection; the nature, extent and fluctuations in disability, as well as any work-relatedness, can guide overall management. Previous consultations with medical practitioners or self-administration of medication, can be used as an indication of severity.

Pain lasting from 0 to 7 days has been defined as 'acute', pain lasting 7 days to 3 months 'subchronic', and anything of a duration greater than 3 months as 'chronic' (Frank, 1993); whilst there is some debate about the point at which chronicity can be said to be established, these definitions are a practical classification for the purposes of osteopathic management. The temporal pattern, both diurnal and long term, can help in diagnosis and management. There are certain pain patterns that are believed to be a common feature of specific conditions, but they have not, in large part, been validated by clinical experimentation. However, pain that is worse first thing in the morning, and eases on movement, may suggest some value will be gained from, say, the use of exercises; pain that is worse at night may require advice on sleeping arrangements. Pain which is getting steadily worse, or remaining static, indicates the presence of maintaining factors that are preventing recovery, e.g. postural asymmetries, prolonged work postures or repetitive actions, or indeed some psychological overlay.

Symptom modifying factors

Knowledge concerning factors that aggravate or relieve the pain can be useful diagnostic aids, and have been tentatively suggested as criteria for syndrome identification (Burton, 1983), whilst Sweetman *et al.* (1993) found a discrete group of low back pain patients exhibiting a 'contra-bend' sign, where flexion or rotation to one side produced pain on the opposite side. Symptom modifying factors may give an indication of disability and loss of function, and hence the degree of severity of the low back disorder (Waddell and Main, 1984). Commonly, inquiries are made concerning the effects of lying down, standing (both stationary, or from sitting), walking, sitting slumped and supported, bending, lifting, coughing, heat, and cold. Again, the value of such interview details is to guide management as well as in establishing a diagnosis.

Some examples commonly used by osteopaths can be given but not all have been substantiated in clinical studies. Pain originating from the facet joints is usually induced by extension, exacerbated by sitting or standing, and reduced by walking (Fairbank *et al.*, 1981). Discogenic pain is aggravated by sitting, straining and flexion, and relieved by lying, especially prone. A postural or stabilizing muscle will cause pain after prolonged usage, but a muscle used primarily for movement will cause discomfort at first attempting contraction or during rapid contraction. Neurogenic pain is aggravated by walking or standing, with recovery on sitting, bending, lying or squatting. Inflammatory states are usually worse on initial movement after immobility and then eased by continuation of movement. They are relieved by cold treatments and anti-inflammatory pain killers. Degenerative states tend to favour light, short duration activity.

Previous history

Low back pain is known to have a high recurrence rate, particularly in the first 2 years (Lloyd and Troup, 1983). This has significant implications for management; it may be unrealistic to expect total symptomatic resolution, or to expect that recurrences will not occur.

Inquiries will be made to gain some impression of whereabouts in the natural history the present spell lies; an early age of onset of the first spell seems to be one of the factors predictive of future chronicity (Burton and Tillotson, 1991). Some osteopaths believe that recurrent problems since childhood may point to a congenital disorder, and that a number of fairly minor episodes, occurring during the 20s and 30s, may be related to early disc degeneration and the possibility of a risk of herniation. However, it must be borne in mind that precise quantification of the previous history is at the mercy of amnesia!

Other medical conditions

It is essential, of course, that the patient be deemed suitable for osteopathic treatment. This can be established through questions concerning past medical history and current general health. Enquiries are made as to the occurrence of any serious illness, major operations or accidents as well as forms of treatments given and any ensuing complications, all of which will affect the physiological state of the patient.

Summary

In simple terms the interview will have given an indication of whether the symptoms are of a mechanical nature or from a pathological or extraspinal origin. In addition, the osteopath will have used this interaction to gain a comprehensive, multimodal assessment of the patient, which will be used along with a physical examination to formulate a strategy for management of the individual rather than just the presenting symptoms.

Examination

Observation

Observation is listening to the patient with your eyes. From the first meeting, to reaching a diagnosis, one should be continually observing the patient. When first meeting a patient, a lot of information can be gleaned simply by observation; how they hold themselves, how they move (ease or fluidity of movement, e.g. moving from sitting to standing), the presence of postural asymmetry, a limp, facial expressions (indicating possible overt pain behaviour). From observation a further overview of the patient's physical and psychological state can be formed.

Clinical examination

When examining a patient clinically it is important to consider initially the patient's suitability for osteopathic treatment. A prime concern is to ensure that the neurological system is not compromised and to eliminate any serious or pathological conditions. The signs and symptoms to be aware of from a clinical viewpoint are well outlined elsewhere and are described as 'red flags' (Clinical Standards Advisory Group, 1994). If the patient exhibits any of the following signs or symptoms then urgent referral to hospital is appropriate:

- Difficulty in micturition.
- Loss of anal sphincter control or faecal incontinence.
- Saddle anaesthesia (anus/perineum/genitals).
- Widespread (more than one nerve root involved) or progressive motor weakness.

If the following signs or symptoms are present, further investigation may be required to eliminate serious spinal pathology or systemic illness:

- Constant non-mechanical pain.
- Violent trauma.
- Systemic steroids, drug abuse.
- Weight loss, history of carcinoma.
- Systemically unwell.
- Persisting severe restriction of lumbar flexion.
- Structural deformity.
- Any deep lingering pain after pressure.

The general screening for complications is done using standard clinical tests covering the following: reflexes, myotomes, dermatomes, orthopaedic tests, straight leg raising test, femoral nerve stretch test, root tension signs, neurological tests. Some may be omitted depending on symptoms and history. Assuming that these tests reveal nothing untoward, and that there are no other 'red flags', the rest of the physical examination can be performed.

Standing exam

With the patient standing, it is possible to assess their posture. By looking at the surface anatomy, it becomes apparent, for instance, if a scoliosis or increased/decreased lordosis/kyphosis is present. By observing the skin, it may be possible to detect an underlying anomaly, e.g. a small growth of hair at the base of the lumbar spine can indicate the presence of spina bifida. By looking at the surface contours, changes in muscle size, or shape, can indicate muscle atrophy/hypertrophy or increased/decreased muscle tone. Assimilation of all the various bits of information will give the osteopath a picture of the patient and how their body is used.

Active movement

When examining active movement, an osteopath will examine not only the extent of mobility in the spine, but also that of the joints of the lower limbs, looking at the ease and fluidity of movement, any movements which produce pain, and comparing quality and quantity of movement between left and right sides. This allows the osteopath to determine if there is any mechanical dysfunction in the lower limb joints, which may be predisposing to, or maintaining, the patient's problems in the lumbar spine.

Lumbar spine and sacroiliac joints

With active movement, an osteopath is looking at how the whole spine functions not just the lumbar spine. As part of the standing examination, it is necessary to assess the active movement of the patient's whole spine, looking at flexion, extension, side-bending and rotation, looking at the quality and quantity of movement and for the movements, or combined movements, which cause pain, specifically ones which reproduce or ease the pain of which the patient is complaining. To assess the sacroiliac joints, an osteopath will palpate in the sulcus of the posterior superior iliac spine and ask the patient to forward flex whilst looking for asymmetrical joint movement.

Palpation

Palpation is the osteopath's prime method for assessing passive movement of spinal joints (and indeed the effects such movement has on paraspinal soft tissues). It is very much an individual art; what each osteopath palpates ostensibly is the same, but the interpretation varies and interobserver variance is known to be great (Burton *et al.*, 1990). Nevertheless, osteopaths rely on their palpatory ability and use it to detect joint movement and tissue changes. It is this use of palpation to 'quantify' joint movement and tissue changes that, arguably, differentiates oste-opathy from some of the other manual therapies.

There are four common parameters examined when palpating either spinal or peripheral joints. In the lumbar spine, the following parameters are considered:

1. *Relative joint movement*. By palpating on the spinous processes, movement of individual motion segments (in flexion, extension, side-bending and rotation, or their combinations) can be assessed relative to the segments above and below.
2. *Joint crepitus/tenderness*. By palpating over the zygapophysial joints the quality of joint movement can be appraised, any crepitus detected, and whether or not the paraspinal structures are tender to touch/movement. Though an osteopath will palpate the joint for tenderness, the inter-pretation of this sign is problematic; many low back pain patients will display residual lumbar tenderness up to a year after consultation, despite having recovered from their presenting problem (Burton *et al.*, 1993).
3. *Muscle tone*. The osteopath will also palpate the muscle masses, feeling for hyper- or hypotonicity, fibrotic tissue, atrophy and hypertrophy. The reaction of the muscles to movement, whether or not it contracts and relaxes, will be assessed.
4. *Skin*. Local changes in skin temperature will be noted, e.g. an increase in temperature indicating possible inflammation.

Some osteopaths will routinely do a palpatory exam-ination of the joints of the lower limb, and indeed other spinal regions, in all cases of low back pain, but many would argue that this is only necessary if other elements of the examination and interview indicate that there may be a problem which could be having an influence on the symptoms from the low back.

The use of sophisticated diagnostic methods such as radiography or blood tests have not been discussed here. Their value is not in question; rather, access to these procedures will depend on local availability, and in many instances, the suspicion of a condition requiring such investigation will be reason for referral to the appropriate medical authority.

Summary

The osteopath, then, first carefully explores the patient's physical well-being and performs the normal clinical tests, to establish suitability for physical treatment. Palpatory findings will contribute to the eventual conclusions. Although osteopaths do make specific diagnoses (often based on the structures supposedly involved), the terminology varies sig-nificantly between practitioners and is outside the scope of this overview. Having thoroughly inter-viewed and examined the patient, the osteopath should now be in a position to offer a management strategy based on the findings from that individual as opposed to being based solely on a diagnostic label.

Management

The management strategies outlined here are those that a typical osteopath might use in office-practice, but the principles would apply similarly, though with suitable modification, in a hospital or industrial environment.

Aims

The principal aim of osteopathic treatment, when applied to mechanical low back pain, is the restora-tion of normal function to the lumbar spine and its surrounding tissues. Traditionally, the main focus is lumbar mobility, or more specifically an increase in the range of mobility at one or more intervertebral joints. It is well accepted that there is, on average, a reduction in the extent of lumbar mobility in the presence of low back pain, and there is evidence that improvement of biomechanical function is, on aver-age, associated with improvement in mechanical low back pain conditions (Doran and Newell, 1975; Koes *et al.*, 1992; Greenough and Fraser, 1994; Mitchell and Carmen, 1994). However, it has also been shown, on an individual basis, that symptomatic improve-ment is as common in patients with unaltered or reduced extent of lumbar flexibility (Burton *et al.*, 1990). It may be that the focus of treatment should be on dynamic qualities of movement rather than just the (static) range. There is little scientific evidence to support this view, but it is one which osteopaths intuitively follow. The tissues likely to be directly affected by osteopathic manipulative treatment are the lumbar musculature, ligaments, joint capsules, and possibly synovial fluid or local vascular/lym-phatic systems. Indirectly, the nutritional pathways to the intervertebral disc may be influenced, and there may also be an indirect effect on neuromuscular performance from afferent stimulation. In short, the effects are likely to be on the structures concerned with dynamic function.

There is much discussion in osteopathic circles regarding natural healing mechanisms within the body, though traditionally treatment is applied with the intention of enhancing such repair and recovery. All human bodily functions rely on a 'homeostatic' balance within the physiology of the tissues; if this situation alters, pathological change may then take place in the tissues. Therefore, it follows that abnor-mal function is a step towards pathological change within tissues. Such changes may occur in the soft tissues of the lumbar spine (e.g. fibrotic infiltration of muscle, ligament, fascia, synovium, and joint capsules, or degenerative changes in hyaline cartilage). Medication and surgery will often be incompatible with such changes, leaving physical approaches such as manipulative treatment as an alternative. If no treatment is offered in these circumstances, does the functional state of the lumbar spine continue to deteriorate leading to irreversible structural changes and chronic pain and disability?

If it is accepted that the lumbar spine should have certain qualities, and/or ranges, of movement, then the goal is achieving as near to normal (for that individual) as possible. There is much uncertainty regarding whether or not mobility of the sacroiliac joints contribute to lumbar dysfunction. It is believed by many osteopaths that positional malalignment of a sacroiliac joint can contribute to mechanical low back pain, but there is conflicting evidence in the literature (Vleeming *et al.*, 1990). Tissues which may influence lumbar movement are the target for treatment; attempts may be made to reduce muscle tone, stretch fibrotic areas, and increase elasticity of joint capsules and intersegmental ligaments. If movement, and therefore function, is improved, then normal repair mechanisms should ensue. The notion proposed by osteopaths is that subtle impairments of movement at a segmental level are of paramount importance for correct function. This theory is not proposed as an alternative to so-called 'orthodox' physiology, osteopaths simply believe that much management of mechanical low back pain often overlooks consideration of intersegmental movement.

When considering the subject of mobility, the osteopath will go further and suggest that impaired movement in other areas of the musculoskeletal system can influence the lumbar spine. If there is a fault at the ankle, knee, hip or thoracic spine, then abnormal stresses may be exerted on the lumbar spine tissues, causing dysfunction. Poor thoracic movement will result in an increased strain on the lumbar spine during bending/lifting. An ankle, knee or hip condition which alters gait may result in abnormal strain on the lumbar spine. It may be considered that these other areas are the locus of the primary fault which, if not addressed, will result in treatment to the lumbar spine being suboptimal and only a temporary measure; in time, the lumbar dysfunction will recur.

The osteopath's approach will go beyond the mechanical consequences of impaired mobility. It is recognized that fear of pain, and negative attitudes, may prolong an episode of low back pain and may also be a factor in the progression to chronicity (Lee *et al.*, 1989; Burton *et al.*, 1995; Symonds *et al.*, 1995). Thus, a vital component of the management process is to alter any inappropriate attitudes and beliefs. Chronic pain is a complex phenomenon, involving not only tissue damage but attitudes to pain, coping strategies, previous experience of pain, and alteration of the central processing mechanisms. It should be a paramount aim in the management of acute patients to avoid progression to chronicity.

Treatment

In order to achieve the stated aims, a variety of technical approaches may be utilized, depending on the individual needs of the patient. Three broad classes of manual procedures are used more or less universally, but there are other techniques, beyond the scope of this chapter, that are used by some osteopaths. Advice, in its various forms, should be considered a part of the therapeutic process.

Classification

Soft tissue

This term refers to direct contact techniques applied to muscle and ligamentous tissue. Three types of muscle techniques are used; cross-fibre stretch, longitudinal stretch, and deep pressure. Cross-fibre stretch is force applied at right angles to the muscle fibres in order to relax the muscle, or increase the elasticity of the muscle fibres. The mechanism by which muscle tone is reduced is not fully understood, but it is thought that the Golgi tendon apparatus has a role to play in adjusting muscle tone. Longitudinal stretch is force applied along the length of the muscle in order to increase elasticity by breaking cross-linkages and stretching fibrous tissue. Deep pressure is applied to so-called 'trigger points', to specific muscles and to areas of fibrosis, to increase local circulation and alter afferent input to the neuromuscular reflex. Ligamentous tissue can also be stretched either across the fibres, longitudinally, or with deep pressure.

Articulation

This term refers to passive joint movement. The joint involved (zygapophysial) is moved within its normal physiological range; in practice, articulation may be combined with soft tissue techniques. If the joint capsule or inter-segmental ligaments are to be stretched, then the joint can be moved beyond its resistance. Joint movement can be carried out with the patient side lying, supine, or prone; flexion, extension, lateral flexion and rotation (or combinations thereof) are possible. A swing-leaf plinth allows the patient to lie prone and passive lateral flexion to be carried out with ease; considerable amplitude can be achieved with a surprising degree of control, and soft tissue stretch is possible at the same time. The effect of articulation is believed to be an alteration of neuromuscular control, allowing improved intersegmental mobility (with resultant pain free movement) and an increase in the local circulation adjacent to the joint, thus aiding the reduction of inflammation.

High velocity thrust

This term refers to a specific joint manipulation. The zygapophysial joint is the focus of the thrust. The aim of high velocity thrust techniques (HVT) is to separate the joint surfaces at right angles to the plane of the facets. The joint is brought to a point of tension using a combination of movements, flexion/rotation and side-bending with or without compression/traction. If a left lumbar joint is to be thrust, the patient would be lying on the right side with the lower leg straight and the upper leg flexed at hip and knee; the thorax would be rotated left and flexed; the pelvis and lumbar spine are rotated right. The intention is to focus the rotational forces from thoracic and lumbar 'levers' to a single spinal level; careful palpation is used to guide the leverage and bring the joint concerned to that point of tension where the soft tissues begin to limit motion; this will always be within the normal physiological range of the joint. At this point of tension, a force is applied at right angles to the joint surface with high velocity but a very small amplitude, thus gapping the joint surfaces and producing 'cavitation'. It is emphasized that the joint should not be moved outside its normal physiological range. The process of cavitation produces a temporary separation of the joint surfaces allowing an increase in the range of movement available (Unsworth *et al.*, 1971). A longer lasting effect is thought to be brought about by afferent input altering the feedback in the neuromuscular reflex arc, thus changing the efferent message to the muscle spindles, resulting in a reduction of muscle tone. Any of the lumbar zygapophysial joints can be manipulated in this way. The sacroiliac joint may also be manipulated, but opinion differs as to efficacy; at what age the joint may fuse is also the subject of some debate (Vleeming *et al.*, 1990).

Advice

Contact time with the practitioner occupies a small proportion of the recovery period; advice is required to supplement the manual therapy. It seems to be increasingly clear that management, rather than just prescribed treatment for mechanical low back pain, is an important distinction. In acute cases, there may be some value to be gained from the use of non-steroidal anti-inflammatory preparations (NSAIDs). A knowledge of the patient's work or sport is necessary, and simple effective advice given and reinforced; the various national, and international, guidelines on work practices and workstations should be considered. Having said this, it should be recognized that prolonged work loss is detrimental, and that exercise in the form of sports can contribute to recovery. Thus, sickness absence is only suggested if absolutely necessary, and return to gentle exercise and sports pursuits should be advised at the earliest opportunity. Prescription of rehabilitation exercises which have a dynamic (rather than passive) component is seen as a fundamental part of the management process, particularly in chronic cases. There is strong evidence that the psychosocial factors are of paramount importance in recovery from low back pain (Burton *et al.*, 1995). Encouragement of movement and everyday activities is important for reduction of fear avoidance behaviours. Bed rest is used only when essential, and restricted to a maximum of 3 days for mechanical low back pain.

Frequency

How often should a patient be treated? This will vary quite considerably between practitioners, but the condition being treated will obviously influence the decision. A wide range for the number of treatments has been reported for osteopathic practice, but the average of six treatments is probably typical (Burton *et al.*, 1995). In cases with acute tissue damage, treatment twice a week seems necessary; support for the patient is essential in alleviating their fears and concerns. Some considerable encouragement will be needed to help them return to normal activities as quickly as possible. Table 23.1 gives general guidelines of treatment frequencies likely to be performed by osteopaths for different forms of low back trouble.

Table 23.1 *Osteopathic treatment for mechanical low back pain – frequency of visits*

Condition	Treatment frequency				
	Weekly sessions	Fortnightly sessions	Monthly sessions	Average number of sessions	Follow-up sessions
Acute low back pain	2–4	2–4	1–3	5–6	no
Acute low back pain and sciatica	2–4	2–4	1–6	6–10	yes
Subchronic low back pain	2–4	2–4	1–3	5–6	no
Subchronic low back pain and sciatica	2–4	2–4	1–6	6–10	yes
Chronic low back pain	2–4	2–4	1–6	5–10	no
Chronic low back pain and sciatica	2–4	2–4	1–6	6–12	yes

Maintenance visits, particularly in chronic or recurrent cases, are used by many osteopaths to monitor a patient over time. The interval may be 2–4 months, and the visit may consist of an assessment only, or may involve some treatment. Whether this helps or hinders is unknown.

Outcome

The success of a treatment should be considered in the light of the natural history of the condition (Weber and Burton, 1986), which for, say, disc herniation is possible to predict with reasonable accuracy (Saal *et al.*, 1990; Weber, 1995). However, the natural history of much mechanical low back trouble is essentially unknown and typically follows a fluctuating course both within and between spells. Thus the apparent effectiveness of treatment may depend more on when outcome is measured, than on any alteration of the natural history (Weber and Burton, 1986; Deyo, 1994). A further question arises when deciding on when therapy or management should end; up to 50% of patients will still have residual symptoms on return to work (Lloyd and Troup, 1983). It is extremely important that these issues are recognized, for they will influence not only clinical management but also what information can be given about likely outcomes to adjust patient expectations. Definition of outcome status is based not only on symptomatic change but should also include change in disability (improvements in ability to perform activities of daily living) and recurrence patterns. Realistic goals should be set out at an early stage of management; they should include both short- and long-term outcomes, and will involve warning the patient about fluctuations in symptoms during the course of treatment. A positive but believable approach is vital from a psychological point of view

for the patient's hope and attitude to recovery; unreasonable expectations can only bring despair and loss of trust. Goals and targets can, of course, act as a monitor for both patient and practitioner.

Functional management

Table 23.2 presents a simple starting point from which to view osteopathic management principles of acute, subchronic and chronic mechanical low back pain. For conditions with no significant structural abnormalities, the specific aims can be summarized as follows:

1. to reduce muscle spasm and to influence neuro-muscular reflexes;
2. to increase segmental mobility;
3. to reduce fear and anxiety and to promote a positive outlook;
4. to advise exercises which will encourage or maintain dynamic spinal movement;
5. to advise on work practices and sports participation in order to reduce risks of recurrence.

Acute low back pain

When acute low back pain is of mechanical origin, it is thought to be a benign, self-limiting condition, but chronicity (symptoms lasting more than 3 months) is common, and many patients do not actually become symptom free (at 1 year), even when treated (Hickman and Mason, 1993; Burton *et al.*, 1995). Osteopathic treatment should attempt to return the patient to normal activities as soon as possible, with particular attention to fear of pain and attitudes to movement or exercises. Treatment focuses on muscle relaxation, joint mobilization,

Table 23.2 *Summary of osteopathic management of low back pain*

Type	Soft tissue	Articulation	HVT	Pain relief	Activity/exercises	Advice
Acute ± leg pain	paraspinal cross-fibre, inhibition	small amplitude	short leverage	ice packs	encourage walking	limit sitting and over-exertion; encourage general exercise/sport
Subchronic ± leg pain	cross-fibre, stretching, friction	larger amplitude	normal leverage	–	encourage general exercise/activity	early uptake of sport; ?alter work practices; promote +ve attitudes
Chronic ± leg pain	stretching	larger amplitudes	normal leverage	–	encourage daily walk and general exercise	progressive uptake of sport; reduce fear-avoidance behaviours
Root compromise acute or subchronic	inhibition, cross-fibre	small amplitude side-bending, traction	minimal	ice packs	encourage mobility	limit sitting, driving and lifting; gradual return to activity; promote +ve attitudes

anti-inflammatory measures, and encouragement of movement and activity. High velocity thrust techniques, articulation and soft tissue techniques, are all felt to be effective in the acute phase. Bed rest should be avoided if at all possible. Walking should be encouraged from the start, sitting still should be limited to 10 minutes maximum, driving should be only in short spells, gentle exercises to encourage soft tissue stretch are appropriate (flexion, rotation and side-bending). Anti-inflammatory measures and analgesics can be useful to control symptoms. A patient would normally be seen twice during the first week, then weekly for approximately 2–4 weeks. Discharge from treatment would depend on likelihood of recurrence.

Subchronic low back pain

This is an intermediate time between 1 week and 3 months. A patient in the subchronic phase will have soft tissue changes (fibrosis) and altered neuromuscular activity which should respond to manual treatment. Larger amplitude movement during treatment will encourage joint mobility, and all techniques of osteopathic treatment are appropriate. Daily exercises will be needed to maintain any changes brought about from treatment; swimming and use of a gymnasium may be advised. A patient would normally be seen on a weekly basis for approximately 1 month, with regular check ups at perhaps monthly intervals for 3–4 months.

Chronic low back pain

This is classed as a condition with a 3-month or more history. Considerable tissue changes may have taken place within the lumbar musculature and ligaments. Chronic low back pain is a complex disorder involving not just physical changes in soft tissues, but also frequently is accompanied by psychological distress (Main *et al.*, 1992), and there may be disturbance of the central processing of pain. All the osteopathic techniques are relevant to help the mechanical aspect of the condition, soft tissue techniques may concentrate on deep friction and articulation will be large amplitude. Much encouragement and support is needed to overcome fear that activity will do further damage or aggravate the condition. Exercises, or regular sport/activity, are vital. Advice on work practices, or sport training schedules, can help prevent the ongoing nature of a condition. Regular 'check-up' visits are thought by some to be worthwhile in monitoring the condition. This does give the osteopath the chance to maintain the emphasis on activity and exercise and avoids the patient being left alone with no advice, perhaps becoming confused about what to do next. Compliance with treatment and advice is perceived to have a large influence on recovery.

Structural management

Some mechanical low back conditions will have a concomitant primary or acquired alteration to spinal structure; the relationship between many structural faults and symptoms is mostly speculative unless the abnormalities are gross. Some of the conditions which fall into this category are:

1. Degenerative zygapophysial joint disease.
2. Degenerative intervertebral disc disease with or without herniation.
3. Lateral scoliosis.
4. Congenital anomalies.
5. Spondylolisthesis.
6. Facet tropism.

Moderate spinal degeneration does not preclude osteopathic treatment. The general treatment principles outlined above will apply, but care should be taken to observe any nerve root compression which could result from osteophytic outgrowth. Extension exercises, and unnecessary extension during treatment, should be avoided, as the compressive force on the facet joints may result in inflammatory reaction. Degenerative changes can be quite severe without any apparent pain, or may only cause pain periodically. The compensatory changes which develop over time often allow for relatively good function. Once the patient is comfortable, treatment should probably cease; attempts to reverse the condition are futile. Appropriate surgical/medical opinion should be sought if response to treatment is poor, or deterioration is evident.

A herniated intervertebral disc may, or may not, produce nerve root irritation. As long as there are no signs suggesting a need for urgent surgical intervention, then manipulation can be justified (Cassidy *et al.*, 1993). A lack of improvement over the first 6–8 weeks (or earlier progressive deterioration) will indicate a need for (orthopaedic) referral. Again all classes of osteopathic treatment are appropriate; sitting should be limited, walking should be encouraged, lifting should be avoided, extension exercises may be helpful (Magnusson *et al.*, 1995). Return to normal activities should begin as soon as possible. A structural lateral scoliosis of the spine causing pain can respond to osteopathic treatment; any attempt to reverse the scoliosis is inadvisable. The aim of treatment is to encourage good mobility within the structural limits. All manipulative techniques may be used in most cases.

Congenital anomalies of the lumbosacral spine are often not identified during the examination, and rarely have any relationship to the back pain. A mechanically unstable spondylolisthesis is an obvious exception, but stable anterior shifts may gain considerable symptomatic relief from osteopathic treatment (though high velocity thrusts and vigorous articulatory manoeuvres would not be used).

Summary

What has been presented here is a pragmatic approach to the osteopathic management of back pain; for detailed descriptions of particular aspects of theory and technique, the reader will need to consult osteopathic texts. Doubtless, much of what has been detailed here will be common to the other 'manual' professions, and equally doubtless is the fact that not all osteopaths will agree with what has been written under their banner. Some of what has been proposed is what osteopaths typically do and believe to be effective, despite the limited support in the literature for the efficacy of osteopathic methods or any other manipulative therapy (MacDonald and Bell, 1990; Koes *et al.*, 1991). The other aspects introduced have been an attempt to focus on restoration of function not only for chronic cases (where functional restoration has been shown to be helpful (Kohles *et al.*, 1990)), but also to conform with emerging guidelines for management of acute cases (Clinical Standards Advisory Group, 1994).

References

Agency for Health Policy and Research, UD (1994) *Management Guidelines For Acute Low-Back Pain*. US Government Printing Office, Washington, DC.

Bolton, J. and Christensen, M. (1994) Back pain distribution patterns: relationship to subjective measures of pain sensitivity and disability. *J. Manipulative Physiol. Ther.,* **17**, 211-218.

Burton, A.K. (1981) Back pain in osteopathic practice. *Rheumatol. Rehabil.,* **20**, 239-246.

Burton, A.K. (1983) Sciatic syndromes: a preliminary report of a search for criteria for identification and assessment. *Br. Osteopath. J.,* **15**, 87-94.

Burton, A.K., Bennett, G. and Sykes, D. (1993) Persistence of lumbar tenderness after resolution of low back trouble symptoms. *Br. Osteopath. J.,* **11**, 11-13.

Burton, A.K. and Tillotson, K.M. (1991) Prediction of the clinical course of low-back trouble using multivariable models. *Spine*, **16**, 7-14.

Burton, A.K., Edwards, V.A. and Sykes, D.A. (1990a) Invisible skin marking for testing palpatory reliability. *Manip. Med.,* **5**, 27-29.

Burton, A.K., Tillotson, K.M., Edwards, V.A. and Sykes, D.A. (1990b) Lumbar sagittal mobility and low back symptoms in patients treated with manipulation. *J. Spinal Disord.,* **3**, 262-268.

Burton, A.K., Tillotson, K.M., Main, C.J. and Hollis, S. (1995) Psychosocial predictors of outcome in acute and sub-chronic low back trouble. *Spine,* **20**, 722-728.

Cassidy, J.D., Thiel, H.W. and Kirkaldy-Willis, W.H. (1993) Side-posture manipulation for lumbar intervertebral disk herniation. *J. Manipulative Phys. Ther.,* **16**, 96-103.

Clinical Standards Advisory Group (1994) *Back Pain*. Report of a CSAG committee on back pain. HMSO, London, pp. 3-89.

Deyo, R.A. (1994) Practice variations, treatment fads, rising disability: do we need a new clinical research paradigm? *Spine,* **18**, 2153-2162.

Doran, D.M.L. and Newell, D.J. (1975) Manipulation in treatment of low back pain: a multicentre study. *Br. Med. J.,* **2**, 161-164.

Fairbank, J.C.T., Park, W.M., McCall, I.W. and O'Brien, J.P. (1981) Apophyseal injection of local anaesthetic as a diagnostic aid in primary low-back pain syndromes. *Spine,* **6**, 598-604.

Frank, A. (1993) Low back pain. *Br. Med. J.,* **306**, 901-909.

Greenough, C.G. and Fraser, R.D. (1994) Aetiology diagnosis and treatment of low back pain. *Eur. Spine J.,* **3**, 22-27.

Hickman, M. and Mason, V. (1993) *The Prevalence of Back Pain*. A report prepared for the Department of Health. Office of Population Censuses Surveys, London.

Koes, B.W., Assendelft, W.J.J., Van der Heijden, G.J., Bouter, L.M. and Knipschild, P.G. (1991) Spinal manipulation and mobilisation for back and neck pain: a blinded review. *Br. Med. J.,* **303**, 1298-1303.

Koes, B.W., Bouter, L.M., Van Mameren, H. *et al.* (1992) The effectiveness of manual therapy and treatment by the general practitioner for non-specific back and neck complaints: a randomised clinical trial. *Spine,* **17**, 28-35.

Kohles, S., Barnes, D., Gatchel, R.J. and Mayer, T.G. (1990) Improved physical performance outcomes after functional restoration treatment in patients with chronic low-back pain: early versus recent training results. *Spine,* **15**, 1321-1324.

Lee, P.W.H., Chow, S.P., Lieh-Mak, F., Chan, K.C. and Wong, S. (1989) Psychosocial factors influencing outcome in patients with low-back pain. *Spine,* **14**, 838-843.

Lloyd, D.C.E.F. and Troup, J.D.G. (1983) Recurrent back pain and its prediction. *J. Soc. Occup. Med.,* **33**, 66-74.

MacDonald, R.S. and Bell, C.M.J. (1990) An open controlled assessment of osteopathic manipulation in nonspecific low-back pain. *Spine,* **15**, 364-370.

Magnusson, M.L., Pope, M.H. and Hansson, T. (1995) Does hyperextension have an unloading effect on the intervetebral disc. *Scand. J. Rehabil. Med.,* **27**, 5-10.

Main, C.J., Wood, P.L., Holis, S., Spanswick, C.C. and Wadell, G. (1992) The distress and risk assessment method: a simple patient classification to identify distress and evaluate the risk of poor outcome. *Spine,* **17**, 42-52.

Mitchell, R.I. and Carmen, G.M. (1994) The functional restoration approach to the treatment of chronic pain in patients with soft tissue and back injuries. *Spine,* **19**, 633-642.

Saal, J.A., Saal, J.S. and Herzog, R.J. (1990) The natural history of lumbar invertebral disc extrusions treated nonoperatively. *Spine,* **15**, 683-686.

Sweetman, B.J., Heinrich, I. and Anderson, J.A. (1993) Review of selected tests that help distinguish common patterns of low back pain and some possible implications. *J. Orthop. Rheumatol.,* **6**, 3-9.

Symonds, T.L., Burton, A.K., Tillotson, K.M. and Main, C.J. (1995) Absence due to low back trouble can be reduced by psychosocial intervention at the workplace. *Spine*, in press.

Unsworth, A., Dowson, D. and Wright, V. (1971) Cracking joints: a bioengineering study of cavitation in the metacarpophalangeal joint. *Ann. Rheum. Dis.,* **30**, 348-358.

Vleeming, A., Stoeckart, R., Snijders, C.J., Van Wingerden, J. and Dijkstra, P. (1990) The sacroiliac joint - anatomical, biomechanical and radiological aspects. *J. Manip. Med.,* **5**, 100-102.

Waddell, G. and Main, C.J. (1984) Assessment of severity in low-back disorders. *Spine,* **9**, 204-208.

Weber, H. (1995) The natural history of disc herniation and the influence of intervention. *Spine,* **19**, 2234-2238.

Weber, H. and Burton, A.K. (1986) Rational treatment of low back trouble? *Clin. Biomech.,* **1**, 160-167.

24

Physiotherapy management of low back pain of mechanical origin

Stephen J. Edmondston and Robert L. Elvey

Introduction

The use of manual treatment for low back pain has evolved from massage and basic exercise, to the present, where manual therapy is a recognized specialization within the physiotherapy profession. The role of the manual therapist is to assess pain and function, detect movement abnormalities, test anatomical structures and design a treatment programme which is related to realistic goals (Farrell and Jensen, 1992). In the process of learning clinical manual therapy, the physiotherapist is presented with what is at times a bewildering array of examination and treatment techniques. These may follow one or more of the popular 'approaches' to manual therapy (Twomey and Taylor, 1987) and generally provide a framework around which a clinical diagnosis can be achieved and an appropriate treatment plan devised. While this may appear to be a suitable model for teaching purposes, in the reality of the clinical situation, the clinician with little experience to draw on is likely to run into trouble on a number of fronts. It is with this problem in mind that this chapter is based. It is not the intention to reiterate detailed descriptions of clinical techniques which are well documented in numerous contemporary manual therapy texts. Rather it is to guide the inexperienced clinician in the use and interpretation of these methods, and to help bridge the gap between manual therapy theory and practice.

The physiotherapy approach to managing low back pain is largely based on the methods described by individuals working in this area of the profession. While differences exist, the common thread between these methods is that they seek to determine the quality and range of spinal mobility, in relation to the presenting symptoms, as a basis for treatment pre-

scription. It is the purpose of this chapter to integrate these examination procedures further and to provide some guidelines and rationales to assist in formulating an appropriate treatment. The primary focus for treatment is on methods of spinal joint mobilization and associated exercise. While the assessment of muscle imbalance and neural tissue involvement are recognized as important aspects of mechanical therapy for the lumbar spine, these will not be specifically covered in relation to the treatment methods described here and readers are referred to the primary sources for details (Jull and Janda, 1987; Butler, 1991; Norris, 1995a). The management of chronic low back pain is another area in which physiotherapists are having an increasing role. However, the complexity of chronic pain and the diversity of the approaches to treatment are beyond the scope of this chapter.

The first part of this chapter provides an overview of the subjective examination with some explanation of possible responses and situations where a modified or abbreviated examination may be required. Some factors to consider prior to performing a physical examination are described as a preface to a summary of the examination procedures. The interpretation of the examination findings and factors to consider in planning an appropriate treatment are discussed briefly. The second part of the chapter describes the various approaches to the treatment of low back pain and the rationale for technique selection in various clinical presentations. There is no attempt to describe treatment methods for specific clinical 'syndromes' (McKenzie, 1981) or to provide 'recipe' treatments for specific presentations. Rather, we have attempted to provide a framework for a problem-solving approach to treatment which is based on movement abnormalities, and the severity and irritability of the associated symptoms.

Examination

Subjective examination

Many patients will report with little prompting a good description of the nature and history of their problem. The patient must be given an opportunity to tell their story but should be guided, with careful questioning, towards providing the information which is required. It is important not to interrogate the patient with a long series of structured questions. Some patients may have difficulty in interpreting the questions and should be assisted by rephrasing the question or suggesting possible responses. The questions should be kept open and free of bias so as not to influence the response. On occasions, particularly in recent cases, acute pain elements of the subjective examination may not be relevant and can be omitted or modified as is appropriate.

Most patients present with pain or discomfort as their primary problem (Grieve, 1991) and the general format of the subjective examination is structured accordingly. It is important to determine at the beginning of the examination whether it is pain or some other factor (usually stiffness) which is the patient's principal problem. In the case of the lumbar spine, it is unusual for patients to present with stiffness, which is not associated with some degree of discomfort during movement or with certain activities or postures. The essential elements of the subjective examination where pain (together with functional limitation) is the primary complaint are described in Table 24.1 (modified from Maitland, 1986).

Pain

A clear description of the location, nature, intensity and frequency of the symptoms is essential. Pain in the lumbar spine and any referred pain should be noted as well as areas of paraesthesia and numbness. Pain which is constant in nature is indicative of an inflammatory process, while intermittent pain is more likely to be mechanical in origin (Bogduk, 1984). Many patients, particularly those with acute back pain, may have pain which is both chemical and mechanical in nature. The location of the pain is unlikely to be helpful in determining the pathological spinal level (McCall *et al.*, 1979) but the nature and severity of the referred symptoms may help differentiate somatic pain from that caused by nerve root compression. Radicular symptoms have a lancinating or shooting quality, are often clearly defined and associated with other neurological symptoms such as paraesthesia and numbness. Conversely, pain referred from other spinal structures is more likely to be perceived as a dull, poorly

Table 24.1 *Summary of the subjective examination for the lumbar spine*

1. Area of symptoms – record on body chart

   For each pain area determine:

   (i)   Constant or intermittent (variable if constant?)
   (ii) Nature of the pain(s), e.g. dull, sharp
   (iii) Location, e.g. deep or superficial

   Record:

   (iv) areas of paraesthesia
   (v) areas of anaesthesia

   Check:

   (vi) other areas which are relevant to the lumbar spine
   (vii) temporal relationships between the symptomatic areas

2. Behaviour of the symptoms
   (i)   Aggravating factors or activities – time for pain to develop/increase and prevent continuation
   (ii) Easing factors – how long for the symptoms to settle. Effect of rest, especially lying and in which position
   (iii) Behaviour of symptoms over the course of the day
   (iv) Behaviour of symptoms at night – effect on sleep – difficulty getting to sleep, waking with pain, need to get up during the night, type of bed
   (v)   Symptom behaviour in the morning – presence of pain and stiffness, time to ease
   (vi) Effects of sustained flexion activities or postures, effect of sitting, difficulty rising from sitting
   (vii) Effect of coughing or sneezing on the back and/or leg pain

3. Special questions
   (i)   General health – recent or on-going medical problems, recent surgery, recent unexplained weight loss, increased weight, normal recreational activities, exercise, work activities
   (ii) Medications for this and other conditions, present or previous steroid or anticoagulant medications
   (iii) Recent radiological examination, e.g. plain radiographs, CT, MRI
   (iv) Disturbance of bowel or bladder function or 'saddle' anaesthesia (suggestive of cauda equina compression)

4. History
   (i)   Current history – when did the symptoms develop, sudden/gradual onset, trauma (direct/indirect), progression of symptoms (better or worse), any treatment for this episode and effect
   (ii) Past history – previous episodes of back pain, similarities/differences with current episode, time to ease, any treatment and effect

localized ache and not associated with other neurological symptoms. It should be remembered that some patients may present with pain which is both radicular and somatic in origin. The location of any leg pain will guide the clinician as to which peripheral joints should be screened as part of the physical examination. The frequency and intensity of the pain should be assessed either descriptively or with the assistance of a visual analogue scale (Price *et al.*, 1983).

Symptom behaviour

An important function of the subjective examination is to assess the severity and irritability of the symptoms, and to determine the effect of functional activities. This information is essential in planning the physical examination and treatment, and to assist in evaluating the results of subsequent treatment. This can only be achieved by determining the behaviour of the symptoms over time, and in relation to posture and activity (Grieve, 1991). The associated behaviour of any referred pain, paraesthesia or numbness should also be determined. A suggested framework to assist in evaluating the behaviour of the symptoms is described in Figure 24.1.

Constant pain is usually inflammatory or chemical in origin and is most commonly associated with a recent injurious event, trauma or more serious pathologies such as inflammatory arthritis, tuberculosis or neoplasm. Pain at night which causes persistent sleep disturbance and necessitates getting out of bed is suggestive of this type of non-mechanical pathology. With the exception of some acute mechanical disorders, individuals with these symptoms are often unsuitable for mechanical therapy. The patients who are more suited to mechanical therapy are those who have pain which is mechanical in origin. With the exception of the less common hypermobility conditions, e.g. spondylolisthesis, most patients have pain which is associated with hypomobility or movement limitation. Morning stiffness is a characteristic feature of joint hypomobility. The behaviour of the symptoms helps to differentiate between chemical and mechanical pain and guides the clinician as to the irritability of the symptoms, and how easy or difficult it might be to reproduce the patient's symptoms during the

physical examination. The behaviour of the symptoms in relation to activity or posture may also reflect the site and nature of the pathology. This concept is developed by Jull (1986). Finally, where possible, subjective criteria should be determined which can be used to assess improvement (or deterioration) of the symptoms over time. These are termed subjective reassessment criteria.

History and progression of the symptoms

The purpose of this part of the subjective examination is to determine the duration and progression of the symptoms. This helps to differentiate pain which has developed acutely from that which has a more progressive onset. In the latter case it is important to determine whether there were any factors which may have contributed to the development of the problem, e.g. past trauma, change of occupation, different recreational activities. In some cases of gradual onset pain, the patient may not be able to account for the development of the symptoms which may have been present to some extent (often episodic) for a number of years. This is usually indicative of what McKenzie (1981) describes as 'adaptive shortening' of periarticular soft tissue structures and may be associated with mild degenerative changes in the symptomatic joints. The patient should be asked to assess whether the symptoms are getting worse, are stable or improving.

The patient should also be asked about previous episodes of low back pain or pain in other regions of the spine. Comparisons with the present symptoms should be sought particularly in terms of onset, location and severity. The time for recovery from previous episodes should be determined as this may be becoming longer with each episode. It is also important to determine the nature, duration and results of previous treatment for this and other episodes of low back pain.

Other information

The final section of the subjective examination is what Maitland (1986) refers to as 'special questions'. The purpose is to find out additional information about the patient's condition and its management and to screen the patient for specific factors which may be indicative of serious pathology. These questions are listed in Table 24.1 but this important part of the examination is worthy of some additional comment. Although clinical trials have found that radiological findings are poorly correlated with the patient's symptoms (Torgerson and Dotter, 1976), the value of plain X-rays and other imaging methods, e.g. CT and

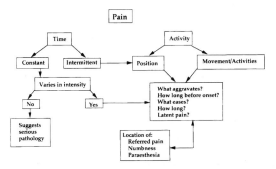

Figure 24.1 A framework for the evaluation of pain and other sensory symptoms in relation to time and activity.

MRI, should not be understated. These techniques provide valuable information about the general condition of, and spacial relationships between, the skeletal structures in the lumbar spine. This allows a direct assessment of spinal curvature and an evaluation of possible changes in load transfer through the intervertebral and zygapophysial joints. When available, the radiological images should be viewed by the clinician and the radiologist's report obtained.

In addition to determining what medication the patient is taking for this condition, a knowledge of other medications helps to establish a picture of the long and short-term general health of the patient. Steroid and anticoagulant therapies are of particular importance due to their regulatory effects on bone density (and consequently strength), and blood clotting mechanisms, respectively. Poor recent general health together with poor appetite, unexplained weight loss and severe night pain is indicative of serious pathology, such as metastatic disease. A personal or family history of rheumatoid arthritis should also be determined.

It is important to establish whether there is any possible pathological involvement of the spinal cord or cauda equina. This includes abnormal bowel or bladder function, altered or loss of sensation in the perineal region, gait or balance disturbances and abnormal sensation in the plantar aspect of the feet. In the presence of bladder retention, the clinician is obligated to transfer the patient to emergency medical care. In the presence of other symptoms suggestive of spinal cord or cauda equina involvement, the clinician must communicate with the referring medical practitioner or refer the patient for medical examination.

Planning the physical examination

Before commencing the physical examination, some time should be taken to consider how much assessment the patient can tolerate and what structures should be examined. Some factors which will influence these decisions are described in Table 24.2.

Having considered these factors, the therapist must then plan which structures need to be examined at the first visit. These can be divided into those which require a detailed examination and those which require only active movement screening. Maitland (1986) uses the following criteria to help with these decisions:

i) Joints which lie under the painful area.
ii) Joints which refer pain into the painful area.
iii) Muscles which lie under the painful area.

In some cases, this may involve a lengthy examination and this must be offset against some of the factors outlined above. In other words, while there is an ideal

Table 24.2 *Factors to consider when planning the physical examination of the lumbar spine*

1. The severity and irritability of the symptoms

2. Is the pain likely to be easy or difficult to reproduce?

3. The age and general condition of the patient

4. Radiological findings

5. The need for modified patient positions during the examination due to pain or other factors, e.g. the patient may not be able to lie prone

6. Are there factors which suggest caution is required?

7. Is a neurological examination required?

8. Are there features which suggest lumbar instability/hypermobility may be present?

physical examination format, the examination performed must be modified in accordance with the patient's presentation.

Physical examination

The primary purpose of the physical examination is to determine which spinal segments or other structures are producing the pain, and to find active movements which can be used for reassessment. To achieve this requires elements of observation, movement testing and joint palpation. The format for examination of the lumbar spine is set out in Table 24.3 and is followed by further description and comment on these procedures. Examination of the sacroiliac joints may be required as part of the examination but for convenience this will be considered separately. Pain which is perceived in the region of the sacroiliac joints may be coming from

Table 24.3 *Summary of the physical examination procedures for the lumbar spine*

1. Observation

2. Active movements
   - Flexion
   - Extension
   - Lateral flexion (L) and (R)
   - Side gliding (L) and (R) (McKenzie, 1981)
   - Other joints as necessary, e.g. hip, knee

3. Palpation

4. Passive movement tests
   - Physiological passive movements
   - Passive accessory intervertebral movements
   - Passive physiological intervertebral movements

5. Neurological tests

these structures, but the sacroiliac region is also a common site of referred pain from the lumbar spine (Bogduk and Twomey, 1991). In general, it is best to exclude the lumbar spine as a source of the symptoms before testing the sacroiliac joints (Grieve, 1991).

Observation

General willingness to move:

- Getting out of a chair
- Gait
- Undressing

From behind:

- Leg length
- Iliac crest levels
- Posterior superior iliac spine (PSIS) levels
- Alignment of the spine in the frontal plane, e.g. scoliosis, lateral shift

From the side:

- Thoracic kyphosis
- Lumbar lordosis
- Pelvic tilt
- Hip and knee position, e.g. hip flexion, knee hyperextension

When assessing spinal posture it is important to remember that significant gender differences exist (Pearsall and Reid, 1992). Furthermore, postural asymmetry and mild scoliosis are relatively common in a normal, unselected population and 'normal' sagittal plane curvatures span a wide range (Stagnara *et al.*, 1982; Singer *et al.*, 1990). Hansson *et al.* (1985) found no difference in the magnitude of the lumbar lordosis in patients with back pain compared to asymptomatic subjects. Consequently, not all apparent postural 'abnormalities' may be related to the condition for which the patient is seeking treatment.

Active movements

Possibly the most important part of the examination is that of active movement testing as it allows for an assessment of the range and quality of movement in relation to pain. The most important objective is to determine specific movements or combinations of movement which reproduce or, in the case of rest pain, increase the symptoms. This allows for an objective reassessment of the patient's condition over time.

Numerous methods have been advocated of measuring spinal mobility (Twomey and Taylor, 1979; Mayer *et al.*, 1984). Most however, have been developed and used for research purposes and are too impractical or time consuming for routine clinical use. Simple objective measurement of spinal movement remains an unsolved problem in clinical practice. However, two common approaches are to estimate the range as a proportion of the expected 'normal' range for that individual, and to use anatomical landmarks as a reference.

A checklist of points to note in association with active movement testing comprises:

- Pain before movement
- Point at which pain is first noted or increases
- Point of movement limitation, i.e. range
- What limits the movement, e.g. pain, stiffness
- Quality of the movement, i.e. speed, rhythm, deviation from normal movement plane, obvious segmental restrictions
- Pain associated with the return movement to the starting position.

In some cases, the patient's pain may not be reproduced by simple active movements in the anatomical planes. A suggested sequence of strategies to assist in reproducing the patient's symptoms is set out in Figure 24.2. Movement testing can be extended to combine movements in different sequences in order to evaluate multidirectional movement patterns in relation to the patient's symptoms (Edwards,

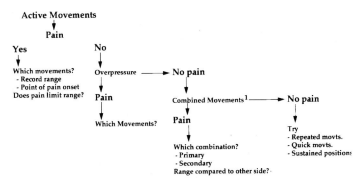

Figure 24.2 A sequence of strategies which can be employed during the physical examination to reproduce the patient's symptoms. (See Edwards (1992)).

1992). Repetition of active movements may be required to reproduce the symptoms in less irritable cases (McKenzie, 1981). At least one active movement or combined movement is required which can be used for reassessment during and between treatment sessions.

Passive movements

The assessment of physiological passive movements in the sagittal plane is advocated by McKenzie (1981). The obvious advantage of this is that it allows for an assessment of pain and range of movement. McKenzie (1981) also suggests that flexion in lying may help differentiate between intervertebral joint restriction and abnormal tension in the hamstring muscles or neural tissues as the cause of pain or limitation of flexion in standing. Passive lateral flexion and rotation may also be assessed but in general it is not essential to incorporate gross passive movements of the lumbar spine as part of the physical examination.

Palpation

Prior to testing intervertebral joint mobility, a brief assessment of the skin quality and temperature should be performed using the dorsal surface of the hand. Gentle palpation of the paravertebral musculature to detect any increase in resting tension or spasm should also be performed. The spinous processes should be palpated for abnormal tenderness, and prominence. Palpation of the supraspinous ligament may reveal areas of undue tenderness or thickening. The palpation findings must be assessed in relation to the symptoms reported and movement signs previously observed (Grieve, 1991).

Passive accessory intervertebral movement

These tests seek to determine the segmental range of accessory intervertebral movement in relation to pain and spasm or other resistance. As with peripheral joint testing it also allows for an assessment of the 'end-feel' of the movement (Kaltenborn, 1980). Postero-anterior (P/A) pressures are applied to each vertebral segment, both centrally over the spinous process, then unilaterally over the articular 'pillar'. Pressures are also applied transversely against the spinous processes. These procedures have been described in detail in other texts (Maitland, 1986; Grieve, 1991). The purpose is to determine the movement (displacement) of the joint and associated pain, relative to the magnitude of the applied pressure (force). Since stiffness is defined by the force/displacement relationship (White and Panjabi, 1990), the therapist is obtaining a tactile impression of joint stiffness in relation to pain. This mental picture of the force/displacement relationship can be expressed as a movement diagram (Maitland, 1986)

or joint picture (Grieve, 1991). In the clinical situation where multiple joints may be assessed in different directions, the use of movement diagrams can be time-consuming and cumbersome. The method of recording accessory intervertebral movement findings described by Grieve (1991) is more practical for routine clinical practice.

These tests appear relatively simple to perform, however, useful information will only be derived if the following points are kept in mind. Most importantly, maximizing the comfort of the application of pressure will maximize the quality and accuracy of the information obtained.

(i) Passive movement tests are subjective in their interpretation and there are no normal values for joint stiffness. The therapist must compare the perceived stiffness in the symptomatic joint with that at other levels, or in relation to his or her memory of a normal joint. This may be difficult, especially for the inexperienced therapist, as studies have shown that the subjective impression of the response to joint pressure is unreliable (Matayas and Bach, 1986; Maher and Adams, 1994). However, Keating *et al.* (1993) have shown that the ability to quantify an applied force can be improved with training. Furthermore, in normal subjects, P/A stiffness of the lumbar spine varies significantly between segments (Lee and Liversidge, 1994). Consequently, both pain and movement are important cues for spinal joint dysfunction (Maher and Latimer, 1992).

(ii) Hand placement should be purposeful and applied as accurately as possible over the structure to which pressure is being applied. Pressure can be applied with the thumb but, in the lumbar spine, increased comfort may result for the patient and therapist if pressure is applied via the medial border of the hand with contact pressure immediately distal to the pisiform. For increased comfort with unilateral P/A pressure, the paravertebral musculature should be pushed laterally so that the bulk of this muscle is not being squashed against the underlying articular 'pillar'.

(iii) Grieve (1991) suggests that the orientation of the facet joint planes is not an important consideration when applying accessory movement tests (or treatments). However, as is the case with peripheral joints, it seems appropriate to consider the morphology and orientation of the joint being examined. The reciprocal angulation of vertebral segments (Stagnara *et al.*, 1982) suggests that P/A pressures should be directed cranially in the upper lumbar spine (L1–L3) and caudally in the lower segments (L4 and L5). This is consistent with the results of Lee (1989), who found that a pressure applied perpendicular to the spinal curvature minimized the axial displacement and rotation moment associated with the anterior translation of the vertebral segment.

(iv) Pressures should initially be applied very gently with two or three oscillations per segment. This allows the patient time to report any discomfort experienced and avoids undue aggravation of the symptoms. Single, sustained pressures do not allow for this and reduce the appreciation of movement. Furthermore, the speed of application and the presence of increased muscle activation may increase the perceived stiffness of the joint (Lee and Svensson, 1993; Lee *et al.*, 1993).

Passive physiological intervertebral movement

Following the assessment of accessory joint movement, these tests are applied to joints which have been found to be restricted and painful. Joints adjacent to the symptomatic joints should also be examined to allow for a comparison with a relatively 'normal' joint. As with accessory movement tests, the joint is moved slowly through its range to assess the available range and 'end-feel'. This information may also be used to reassess changes in the range of movement in response to treatment. However, these are possibly the most difficult movements to obtain a 'feel' for and considerable practice is required to gain confidence in their use. Detailed descriptions of the testing procedures for the lumbar joints are described by Maitland (1986). For recording purposes, segmental motion may be graded using an ordinal scale such as that proposed by Grieve (1991):

```
0 = ankylosed
1 = trace
2 = reduced
3 = normal
4 = hypermobile
```

Examination of the sacroiliac joint

Examination of the sacroiliac joint is required when this joint is implicated by the patient's description of the nature and behaviour of the symptoms, and where examination of the lumbar spine does not reveal movement dysfunction which correlates with the presenting symptoms. Specific tests include:

Positional tests (Woerman, 1989)

(i) Leg length assessment (supine) to establish the presence of fixed innominate rotation.
(ii) Leg length assessment in long sitting to confirm innominate rotation.

Changes in the relative leg lengths in these two positions suggest a fixed innominate rotation. For

example, a posterior rotated innominate will result in apparent leg shortening on the affected side. In long sitting, the leg length will appear to increase on the affected side while the leg on the non-fixated side will remain in the same position.

Active movement tests

(i) Relative movement of the two PSISs during flexion. Earlier movement will occur on the restricted side.
(ii) Relative movement of the sacrum (S2 tubercle) and the PSIS during flexion (in standing or sitting). The sacrum should move slightly earlier than the PSIS. Simultaneous movement is indicative of fixation or hypomobility of the joint being tested.
(iii) Active hip flexion with bony palpation as above. The PSIS should move before the sacrum in a normally mobile joint.

Passive movement (or stress) tests

(i) Anterior rotation of the innominate on the sacrum with joint line palpation.
(ii) Posterior rotation of the innominate on the sacrum with joint line palpation.
(iii) Sacroiliac joint compression.
(iv) Sacroiliac distraction.

These tests can only be considered positive if they elicit a painful response.

Palpation

This is used to confirm the sacroiliac joint as a primary source of pain. Palpation should include the interosseous ligament in the posterior aspect of the joint, the joint line immediately below the PSIS, the sacrotuberous ligament and the sacrospinous ligament.

Neurological tests

Neurological testing consists of three phases: (i) muscle power, (ii) reflex testing and (iii) skin sensation. Also included in this section are tests of neuromeningeal movement or what Maitland (1986) has called 'movement of pain sensitive structures in the vertebral canal and intervertebral foramen'. Specific indications for neurological testing include subjective reports of altered sensation, paraesthesia, muscle weakness and severe, well-defined radiating pain.

Muscle power

These are tests of the power and endurance of muscles innervated predominantly by specific spinal nerve trunks. With the exception of the toe-raise test for the S1 nerve root, these tests should be performed isometrically with the associated joint positioned so that the muscle is working in mid-range. Where pain is produced by the resisted contraction it may be indicative of a lesion within the muscle and help differentiate contractile from non-contractile structures as the cause of the pain (Cyriax, 1993). The patient is asked for a maximal effort which should be sustained for at least 5 seconds. The following tests should be performed:

In standing:
  Toe raise (S1–S2)

In supine:
  Iliopsoas (L2)
  Quadriceps (L3/4)
  Tibialis anterior (L4)
  Extensor hallucies longus (L5)

In prone:
  Gluteus maximus/medius (S1)
  Hamstrings (S2)

Reflexes

Reflex testing is performed easily with the patient positioned comfortably in side lying. The reflexes are tested with reference to their presence and briskness, and comparison is made between the two limbs. Each reflex should be tested 5–6 times consecutively. Diminution of the response with repeated tests is suggestive of early nerve root compression and consequent impairment of innervation. Total loss of the reflex indicates a significant nerve root compression, while bilateral reflex loss may be indicative of a central disc protrusion. It is important to consider that the response to reflex testing may vary considerably between individuals. The inability to elicit a particular reflex does not necessarily indicate neurological pathology. The reflexes routinely tested in the lower limb are:

● Adductor magnus (L2,3,4)
● Patella tendon (L3–L4)
● Gluteus minimus/tensor fascia latae (L4–L5)
● Semitendionosis (L5,S1)
● Achilles tendon (S1)
● Plantar cutaneous reflex (S2)

In addition, screening tests for spinal cord or cauda equina involvement should be performed. These are:

(i) Babinski reflex.
(ii) Test for ankle clonus.

Sensation

Pain which is due to nerve root compression may be associated with altered cutaneous sensation in the associated dermatome. Where symptoms of paraesthesia or numbness are present, sensory testing is indicated to map the affected area. While there may be some overlap of dermatomes and variation between individuals, the area of altered sensation may be a guide in identifying the symptomatic vertebral segment. While somatic and radicular pain may coexist (Bogduk and Twomey, 1991), altered sensation will only occur in the presence of nerve root compression. Light touch and sharp/blunt sensation should be tested to differentiate large and small fibre involvement. Circumferential tests are applied around the thigh, knee and lower leg, followed by a careful examination of the foot.

Tests of neuromeningeal movement

When pain is referred into the buttock or leg, these tests are used to determine the relative mobility of neural tissues in the vertebral canal, the intervertebral foramen and along their peripheral pathway. They include:

(i)   Straight leg raise.
(ii) Prone knee flexion.
(iii) Passive neck flexion.

Detailed methods for testing neuromeningeal movement are described by Butler (1991).

Integration and analysis of examination findings

Having completed the physical examination it is important to summarize the principal findings. It is not always possible nor necessary to know which spinal structures are responsible for producing the patient's symptoms. While there may be many causes of low back pain, treatments which are prescribed according to aetiological factors or clinical diagnosis are likely to help only a small percentage of patients in any given group. Grieve (1988) summarizes some of the common clinical presentations of low back pain, categorized according to typical presentations and examination findings. Although this is not a scientific approach to disease classification or diagnosis, it is now recognized that the prescription of treatment according to the presenting clinical features is the cornerstone for the successful application of mechanical therapy. The choice of treatment is based on the severity and irritability of the symptoms, the relationship between the range and pain of the active movements, and tests of physiological and accessory intervertebral movements. In planning treatment and selecting mobilization techniques it is important to consider the following factors.

1. The irritability of the symptoms – important in planning what type of technique and how much treatment should be attempted on the first treatment session.
2. Comparable active movement signs – at least one active movement or combined movement should be selected in order to assess the response to treatment.
3. The relationship between pain and movement with intervertebral movement testing. This is essential in order to select an appropriate technique and grade of movement when applying spinal mobilization.
4. The effect of patient position on the pain. The patient may not be able to tolerate certain positions which will influence the choice of treatment technique or require a modified technique.
5. The presence of referred leg pain and neurological symptoms which should be monitored closely throughout the treatment session.

Treatment

Treatment technique

Passive mobilization and manipulation

The joint mobilization and manipulative techniques used in treating the lumbar spine are graded modifications or combinations of the accessory and physiological intervertebral movement tests (Maitland, 1986). Traction is included as a mobilization technique. The mobilization and manipulative techniques referred to in this section are described in detail by McKenzie (1981), Maitland (1986) and Grieve (1991). Mobilization techniques can be categorized as localized or regional. Localized techniques are performed such that movement preferentially occurs at one intervertebral segment. Regional techniques are applied as a more generalized movement of two or more segments. The factors which guide technique selection are (i) the comparable active movement restrictions found on examination, (ii) the onset, rate of increase and severity of the associated pain, (iii) the irritability of the symptoms, and most importantly (iv), the relationship between range, pain and resistance of the symptomatic segment as determined from the passive intervertebral movement tests. In summary, the choice of technique and grade of movement is determined by accurate assessment of the patient's signs and symptoms before and after each repetition of a technique. Mobilization techniques (grades I–IV) are applied as even, rhythmical oscillations at a rate of about two cycles per second.

Mobilization with movement

An innovative approach to the treatment of joint pain and restriction has been described by Mulligan (1989). These techniques combine the principles of accessory glides with active movement. In other words, these are patient-assisted mobilizations. The advantages of these techniques are (i) that the mobilization is applied with the joint in a weight-bearing position, (ii) the patient has control over how far into range the movement is performed, (iii) the technique is applied as a sustained stretch at the extreme of the available range and (iv) reassessment can be quickly performed without moving the patient on and off the treatment bed. These techniques are known as 'SNAGS' (sustained natural apophysial glides) and may be incorporated as part of a treatment regime either alone, or in conjunction with other techniques. However, as these are weight-bearing techniques they are generally not appropriate for use in acute pain conditions.

Grades of movement

Grades of movement describe how far into the available range the joint is moved. These are depicted for a normal and a restricted joint in Figure 24.3. In a joint which is not normally mobile, the movement grades are described in relation to the pathological limit. Each grade has position on the available range of movement and amplitude, which is a proportion of it (Grieve, 1991). The grade of movement chosen for treatment is determined by the factor limiting movement, and relationship between pain and resistance through range as determined from the tests of passive intervertebral movement. In general, where pain occurs early in range and is the factor-limiting movement, a low-grade technique is performed (grade I–II). Where pain occurs later in range and is secondary to resistance, grade III or IV techniques should be used to improve joint range. Consequently, the initial decision in selecting a grade of movement

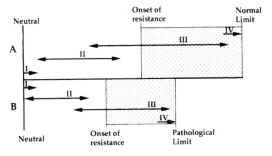

Figure 24.3 A diagrammatic representation of grades of joint movement in relation to the available range in a normal joint (A), and a joint with pathological movement restriction (B).

is whether pain or restriction is the primary factor being treated. Muscle spasm which results from joint movement can be treated with movement up to the point at which the spasm is provoked. In other words, spasm is used as a guide to the depth of the technique. *No attempt should ever be made to mobilize through muscle spasm.*

Manipulation

Manipulative techniques (grade V) are applied as a localized, low amplitude, high velocity thrust at the end of the available range. Indications for the use of grade V techniques are:

1. Minimal pain which is only apparent at end-range.
2. Where mobilization has been progressed to grade IV but is no longer achieving improvement.
3. Localized symptoms of sudden onset where the joint can be positioned at end-range without provoking muscle spasm.

As these thrust techniques are not under the control of the patient some specific precautions (additional to the recognized contraindications) should be observed (Grieve, 1991). These include:

1. Hypermobility of the involved segment.
2. Joint irritability and the presence of protective spasm.
3. Irritability or hypermobility in the segments adjacent to the symptomatic joint which may be aggravated by positioning for manipulation.
4. Inability of the patient to relax.

Application of treatment techniques

The importance of patient comfort in the application of spinal mobilization cannot be over-emphasized. This includes the position of the patient on the treatment plinth and the manner in which the technique is applied. A patient position should be chosen which is comfortable and will allow maximal relaxation during treatment. In some cases, it may be necessary or desirable to apply a treatment with the lumbar spine in a weight-bearing position such as sitting or standing (Mulligan, 1989). Accurate hand placement is important to ensure good contact with the required part of the vertebrae being moved. Where direct pressure techniques are employed, increased comfort may be achieved with modified pressure application (e.g. the ulnar border of the hand rather than the thumb tips). Pressures should not be applied through the bulk of the paravertebral muscles which may be very tender. These muscles should be pushed laterally when performing unilateral pressures to obtain a better contact with the articular 'pillar'. Vertebral pressures should be applied through a relaxed hand with the pressure being produced by the therapist's body weight rather than the muscles of the arm or hand. Careful attention to comfort when performing spinal mobilization will make the technique more effective, as the patient is able to relax and the response of the patient's symptoms to the technique is less confused with local discomfort associated with its application. Modified grades of movement can be used to good effect to improve patient comfort. Techniques performed at end-range to treat stiffness are generally more comfortable when a large amplitude is used. A grade III+ technique may not improve joint range as quickly as a grade IV but it may help overcome problems with treatment soreness. Finally, the orientation of the zygapophysial joints and the effect of this on joint movement should be considered when applying mobilization techniques.

Treatment protocol

Having identified at least one active movement for reassessment, the therapist decides on a mobilization technique, grade and duration of application. Once the patient is positioned they should be asked about their symptoms prior to initiating treatment. The mobilization technique is then applied at the chosen grade and the patient should be questioned regularly as to the effect on their symptoms. Local discomfort and symptom reproduction in the low back during treatment is acceptable, however, techniques which increase the referred symptoms should be discontinued. Having applied the technique for the chosen time, the patient is asked to stand up and is questioned about their pain prior to reassessment of the chosen active movements. Depending on the outcome, the following action may be taken.

Reassessment movement

Worse:

1. Repeat technique at a reduced grade.
2. Repeat technique for a shorter duration.

Reassess – if still worse change to a different technique.

Unchanged:

1. Increase technique grade.
2. Increase duration of repetition.

Better:

1. Continue with chosen technique until no further improvement is obtained.
2. Increase grade of movement.
3. Add a new technique according to the change in active movement signs.

Careful reassessment of active movements and appropriate modification or change of technique, is the key to systematic application of joint mobilization.

Treatment of acute pain

One of the most challenging presentations for the clinician is that of acute low back pain. Acute pain is usually rapid in onset and can be attributed to a particular movement or activity. All movements are usually painful and the pain may not be relieved completely by rest. The patient may adopt postures which reduce pressure on the symptomatic joints. Trunk flexion, lateral deviation of the trunk on the pelvis and reluctance to weight-bearing through the leg on the painful side are typical presentations. The scope of physical examination which can be performed may be limited by the irritability of the symptoms. However, careful observation and a limited active movement examination may provide sufficient information on which to plan and initiate treatment. The treatment concepts of McKenzie (1981) are most useful in the initial stages of treatment of acute low back pain as they use active movements over which the patient has complete control.

The following section outlines the initial treatment aims and associated treatment methods. Any movement or technique which increases pain laterally or distally into the leg(s) should be ceased and time allowed for the pain to ease. An increase in back pain is considered acceptable if it is associated with a reduction in the more distal symptoms (McKenzie, 1981).

1. Correct any lateral shift of the trunk

Method: active, repeated side-glide in standing (SGIS) to the restricted side or where unable to correct with active movements, active-assisted or passive correction should be attempted (McKenzie, 1981). Over vigorous lateral shift correction should be avoided as it may cause the patient to feel light-headed or faint.

2. Obtain extension to neutral and work into the extension range as pain allows

Method: having corrected the lateral shift, active extension in standing is encouraged while assisting the patient in maintaining the corrected posture. If the lateral shift has not been eliminated, attempts to extend the spine will fail and result in an exacerbation of the symptoms. It is often necessary to unload the spine to assist in restoring extension. If the patient is able to lie prone they should progress to forearm support prone lying and then to half 'push-ups' into extension (McKenzie, 1981). If increased pain results from these movements the patient should rest then move the pelvis laterally, in the direction of the shift correction, and attempt the extension exercises again. Unilateral or central pressure over the symptomatic segments may help restore passive extension. It is important not to over-treat with extension in patients who have very acute pain. Full extension may not be restored on the initial visit and if it is, the patient should move very carefully into the upright position as an exacerbation of symptoms can result on initial weight-bearing.

3. Retain lateral shift correction and lumbar extension until the next treatment session

Method: teach self-correction of lateral shift (McKenzie, 1981) and continue this with short sessions of prone lying and passive extension (half push-ups). Explain the importance of these movements and the effect they should have on their symptoms. The patient should avoid sitting and activities which require lumbar flexion, as much as possible. Rest in lying will relieve pressure on deformed or inflamed tissues but short spells of standing and walking are also important. When resuming an upright posture after lying, self-correction of the lateral shift should be performed.

Most importantly, lumbar flexion should be avoided as this will increase intervertebral disc pressure due to the associated compressive loading and shear stress, and increase the tensile stress in the posterior ligaments.

The patient can be reviewed daily during the acute episode to monitor the progress of symptoms and to ensure that the shift correction and lumbar extension are being maintained. The progression of treatment for resolving acute pain is considered in the next section.

Joint mobilization for acute low back pain

In some cases shift correction and restoration of extension may not be achieved using the active and assisted movement techniques described. Where local pain and spasm allow, mobilization can be used to help achieve these goals. Useful techniques at this stage are:

To correct the lateral shift:

1. Lateral flexion away from the side of the lateral shift of the trunk combined with transverse vertebral pressure on the spinous process of the symptomatic level(s). This may be performed up to grade III+ (see previous definitions) as pain allows. The transverse pressure should be angled slightly caudad to minimize zygapophysial joint compression.

2. Lumbar rotation (Maitland, 1986) with the patient lying on the side to which the trunk is shifted. Rotation may be attempted up to grade III+ as long as the low back or referred pain is not increased and the movement does not produce spasm. Following reassessment the technique may be progressed to grade V if improvement has been effected and the joint can be moved to end-range with minimal pain and no spasm. Sustained rotation in flexion (towards the side of pain and/or straight leg raise limitation) may also be useful (McKenzie, 1981).

To restore extension:

1. Where pain is central, or bilateral and symmetrical – P/A central vertebral pressures (centrally through the spinous process or bilaterally over the articular pillars).
2. Where pain is unilateral – P/A unilateral vertebral pressures.

Resolving acute pain

As the symptoms associated with acute low back pain settle, persisting discomfort may still be present when weight-bearing and moving, depending on the degree of residual restriction. The principal objective of treatment now is to restore full range of movement and normal function. In this regard, the sagittal plane movements, particularly flexion, are most important. However, in order to achieve normal sagittal movement, symmetrical frontal plane movement must also be restored. If this is not achieved, asymmetrical facet joint movement may result in a mechanical block (and pain) at some point during the movement (Cailliet, 1981). The progression of treatment is to:

(i) obtain full-range lateral flexion and side-glide to both sides; then
(ii) improve extension in lying and in standing;
(iii) gradually progress into flexion and improve the flexion range.

Mobilization technique selection should be based on the direction of active movement restriction and the associated passive intervertebral movement test findings. Table 24.4 describes some guides for technique selection for some common clinical presentations of movement restriction. The grade of movement chosen must always be guided by the relationship between movement and pain in the active and intervertebral movement tests. Weight-bearing techniques should be used when pain occurs due to restriction at the limit of range. These techniques are often less useful when movement is limited by pain early in range.

Table 24.4 *Suggested mobilization techniques to restore specific movement restrictions in the lumbar spine*

Lateral flexion or side-gliding

Unilateral intervertebral movement restriction/pain

(i) P/A unilateral vertebral pressure
(ii) Lateral flexion localized with transverse vertebral pressure to the restricted segment
(iii) Lateral flexion 'SNAG' (Mulligan 1989) with pressure over articular pillar or transverse pressure on spinous process

Bilateral intervertebral movement restriction/pain

(i) P/A central vertebral pressure
(ii) Lateral flexion 'SNAGS' with pressure over the spinous process

Extension

Unilateral intervertebral movement restriction/pain

(i) P/A unilateral vertebral pressure
(ii) Rotation with the patient lying on the restricted side
(iii) Extension 'SNAGS' (sitting or standing) with unilateral or transverse pressure

Bilateral intervertebral movement restriction/pain

(i) P/A central vertebral pressure
(ii) Extension 'SNAG' with central pressure

Flexion

Unilateral intervertebral movement restriction/pain

(i) Rotation with the restricted side up
(ii) Rotation with the restricted side down
(iii) P/A unilateral vertebral pressure
(iv) Flexion 'SNAG' with unilateral pressure

Bilateral intervertebral movement restriction/pain

(i) Rotation to both sides
(ii) P/A central vertebral pressures
(iii) Flexion 'SNAG' with central pressure
(iv) Flexion in lying as a self-assisted (McKenzie, 1981) or therapist-assisted (Maitland, 1986) technique.

Clinically, lumbar rotation is a technique which can be useful to improve mobility in all planes of movement. However, recent *in vitro* modelling studies suggest that axial torsion of the whole lumbar spine is coupled with upward translation and flexion rotation at all segments (Shirazi-Adl, 1994). Although approximation of the articular facets will permit only 2–3 degrees of pure lumbar rotation, the associated flexion rotation provides a strong theoretical basis for the use of rotation mobilization to restore restricted lumbar flexion.

These techniques may be progressed by modifying the patient position and consequently applying the technique with the joint positioned further into the available range. For example, the patient may be positioned in a degree of lateral flexion prior to performing a lateral flexion or P/A unilateral vertebral pressure technique, to restore an end-range limitation of side-flexion. This concept is developed as the fundamental principle in the treatment of joint pain and restriction using combined movements (Edwards, 1992). The reader should refer to that text for details of the combined movement approach to spinal manual therapy. Manipulative techniques can be applied during the resolving phase and may increase the rate of movement restoration. The only limitation on manipulation is that the joint must be able to be positioned in the pre-manipulative position with minimal reproduction of the prevailing symptoms. The frequency of treatment can be reduced for resolving conditions but the patient must be instructed in appropriate exercises to help maintain and improve their mobility between treatments. The final objective is to restore full-range, pain-free movement in all directions. Where this has been met but there are persisting joint signs (either tenderness or restricted segmental motion) the treatment should be discontinued and the patient reviewed after a week or 10 days.

Treatment of neural tissue restriction following acute back pain

Restriction of neural tissue mobility such as a limitation of straight-leg raise (SLR), may persist following an episode of acute pain. Conversely, such a restriction may develop progressively in the absence of acute pain, with altered lumbar movement patterns and leg symptoms. McKenzie (1981) describes this restriction, together with the associated problems of persisting leg pain and abnormal movement patterns, as being due to nerve root adherence. Maitland (1986) refers to this problem as restricted mobility of pain sensitive structures in the intervertebral foramen, while Butler (1991) suggests that the movement restriction can occur anywhere along the neuromechanical interface. In the absence of associated intervertebral joint signs, the common clinical presentation is that of a painful restriction of SLR and deviation towards the painful/restricted side during flexion in standing.

The treatment principles and techniques have been described in detail in the previously cited texts (McKenzie, 1981; Maitland, 1986; Butler, 1991).

Spinal joint 'dysfunction' – gradual onset pain and stiffness

Typically, the pain associated with this presentation is of gradual onset and not usually (but can be) associated with a specific event or trauma. The patient describes a dull ache which may be referred into the buttocks or legs. Often, there is increased stiffness on rising in the morning or after a period of sitting. The pain tends to increase during the day particularly if prolonged sitting or repeated or sustained flexion are required. Most importantly, the patient is often less aware of the pain when moving and the ache may be eased by gentle, non-weight-bearing exercises. This presentation is typical of what McKenzie (1981) describes as joint 'dysfunction', where pain is produced by mechanical deformation of 'adaptively shortened' soft tissue structures.

On examination, movement is restricted in all directions but typically conforms to the capsular pattern described by Cyriax and Cyriax (1993), in which lateral flexion (or side-glide), and extension, are the earliest and more severely restricted movements. Pain is produced at the extremes of the range, relieved on returning to the upright position and does not get worse with repeated movements. Straight-leg raise is commonly limited bilaterally by hamstring muscle tightness. Intervertebral movement testing often reveals a more generalized restriction of accessory and physiological movement with increased resistance to movement and tenderness at end-range. The restrictions are often greater in the lower than the upper lumbar segments.

The approach to treatment is to treat the movement restrictions with mobilization techniques which will stretch the shortened joint structures at the end of the available range. Technique selection should follow the guidelines set out in the previous section (Table 24.4) with the objective of restoring symmetrical side-gliding and then increasing extension. Grade III+ techniques will help reduce treatment soreness initially but this can be progressed to grade IV once the response to treatment has been determined. The duration of each repetition can be extended to 3 or 4 minutes. Grade V techniques can be attempted but end-range tightness may be too great for the manipulation to be successful.

Due to the insidious and often chronic nature of these problems, the patient must be given a clear explanation of the problem, the treatment and its objectives and the time frame for improvement and resolution. Since these problems may have developed over months or even years, the improvement is expected to be slow and gradual. Initially the patient may be treated two or three times over a week or 10 days to monitor the response. The frequency of treatment may then be reduced to once or twice per week as long as the patient is provided with the appropriate mobility exercises to continue at home. The exercises should be performed into the restricted part of the range to stretch the shortened soft tissues. Some local discomfort must be experienced during these exercises in order for them to be effective and they should be performed several times throughout the day.

One important consideration with the treatment of lumbar spine 'dysfunction' is that of the effect of changes in skeletal structure and joint degeneration on intervertebral mechanics, particularly extension. This issue will be examined in the next section but the important point here is the effect of these changes on the range, and factors limiting movement. In some cases, extension may be limited more by approximation of the posterior skeletal structures rather than soft tissue tension (Cailliet, 1981). The resulting loads transferred through the laminae and articular surfaces of the zygapophysial joints may aggravate the patient's condition even though the initial movement pattern is consistent with that of soft tissue adaptive shortening. A cautious approach to the treatment of extension dysfunction in individuals with radiological evidence of degenerative changes in either the anterior or posterior column is recommended.

Degenerative joint disease/spondylosis

Many patients, of all ages, who present with low back pain may have radiological anomalies of some kind. These may be normal variations in structure such as an extra lumbar vertebra or the presence of Schmorl's nodes. The radiographs may also reveal important clinical information such as changes in vertebral body shape, osteophyte development, zygapophysial joint degeneration and apparent change in height of the intervertebral disc spaces. Although these factors may not be directly related to the pain for which the patient is seeking treatment, it is important to be aware of their presence (Grieve, 1991). This is because degenerative changes affecting the intervertebral disc and zygapophysial joints may limit the quality and range of movement in these segments.

Moderate or severe degenerative changes in the elderly are a common and important consideration irrespective of their relationship to the patient's symptoms. The physical examination should be modified to account for these factors, although the general scheme is consistent with that previously described. Abnormal spinal alignment in the frontal plane may not be due to a mobile lateral shift, but to a structural deformity resulting from changes in vertebral body and intervertebral disc shape. The sagittal plane curvatures may be exaggerated or reduced, and relatively fixed (Singer *et al.*, 1994), due to their dependence on vertebral body shape, and the greater stiffness of the intervertebral disc (Bogduk and Twomey, 1991). When testing active movements, overpressure should not be applied at end-range and extra care is required when using combined movement tests. A loss of hip or lumbar spine extension may make prone lying uncomfortable such that

accessory intervertebral movement tests may need to be performed in sitting or side-lying. Relatively less passive physiological intervertebral movement can be expected compared to younger individuals due to a combination of structural changes and increased stiffness in the structures which limit joint movement.

Some patients with degenerative joint disease may never have needed to seek treatment for back pain yet present having been told they have 'arthritis' and there is no cure. However, in many cases the pain is due to restricted joint movement and can therefore respond well to appropriate and carefully applied manual therapy. However, extra care should be taken to exclude serious pathology such as compression fracture, ankylosing spondylitis or neoplasm as the cause of the symptoms. The treatment approach is guided by the history of the symptoms and the examination findings. One of the following presentations will often emerge:

(i) Acute onset pain and restriction with localized, more specific joint signs superimposed on a more generalized movement restriction.
(ii) Gradual onset pain and stiffness with generalized joint restriction.

Acute pain in older patients with degenerative joints requires a different approach to that previously described. Severe nerve root pain referred to the leg is more likely to be due to osteophytic irritation than to disc protrusion, and is recognized as the most common cause of sciatica in mature patients (Grieve, 1988). The lateral shift/extension principle is generally not appropriate due to the structural limitation of extension. In the acute stage, rest is most important to relieve the symptomatic joints of the compressive loads of weight-bearing. Mobilization techniques which relieve pressure across the symptomatic joints are the first choice for treatment.

Techniques such as rotation and lateral flexion away from the side of pain are often more useful than vertebral pressures. In the absence of specific, localized joint signs, regional techniques are useful, particularly when primarily treating pain. Where vertebral pressure techniques are used they may be more effective with the patient positioned in side-lying rather than prone. The movement should be performed only to the point where pain is first felt and spasm should be avoided. These techniques can be progressed up to grade III+ as the symptoms settle but strong techniques at end-range (grade IV and V) should be avoided in patients with moderate or severe degenerative changes. When the acute symptoms have settled, lumbar 'SNAGS' are helpful to restore movement. The advantage is that the patient is in a functional, weight-bearing position and is in control of the movement. This approach is particularly useful for restoring lateral flexion and flexion. The restoration of end-range extension is not an important or immediate goal and P/A vertebral pressures at end-range and passive extension exercises should be applied with extreme caution.

An alternative approach to treatment of low back pain associated with joint degeneration is that of lumbar traction. The possible physiological effects of traction and the literature reporting its therapeutic value have been summarized by Grieve (1991). The most obvious advantage in patients with degenerative changes in the lumbar spine is that it reverses the compressive loads on the intervertebral disc and zygapophysial joints. Mechanical traction has the advantage of being able to apply a controlled, sustained (static) force for a fixed period or intermittent periods of traction and rest. For acute pain conditions, static traction is recommended as movement of the irritable joint structures is minimized. For non-acute conditions where less specific pain is associated with general movement restriction, intermittent traction is preferred. The oscillatory nature of intermittent traction may improve joint nutrition, and relieve pain due to increased activation of afferent joint mechanoreceptors. Lumbar traction is usually applied with the lordosis eliminated and with the patient positioned either supine or prone.

Maitland (1986) recommends the following protocol when using mechanical traction.

(i) Use 13 kg as the initial traction force (however, this is somewhat dependent on the physique of the patient).
(ii) Apply an initial force for 10 seconds then reassess the symptoms.
(iii) If the symptoms are completely relieved the force is halved and treatment time reduced. If this is not done an exacerbation of the pain may result when the traction is released.
(iv) If the symptoms are minimally relieved the force is increased slightly and treatment continued for 10 minutes on the first occasion.
(v) If the symptoms are worse, the force should be reduced until the symptoms return to the baseline level and the traction applied for 5 minutes.
(vi) Following treatment the patient should rest for a minute or two before getting up slowly.
(vii) Reassessment of symptoms and comparable movement signs. There may not be an immediate change in the active movements and flexion may be worse after treatment (Maitland, 1986).

Traction is progressed according to the severity of pain and response to the previous treatment. Where symptoms are improved with static traction, the duration is increased until improvement plateaus, at which point the traction force is increased slowly. Traction should be progressed more slowly when treating acute conditions. Fifteen minutes is the recommended maximum treatment time. When using intermittent traction, initially a shorter traction time is used with a similar rest time. Treatment is progressed as for static traction but with increasing hold and decreasing rest times. The maximum treatment time can be increased up to 20–25 minutes in non-irritable conditions where stiffness is the predominant problem. Changes in symptoms or movement signs due to the application of traction may be harder to assess than with other mobilization techniques. Maitland (1986) suggests that a trial of four treatments is necessary before a decision on its effectiveness can be made.

The frequency of treatment is dependent on the severity and duration of the presenting symptoms. Patients with acute pain may require daily treatment initially to monitor the response to treatment and help settle the acute symptoms and movement restriction more rapidly. The treatment frequency for non-acute conditions is as described for patients with movement 'dysfunction'.

Lumbar instability

Lumbar instability is a controversial and challenging condition for all clinicians involved in the management of low back pain. In contrast to the clinical presentations previously described, the main feature in these patients is excessive intersegmental motion due to a deficiency in the passive, non-contractile tissues (Panjabi, 1992). Instability is present when there is an abnormal range of movement for which there is no protective muscular control (Maitland, 1986). Hypermobility differs from instability in that muscular control is retained throughout the excessive range of movement (Norris, 1995a). Stoddard (1983) suggests that the aetiology of lumbar instability includes:

(i) Severe strain or trauma associated with a hyperflexion injury.
(ii) Chronic, habitual ligamentous strain due to faulty or abnormal postures or structural anomalies, e.g. leg length difference.·
(iii) Joint degeneration involving the joints and ligaments of the vertebral complex.

In some cases the instability may be due to an identifiable structural abnormality such as a spondylolisthesis. However, in others, no radiological abnormality may be visible and diagnosis can only be made on the basis of the history, clinical features and examination findings. Criteria which suggest lumbar instability are described by Grieve (1986).

The physical examination format is as previously described but attention should be focused on the following areas:

(i) Active movements: may be full and pain-free although extreme mobility may be a feature. On extension, the lumbar spine may hinge at one segment and movements may be performed slowly or cautiously. A momentary catch of pain may occur during the movement, usually flexion. A transient deviation from the path of movement may accompany the mid-range pain. In more severe cases, the spine may be held in lordosis during flexion and there is a tendency to push off the thighs when returning to neutral.

(ii) Palpation findings may include: (a) local tenderness between spinous processes in the affected segment, (b) increased resting tension and prominence of the lumbar paravertebral muscles adjacent to the affected segment, (c) a palpable 'step' between spinous processes, (d) a 'boggy' feel on accessory movement testing, (e) excessive segmental intervertebral movement especially in flexion, and (f) increased antero-posterior shear at the affected segment. Hypomobility in segments adjacent to the hypermobile joint may be detected.

(iii) Although pain may be referred into the leg, neurological deficit is uncommon. Straight-leg raise may be limited by tight hamstrings rather than pain associated with nerve root tension.

Treatment for lumbar instability

Mobilization

Mobilization may be applied in those patients with a normal end-feel to accessory movement. Techniques within range (grade II–III) may be useful to relieve local joint discomfort. Mobilization of hypomobile joints can still be performed as long as the techniques are applied carefully and localized accurately to the affected joints. Mobilization is not appropriate in joints with a 'boggy', unphysiological movement and no palpable end-range (Grieve, 1986).

Stabilization

The logical approach to the treatment of hypermobility is stabilization. A lumbar support or corset may be useful to help relieve acute symptoms, but the long-term aim is to provide dynamic stabilization by strengthening the regional and segmental trunk musculature (Grieve, 1986). This may help to compensate for the reduced support provided by the passive stabilizing structures. Dynamic stabilization of the lumbar spine is enhanced by contraction of the abdominal and erector spinae muscles due to their influence on intra-abdominal pressure and the thoracolumbar fascia mechanism (Gracovetsky *et al.*, 1985; Tesh *et al.*, 1987). According to Valencia and Munro (1985), the lumbar multifidus also has an important role in providing intersegmental stability.

Consequently, dynamic stabilization of the lumbar spine is best achieved with abdominal bracing and hollowing exercises together with isometric retraining of the lumbar multifidus (Grieve, 1986; Richardson *et al.*, 1992). The abdominal exercises are initially taught in supine lying with the aid of pressure or EMG biofeedback and progressed into the more functional positions of sitting and standing. Jull and Richardson (1994) and Norris (1995b) provide a detailed description of abdominal bracing exercises and their use in retraining lumbar spine stabilization.

Treatment of the sacroiliac joint

The involvement of the sacroiliac joint in patients presenting with low back pain can only be determined by careful correlation of the symptoms with the previously described tests of sacroiliac position, movement and palpation. Sacroiliac joint symptoms may be acute, associated with a recent fall or twisting injury. Chronic or gradual onset problems are often seen in younger individuals participating in sporting activities which require strong and repeated torsional stresses such as athletics and golf (Wells, 1986). It is important to consider the possibility of inflammatory conditions such as ankylosing spondylitis and sacroiliitis, and when suspected, medical referral is necessary. During pregnancy and for a variable period postpartum, sacroiliac dysfunction may be due to hypermobility in which case stabilization is advisable. This can be achieved with the use of an appropriately fitted belt support together with advice on intermittent bed rest in severe cases. Pelvic support may also assist in the management of other sacroiliac hypermobility problems. Pain relief in such cases may assist in confirming the diagnosis.

In cases of hypomobility or positional innominate fixation, passive movement is the treatment of choice. The direction of passive movement is determined by the physical examination findings. Hypomobility is treated with a direction and grade of movement which eases the pain. If an innominate is fixed in an anterior or posterior position, passive movement is performed in the opposite direction. The passive movement treatment techniques are modifications of the examination tests. Anterior or posterior innominate rotation is used to restore motion and relieve pain and the leg can be used as a lever when stronger force is required. For example, with the patient prone, the thigh can be used as a lever at the extreme of hip extension to rotate the innominate anteriorly. The opposite leg can be fixed with a belt to increase the force on the innominate. To rotate the innominate posteriorly, the thigh is used as a lever in full hip extension while the rotation is reinforced by pressure through the ischial tuberosity. Strong isometric contraction of the hip extensor muscles can be used to correct anterior innominate rotation and this can be continued as a home exercise (DonTigny, 1993).

In addition to manual therapy treatment, home exercises and back care are required to maintain and correct sacroiliac joint position and movement. Direct stretching or isometric exercises can be used to correct innominate position, while strengthening the abdominals, gluteus maximus and hamstring muscles will improve dynamic support for the joints. Lumbar support in sitting will help maintain a correct sacroiliac position and correct standing posture is also important to prevent excessive anterior pelvic rotation. At night, support for the sacroiliac joint can be achieved by placing a pillow under the knees when supine, or between the knees in side-lying.

Outcome measures in manual therapy

Identifying and measuring appropriate outcome measures for manual therapy treatment is an increasingly important part of patient management and clinical practice. Outcome measures provide a means of assessing the effectiveness of treatment over time. This information can be used to support the continuation or cessation of treatment, and to provide consistent and reliable outcome data for clinical trials which examine the effectiveness of manual therapy. Structural pathology in the low back is associated with movement impairment, functional limitation and consequently disability (Fitzgerald *et al.*, 1994). Manual therapy intervention is directed towards changing the physical impairments and functional limitations that are related to the disability (Guccione, 1991). The severity and frequency of pain is an obvious additional outcome measure and numerous pain and disability scales are available which measure the effect of pain on function (Millard, 1991). However, specific impairments such as active movement restriction and the ability to perform functional activities are outcomes which are most appropriate when treating musculoskeletal disabilities.

Summary

This chapter has outlined the physiotherapy approach to the assessment and management of low back pain. The key elements of this approach are a systematic examination of active and passive spinal mobility and the effect of these manoeuvres on the presenting symptoms. The objective is not specifically to identify the pain producing structures, but to develop a treatment hypothesis based on the relationship between the functional limitation, and the signs and symptoms. The loss of function, which is usually manifested as abnormalities of movement, is treated with joint mobilization and/or muscle re-education as indicated from the examination findings. When treating joint restriction, the mobilization techniques are graded according to the relationship between pain and movement. Guidelines for technique selection in common clinical presentations are provided to assist the inexperienced clinician. However, the underlying principle remains that the choice of treatment technique is based on the examination findings and the severity and irritability of the symptoms.

The emphasis in this chapter has been on the use of manual therapy to treat low back pain, with an attempt to integrate the treatment concepts described by individuals working in this area of the profession. The limited scope of this chapter does not allow for a detailed description of their methods or for an integration of other complementary approaches to treatment. It is stressed that this chapter is a summary of the physiotherapy approach to the management of low back pain and it is strongly recommended that the reader refers to the clinical texts listed in the reference section.

References

Bogduk, N. (1984) The rationale for patterns of neck and back pain. *Patient Management*, **13**, 17–28.

Bogduk, N. and Twomey, L.T. (1991) *Clinical Anatomy of the Lumbar Spine*. Churchill Livingstone, New York.

Butler, D.S. (1991) *Mobilisation of the Nervous System*. Churchill-Livingstone, New York.

Cailliet, R. (1981) *Low Back Pain Syndrome*. F. A. Davis, Philadelphia.

Cyriax, J.H. and Cyriax, P.J. (1993) *Cyriax's Illustrated Manual of Orthopaedic Medicine*. Butterworth Heinemann, Oxford.

DonTigny, R.L. (1993) Mechanics and treatment of the sacroiliac joint. *J. Man. Manip. Ther.*, **1**, 3–12.

Edwards, B.C. (1992) *Manual of Combined Movements*. Churchill Livingstone, New York.

Farrell, J.P. and Jensen, G.M. (1992) Manual therapy: a critical assessment of role in the profession of physical therapy. *Phys. Ther.*, **72**, 843–852.

Fitzgerald, G.K., McClure, P.W., Beattie, P. *et al.* (1994) Issues in determining effectiveness of manual therapy. *Phys. Ther.*, **74**, 227–233.

Gracovetsky, S., Farfan, H. and Helleur, C. (1985) The abdominal mechanism. *Spine*, **10**, 317–324.

Grieve, G.P. (1988) Common patterns of clinical presentation. In *Common Vertebral Joint Problems* (G.P. Grieve, ed.). Churchill Livingstone, New York, pp. 355–457.

Grieve, G.P. (1991) *Mobilisation of the Spine*. Churchill Livingstone, New York.

Guccionne, A.A. (1991) Physical therapy diagnosis and the relationship between impairments and function. *Phys. Ther.*, **71**, 499–503.

Hansson, T., Bigos, S., Beecher, P. *et al.* (1985) The lumbar lordosis in acute and chronic low-back pain. *Spine*, **10**, 154–155.

Jull, G.A. (1986) Examination of the lumbar spine. In *Modern Manual Therapy of the Vertebral Column* (G.P. Grieve, ed.). Churchill Livingstone, New York, pp. 547–560.

Jull, G.A. and Janda, V. (1987) Muscles and motor control in low back pain: assessment and management. In *Physical Therapy of the Low Back* (L.T. Twomey and J. R. Taylor, eds). Churchill Livingstone, New York, pp. 253–278.

Jull, G.A. and Richardson, G.A. (1994) Rehabilitation of active stabilisation of the lumbar spine. In *Physical Therapy of the Low Back* (L.T. Twomey and J.R. Taylor, eds). Churchill Livingstone, New York, pp. 251–273.

Kaltenborn, F.M. (1989) *Manual Mobilization of the Extremity Joints*. Bokhandel, Oslo.

Keating, J., Matyas, T. and Bach, T. (1993) The effect of training on physical therapists ability to apply specified forces of palpation. *Phys. Ther.*, **73**, 38–46.

Lee, M. (1989) Mechanics of spinal joint manipulation in the thoracic and lumbar spine: a theoretical study of posteroanterior force techniques. *Clin. Biomech.*, **4**, 249–251.

Lee, M. and Liversidge, K. (1994) Posteroanterior stiffness at three locations in the lumbar spine. *J. Manipulative Physiol. Ther.*, **17**, 511–516.

Lee, M. and Svensson, N.L. (1993) Effect of loading frequency on response of the spine to lumbar posteroanterior forces. *J. Manipulative Physiol. Ther.*, **16**, 439–446.

Maher, C. and Adams, R. (1994) Reliability of pain and stiffness assessments in clinical manual lumbar spine examination. *Phys. Ther.*, **74**, 801–811.

Lee, M., Esler, M-A., Mildren, J. *et al.* (1993) Effect of extensor muscle activation on the response to lumbar posteroanterior forces. *Clin. Biomech.*, **8**, 115–119.

Maher, C. and Latimer, J. (1992) Pain or resistance – the manual therapists' dilemma. *Aust. J. Physiol.*, **38**, 257–260.

Maitland, G.D. (1986) *Vertebral Manipulation*. Butterworth Heinemann, London.

Matyas, T. and Bach, T. (1985) The reliability of selected techniques in clinical arthrometrics. *Aust. J. Physiol.*, **31**, 175–199.

Mayer, T.G., Tencer, A.F., Kristoferson, S. *et al.* (1984) Use of non-invasive techniques for quantification of spinal range of motion in normal subjects and chronic low-back dysfunction patients. *Spine*, **9**, 588–595.

McCall, I.W., Park, W.M. and O'Brien, J.P. (1979) Induced pain referral from posterior lumbar elements in normal subjects. *Spine*, **4**, 441–446.

McKenzie, R.A. (1981) *The Lumbar Spine: Mechanical Diagnosis and Therapy*. Spinal Publications, Wellington.

Millard, R.W. (1991) A critical review of questionnaires for assessing pain-related disability. *J. Occup. Rehabil.*, **1**, 289–302.

Mulligan, B.R. (1989) *Manual Therapy – NAGS, 'SNAGS', 'PRP's etc.* Plane View Services, Wellington.

Norris, C.M. (1995a) Spinal stabilisation. 1. Active lumbar stabilisation – concepts. *Physiotherapy*, **81**, 61–64.

Norris, C.M. (1995b) Spinal stabilisation. 5. An exercise programme to enhance lumbar stabilisation. *Physiotherapy*, **81**, 138–146.

Panjabi, M.M. (1992) The stabilizing system of the spine. Part II. Neutral zone and instability hypothesis. *J. Spinal Dis.*, **5**, 390–397.

Pearsall, D.J. and Reid, J.G. (1992) Line of gravity relative to upright vertebral posture. *Clin. Biomech.*, **7**, 80–86.

Price, D.D., McGrath, P.A., Rafii, A. *et al.* (1983) The validation of visual analogue scales as ratio scale measures for chronic and experimental pain. *Pain*, **17**, 46–56.

Richardson, C., Jull, G., Toppenberg, R. *et al.* (1992) Techniques for active lumbar stabilisation for spinal protection: a pilot study. *Aust. J. Physiol.*, **38**, 105–112.

Sharazi-Adl, A. (1994) Nonlinear stress analysis of the whole lumbar spine in torsion – mechanics of facet articulation. *J. Biomech*, **27**, 289–299.

Singer, K.P., Jones, T.J. and Breidahl, P.D. (1990) A comparison of radiographic and computer-assisted measurements of thoracic and thoracolumbar sagittal curvature. *Skeletal Radiol.*, **19**, 21–26.

Singer, K.P., Edmondston, S.J., Day, R.E. *et al.* (1994) Computer-assisted curvature assessment and Cobb angle determination of the thoracic kyphosis: an *in vivo* and *in vitro* comparison. *Spine*, **19**, 1381–1384.

Stagnara, P., De Mauroy, J.C., Dran, G. *et al.* (1982) Reciprocal angulation of vertebral bodies in a sagittal plane: approach to references for the evaluation of kyphosis and lordosis. *Spine*, **7**, 335–342.

Stoddard, A. (1983) *Manual of Osteopathic Practice*. Hutchinson, London.

Tesh, K.M., Shaw Dunn, J.S. and Evans, J.H. (1987) Abdominal muscles and vertebral stability. *Spine*, **12**, 501–508.

Torgerson, W.R. and Dotter, W.E. (1976) Comparative roentgenographic study of the asymptomatic and symptomatic lumbar spine. *J. Bone Joint Surg.*, **58A**, 850–853.

Twomey, L.T. and Taylor, J.R. (1979) A description of two new instruments for measuring sagittal and horizontal plane motions in the lumbar region. *Aust. J. Physiol.*, **25**, 201–203.

Twomey, L.T. and Taylor, J.R. (1987) *Physical Therapy of the Low Back*. Churchill Livingstone, New York.

Valencia, F.P. and Munro, R.R. (1985) An electromyographic study on the lumbar multifidus in man. *Electro. Clin. Physiol.*, **25**, 205–221.

Wells, P.E. (1986) Examination of the pelvic joints. In *Modern Manual Therapy of the Vertebral Column* (G.P. Grieve, ed.). Churchill Livingstone, New York, pp. 590–602.

White, A.A. and Panjabi, M.M. (1990) *Clinical Biomechanics of the Spine*. J.B. Lippincott, Philadelphia.

Woerman, A.L. (1989) Evaluation and treatment of the lumbar–pelvic–hip complex. In *Orthopaedic Physical Therapy* (R. Donatelli and M. J. Wooden, eds) Churchill Livingstone, New York, pp. 403–484.

25

Contraindications to spinal manipulation

K.P. Singer

Summary

Reported complications following manipulation of the lumbar spine are few. In general, more forceful manipulative techniques, often incorporating rotation or hyper-extension, have been associated with problems. The most frequently recorded injury is to the intervertebral disc, resulting in cauda equina compromise. Careful assessment of the presenting signs and symptoms, and monitoring responses between treatments should prevent serious complications.

Inadequate clinical examination, improper interpretation of imaging films, and lack of knowledge can lead to incorrect diagnosis and, therefore, to inappropriate indications for spinal manipulation. Bilateral radiculopathies, with distal paralysis of the lower limbs, sensory loss in the sacral distribution, and sphincter paralysis should be regarded as a surgical emergency.

In this chapter a clinical reasoning approach is provided to guide the practitioner in determining the appropriateness of mechanical therapy.

Spinal manipulation therapy (SMT) is administered to millions of patients each year. Despite this, there has been little study of the full incidence of risks associated with such therapy. In their analysis of 138 cases cited in the literature, Powell *et al.* (1993) suggested five main factors relating to complications of SMT. These included: misdiagnosis; failure to correctly identify the onset or progression of neurological signs or symptoms; inappropriate technique; and SMT performed in the presence of a herniated nucleus pulposus or a coagulation disorder. Given the acceptance and use by practitioners of SMT, the risk of complication is placed by Haldeman and Rubinstein (1993) at one per many millions of manipulations.

The order of frequency of lumbar spine complications arising from SMT showed that: disc injury; diagnostic error; vascular accidents; excessive force; rib fracture; abdominal and inguinal hernia; and neoplasm were the major problems (Figure 25.1). A full case description of reported cases is presented in the reviews by Gatterman (1981), Ladermann (1981), and Terrett and Kleynhans (1992). Further reviews and analysis of literature may be found in reports by Dvorak (1991) and Patijn (1991).

The exact incidence and prevalence of complications during manipulative therapy are unknown, in part due to a lack of standardized reporting systems, either within hospitals or coronial offices (C. Maher, personal communication, 1995), as not all problems reach the clinical literature. There are no known prospective studies which seek to record the true nature of complications from SMT. Such information is an important element in substantiating the risk/benefit ratio (Shekelle *et al.*, 1992; Powell *et al.*, 1993; Ryan, 1993).

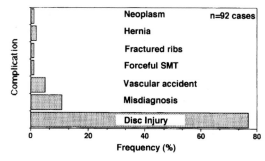

Figure 25.1 Frequency of reported complications arising from lumbar SMT (updated from Terrett and Kleynhans, 1992).

For this reason, practitioners accept full responsibility for providing careful and appropriate mechanical therapy to their patients. It must be assumed that all practitioners of SMT have received carefully supervised training where the issue of contraindications to mechanical therapy have been elaborated.

Diagnostic procedures, such as clinical history, examination and imaging, are important in screening the patient and selecting the most appropriate therapy. A full description of the diagnostic assessment process is presented in Chapter 20.

The indications and contraindications for manipulation

The indication for SMT is a diagnosis of mechanical low back pain and may include the conditions listed in Table 25.1. With experience, the clinician is able to

Table 25.1 *Indications and contraindications for spinal manipulative therapy are dependent upon the patient's presenting signs and symptoms*

Indications for manipulative therapy

- Zygapophysial and sacroiliac joint dysfunction
- Paraspinal muscle syndromes
- Joint dysfunction in lateral and central stenosis
- Joint dysfunction in spondylolisthesis
- Sacroiliac syndrome in post-operative low back pain

Contraindications for manipulative therapy

Relative

- Osteopenia
- Advanced arthopathies
- Spinal anomalies
- Patients on anticoagulant medication
- Vascular disorders
- Psychological overlay and undiagnosed pain
- Pregnancy*

Absolute (often due to coexisting disease)

- Neoplastic lesions of the spine, ribs, and pelvis
- Non-neoplastic bone disease (e.g. osteomyelitis, tuberculosis, osteoporosis)
- Inflammation (e.g. rheumatoid arthritis, ankylosing spondylitis, septic arthritis)
- Healing fracture or dislocation
- Gross segmental instability and spinal anomalies
- Cauda equina syndrome (spinal cord compromise signs in limbs)
- Large abdominal aneurysm
- Visceral referred pain
- Obvious spinal deformity
- Congenital generalized hypermobility
- Joint irritability, spasm and pain; client unable to relax

(Modified from Grieve (1981), Dvorak (1991) and Terrett and Kleynhans (1992.)

* SMT should not be used if there is possibility of miscarriage. Techniques involving compression and rotation of the thoracolumbar spine are probably best avoided in the latter stages of pregnancy.

differentiate between the those signs and symptoms which suggest caution and those which permit careful application of SMT techniques.

Contraindications can be divided into two categories: relative and absolute. Relative contraindications may suggest a modification of the technique and must be considered on a case-by-case basis. In the presence of an absolute contraindication, however, no manipulative therapy should be administered.

In the following section, the major contraindications are discussed.

Lumbar spine disc lesions

The most frequently reported complication from SMT in the lumbar region is compression of the cauda equina by a large disc herniation of the lower lumbar intervertebral discs. These injuries often result from forceful rotatory SMT techniques with, or without, lumbar extension (Figure 25.2). The resultant syndrome is characterized by paralysis, weakness, pain, reflex change, and a neurogenic bowel and bladder. Although there is a risk of precipitating a cauda equina compression syndrome using SMT, the general concensus is that an uncomplicated herniated disc lesion can be effectively treated conservatively with manipulative therapy (Haldeman and Rubinstein, 1993). The risk of inducing cauda equina compromise is estimated by Shekelle *et al.* (1992) at between 10 and 100 million to one. However, the practitioner is reminded that bilateral radiculopathies with distal paralysis of the lower limbs, sensory loss in the sacral distribution, and sphincter paralysis should be considered a surgical emergency. In the acute stage, SMT, using high velocity thrust techniques, is almost always inappropriate, especially, if radicular symptoms and signs indicating a nerve root compression are present.

A surgical opinion should be recommended to the patient if progressive neurological deficit occurs and radiological imaging (MRI, CT, myelo-CT) confirm nerve root compression (Lehmann *et al.*, 1991) (refer to Chapter 18).

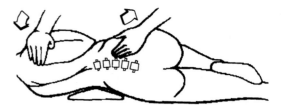

Figure 25.2 Rotation posture manipulation coupled with excessive force application has been implicated in lumbar disc complications. (Adapted from Kirkaldy-Willis and Cassidy, 1985.)

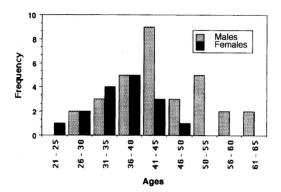

Figure 25.3 Incidence by age and gender of serious lumbar spinal complications following SMT (updated from Terrett and Kleynhans (1992)).

Of the 65 disc injuries reviewed by Terrett and Kleynhans (1992), manipulation under anaesthesia was implicated in almost half of those reported. This practice would appear to have declined in popularity since the early 1980s.

The incidence of discal injury for males and females following manipulation is shown in Figure 25.3. Greater susceptibility appears between 30 and 50 years of age for both genders.

Misdiagnosis of low back pain

Misdiagnosis refers to the unidentified presence of disease processes which may mimic low back pain symptoms. As a result of misdiagnosis, complications arise through delays in initiating appropriate treatment via referral. In the extreme case, paraplegia may be induced. Primary and secondary tumours of the spinal column and neural structures are contraindications for SMT. Manipulation of diseased vertebrae can potentially induce spinal fractures, or dislocations, resulting in acute compression syndromes of the spinal cord or nerve roots.

Vascular accident

Practitioners must establish the medications used by their patients and recognize the potential risk to those on anticoagulant therapy. Vascular problems include aortic occlusion, haematoma, and thrombosis.

Trauma of the lumbar spine

Direct and indirect trauma of the lumbar spine, leading to functional disorders, are few. However, traumatically induced disc herniations, vertebral instability, as well as bony lesions with neurogenic signs, should be considered as contraindications for SMT.

Unnecessary force application during SMT

Fortunately, few cases have been reported where excessive force has resulted in long-term complications. However, the production of rib fractures, vertebral fractures, femoral compression neuropathy, and both inguinal and abdominal hernias have been documented (Patijn, 1991; Terrett and Kleynhans, 1991).

Grieve (1981) reminds practitioners not to manipulate spinal joints that produce a rubbery resistance to pre-testing.

Osteoporosis

Spinal manipulative therapy is contraindicated in the presence of pathological vertebral fractures, as these fractures may be exacerbated by manipulation (Haldemann and Rubinstein, 1993). Assessment of fracture risk using bone density measurements is the preferred management strategy. There may be a role for gentle SMT, but this must be considered on a case-by-case basis.

Inflammatory disease of the spine and degenerative spondylosis

Rheumatoid arthritis may present with signs of spinal instability and must be assessed cautiously by the practitioner. In the acute inflammatory stage of ankylosing spondylitis, SMT is contraindicated. Chronic degenerative osteoarthritis and spondylosis osteochondrosis, are relative indications for SMT. Mobilization is, however, recommended in place of high velocity thrust techniques. Radiological evaluation is recommended to avoid inappropriate manipulation. Cases with advanced osteoarthritis of the intervertebral joints may not benefit from manipulation. Ossification of intervertebral ligaments, as in diffuse idiopathic skeletal hyperostosis, are relative contraindications for manipulation and mobilization (Arnold, 1994). Degenerative disorders with resultant soft tissue hypertrophy of the intervertebral joints and the ligamentum flavum can induce spinal stenosis. These clients often do not benefit from SMT (Grieve, 1981).

Progressive osteoarthritis resulting in complete fusion of the sacroiliac joints is a contraindication for repeated manipulation, particularly if SMT increases pain. Manipulation is unlikely to reduce spondylolisthesis, but commonly the adjacent spinal segments and/or sacroiliac joints can be treated successfully by manipulation or mobilization. Progressive unstable spondylolisthesis, especially where radicular signs are present, is a contraindication to SMT, as the symptoms may be exacerbated.

Congenital or acquired spinal hypermobility should be assessed with functional radiological studies to determine the instability of a particular spinal region. In such cases, mobilization techniques are not indicated.

Spinal manipulative therapy in patients with psychogenic disorders

Patients who present with psychogenic disorders must be evaluated carefully, preferably by a psychologist and/or psychiatrist, before an indication for SMT is recommended (refer to Chapter 19). Such an indication should indicate a reproducible functional disorder of the spine. Patients with psychogenic disorders can develop an 'addiction for manipulation' and coerce the practitioner into administering such therapy.

Clinical reasoning algorithm for continuing or abandoning mechanical therapy of the low back

Spinal manipulative therapy may be continued or discontinued according the presenting signs and symptoms relating to pre-testing or follow-up examination. An exacting history is mandatory in determining the appropriateness of mechanical therapy. A clinical guide is outlined in Table 25.2, which provides a logical sequence for considering or re-evaluating the role of SMT.

Conclusions

Despite the lack of any systematic study into lumbar complications following SMT, the reported incidence is low. The true rate of complications requires prospective surveys and honest reporting before full appreciation of the problems are known. The major complications which arise from SMT reflect misdiagnosis, failure to correctly identify the onset or progression of neurological signs or symptoms, the choice of inappropriate technique, and SMT performed in the presence of a herniated nucleus pulposus or a blood coagulation disorder.

Careful history taking, assessment, awareness of the major risk factors, and judicious selection of SMT techniques, would appear to markedly lessen the already low incidence of lumbar complications.

Table 25.2 *Clinical reasoning for continuing or abandoning mechanical therapy of the low back*

(i) **The patient reports improvement following treatment:**

- Treatment is repeated until the client is symptom free or until the treatment goal has been attained

(ii) **The patient's symptoms are exacerbated hours following treatment but improve the day after treatment:**

- Continue treatment

(iii) **The patient's symptoms are exacerbated immediately after treatment:**

- The client should be reassured
- Re-evaluation of the previous findings
- Consider substituting treatment using electrophysical therapeutics
- Gentle traction of the treated spinal segments or possibly massage of the paravertebral muscles
- Detailed documentation of the physical findings, including neurological assessment and history

(iv) **Progressively worsening symptoms over days, week to months:**

- Reassessment of previous diagnostic findings
- Manipulative treatment should be discontinued
- Consider substituting treatment using electrophysical therapeutics
- Consider medical referral for local infiltration
- Neurological, rheumatological or orthopaedic consultations may become necessary and should not be postponed

(v) **In case of neurological complications: anaesthesia, tingling, weakness:**

- Urgent reassessment
- Consider immediate hospitalization
- Complete documentation of the incident and all findings

(vi) **The patient's status remains unchanged (i.e. neither improvement nor worsening of the initial symptoms) after several (9–10) treatments**

- Reassessment of diagnostic findings
- Change mechanical therapy approach
- Consider the client's psychosocial situation
- Appropriate referral of patient

(vii) **In every situation the following guide applies:**

- Economy of vigour in technique
- Treatment guided by assessment and reassessment

(Modified from Dvorak (1991) and Terrett and Kleynhans (1992).)

References

Arnold, M. (1994) Thoracic spine problems: the rheumatologist's perspective. In *Proceedings of The Forgotten Thoracic Spine Conference*. MPAA (NSW) University of Sydney, November 26, pp. 7-12.

Dvorak, J. (1991) Inappropriate indications and contra-indications for manual therapy. *Man. Med.*, **6**, 85-88.

Gatterman, M.I. (1981) Contraindications and complications of spinal manipulative therapy. *J. Chiro.*, **15**, S75-86.

Grieve, G. (1981) *Common Vertebral Joint Problems*. Churchill Livingstone, Edinburgh, pp. 465–466.

Haldemann, S. and Rubinstein, S.M. (1993) Cauda equina syndrome in patients undergoing manipulation of the lumbar spine. *Spine*, **17**, 1469–1473.

Kirkaldy-Willis, W. and Cassidy, J. (1985) Spinal manipulator in the treatment of low back pain. *Can. Fam. Phys.* **31**, 535–540.

Ladermann, S.P. (1981) Accidents of spinal manipulation. *Ann. Swiss. Chiropract. Assoc.*, **7**, 161–208.

Lehmann, O.J., Mendoza, N.D. and Bradford, R. (1991) Beware the prolapsed disc. *Br. J. Hosp. Med.*, **46**, 61.

Patijn, J. (1991) Complications in manual medicine; a review of the literature. *Man. Med.*, **6**, 89–92.

Powell, F.C, Hanigan, W.C. and Olivero, W.C. (1993) A risk/benefit analysis of spinal manipulation therapy for relief of lumbar or cervical pain. *Neurosurgery*, **33**, 73–78.

Ryan, M.D. (1993) Massive disc sequestration after spinal manipulation (letter). *Med. J. Aust.*, **158**, 61.

Shekelle, P.G., Adams, A.H., Chassin, M.R. *et al.* (1992) Spinal manipulation for low back pain. *Ann. Int. Med.*, **117**, 590–598.

Terrett, A.G.J. and Kleynhans, A.M. (1992) Complications from manipulation of the low back. *Chiro. J. Aust.*, **22**, 129–140.

Definitions and Abbreviations

Definitions and abbreviations

L.G.F. Giles

Anatomical planes of the body – the descriptive planes of the body are shown in Figure 1.

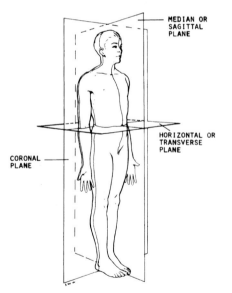

Figure 1 The descriptive planes of the body. (Reproduced with permission from Davies, D.V. and Davies, F. (1964) *Gray's Anatomy. Descriptive and Applied*, edn 33. Longmans, Green, London, p. xix.)

Antalgic posture – a posture assumed by patients experiencing acute low back pain, with or without leg pain, in which they lean away from the painful area.

Antero-posterior (A-P) – the *position* of patients when an X-ray beam is directed to their anterior surface and an X-ray plate is positioned behind them. In this text, the A-P radiographs are *viewed* from behind the patient; the patient's right side is indicated by a right marker (R).

Articular triad – the intervertebral joint and the two zygapophysial joints at any given level of the spine (Lewin *et al.*, 1961; Hirsch *et al.*, 1963) (below the second cervical vertebra).

Cobb's method (1948) – method for measuring the angle of scoliotic spinal curvature. The angle of curvature is measured by drawing lines parallel to the superior surface of the most upper vertebral body of the curvature and to the inferior surface of the lowest vertebra of the curvature (Figure 2).

Intra-articular synovial fold – a fibrous or highly vascular fat-filled zygapophysial joint synovial fold, which is covered by the synovial lining membrane.

Intervertebral disc –

  Contained herniation is when nuclear material does not escape from the confines of the anular fibres.

  Extrusion is when nuclear material escapes beyond the confines of the anular fibres.

'Leg length' inequality – the absolute inequality in length of the lower limbs. In this text a 'significant leg length inequality' is referred to when an inequality of 9 mm or more is found using an accurate method for erect posture radiography (Figure 2).

Low back pain –

  Acute low back pain refers to severe pain of recent onset (less than 3 weeks) with marked limitation of lumbar spine movements and antalgic posture.

  Chronic low back pain refers to low back pain of long duration (13 weeks or more) without marked limitation of lumbar spine movements.

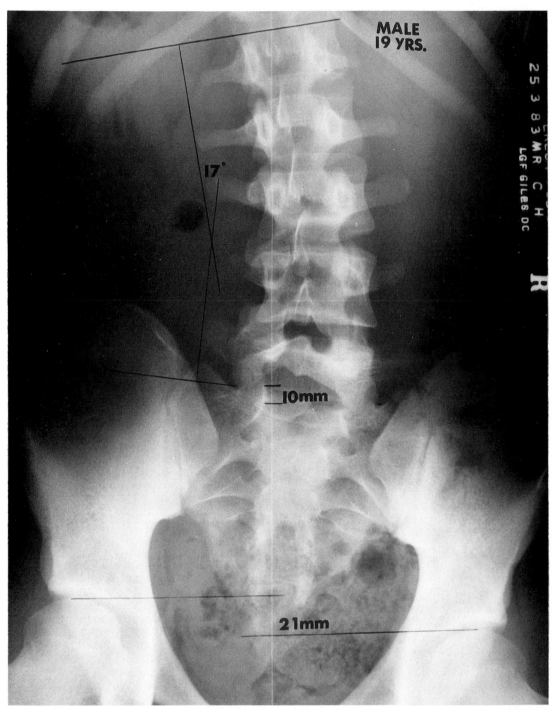

Figure 2 An erect posture radiograph of a 19-year-old male showing a right leg length deficiency of 21 mm, sacral base obliquity and postural scoliosis with a 17 degree angle of curvature. R = right side of the patient. Note the vertical plumb-line shadow which is used for measuring leg lengths by drawing a horizontal line from the top of each femur head to meet the plumb-line at right angles. Sacral base obliquity is measured by drawing a horizontal line from each superior sacral notch to meet the plumb-line at right angles. The vertical difference between paired horizontal lines gives the difference in leg lengths and the difference in height between the superior sacral notches. (Reproduced with permission from Giles, L.G.F. (1989) *Anatomical Basis of Low Back Pain*. Williams and Wilkins, Baltimore.)

Manipulation – (Cassidy and Kirkaldy-Willis, 1988)

The definition given by Sandoz (1976, 1981) is both clear and concise. A manipulation or lumbar intervertebral joint adjustment is a passive manual manoeuvre during which the three-joint complex is suddenly carried beyond the normal physiological range of movement without exceeding the boundaries of anatomical integrity. The usual characteristic is a thrust – a brief, sudden, and carefully administered 'impulsion' that is given at the end of the normal passive range of movement. It is usually accompanied by a cracking noise.

The stages of a manipulation are illustrated in Figure 22.1. When mobilization is forced beyond the elastic barrier, a sudden yielding is felt; a cracking noise is perceived; and the range of movement is slightly increased beyond the physiological limit into the paraphysiological space. At this point a second final barrier of resistance is encountered, formed by the stretched ligaments and capsule; it is called the limit of anatomical integrity. Forcing movement beyond this point would damage the ligaments and capsule. Characteristically, chiropractic manipulation involves the use of a high velocity, low amplitude thrust to a joint (Meade *et al.*, 1990).

Mobilization – (McQuarrie, 1988)

Specific passive mobilization techniques are frequently used in physical therapy to assess joint movement, to restore joint movement, to provide for pain control, to improve joint lubrication, and to relax muscle spasm (Paris, 1979). The patient is positioned carefully to allow for movement to be directed at a specific spinal segment. The therapist may choose to reproduce passively a single movement or combinations of flexion, extension, rotation, and lateral flexion at that spinal segment. The amount of movement is carefully graded to reproduce the range of movement desired at a specific spinal segment. The mobilization chosen may use gentle oscillations or stretching techniques depending on the specific joint dysfunction.

Characteristically, mobilization uses low velocity passive movements within or at the limit of joint range (Ottenbacher and Di Fabio, 1985; Spitzer *et al.*, 1987).

Motion (mobile) segment of Junghanns – all the space between two vertebrae where movement occurs; the intervertebral disc with its cartilaginous plates, the anterior and posterior longitudinal ligaments, the zygapophysial joints with their fibrous joint capsules and the ligamenta flava, the contents of the spinal canal and the left and right intervertebral canal, and the supraspinous and interspinous ligaments (Schmorl and Junghanns, 1971) (Figure 1.6).

Neuro-orthopaedic tests

Gaenslen's sign – The patient lies supine on the table, and is asked to draw both legs onto the chest. The patient is then shifted to the side of the table to enable one buttock to extend over the edge of the table. Allow the unsupported leg to drop over the edge, while the opposite leg remains flexed. Complaints of subsequent pain in the sacroiliac joint area gives an indication of pathology in that area.

Hoover test – This test helps to determine whether the patient is malingering when stating that the leg cannot be raised. It should be performed in conjunction with a straight leg raising test. The examiner's hands are put under the patient's heels and, as the patient tries to raise one leg, the opposite heel is used to gain leverage; this causes his downward pressure to be felt on the examiner's hand. If the patient does not bear down while attempting to raise one leg, he is probably not really trying.

Kernig test – This procedure applies tension to the spinal cord and can reproduce pain. Ask the patient to lie supine, then to place both hands behind the head to forcibly flex the head onto the chest. The patient may complain of pain in the cervical spine, and, occasionally, in the low back or down the legs, an indication of meningeal irritation, nerve root involvement, or irritation of the dural coverings of the nerve roots. Ask the patient to locate the area from which the pain originates.

Milgram test – The patient lies supine on the examining table with legs straight, then raises them to a position about two inches from the table. The patient is asked to hold this position as long as possible. This manoeuvre stretches the iliopsoas muscle, the anterior abdominal muscles, and increases the intrathecal pressure. If the patient can maintain this position for 30 seconds without pain, intrathecal pathology may be ruled out. If the patient cannot hold the position, or cannot lift the legs at all, or experiences pain in the attempt, there may be intrathecal or extrathecal pathology (herniated disc).

Naffziger test – A compression test designed to increase intrathecal pressure by increasing the intraspinal fluid pressure. The jugular veins are gently compressed for about 10 seconds until the patient's face begins to flush. The patient is asked to cough; if coughing causes pain, there is probably pathology pressing upon the theca. The patient is asked to locate the painful area.

Patrick or Fabere test – A test for detecting pathology in the hip, as well as in the sacroiliac joint. The patient lies supine on the table and places the foot of the painful side on the opposite knee. This causes the hip joint to be flexed, abducted, and externally rotated. In this position, inguinal pain gives a general indication of pathology in the hip joint or the surrounding muscles. At full ranges of flexion, abduction, and external rotation, the femur is fixed in relation to the pelvis. To stress the sacroiliac joint, place one hand on the flexed knee joint and the other hand on the opposite anterior superior iliac spine. Press down on each of these points and if the patient complains of increased pain, there may be sacroiliac joint pathology.

Valsalva manoeuvre - The patient is asked to bear down as if trying to move the bowels. This increases the intrathecal pressure. If bearing down causes pain in the back, or radiating pain down the legs, there is probably pathology either causing intrathecal pressure or involving the theca itself.

Obliquity -
> *Pelvic obliquity* - this is a lateral inclination of the pelvis which is tilted downward to the short leg side (Figure 2).
> *Sacral base obliquity* - a lateral inclination of the sacral base (Figure 2).

Osteoarthritis - (degenerative joint disease, degenerative arthritis, hypertrophic arthritis) - characterized by degeneration of articular cartilage, hypertrophy of bone at joint margins, and synovial membrane changes; usually associated with pain and stiffness (Hellmann, 1992).

Osteoarthrosis - Chronic non-inflammatory arthritis.

Scoliosis -
> *Angle of curvature* - the angle between lines drawn parallel to the superior surface of the upper vertebra of the curvature and to the inferior surface of the lowest vertebra of the curvature.
> *Postural (compensatory)* - this is a lumbar or thoracolumbar scoliosis (lateral curvature) which is an adaptation of the vertebral column to pelvic obliquity and which is convex on the short leg side. The intervertebral discs are wedged from the concave to the convex sides on the A-P radiograph with the discs being wider on the convex side of the scoliosis (Figure 2).
> *Structural idiopathic* - a lateral curvature with fixed rotational deformity of the spine.

Shoe-raise therapy - the provision of a shoe-raise on the side of the short leg. The raise on the heel is equal to the difference in leg lengths and the raise on the sole is 5 mm less.

Slump test - the patient sits with the back straight and the legs hanging over the edge of the examination table then slumps the cervical and thoracic spines forward then straightens one leg at a time to traction the dura. If further dural traction is necessary, dorsiflex the foot. Ask the patient to extend the neck and, if low back or leg pain is relieved, the pain arises from the spine (Kenna and Murtagh, 1989).

Spondylosis - osteophytosis secondary to degenerative intervertebral disc disease (Weinstein *et al.*, 1977).

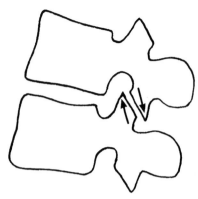

Figure 3 Note the subluxation (imbrication telescoping) of the zygapophysial joint facet surfaces as indicated by the arrows. (Reproduced with permission from Giles, L.G.F. (1989) *Anatomical Basis of Low Back Pain*. Williams and Wilkins, Baltimore.)

Subluxation - the alteration of the normal dynamics, anatomical or physiologic relationships of contiguous articular structures (Schafer, 1980). In this text, the term is used when apposing facet surfaces of the zygapophysial joint are no longer congruous, as demonstrated by imbrication (telescoping) of the zygapophysial joint facet surfaces (Hadley, 1964) (Figure 3).

Tropism - asymmetry in the horizontal plane of paired left and right zygapophysial joints.

Zygapophysial joint - the diarthrodial synovial joint between adjacent vertebral arches (apophysial joint, 'facetal' joint, interlaminar joint).

Zygapophysial joint cartilage - According to Hadley (1964), this is of the hyaline articular cartilage variety and it lines the facet surfaces; extensions of cartilage beyond the facet surface, known as 'bumper-fibrocartilage', are not composed of hyaline cartilage (Hadley, 1964).

References

Cassidy, J.D. and Kirkaldy-Willis, W.H. (1988) Manipulation. In *Managing Back Pain*, (W.H. Kirkaldy-Willis, ed.) 2nd edition. Churchill Livingstone, New York, pp. 287-296.

Cobb, J.R. (1948) Outline for the study of scoliosis. Instructional course lectures. *Am. Acad. Orthop. Surg.*, **5**, 261-275.

Davies, D.V. and Davies, F. (1964) *Gray's Anatomy. Descriptive and Applied*, 33rd edition. Longmans, Green, London, p. xix.

Giles, L.G.F. (1989) *Anatomical Basis Of Low Back Pain*. Williams and Wilkins, Baltimore.

Hadley, L.A. (1964) *Anatomico-Roentgenographic Studies of the Spine*. Charles C. Thomas, Springfield, IL, pp. 178, 183.

Hellmann, D.B. (1992) Arthritis and musculoskeletal disorders. In *Current Medical Diagnosis and Treatment*

(S.A. Schroeder, L.M. Tierney, Jr, S.J. McPhee *et al.*, eds). Appleton and Lange, Connecticut.

Hirsch, C., Ingelmark, B.E. and Miller, M. (1963) The anatomical basis for low back pain. *Acta Orthop. Scand.*, **33**, 1-17.

Kenna, C. and Murtagh, J. (1989) *Back Pain and Spinal Manipulation: A Practical Guide*. Butterworth-Heinemann, Oxford, pp. 98-101.

Lewin, T., Moffet, B. and Viidik, A. (1961) The morphology of the lumbar synovial intervertebral joints. *Acta Morphol. Neerl. Scand.*, **4**, 299-319.

McQuarrie, A. (1988) Physical therapy. In *Managing Low Back Pain*, (W.H. Kirkaldy-Willis, ed.). 2nd edition. Churchill Livingstone, New York, pp. 345-354.

Meade, T.W., Dyer, S. and Browne, W. (1990) Low back pain of mechanical origin: randomised comparison of chiropractic and hospital outpatient treatment. *Br. Med. J.*, **300**, 1431-1437.

Ottenbacher, K. and De Fabio, R.P. (1985) Efficacy of spinal manipulation/mobilisation therapy; a meta-analysis. *Spine*, **10**, 833-837.

Paris, S.V. (1979) Mobilisation of the spine. *Phys. Ther.*, **59**, 988.

Sandoz, R. (1976) Some physical mechanisms and effects of spinal adjustments. *Ann. Swiss Chirop. Assoc.*, **6**, 91.

Sandoz, R. (1981) Some reflex phenomena associated with spinal derangements and adjustments. *Ann. Swiss Chirop. Assoc.*, **7**, 45.

Schafer, R.C. (1980) *Chiropractic Physical and Spinal Diagnosis*. Oklahoma Associated Chiropractic Academic Press, Oklahoma City.

Schmorl, G. and Junghanns, H. (1971) *The Human Spine in Health and Disease*, 2nd edn. Grune and Stratton, New York, p. 37.

Spitzer, W.O., LeBlanc, F.E. and Dupuis, M. (1987) Scientific approach to the assessment and management of activity-related spinal disorders. *Spine*, **12**: S29, S37-S39.

Weinstein, P.R., Ehni, G. and Wilson, C.B. (1977) Clinical features of lumbar spondylosis and stenosis. In *Lumbar Spondylosis, Diagnosis, Management and Surgical Treatment* (P.R. Weinstein, G. Ehni and C.B. Wilson, eds). Year Book Medical Publishers, Chicago, pp. 115-133.

Index